4th EDITION

Programming and Problem Solving

with

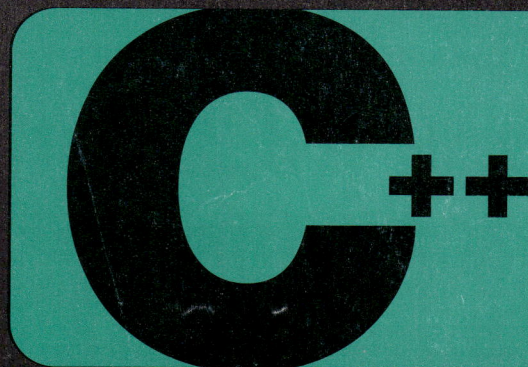

Nell Dale

University of Texas, Austin

Chip Weems

University of Massachusetts, Amherst

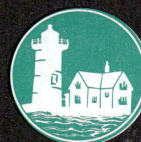

JONES AND BARTLETT PUBLISHERS

Sudbury, Massachusetts

BOSTON   TORONTO   LONDON   SINGAPORE

World Headquarters

Jones and Bartlett Publishers
40 Tall Pine Drive
Sudbury, MA 01776
978-443-5000
info@jbpub.com
www.jbpub.com

Jones and Bartlett Publishers
Canada
2406 Nikanna Road
Mississauga, ON L5C 2W6
CANADA

Jones and Bartlett Publishers
International
Barb House, Barb Mews
London W6 7PA
UK

Cover image © Image 100 Ltd.

Library of Congress Cataloging-in-Publication Data

Dale, Nell B.
  Programming and problem solving with C++ / Nell Dale, Chip Weems.— 4th ed.
    p. cm.
  Includes index.
  ISBN 0-7637-0798-8 (pbk.)
  1. C++ (Computer program language) I. Weems, Chip. II. Title.
  QA76.73.C153D34 2004
  005.13'3—dc22

                    2004003715

Chief Executive Officer: Clayton Jones
Chief Operating Officer: Don W. Jones, Jr.
Executive V.P. and Publisher: Robert Holland
V.P., Design and Production: Anne Spencer
V.P., Manufacturing and Inventory Control: Therese Bräuer
Acquisitions Editor: Stephen Solomon
Production Manager: Amy Rose
Marketing Manager: Matthew Bennett
Editorial Assistant: Caroline Senay
Production Assistant: Tracey Chapman
Production Coordination: Jennifer Bagdigian
Cover Design: Kristin E. Ohlin
Text Design: Anne Spencer
Composition: Northeast Compositors
Illustrations and Technical Art: Dartmouth Publishing
Printing and Binding: Courier Westford
Cover Printing: John Pow Company

Printed in the United States of America
08 07 06 05 04   10 9 8 7 6 5 4 3 2

To Al, my husband and best friend, and to our children and our children's children.

N.D.

To Lisa, Charlie, and Abby with love.

C.W.

To quote Mephistopheles, one of the chief devils, and tempter of Faust,

...My friend, I shall be pedagogic,
And say you ought to start with Logic...
...Days will be spent to let you know
That what you once did at one blow,
Like eating and drinking so easy and free,
Can only be done with One, Two, Three.
Yet the web of thought has no such creases
And is more like a weaver's masterpieces;
One step, a thousand threads arise,
Hither and thither shoots each shuttle,
The threads flow on, unseen and subtle,
Each blow effects a thousand ties.
The philosopher comes with analysis
And proves it had to be like this;
The first was so, the second so,
And hence the third and fourth was so,
And were not the first and second here,
Then the third and fourth could never appear.
That is what all the students believe,
But they have never learned to weave.

J. W. von Goeth, *Faust*, Walter Kaufman trans., New York, 1963, 199.

As you study this book, do not let the logic of algorithms bind your imagination, but rather make it your tool for weaving masterpieces of thought.

Preface

The first three editions of *Programming and Problem Solving with C++* consistently have been among the best-selling computer science textbooks in the United States. These editions, as well as the Pascal and Ada versions, have been accepted widely as model textbooks for ACM/IEEE-recommended curricula for the CS1/C101 course, and for the Advanced Placement A exam in computer science.

Throughout the successive editions of this book, one thing has not changed: our commitment to the student. As always, our efforts are directed toward making the sometimes difficult concepts of computer science more accessible to all students.

This edition of *Programming and Problem Solving with C++* continues to reflect our philosophy that topics once considered too advanced can be taught in the first course. For example, we address metalanguages explicitly as the formal means of specifying programming language syntax. We introduce Big-*O* notation early, and use it to compare algorithms in later chapters. We discuss modular design in terms of abstract steps, concrete steps, functional equivalence, and functional cohesion. Preconditions and postconditions are used in the context of the algorithm walk-through, in the development of testing strategies, and as interface documentation for user-written functions. The discussion of function interface design includes encapsulation, control abstraction, and communication complexity. Data abstraction and abstract data types (ADTs) are explained in conjunction with the C++ class mechanism, creating a natural lead-in to object-oriented programming.

ISO/ANSI-standard C++ is used throughout the book, including relevant portions of the new C++ standard library.

Changes to the Fourth Edition

The fourth edition does not introduce additional C++ syntax nor change the order of the content. What we have done is completely revamp the goals, the case studies, and the exercises. In addition, beginning with Chapter 13, the language of the material has become more object oriented.

Goals The chapter goals have been reorganized to reflect two aspects of learning: knowledge and skills. Thus, the goals are divided into two sections. The first lists the knowledge goals, phrased in terms of what the student should know after reading the chapter. The second lists what the student should be able to do after reading the chapter.

Problem-Solving Case Studies Each chapter has a completely new case study. Case studies that begin with a problem statement and end with a tested program have been the hallmark of our books. In this edition, we have added screen shots of the output for each of the case studies.

The case study for Chapter 14 begins the construction of an appointment calendar. The project is completed in Chapter 16. In Chapter 17, the implementation of one class is changed, emphasizing that such changes do not affect the user. The program also is made more robust by adding and handling exceptions. At each stage of the project, drivers are written to test the classes as they are created. This organization shows object-oriented design and programming in action.

Because some of the small examples used in a chapter find their way into the case study code, these examples have been changed to be consistent with the new case studies.

Exercises With the exception of Chapter 17, all of the exercises are new in this edition. The number of exercises has been expanded by between twenty and thirty percent. All of the programming problems are new.

Object-oriented language The List ADT in Chapter 13 has been changed by removing the Print operation and introducing an iterator pair, `Reset` and `GetNextItem`. This change provides better encapsulation. The list does not need to know anything about the items that it contains. The list simply returns objects to the client program, which should know what the objects are. The flaw in this design is pointed out in Chapter 14: The `Delete` and `BinSearch` operations use the relational operators, limiting the type of item to built-in types. In this chapter, the relational operators are replaced by operations `LessThan` and `Equal`; the documentation states that `ItemType` must implement these operations. The concepts of action responsibilities and knowledge responsibilities also are discussed.

The use of classes to build increasingly complex items is stressed in the case studies. Each class is independently tested, stressing the importance of testing.

C++ and Object-Oriented Programming

Some educators reject the C family of languages (C, C++, Java) as too permissive and too conducive to writing cryptic, unreadable programs. Our experience does not support this view, *provided that the use of language features is modeled appropriately.* The fact that the C family permits a terse, compact programming style cannot be labeled simply as "good" or "bad". Almost any programming language can be used to write in a style that is too terse and clever to be easily understood. The C family indeed may be used in this manner more often than are other languages, but we have found that with careful instruction in software engineering, and a programming style that is straightforward, disciplined, and free of intricate language features, students can learn to use C++ to produce clear, readable code.

It must be emphasized that although we use C++ as a vehicle for teaching computer science concepts, the book is not a language manual and does not attempt to cover all of C++. Certain language features—operator overloading, default arguments, run-time type information, and mechanisms for advanced forms of inheritance, to name a few—are omitted in an effort not to overwhelm the beginning student with too much, too fast.

There are diverse opinions about when to introduce the topic of object-oriented programming (OOP). Some educators advocate an immersion in OOP from the very beginning, whereas others (for whom this book is intended) favor a more heterogeneous approach, in which both functional decomposition and object-oriented design are presented as design tools. The chapter organization of *Programming and Problem Solving with C++* reflects a transitional approach to OOP. Although we provide an early preview of object-oriented design in Chapter 4, we delay a focused discussion until Chapter 14, after students have acquired a firm grounding in algorithm design, control abstraction, and data abstraction with classes.

Synopsis

Chapter 1 is designed to create a comfortable rapport between students and the subject. The basics of hardware and software are presented, issues in computer ethics are raised, and problem-solving techniques are introduced and reinforced in a problem-solving case study.

Instead of overwhelming the student right away with the various numeric types available in C++, Chapter 2 concentrates on only two types: char and string. (For the latter, we use the ISO/ANSI string class provided by the standard library.) With fewer data types to keep track of, students can focus on overall program structure and get an earlier start on creating and running a simple program. Chapter 3 follows with a discussion of the C++ numeric types and proceeds with material on arithmetic expressions, function calls, and output. Unlike many books that detail *all* of the C++ data types and *all* of the C++ operators at once, these two chapters focus on only the int, float, char, and string types, and the basic arithmetic operators. Details of the other data types, and the more elaborate C++ operators, are postponed until Chapter 10.

Functional decomposition and object-oriented design methodologies are a major focus of Chapter 4, and the discussion is written with a healthy degree of formalism. The treatment of object-oriented design this early in the book is more superficial than that of functional decomposition. However, students gain the perspective early that there are two—not just one—design methodologies in widespread use and that each serves a specific purpose. Object-oriented design is covered in depth in Chapter 14. Chapter 4 also covers input and file I/O. The early introduction of files permits the assignment of programming problems that require the use of sample data files.

Students learn to recognize functions in Chapters 1 and 2, and they learn to use standard library functions in Chapter 3. Chapter 4 reinforces the basic concepts of function calls, argument passing, and function libraries. Chapter 4 also relates functions to the implementation of modular designs, and begins the discussion of interface design that is essential to writing proper functions.

Chapter 5 begins with Boolean data, but its main purpose is to introduce the concept of flow of control. Selection, using If-Then and If-Then-Else structures, is used to demonstrate the distinction between physical ordering of statements and logical ordering. We also develop the concept of nested control structures. Chapter 5 concludes with a lengthy Testing and Debugging section that expands on the modular design discussion by introducing preconditions and postconditions. The algorithm walk-through and code walk-through are introduced as means of preventing errors, and the execution trace is used to find errors that may have made it into the code. We also cover data validation and testing strategies extensively in this section.

Chapter 6 is devoted to loop control strategies and looping operations using the syntax of the While statement. Rather than introducing multiple syntactical structures, our approach is to teach the concepts of looping using only the While statement. However, because many instructors have told us that they prefer to show students the syntax for all of C++'s looping statements at once, the discussion of For and Do-While statements in Chapter 9 can be covered after Chapter 6.

By Chapter 7, students are already comfortable with breaking problems into modules and using library functions, and they are receptive to the idea of writing their own functions. Thus Chapter 7 focuses on passing arguments by value and covers flow of control in function calls, arguments and parameters, local variables, and interface design. Coverage of interface design includes preconditions and postconditions in the interface documentation, control abstraction, encapsulation, and physical versus conceptual hiding of an implementation. Chapter 8 expands the discussion to include reference parameters, scope and lifetime, stubs and drivers, and more on interface design, including side effects.

Chapter 9 covers the remaining "ice cream and cake" control structures in C++ (Switch, Do-While, and For), along with the Break and Continue statements. These structures are useful but not necessary. Chapter 9 is a natural ending point for the first quarter of a two-quarter introductory course sequence.

Chapter 10 begins the transition between the control structures orientation of the first half of the book and the abstract data type orientation of the second half. We examine the built-in simple data types in terms of the set of values represented by each type and the allowable operations on those values. We introduce additional C++ operators and discuss at length the problems of floating-point representation and precision. User-defined simple types, user-written header files, and type coercion are among the other topics covered in this chapter.

We begin Chapter 11 with a discussion of simple versus structured data types. We introduce the record (struct in C++) as a heterogeneous data structure, describe the syntax for accessing its components, and demonstrate how to combine record types into a hierarchical record structure. From this base, we proceed to the concept of data abstraction and give a precise definition to the notion of an ADT, emphasizing the separation of specification from implementation. The C++ class mechanism is introduced as a programming language representation of an ADT. The concepts of encapsulation, information hiding, and public and private class members are stressed. We describe the separate compilation of program files, and students learn the technique of placing a class's declaration and implementation into two separate files: the specification (.h) file and the implementation (.cpp) file.

In Chapter 12, the array is introduced as a homogeneous data structure whose components are accessed by position rather than by name. One-dimensional arrays are examined in depth, including arrays of structs and arrays of class objects. Material on multidimensional arrays completes the discussion.

Chapter 13 integrates the material from Chapters 11 and 12 by defining the list as an ADT. Because we have already introduced classes and arrays, we can clearly distinguish between arrays and lists from the beginning. The array is a built-in, fixed-size data structure. The list is a user-defined, variable-size structure, represented in this chapter as a length variable and an array of items bound together in a class object. The elements in the list are those elements in the array from position 0 through position *length* − 1. In this chapter, we design C++ classes for unsorted and sorted list ADTs, and we code the list algorithms as class member functions. We use Big-O notation to compare the various searching and sorting algorithms developed for these ADTs. Finally, we examine C strings in order to give students some insight into how a higher-level abstraction (a string as a list of characters) might be implemented in terms of a lower-level abstraction (a null-terminated char array).

Chapter 14 extends the concepts of data abstraction and C++ classes to an exploration of object-oriented software development. Object-oriented design, introduced briefly in Chapter 4, is revisited in greater depth. Students learn to distinguish between inheritance and composition relationships during the design phase, and C++'s derived classes are used to implement inheritance. This chapter also introduces C++ virtual functions, which support polymorphism in the form of run-time binding of operations to objects.

Chapter 15 examines pointer and reference types. We present pointers as a way of making programs more efficient and of allowing the run-time allocation of program data. The coverage of dynamic data structures continues in Chapter 16, in which we present linked lists, linked-list algorithms, and alternative representations of linked lists.

Chapter 17 introduces C++ templates and exception handling, and Chapter 18 concludes the text with coverage of recursion. There is no consensus as to the best place to introduce these subjects. We believe that it is better to wait until at least the second semester to cover them. However, we have included this material for those instructors who have requested it. Both chapters have been designed so that they can be assigned for reading along with earlier chapters. We suggest the following prerequisite reading for the topics in Chapters 17 and 18:

Section(s)	Topic	Prerequisite
17.1	Template functions	Chapter 10
17.2	Template classes	Chapter 13
17.3	Exceptions	Chapter 11
18.1–18.3	Recursion with simple variables	Chapter 8
18.4	Recursion with arrays	Chapter 12
18.5	Recursion with pointer variables	Chapter 16

Additional Features

Web Links Special Web icons found in the Special Sections (see below) prompt students to visit the text's companion website, located at `www.problemsolvingcpp.jbpub.com` for additional information about selected topics. These Web links give students instant access to real-world applications of material presented in the text. The Web links are updated on a regular basis to ensure that students receive the most recent information available on the Internet.

Special Sections Five kinds of features are set off from the main text. Theoretical Foundations sections present material related to the fundamental theory behind various branches of computer science. Software Engineering Tips discuss methods of making programs more reliable, robust, or efficient. Matters of Style address stylistic issues in the coding of programs. Background Information sections explore side issues that enhance the student's general knowledge of computer science. May We Introduce sections contain biographies of computing pioneers such as Blaise Pascal, Ada Lovelace, and Grace Murray Hopper. Web links appear in most of these Special Sections prompting students to visit the companion website for expanded material.

Goals As described earlier, each chapter begins with a list of goals for the student, broken into two categories: knowledge goals and skill goals. They are reinforced and tested in the end-of-chapter exercises.

Problem-Solving Case Studies Problem solving is best demonstrated through case studies. In each case study, we present a problem and use problem-solving techniques to develop a manual solution. Next, we expand the solution to an algorithm, using functional decomposition, object-oriented design, or both; then we code the algorithm in C++. We show sample test data and output and follow up with a discussion of what is involved in thoroughly testing the program.

Testing and Debugging Testing and debugging sections follow the case studies in each chapter and consider in depth the implications of the chapter material with regard to thorough testing of programs. These sections conclude with a list of testing and debugging hints.

Quick Checks At the end of each chapter are questions that test the student's recall of major points associated with the chapter goals. Upon reading each question, the student immediately should know the answer, which he or she can then verify by glancing at the answers at the end of the section. The page number on which the concept is discussed appears at the end of each question so that the student can review the material in the event of an incorrect response.

Exam Preparation Exercises These questions help the student prepare for tests. The questions usually have objective answers and are designed to be answerable with a few minutes of work. Answers to selected questions are given in the back of the book, and the remaining questions are answered in the *Instructor's Guide*.

Programming Warm-Up Exercises This section provides the student with experience in writing C++ code fragments. The student can practice the syntactic constructs in each chapter without the burden of writing a complete program. Solutions to selected questions from each chapter appear in the back of the book; the remaining solutions can be found in the *Instructor's Guide.*

Programming Problems These exercises, drawn from a wide range of disciplines, require the student to design solutions and write complete programs.

Case Study Follow-Up Much of modern programming practice involves reading and modifying existing code. These exercises give the student an opportunity to strengthen this critical skill by answering questions about the case study code or by making changes to it. All of the solutions to these exercises are in the *Instructor's Guide*, rather than the text, allowing the instructor the flexibility of assigning them as programming problems.

Supplements

Instructor's Guide and Test Bank The *Instructor's Guide* features chapter-by-chapter teaching notes, answers to the balance of the exercises, and a compilation of exam questions with answers. The *Instructor's Guide*, included on the *Instructor's ToolKit,* is available to adopters on request from Jones and Bartlett.

Instructor's ToolKit The *Instructor's ToolKit* is a powerful teaching tool available to adopters upon request from the publisher. It contains an electronic version of the *Instructor's Guide,* a computerized test bank, PowerPoint lecture presentations, and the complete programs from the text.

Programs The programs contain the source code for all of the complete programs that are found within the textbook. They are available on the *Instructor's ToolKit,* and also as a free download for instructors and students from the publisher's website (www.problemsolvingcpp.jbpub.com). The programs from all of the case studies, plus complete programs that appear in the chapter bodies, are included. (Fragments or snippets of program code are not included nor are the solutions to the chapter-ending "Programming Problems.") The program files can be viewed or edited using any standard text editor, but a C++ compiler must be used in order to compile and run the programs. The publisher offers compilers bundled with this text at a substantial discount.

Companion Website This website (www.problemsolvingcpp.jbpub.com) features integrated Web links from the textbook, the complete programs from the text, and Appendix D, entitled "Using this Book with a Prestandard Version of C++," which describes the changes needed to allow the programs in the textbook to run successfully with a prestandard compiler.

A Laboratory Course in C++, Fourth Edition Written by Nell Dale, this lab manual follows the organization of this edition of the text. The lab manual is designed to allow the instructor maximum flexibility and may be used in both open and closed laboratory settings. Each chapter contains three types of activities: Prelab, Inlab, and Postlab. Each lesson is broken into exercises that thoroughly demonstrate the concepts covered in the corresponding chapter. The programs, program shells (partial programs), and data files that accompany the lab manual can be found on the website for this book (www.problemsolvingcpp.jbpub.com).

Student Lecture Notebook Based on the design of the PowerPoint presentations developed for this text, the Student Lecture Notebook is an invaluable tool for learning. The notebook is designed to encourage students to focus their energies on listening to the lecture as they fill in additional details. The skeletal outline concept helps students organize their notes and readily recognize the important concepts in each chapter.

Acknowledgments

We would like to thank the many individuals who have helped us in the preparation of this fourth edition. We are indebted to the members of the faculties of the Computer Science Departments at the University of Texas at Austin and the University of Massachusetts at Amherst.

We extend special thanks to Jeff Brumfield for developing the syntax template metalanguage and allowing us to use it in the text.

For their many helpful suggestions, we thank the lecturers, teaching assistants, consultants, and student proctors who run the courses for which this book was written, as well as the students themselves.

We are grateful to the following people who took the time to offer their comments on potential changes for previous editions: Trudee Bremer, Illinois Central College; Mira Carlson, Northeastern Illinois University; Kevin Daimi, University of Detroit, Mercy; Bruce Elenbogen, University of Michigan, Dearborn; Sandria Kerr, Winston-Salem State University; Alicia Kime, Fairmont State College; Shahadat Kowuser, University of Texas, Pan America; Bruce Maxim, University of Michigan, Dearborn; William McQuain, Virginia Tech; Xiannong Meng, University of Texas, Pan America; William Minervini, Broward University; Janet Remen, Washtenaw Community College; Viviana Sandor, Oakland University; Mehdi Setareh, Virginia Tech; Katy Snyder, University of Detroit, Mercy; Tom Steiner, University of Michigan, Dearborn; John Weaver, West Chester University; Charles Welty, University of Southern Maine; Cheer-Sun Yang, West Chester University.

We also thank Mike and Sigrid Wile, along with the many people at Jones and Bartlett who contributed so much, especially Stephen Solomon and Anne Spencer. Our special thanks go to Amy Rose, our Production Manager, whose skills and genial nature turn hard work into pleasure.

Anyone who has ever written a book—or is related to someone who has—can appreciate the amount of time involved in such a project. To our families—all of the Dale clan and the extended Dale family (too numerous to name), and to Lisa, Charlie, and Abby—thanks for your tremendous support and indulgence.

N. D.
C. W.

CONTENTS

5 Conditions, Logical Expressions, and Selection Control Structures 191

13 Array-Based Lists   661

17 Templates and Exceptions   907

Overview of Programming and Problem Solving

Goals

Knowledge Goals

- ■ *To understand what a computer program is.*
- ■ *To understand what an algorithm is.*
- ■ *To learn what a high-level programming language is.*
- ■ *To understand the compilation and execution processes.*
- ■ *To learn the history of the C++ language.*
- ■ *To learn what the major components of a computer are and how they work together.*
- ■ *To learn about some of the basic ethical issues confronting computing professionals.*

Skill Goals

To be able to:

- ■ *List the basic stages involved in writing a computer program.*
- ■ *Describe what a compiler is and what it does.*
- ■ *Distinguish between hardware and software.*
- ■ *Choose an appropriate problem-solving method for developing an algorithmic solution to a problem.*

1.1 Overview of Programming

In the box in the margin is a definition of computer. What a brief definition for something that has, in just a few decades, changed the way of life in industrialized societies! Computers touch all areas of our lives: paying bills, driving cars, using the telephone, shopping. In fact, it would be easier to list those areas of our lives that are not affected by computers.

com•put•er \kəm-'pyüt-ər\ *n. often attrib* (1646): one that computes; *specif*: a programmable electronic device that can store, retrieve, and process data*

It is sad that a device that does so much good is so often maligned and feared. How many times have you heard someone say, "I'm sorry, our computer fouled things up" or "I just don't understand computers; they're too complicated for me"? The very fact that you are reading this book, however, means that you are ready to set aside prejudice and learn about computers. But be forewarned: This book is not just about computers in the abstract. This is a text to teach you how to program computers.

What Is Programming?

Much of human behavior and thought is characterized by logical sequences. Since infancy, you have been learning how to act, how to do things. And you have learned to expect certain behavior from other people.

A lot of what you do every day you do automatically. Fortunately, it is not necessary for you to consciously think of every step involved in a process as simple as turning a page by hand:

1. Lift hand.
2. Move hand to right side of book.
3. Grasp top right corner of page.
4. Move hand from right to left until page is positioned so that you can read what is on the other side.
5. Let go of page.

Think how many neurons must fire and how many muscles must respond, all in a certain order or sequence, to move your arm and hand. Yet you do it unconsciously.

Much of what you do unconsciously you once had to learn. Watch how a baby concentrates on putting one foot before the other while learning to walk. Then watch a group of three-year-olds playing tag.

On a broader scale, mathematics never could have been developed without logical sequences of steps for solving problems and proving theorems. Mass production never would have worked without operations taking place in a certain order. Our whole civilization is based on the order of things and actions.

---

*By permission. From *Merriam-Webster's Collegiate Dictionary*, Tenth Edition. © 1994 by Merriam-Webster Inc.

We create order, both consciously and unconsciously, through a process we call **programming**. This book is concerned with the programming of one of our tools, the **computer**.

Just as a concert program lists the order in which the players perform pieces, a **computer program** lists the sequence of steps the computer performs. From now on, when we use the words *programming* and *program*, we mean **computer programming** and *computer program*.

> **Programming**   Planning or scheduling the performance of a task or an event.
>
> **Computer**   A programmable device that can store, retrieve, and process data.
>
> **Computer program**   A sequence of instructions to be performed by a computer.
>
> **Computer programming**   The process of planning a sequence of steps for a computer to follow.

The computer allows us to do tasks more efficiently, quickly, and accurately than we could by hand—if we could do them by hand at all. In order to use this powerful tool, we must specify what we want done and the order in which we want it done. We do this through programming.

How Do We Write a Program?

A computer is not intelligent. It cannot analyze a problem and come up with a solution. A human (the *programmer*) must analyze the problem, develop a sequence of instructions for solving the problem, and then communicate it to the computer. What's the advantage of using a computer if it can't solve problems? Once we have written the solution as a sequence of instructions for the computer, the computer can repeat the solution very quickly and consistently, again and again. The computer frees people from repetitive and boring tasks.

To write a sequence of instructions for a computer to follow, we must go through a two-phase process: *problem solving* and *implementation* (see Figure 1–1).

Problem–Solving Phase

1. *Analysis and specification.*   Understand (define) the problem and what the solution must do.
2. *General solution (algorithm).*   Develop a logical sequence of steps that solves the problem.
3. *Verify.*   Follow the steps exactly to see if the solution really does solve the problem.

Implementation Phase

1. *Concrete solution (program).*   Translate the algorithm into a programming language.
2. *Test.*   Have the computer follow the instructions. Then manually check the results. If you find errors, analyze the program and the algorithm to determine the source of the errors, and then make corrections.

PROBLEM-SOLVING PHASE   IMPLEMENTATION PHASE

Analysis
and
specification

↓

General solution
(algorithm)

↓

Verify

Concrete solution
(program)

↓

Test

MAINTENANCE PHASE

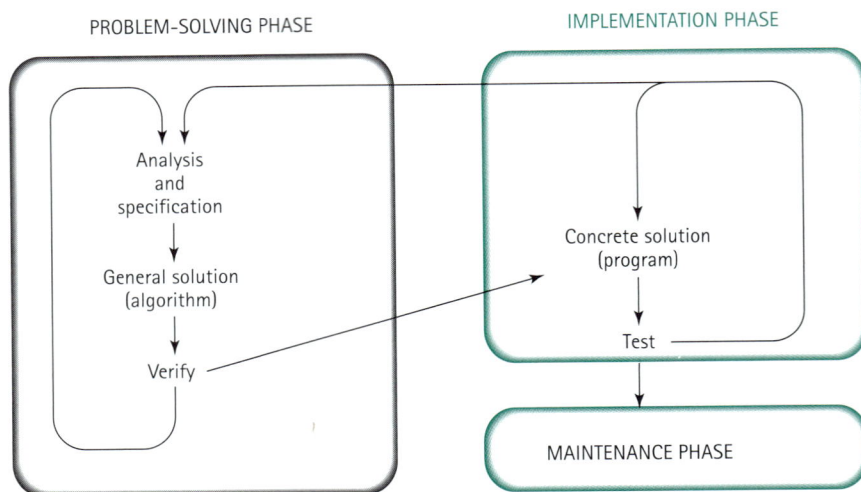

Figure 1–1 *Programming Process*

Once a program has been written, it enters a third phase: *maintenance.*

Maintenance Phase

1. *Use.* Use the program.
2. *Maintain.* Modify the program to meet changing requirements or to correct any errors that show up in using it.

> **Algorithm**   A step-by-step procedure for solving a problem in a finite amount of time.

The programmer begins the programming process by analyzing the problem and developing a general solution called an **algorithm**. Understanding and analyzing a problem take up much more time than Figure 1–1 implies. They are the heart of the programming process.

If our definitions of a computer program and an algorithm look similar, it is because all programs are algorithms. A program is simply an algorithm that has been written for a computer.

An algorithm is a verbal or written description of a logical sequence of actions. We use algorithms every day. Recipes, instructions, and directions are all examples of algorithms that are not programs.

When you start your car, you follow a step-by-step procedure. The algorithm might look something like this:

1. Insert the key.
2. Make sure the transmission is in Park (or Neutral).
3. Depress the gas pedal.
4. Turn the key to the start position.
5. If the engine starts within six seconds, release the key to the ignition position.
6. If the engine doesn't start in six seconds, release the key and gas pedal, wait ten seconds, and repeat Steps 3 through 6, but not more than five times.
7. If the car doesn't start, call the garage.

Without the phrase "but not more than five times" in Step 6, you could be trying to start the car forever. Why? Because if something is wrong with the car, repeating Steps 3 through 6 over and over again will not start it. This kind of never-ending situation is called an *infinite loop*. If we leave the phrase "but not more than five times" out of Step 6, the procedure does not fit our definition of an algorithm. An algorithm must terminate in a finite amount of time for all possible conditions.

Suppose a programmer needs an algorithm to determine an employee's weekly wages. The algorithm reflects what would be done by hand:

1. Look up the employee's pay rate.
2. Determine the number of hours worked during the week.
3. If the number of hours worked is less than or equal to 40, multiply the number of hours by the pay rate to calculate regular wages.
4. If the number of hours worked is greater than 40, multiply 40 by the pay rate to calculate regular wages, and then multiply the difference between the number of hours worked and 40 by $1\frac{1}{2}$ times the pay rate to calculate overtime wages.
5. Add the regular wages to the overtime wages (if any) to determine total wages for the week.

The steps the computer follows are often the same steps you would use to do the calculations by hand.

After developing a general solution, the programmer tests the algorithm, walking through each step mentally or manually. If the algorithm doesn't work, the programmer repeats the problem-solving process, analyzing the problem again and coming up with another algorithm. Often the second algorithm is just a variation of the first. When the programmer is satisfied with the algorithm, he or she translates it into a **programming language**. We use the C++ programming language in this book.

> **Programming language**   A set of rules, symbols, and special words used to construct a computer program.

A programming language is a simplified form of English (with math symbols) that adheres to a strict set of grammatical rules. English is far too complicated a language for today's computers to follow. Programming languages, because they limit vocabulary and grammar, are much simpler.

Although a programming language is simple in form, it is not always easy to use. Try giving someone directions to the nearest airport using a vocabulary of no more than 45 words, and you'll begin to see the problem. Programming forces you to write very simple, exact instructions.

Translating an algorithm into a programming language is called *coding* the algorithm. The product of that translation—the program—is tested by running (*executing*) it on the computer. If the program fails to produce the desired results, the programmer must *debug* it—that is, determine what is wrong and then modify the program, or even the algorithm, to fix it. The combination of coding and testing an algorithm is called *implementation*.

There is no single way to implement an algorithm. For example, an algorithm can be translated into more than one programming language. Each translation produces a different implementation. Even when two people translate an algorithm into the same programming language, they are likely to come up with different implementations (see Figure 1–2). Why? Because every programming language allows the programmer some flexibility in how an algorithm is translated. Given this flexibility, people adopt their own styles in writing programs, just as they do in writing short stories or essays. Once you have some programming experience, you develop a style of your own. Throughout this book, we offer tips on good programming style.

Some people try to speed up the programming process by going directly from the problem definition to coding the program (see Figure 1–3). A shortcut here is very tempting and at first seems to save a lot of time. However, for many reasons that will become obvious to you as you read this book, this kind of shortcut actually takes *more* time and effort. Developing a general solution before you write a program helps you manage the problem, keep your thoughts straight, and avoid mistakes. If you don't take the time at the beginning to think out and polish your algorithm, you'll spend a lot of extra time debugging and revising your program. So think first and code later! The sooner you start coding, the longer it takes to write a program that works.

Once a program has been put into use, it is often necessary to modify it. Modification may involve fixing an error that is discovered during the use of the program or changing the program in response to changes in the user's requirements. Each time the program is modified, it is necessary to repeat the problem-solving and implementation phases for those aspects of the program that change. This phase of the programming process is known as maintenance and actually accounts for the majority of the effort expended on most programs. For example, a program that is implemented in a few months may need to be maintained over a period of many years. Thus, it is a cost-effective investment of time to develop the initial problem solution and program implementation carefully. Together, the problem-solving, implementation, and maintenance phases constitute the program's *life cycle*.

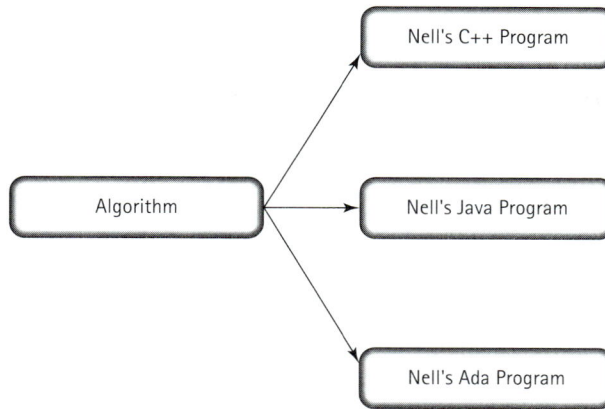

a. Algorithm translated into different languages

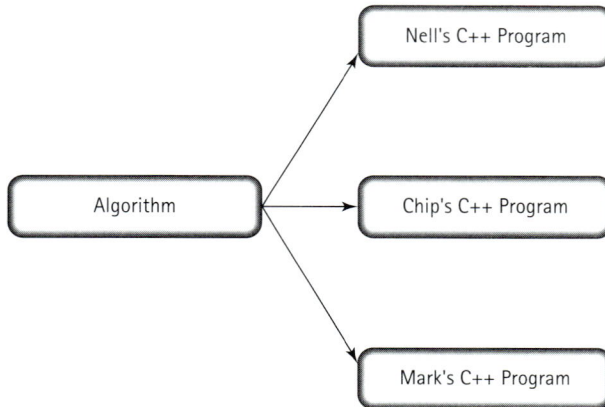

b. Algorithm translated by different people

Figure 1–2 *Differences in Implementation*

In addition to solving the problem, implementing the algorithm, and maintaining the program, **documentation** is an important part of the programming process. Documentation includes written explanations of the problem being solved and the organization of the solution, comments embedded within the program itself, and user manuals that describe how to use the program. Most programs are worked on by many different people over a long period of time. Each of those people must be able to read and understand your code.

> **Documentation** The written text and comments that make a program easier for others to understand, use, and modify.

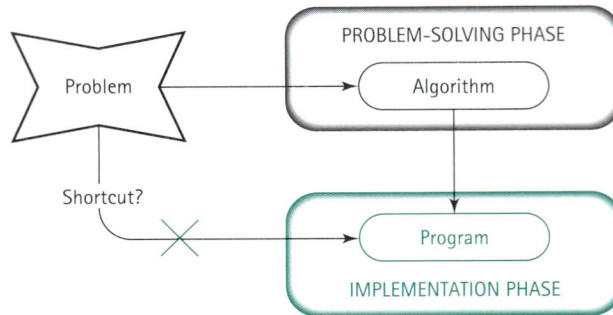

Figure 1-3   *Programming Shortcut?*

After you write a program, you must give the computer the information or data necessary to solve the problem. **Information** is any knowledge that can be communicated, including abstract ideas and concepts such as "the earth is round." **Data** is information in a form the computer can use—for example, the numbers and letters making up the formulas that relate the earth's radius to its volume and surface area. But data is not restricted to numbers and letters. These days, computers also process data that represents sound (to be played through speakers), graphic images (to be displayed on a computer screen or printer), video (to be played on a DVD player), and so forth.

Information   Any knowledge that can be communicated.

Data   Information in a form a computer can use.

Theoretical Foundations

Binary Representation of Data

In a computer, data is represented electronically by pulses of electricity. Electric circuits, in their simplest form, are either on or off. Usually a circuit that is on is represented by the number 1; a circuit that is off is represented by the number 0. Any kind of data can be represented by combinations of enough 1s and 0s. We simply have to choose which combination represents each piece of data we are using. For example, we could arbitrarily choose the pattern 1101000110 to represent the name C++.

Data represented by 1s and 0s is in *binary form*. The binary (base–2) number system uses only 1s and 0s to represent numbers. (The decimal [base–10] number system uses the digits 0 through 9.) The word *bit* (short for **b**inary dig**it**) often is used to refer to a single 1 or 0. The pattern 1101000110 thus has 10 bits. A binary number with 10 bits can represent 2^{10} (1024) different patterns. A *byte* is a

(continued) ▼

Binary Representation of Data

group of 8 bits; it can represent 2^8 (256) patterns. Inside the computer, each character (such as the letter *A*, the letter *g*, or a question mark) is usually represented by a byte. Four bits, or half of a byte, is called a *nibble* or *nybble*—a name that originally was proposed with tongue in cheek but now is standard terminology. Groups of 16, 32, and 64 bits are generally referred to as *words* (although the terms *short word* and *long word* are sometimes used to refer to 16-bit and 64-bit groups, respectively).

The process of assigning bit patterns to pieces of data is called *coding*—the same name we give to the process of translating an algorithm into a programming language. The names are the same because the only language that the first computers recognized was binary in form. Thus, in the early days of computers, programming meant translating both data and algorithms into patterns of 1s and 0s.

Binary coding schemes are still used inside the computer to represent both the instructions that it follows and the data that it uses. For example, 16 bits can represent the decimal integers from 0 to $2^{16} - 1$ (65,535). Characters also can be represented by bit combinations. In one coding scheme, 01001101 represents *M* and 01101101 represents *m*. More complicated coding schemes are necessary to represent negative numbers, real numbers, numbers in scientific notation, sound, graphics, and video. In Chapter 10, we examine in detail the representation of numbers and characters in the computer.

The patterns of bits that represent data vary from one computer to another. Even on the same computer, different programming languages can use different binary representations for the same data. A single programming language may even use the same pattern of bits to represent different things in different contexts. (People do this too. The word formed by the four letters *tack* has different meanings depending on whether you are talking about upholstery, sailing, sewing, paint, or horseback riding.) The point is that patterns of bits by themselves are meaningless. It is the way in which the patterns are used that gives them their meaning.

Fortunately, we no longer have to work with binary coding schemes. Today the process of coding is usually just a matter of writing down the data in letters, numbers, and symbols. The computer automatically converts these letters, numbers, and symbols into binary form. Still, as you work with computers, you will continually run into numbers that are related to powers of 2—numbers such as 256, 32,768, and 65,536—reminders that the binary number system is lurking somewhere nearby.

1.2   What Is a Programming Language?

In the computer, all data, whatever its form, is stored and used in binary codes, strings of 1s and 0s. Instructions and data are stored together in the computer's memory using these binary codes. If you were to look at the binary codes representing instructions and data in memory, you could not tell the difference between them; they are distinguished

Machine language The language, made up of binary-coded instructions, that is used directly by the computer.

Assembly language A low-level programming language in which a mnemonic is used to represent each of the machine language instructions for a particular computer.

only by the manner in which the computer uses them. It is thus possible for the computer to process its own instructions as a form of data.

When computers were first developed, the only programming language available was the primitive instruction set built into each machine, the **machine language**, or *machine code*.

Even though most computers perform the same kinds of operations, their designers choose different sets of binary codes for each instruction. So the machine code for one computer is not the same as for another.

When programmers used machine language for programming, they had to enter the binary codes for the various instructions, a tedious process that was prone to error. Moreover, their programs were difficult to read and modify. In time, **assembly languages** were developed to make the programmer's job easier.

Instructions in an assembly language are in an easy-to-remember form called a *mnemonic* (pronounced ni-MON-ik). Typical instructions for addition and subtraction might look like this:

Assembly Language	Machine Language
ADD	100101
SUB	010011

Although assembly language is easier for humans to work with, the computer cannot directly execute the instructions. One of the fundamental discoveries in computer science is that, because a computer can process its own instructions as a form of data, it is possible to write a program to translate the assembly language instructions into machine code. Such a program is called an **assembler**.

Assembler A program that translates an assembly language program into machine code.

Compiler A program that translates a high-level language into machine code.

Source program A program written in a high-level programming language.

Object program The machine language version of a source program.

Assembly language is a step in the right direction, but it still forces programmers to think in terms of individual machine instructions. Eventually, computer scientists developed high-level programming languages. These languages are easier to use than assembly languages or machine code because they are closer to English and other natural languages (see Figure 1–4).

A program called a **compiler** translates programs written in certain high-level languages (C++, Pascal, FORTRAN, COBOL, Modula–2, and Ada, for example) into machine language. If you write a program in a high-level language, you can run it on any computer that has the appropriate compiler. This is possible because most high-level languages are *standardized*, which means that an official description of the language exists.

A program in a high-level language is called a **source program**. To the compiler, a source program is just input data. It translates the source program into a machine language program called an **object program** (see Figure 1–5). Some compilers also output a *listing*—a copy of the program with error messages and other information inserted.

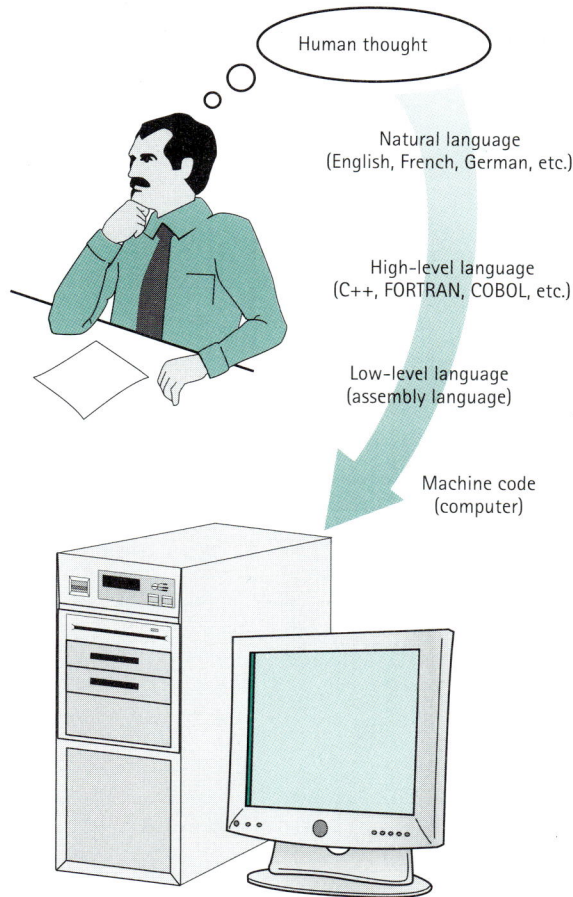

Figure 1–4   *Levels of Abstraction*

A benefit of standardized high-level languages is that they allow you to write *portable* (or *machine-independent*) code. As Figure 1–5 emphasizes, a single C++ program can be used on different machines, whereas a program written in assembly language or machine language is not portable from one computer to another. Because each computer has its own machine language, a machine language program written for computer A will not run on computer B.

It is important to understand that compilation and execution are two distinct processes. During compilation, the computer runs the compiler program. During execution, the object program is loaded into the computer's memory unit, replacing the compiler program. The computer then runs the object program, doing whatever the program instructs it to do (see Figure 1–6).

SOURCE PROGRAM
(C++)

COMPUTER
EXECUTES
TRANSLATOR
PROGRAM
(COMPILER)

OBJECT
PROGRAM
(MACHINE
LANGUAGE
VERSION OF
SOURCE PROGRAM)

COMPUTER
EXECUTES
OBJECT
PROGRAM

Windows PC
C++ compiler

Windows PC
machine
language

Windows PC
computer

C++ Program

UNIX
workstation
C++ compiler

UNIX
workstation
machine
language

UNIX
workstation
computer

Macintosh
C++ compiler

Macintosh
machine
language

Macintosh
computer

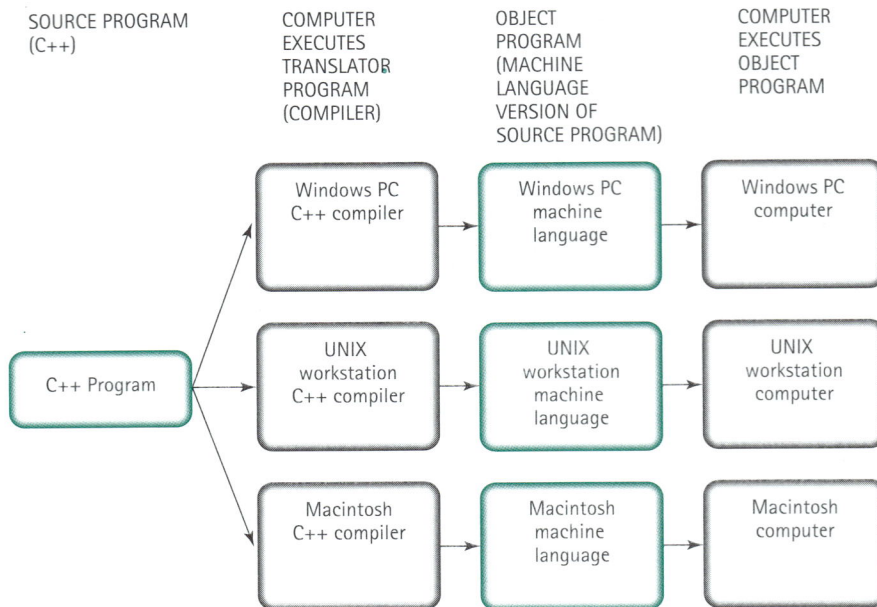

Figure 1–5   *High-Level Programming Languages Allow Programs to Be Compiled on Different Systems*

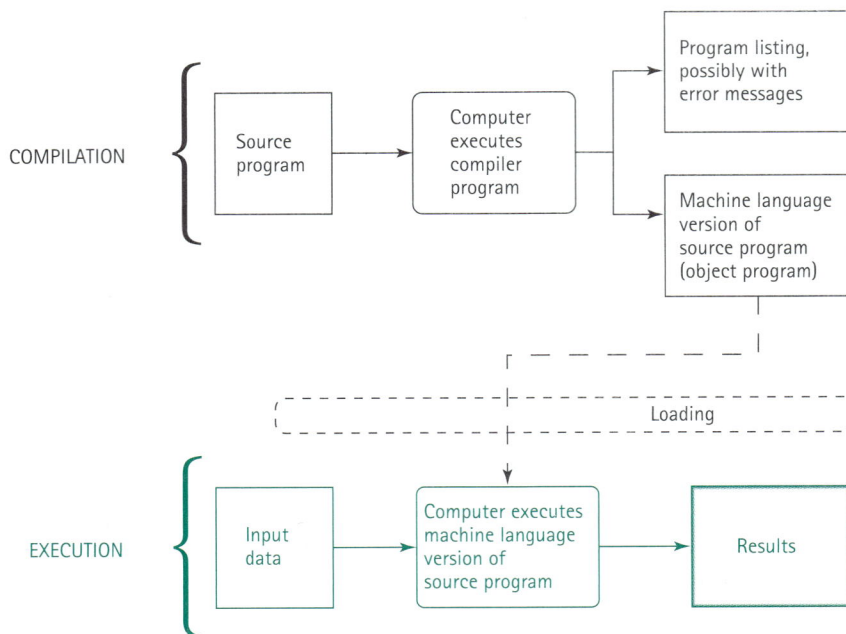

COMPILATION

Source
program

Computer
executes
compiler
program

Program listing,
possibly with
error messages

Machine language
version of
source program
(object program)

Loading

EXECUTION

Input
data

Computer executes
machine language
version of
source program

Results

Figure 1–6   *Compilation and Execution*

Background Information

Compilers and Interpreters

Some programming languages—LISP, Prolog, and many versions of BASIC, for example—are translated by an *interpreter* rather than a compiler. An interpreter translates *and executes* each instruction in the source program, one at a time. In contrast, a compiler translates the entire source program into machine language, after which execution of the object program takes place.

The Java language uses both a compiler and an interpreter. First, a Java program is compiled, not into a particular computer's machine language, but into an intermediate code called bytecode. Next, a program called the Java Virtual Machine (JVM) takes the bytecode program and interprets it (translates a bytecode instruction into machine language and executes it, translates the next one and executes it, and so on). Thus, a Java program compiled into bytecode is portable to many different computers, as long as each computer has its own specific JVM that can translate bytecode into the computer's machine language.

The instructions in a programming language reflect the operations a computer can perform:

- A computer can transfer data from one place to another.
- A computer can input data from an input device (a keyboard or mouse, for example) and output data to an output device (a screen, for example).
- A computer can store data into and retrieve data from its memory and secondary storage (parts of a computer that we discuss in the next section).
- A computer can compare two data values for equality or inequality.
- A computer can perform arithmetic operations (addition and subtraction, for example) very quickly.

Programming languages require that we use certain *control structures* to express algorithms as programs. There are four basic ways of structuring statements (instructions) in most programming languages: sequentially, conditionally, repetitively, and with subprograms (see Figure 1–7). A *sequence* is a series of statements that are executed one after another. *Selection*, the conditional control structure, executes different statements depending on certain conditions. The repetitive control structure, the *loop*, repeats statements while certain conditions are met. The *subprogram* allows us to structure a program by breaking it into smaller units. Each of these ways of structuring statements controls the order in which the computer executes the statements, which is why they are called control structures.

Imagine you're driving a car. Going down a straight stretch of road is like following a sequence of instructions. When you come to a fork in the road, you must decide which way to go and then take one or the other branch of the fork. This is what the

SEQUENCE

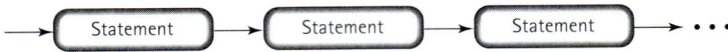

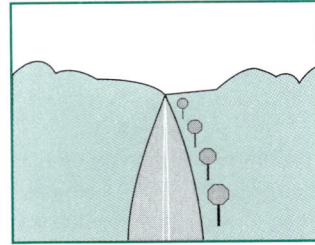

SELECTION   (also called *branch* or *decision*)

IF condition THEN statement1 ELSE statement2

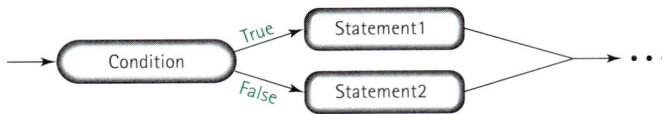

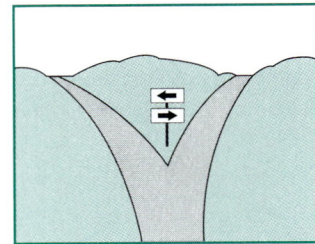

LOOP   (also called *repetition* or *iteration*)

WHILE condition DO statement1

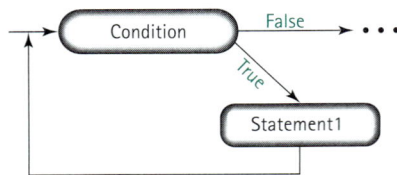

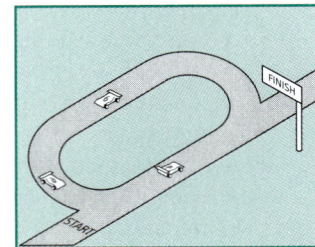

SUBPROGRAM   (also called *procedure, function, method,* or *subroutine*)

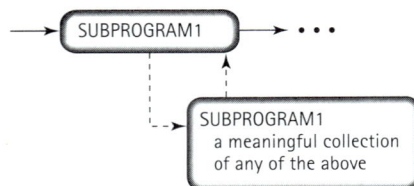

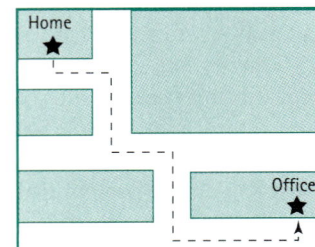

Figure 1–7   *Basic Control Structures of Programming Languages*

computer does when it encounters a selection control structure (sometimes called a *branch* or *decision*) in a program. Sometimes you have to go around the block several times to find a place to park. The computer does the same sort of thing when it encounters a loop in a program.

A subprogram is a process that consists of multiple steps. Every day, for example, you follow a procedure to get from home to work. It makes sense, then, for someone to give you directions to a meeting by saying, "Go to the office, then go four blocks west" without specifying all the steps you have to take to get to the office. Subprograms allow us to write parts of our programs separately and then assemble them into final form. They can greatly simplify the task of writing large programs.

1.3   What Is a Computer?

You can learn a programming language, how to write programs, and how to run (execute) these programs without knowing much about computers. But if you know something about the parts of a computer, you can better understand the effect of each instruction in a programming language.

Most computers have six basic components: the memory unit, the arithmetic/logic unit, the control unit, input devices, output devices, and auxiliary storage devices. Figure 1–8 is a stylized diagram of the basic components of a computer.

The **memory unit** is an ordered sequence of storage cells, each capable of holding a piece of data. Each memory cell has a distinct address to which we refer in order to store

Memory unit   Internal data storage in a computer.

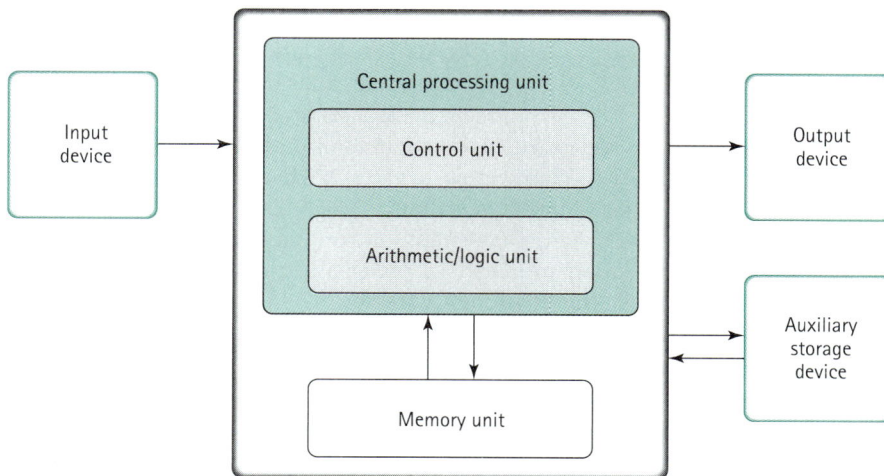

Figure 1–8   *Basic Components of a Computer*

MEMORY

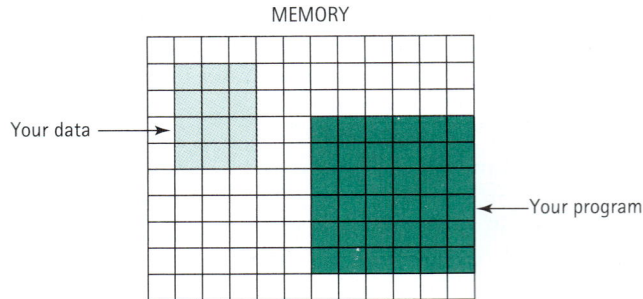

Figure 1-9   *Memory*

data into it or retrieve data from it. These storage cells are called *memory cells*, or *memory locations.** The memory unit holds data (input data or the product of computation) and instructions (programs), as shown in Figure 1-9.

The part of the computer that follows instructions is called the **central processing unit (CPU)**. The CPU usually has two components. The **arithmetic/logic unit (ALU)** performs arithmetic operations (addition, subtraction, multiplication, and division) and logical operations (comparing two values). The **control unit** controls the actions of the other components so that program instructions are executed in the correct order.

For us to use computers, there must be some way of getting data into and out of them. **Input/output (I/O) devices** accept data to be processed (input) and present data values that have been processed (output). A keyboard is a common input device. Another is a *mouse*, a pointing device. A video display is a common output device, as are printers and liquid crystal display (LCD) screens. Some devices, such as a connection to a computer network, are used for both input and output.

For the most part, computers simply move and combine data in memory. The many types of computers differ primarily in the size of their memories, the speed with which data can be recalled, the efficiency with which data can be moved or combined, and limitations on I/O devices.

When a program is executing, the computer proceeds through a series of steps, the *fetch-execute cycle*:

1. The control unit retrieves (*fetches*) the next coded instruction from memory.
2. The instruction is translated into control signals.

Central processing unit (CPU)   The part of the computer that executes the instructions (program) stored in memory; made up of the arithmetic/logic unit and the control unit.

Arithmetic/logic unit (ALU)   The component of the central processing unit that performs arithmetic and logical operations.

Control unit   The component of the central processing unit that controls the actions of the other components so that instructions (the program) are executed in the correct sequence.

Input/output (I/O) devices   The parts of the computer that accept data to be processed (input) and present the results of that processing (output).

---

*The memory unit is also referred to as RAM, an acronym for random-access memory (so called because we can access any location at random).

3. The control signals tell the appropriate unit (arithmetic/logic unit, memory, I/O device) to perform (execute) the instruction.

4. The sequence repeats from Step 1.

Computers can have a wide variety of **peripheral devices** attached to them. An **auxiliary storage device**, or *secondary storage device*, holds coded data for the computer until we actually want to use the data. Instead of inputting data every time, we can input it once and have the computer store it onto an auxiliary storage device. Whenever we need

> **Peripheral device**   An input, output, or auxiliary storage device attached to a computer.
>
> **Auxiliary storage device**   A device that stores data in encoded form outside the computer's main memory.

to use the data, we tell the computer to transfer the data from the auxiliary storage device to its memory. An auxiliary storage device therefore serves as both an input and an output device. Typical auxiliary storage devices are disk drives and magnetic tape drives. A *disk drive* is a cross between a compact disc player and a tape recorder. It uses a thin disk made out of magnetic material. A read/write head (similar to the record/playback head in a tape recorder) travels across the spinning disk, retrieving or recording data. A *magnetic tape drive* is like a tape recorder and is most often used to *back up* (make a copy of) the data on a disk in case the disk is ever damaged.

Other examples of peripheral devices include the following:

- Scanners, which "read" visual images on paper and convert them into binary data
- CD-ROM (compact disc–read-only memory) drives, which read (but cannot write) data stored on removable compact discs
- CD-R (compact disc–recordable) drives, which can write to a particular CD once only but can read from it many times
- CD-RW (compact disc–rewritable) drives, which can both write to and read from a particular CD many times
- DVD-ROM (digital video disc [or digital versatile disc]–read-only memory) drives, which use CDs with far greater storage capacity than conventional CDs
- Modems (modulator/demodulators), which convert back and forth between binary data and signals that can be sent over conventional telephone lines
- Audio sound cards and speakers
- Voice synthesizers
- Digital cameras

Together, all of these physical components are known as **hardware**. The programs that allow the hardware to operate are called **software**. Hardware usually is fixed in design; software is easily changed. In fact, the ease with which software can be manipulated is what makes the computer such a versatile, powerful tool.

> **Hardware**   The physical components of a computer.
>
> **Software**   Computer programs; the set of all programs available on a computer.

Background Information

PCs, Workstations, and Mainframes

There are many different sizes and kinds of computers. *Mainframes* are very large (they can fill a room!) and very fast. A typical mainframe computer consists of several cabinets full of electronic components. Inside those cabinets are the memory, the central processing unit, and input/output units. It's easy to spot the various peripheral devices: Separate cabinets contain the disk drives and tape drives. Other units are obviously printers and terminals (monitors with keyboards). It is common to be able to connect hundreds of terminals to a single mainframe. For example, all of the cash registers in a chain of department stores might be linked to a single mainframe.

At the other end of the spectrum are *personal computers (PCs)*. These are small enough to fit comfortably on top of a desk. Because of their size, it can be difficult to spot the individual parts inside personal computers. Many PCs are just a single box with a screen, a keyboard, and a mouse. You have to open up the case to see the central processing unit, which is usually just an electronic component called an *integrated circuit* or *chip*.

Some personal computers have tape drives, but most operate only with disk drives, CD-ROM drives, and printers. The CD-ROM and disk drives for personal computers typically hold much less data than disks used with mainframes. Similarly, the printers that are attached to personal computers typically are much slower than those used with mainframes.

Laptop or *notebook* computers are PCs that have been reduced to the size of a large notebook and operate on batteries so that they are portable. They typically consist of two parts that are connected by a hinge at the back of the case. The upper part holds a flat, liquid crystal display (LCD) screen, and the lower part has the keyboard, pointing device, processor, memory, and disk drives.

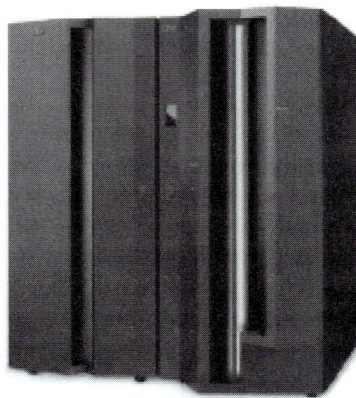

Mainframe Computer   Photo Courtesy of IBM

(continued) ▼

PCs, Workstations, and Mainframes

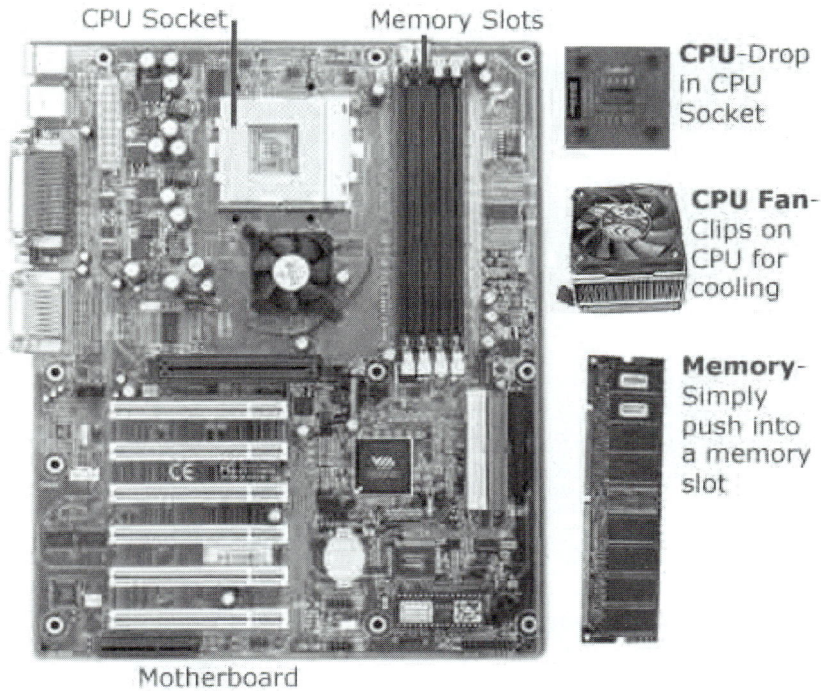

CPU Socket   Memory Slots

CPU-Drop in CPU Socket

CPU Fan-Clips on CPU for cooling

Memory-Simply push into a memory slot

Motherboard

(A) Inside a PC, System Unit Broken Down   Photo Courtesy of UltimaTec

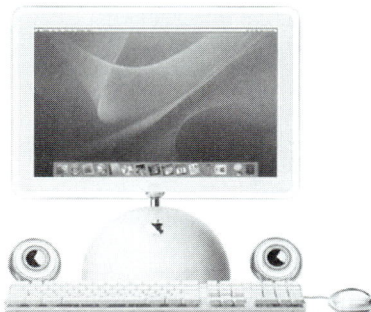

(B) Personal Computer, Macintosh
Photo Courtesy of Apple Computers

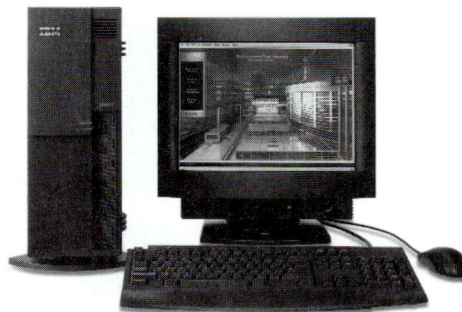

(C) Personal Computer*

*The figures (C) and (G) on pages 19 and 20 are reproduced courtesy of International Business Machines Corporation. Unauthorized use not permitted.

(continued) ▼

PCs, Workstations, and Mainframes

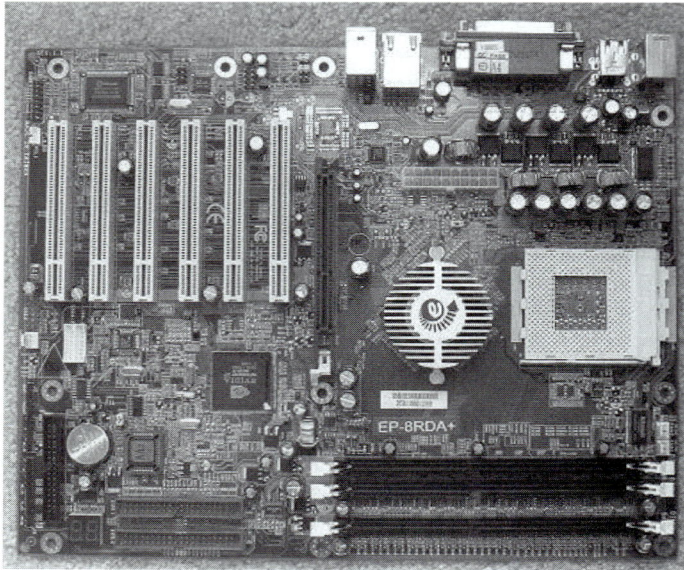

(D) Inside a PC, Close-Up of a System Board   *Photo Courtesy of Rob Williams*

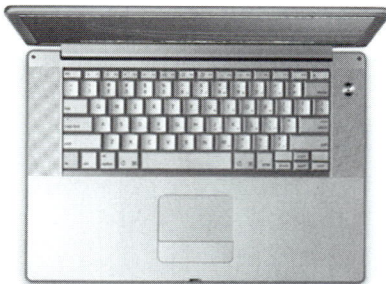

(E) Notebook Computer
Photo Courtesy of Apple Computers

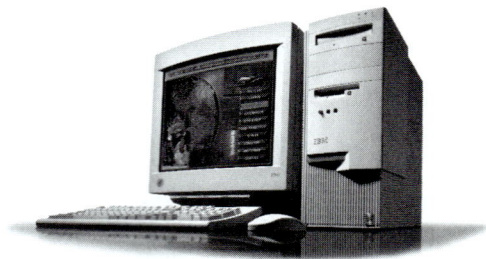

(G) Workstation*

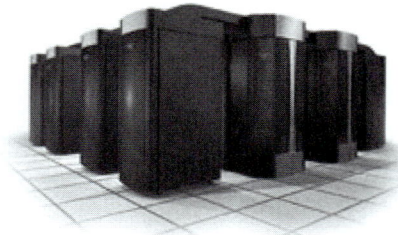

(F) Supercomputer
Photo Courtesy of Cray, Inc.

(continued) ▼

PCs, Workstations, and Mainframes

Between mainframes and personal computers are *workstations*. These intermediate-sized computer systems are usually less expensive than mainframes and more powerful than personal computers. Workstations are often set up for use primarily by one person at a time. A workstation may also be configured to act like a small mainframe, in which case it is called a *server*. A typical workstation looks very much like a PC. In fact, as PCs have grown more powerful and workstations have become more compact, the distinction between them has begun to fade.

One last type of computer that we should mention is the *supercomputer*, the most powerful class of computer in existence. Supercomputers typically are designed to perform scientific and engineering calculations on immense sets of data with great speed. They are very expensive and thus are not in widespread use.

In addition to the programs that we write or purchase, there are programs in the computer that are designed to simplify the user/computer **interface**, making it easier for us to use the machine. The interface between user and computer is a set of I/O devices—for example, a keyboard, mouse, and screen—that allow the user to communicate with the computer. We work with the keyboard, mouse, and screen on our side of the interface boundary; wires attached to these devices carry the electronic pulses that the computer works with on its side of the interface boundary. At the boundary itself is a mechanism that translates information for the two sides.

Interface   A connecting link at a shared boundary that allows independent systems to meet and act on or communicate with each other.

Interactive system   A system that allows direct communication between user and computer.

Operating system   A set of programs that manages all of the computer's resources.

Editor   An interactive program used to create and modify source programs or data.

When we communicate directly with the computer, we are using an **interactive system**. Interactive systems allow direct entry of programs and data and provide immediate feedback to the user. In contrast, *batch systems* require that all data be entered before a program is run and provide feedback only after a program has been executed. In this text we focus on interactive systems, although in Chapter 4 we discuss file-oriented programs, which share certain similarities with batch systems.

The set of programs that simplify the user/computer interface and improve the efficiency of processing is called *system software*. It includes the compiler as well as the operating system and the editor (see Figure 1–10). The **operating system** manages all of the computer's resources. It can input programs, call the compiler, execute object programs, and carry out any other system commands. The **editor** is an interactive program used to create and modify source programs or data.

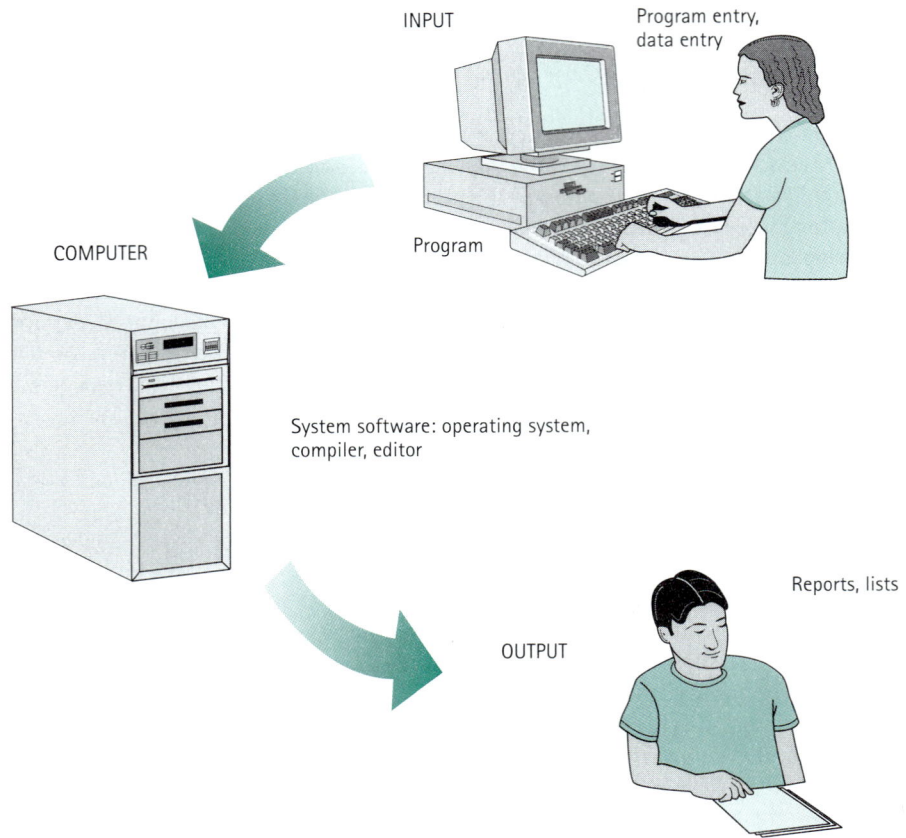

Figure 1–10 *User/Computer Interface*

Although solitary (*stand-alone*) computers are often used in private homes and small businesses, it is very common for many computers to be connected together, forming a *network*. A *local area network* (*LAN*) is one in which the computers are connected by wires and must be reasonably close together, as in a single office building. In a *wide area network* (*WAN*) or *long-haul network*, the computers can be far apart geographically and communicate through phone lines, fiber optic cable, and other media. The most well-known long-haul network is the Internet, which was originally devised as a means for universities, businesses, and government agencies to exchange research information. The Internet exploded in popularity with the establishment of the World Wide Web, a system of linked Internet computers that support specially formatted documents (*Web pages*) that contain text, graphics, audio, and video.

Background Information

The Origins of C++

In the late 1960s and early 1970s, Dennis Ritchie created the C programming language at AT&T Bell Labs. At the time, a group of people within Bell Labs were designing the UNIX operating system. Initially, UNIX was written in assembly language, as was the custom for almost all system software in those days. To escape the difficulties of programming in assembly language, Ritchie invented C as a system programming language. C combines the low-level features of an assembly language with the ease of use and portability of a high-level language. UNIX was reprogrammed so that approximately 90% was written in C, and the remainder in assembly language.

People often wonder where the cryptic name C came from. In the 1960s a programming language named BCPL (Basic Combined Programming Language) had a small but loyal following, primarily in Europe. From BCPL, another language arose with its name abbreviated to B. For his language, Dennis Ritchie adopted features from the B language and decided that the successor to B naturally should be named C. So the progression was from BCPL to B to C.

In 1985 Bjarne Stroustrup, also of Bell Labs, invented the C++ programming language. To the C language he added features for data abstraction and object-oriented programming (topics we discuss later in this book). Instead of naming the language D, the Bell Labs group in a humorous vein named it C++. As we see later, ++ signifies the increment operation in the C and C++ languages. Given a variable x, the expression x++ means to increment (add one to) the current value of x. Therefore, the name C++ suggests an enhanced ("incremented") version of the C language.

In the years since Dr. Stroustrup invented C++, the language began to evolve in slightly different ways in different C++ compilers. Although the fundamental features of C++ were nearly the same in all companies' compilers, one company might add a new language feature, whereas another would not. As a result, C++ programs were not always portable from one compiler to the next. The programming community agreed that the language needed to be standardized, and a joint committee of the International Standards Organization (ISO) and the American National Standards Institute (ANSI) began the long process of creating a C++ language standard. After several years of discussion and debate, the ISO/ANSI language standard for C++ was officially approved in mid–1998. Most of the current C++ compilers support the ISO/ANSI standard (hereafter called *standard* C++). To assist you if you are using a pre–standard compiler, throughout the book we point out discrepancies between older language features and new ones that may affect how you write your programs.

Although C originally was intended as a system programming language, both C and C++ are widely used today in business, industry, and personal computing. C++ is powerful and versatile, embodying a wide range of programming concepts. In this book you will learn a substantial portion of the language, but C++ incorporates sophisticated features that go well beyond the scope of an introductory programming course.

1.4 Ethics and Responsibilities in the Computing Profession

Every profession operates with a set of ethics that help to define the responsibilities of people who practice the profession. For example, medical professionals have an ethical responsibility to keep information about their patients confidential. Engineers have an ethical responsibility to their employers to protect proprietary information, but they also have a responsibility to protect the public and the environment from harm that may result from their work. Writers are ethically bound not to plagiarize the work of others, and so on.

The computer presents us with a vast new range of capabilities that can affect people and the environment in dramatic ways. It thus challenges society with many new ethical issues. Some of our existing ethical practices apply to the computer, whereas other situations require new ethical rules. In some cases, there may not be established guidelines, but it is up to you to decide what is ethical. In this section we examine some common situations encountered in the computing profession that raise particular ethical issues.

A professional in the computing industry, like any other professional, has knowledge that enables him or her to do certain things that others cannot do. Knowing how to access computers, how to program them, and how to manipulate data gives the computer professional the ability to create new products, solve important problems, and help people to manage their interactions with the ever more complex world in which we all live. Knowledge of computers can be a powerful means to effect positive change.

Knowledge also can be used in unethical ways. A computer can be programmed to trigger a terrorist's bomb, to sabotage a competitor's production line, or to steal money. Although these blatant examples make an extreme point and are unethical in any context, there are more subtle examples that are unique to computers.

Software Piracy

Computer software is easy to copy. But just like books, software is usually copyrighted. It is illegal to copy software without the permission of its creator. Such copying is called **software piracy**.

> **Software piracy**   The unauthorized copying of software for either personal use or use by others.

Copyright laws exist to protect the creators of software (and books and art) so that they can make a profit from the effort and money spent developing the software. A major software package can cost millions of dollars to develop, and this cost (along with the cost of producing the package, shipping it, supporting customers, and allowing for retailer markup) is reflected in the purchase price. If people make unauthorized copies of the software, then the company loses those sales and either has to raise its prices to compensate or spend less money to develop improved versions of the software—in either case, a desirable piece of software becomes harder to obtain.

Software pirates sometimes rationalize their software theft with the excuse that they're just making one copy for their own use. It's not that they're selling a bunch of bootleg copies, after all. But if thousands of people do the same, then it adds up to millions of dollars in lost revenue for the company, which leads to higher prices for everyone.

Computing professionals have an ethical obligation to not engage in software piracy and to try to stop it from occurring. You should never copy software without permission. If someone asks you for a copy of a piece of software, you should refuse to supply it. If someone says that he or she just wants to "borrow" the software to "try it out," tell that person that he or she is welcome to try it out on your machine (or at a retailer's shop) but not to make a copy.

This rule isn't restricted to duplicating copyrighted software; it includes plagiarism of all or part of code that belongs to anyone else. If someone gives you permission to copy some of his or her code, then, just like any responsible writer, you should acknowledge that person with a citation in the code.

Privacy of Data

The computer enables the compilation of databases containing useful information about people, companies, geographic regions, and so on. These databases allow employers to issue payroll checks, banks to cash a customer's check at any branch, the government to collect taxes, and mass merchandisers to send out junk mail. Even though we may not care for every use of databases, they generally have positive benefits. However, they also can be used in negative ways.

For example, a car thief who gains access to the state motor vehicle registry could print out a shopping list of valuable car models together with their owners' addresses. An industrial spy might steal customer data from a company database and sell it to a competitor. Although these are obviously illegal acts, computer professionals face other situations that are not so obvious.

Suppose your job includes managing the company payroll database. In that database are the names and salaries of the employees in the company. You might be tempted to poke around in the database to see how your salary compares with your associates; however, this act is unethical and an invasion of your associates' right to privacy, because this information is confidential. Any information about a person that is not clearly public should be considered confidential. An example of public information is a phone number listed in a telephone directory. Private information includes any data that has been provided with an understanding that it will be used only for a specific purpose (such as the data on a credit card application).

A computing professional has a responsibility to avoid taking advantage of special access that he or she may have to confidential data. The professional also has a responsibility to guard that data from unauthorized access. Guarding data can involve such simple things as shredding old printouts, keeping backup copies in a locked cabinet, and not using passwords that are easy to guess (such as a name or word) as well as more complex measures such as *encryption* (keeping data stored in a secret coded form).

Use of Computer Resources

If you've ever bought a computer, you know that it costs money. A personal computer can be relatively inexpensive, but it is still a major purchase. Larger computers can cost millions of dollars. Operating a PC may cost a few dollars a month for electricity and an occasional outlay for paper, disks, and repairs. Larger computers can cost tens of thousands of dollars per month to operate. Regardless of the type of computer, whoever owns it has to pay these costs. They do so because the computer is a resource that justifies its expense.

The computer is an unusual resource because it is valuable only when a program is running. Thus, the computer's time is really the valuable resource. There is no significant physical difference between a computer that is working and one that is sitting idle. By contrast, a car is in motion when it is working. Thus, unauthorized use of a computer is different from unauthorized use of a car. If one person uses another's car without permission, that individual must take possession of it physically—that is, steal it. If someone uses a computer without permission, the computer isn't physically stolen, but just as in the case of car theft, the owner is being deprived of a resource that he or she is paying for.

For some people, theft of computer resources is a game—like joyriding in a car. The thief really doesn't want the resources, just the challenge of breaking through a computer's security system and seeing how far he or she can get without being caught. Success gives a thrilling boost to this sort of person's ego. Many computer thieves think that their actions are acceptable if they do no harm, but whenever real work is displaced from the computer by such activities, then harm is clearly being done. If nothing else, the thief is trespassing in the computer owner's property. By analogy, consider that even though no physical harm may be done by someone who breaks into your bedroom and takes a nap while you are away, such an action is certainly disturbing to you because it poses a threat of potential physical harm. In this case, and in the case of breaking into a computer, mental harm can be done.

Other thieves can be malicious. Like a joyrider who purposely crashes a stolen car, these people destroy or corrupt data to cause harm. They may feel a sense of power from being able to hurt others with impunity. Sometimes these people leave behind programs that act as time bombs, to cause harm long after they have gone. Another kind of program that may be left is a virus—a program that replicates itself, often with the goal of spreading to other computers. Viruses can be benign, causing no other harm than to use up some resources. Others can be destructive and cause widespread damage to data. Incidents have occurred in which viruses have cost millions of dollars in lost computer time and data.

> **Virus** A computer program that replicates itself, often with the goal of spreading to other computers without authorization, and possibly with the intent of doing harm.

Computing professionals have an ethical responsibility never to use computer resources without permission, which includes activities such as doing personal work on an employer's computer. We also have a responsibility to help guard resources to which we have access—by using unguessable passwords and keeping them secret, by watching for signs of unusual computer use, by writing programs that do not provide loopholes in a computer's security system, and so on.

Software Engineering

Humans have come to depend greatly on computers in many aspects of their lives. That reliance is fostered by the perception that computers function reliably; that is, they work correctly most of the time. However, the reliability of a computer depends on the care that is taken in writing its software.

Errors in a program can have serious consequences, as the following examples of real incidents involving software errors illustrate. An error in the control software of the F–18 jet fighter caused it to flip upside down the first time it flew across the equator. A rocket launch went out of control and had to be blown up because there was a comma typed in place of a period in its control software. A radiation therapy machine killed several patients because a software error caused the machine to operate at full power when the operator typed certain commands too quickly.

Even when the software is used in less critical situations, errors can have significant effects. Examples of such errors include the following:

- An error in your word processor that causes your term paper to be lost just hours before it is due
- An error in a statistical program that causes a scientist to draw a wrong conclusion and publish a paper that must later be retracted
- An error in a tax preparation program that produces an incorrect return, leading to a fine

Programmers thus have a responsibility to develop software that is free from errors. The process that is used to develop correct software is known as **software engineering**.

Software engineering has many aspects. The software life cycle described at the begin-

> **Software engineering**   The application of traditional engineering methodologies and techniques to the development of software.

ning of this chapter outlines the stages in the development of software. Different techniques are used at each of these stages. We address many of the techniques in this text. In Chapter 4 we introduce methodologies for developing correct algorithms. We discuss strategies for testing and validating programs in every chapter. We use a modern programming language that enables us to write readable, well-organized programs, and so on. Some aspects of software engineering, such as the development of a formal, mathematical specification for a program, are beyond the scope of this text.

1.5   Problem-Solving Techniques

You solve problems every day, often unaware of the process you are going through. In a learning environment, you usually are given most of the information you need: a clear statement of the problem, the necessary input, and the required output. In real life, the process is not always so simple. You often have to define the problem yourself and then decide what information you have to work with and what the results should be.

After you understand and analyze a problem, you must come up with a solution—an algorithm. Earlier we defined an algorithm as a step-by-step procedure for solving a problem in a finite amount of time. Although you work with algorithms all the time, most of your experience with them is in the context of *following* them. You follow a recipe, play a game, assemble a toy, take medicine. In the problem-solving phase of computer programming, you will be *designing* algorithms, not following them. This means you must be conscious of the strategies you use to solve problems in order to apply them to programming problems.

Ask Questions

If you are given a task orally, you ask questions—When? Why? Where?—until you understand exactly what you have to do. If your instructions are written, you might put question marks in the margin, underline a word or a sentence, or in some other way indicate that the task is not clear. Your questions may be answered by a later paragraph, or you might have to discuss them with the person who gave you the task.

These are some of the questions you might ask in the context of programming:

- With what do I have to work—that is, what is my data?
- What do the data items look like?
- How much data is there?
- How will I know when I have processed all the data?
- What should my output look like?
- How many times is the process going to be repeated?
- What special error conditions might come up?

Look for Things That Are Familiar

Never reinvent the wheel. If a solution exists, use it. If you've solved the same or a similar problem before, just repeat your solution. People are good at recognizing similar situations. We don't have to learn how to go to the store to buy milk, then to buy eggs, and then to buy candy. We know that going to the store is always the same; only what we buy is different.

In programming, certain problems occur again and again in different guises. A good programmer immediately recognizes a subtask he or she has solved before and plugs in the solution. For example, finding the daily high and low temperatures is really the same problem as finding the highest and lowest grades on a test. You want the largest and smallest values in a set of numbers (see Figure 1–11).

Solve by Analogy

Often a problem reminds you of a similar problem you have seen before. You may find solving the problem at hand easier if you remember how you solved the other problem. In other words, draw an analogy between the two problems. For example, a solution to a perspective-projection problem from an art class might help you figure out how to compute the distance to a landmark when you are on a cross-country hike. As you work

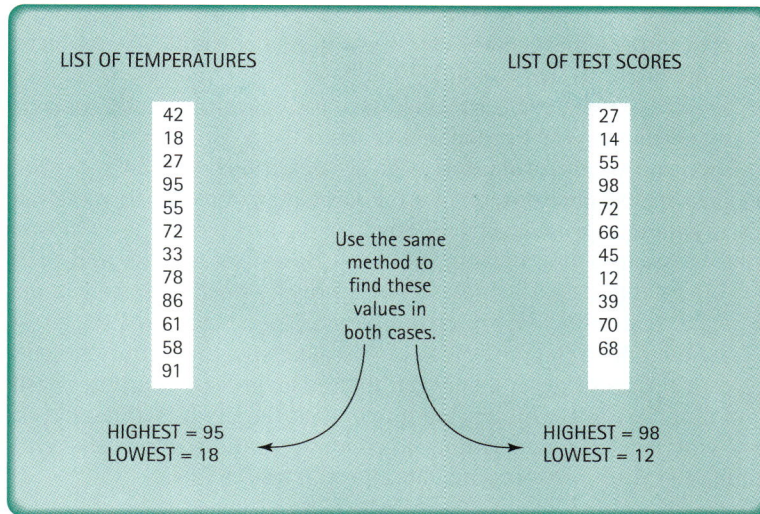

LIST OF TEMPERATURES

42
18
27
95
55
72
33
78
86
61
58
91

HIGHEST = 95
LOWEST = 18

Use the same method to find these values in both cases.

LIST OF TEST SCORES

27
14
55
98
72
66
45
12
39
70
68

HIGHEST = 98
LOWEST = 12

Figure 1–11   *Look for Things That Are Familiar*

your way through the new problem, you come across things that are different than they were in the old problem, but usually these are just details that you can deal with one at a time.

Analogy is really just a broader application of the strategy of looking for things that are familiar. When you are trying to find an algorithm for solving a problem, don't limit yourself to computer-oriented solutions. Step back and try to get a larger view of the problem. Don't worry if your analogy doesn't match perfectly—the only reason for using an analogy is that it gives you a place to start (see Figure 1–12). The best programmers are people who have broad experience solving all kinds of problems.

Means-Ends Analysis

Often the beginning state and the ending state are given; the problem is to define a set of actions that can be used to get from one to the other. Suppose you want to go from

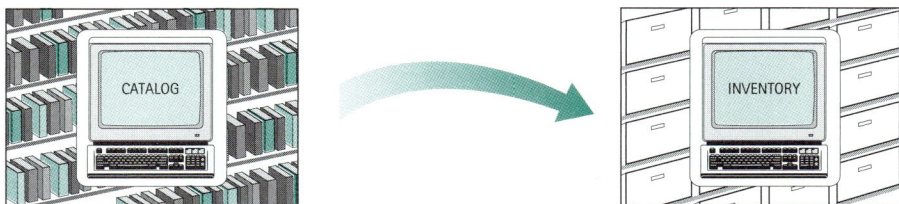

A library catalog system can give insight into how to organize a parts inventory.

Figure 1–12   *Analogy*

Boston, Massachusetts, to Austin, Texas. You know the beginning state (you are in Boston) and the ending state (you want to be in Austin). The problem is how to get from one to the other. In this example, you have lots of choices. You can fly, walk, hitchhike, ride a bike, or whatever. The method you choose depends on your circumstances. If you're in a hurry, you'll probably decide to fly.

Once you've narrowed down the set of actions, you have to work out the details. It may help to establish intermediate goals that are easier to meet than the overall goal. Let's say there is a really cheap, direct flight to Austin out of Newark, New Jersey. You might decide to divide the trip into legs: Boston to Newark and then Newark to Austin. Your intermediate goal is to get from Boston to Newark. Now you only have to examine the means of meeting that intermediate goal (see Figure 1–13).

The overall strategy of means-ends analysis is to define the ends and then to analyze your means of getting between them. The process translates easily to computer programming. You begin by writing down what the input is and what the output should be. Then you consider the actions a computer can perform and choose a sequence of actions that can transform the data into the results.

Divide and Conquer

We often break up large problems into smaller units that are easier to handle. Cleaning the whole house may seem overwhelming; cleaning the rooms one at a time seems much more manageable. The same principle applies to programming. We break up a large problem into smaller pieces that we can solve individually (see Figure 1–14). In fact, the functional decomposition and object-oriented methodologies, which we describe in Chapter 4, are based on the principle of divide and conquer.

The Building-Block Approach

Another way of attacking a large problem is to see if any solutions for smaller pieces of the problem exist. It may be possible to put some of these solutions together end-to-end to solve most of the big problem. This strategy is just a combination of the look-for-

Start: Boston **Goal:** Austin	**Means:** *Fly*, walk, hitchhike, bike, drive, sail, bus
Start: Boston **Goal:** Austin	**Revised Means:** Fly to Chicago and then Austin; *fly to Newark and then Austin;* fly to Atlanta and then Austin
Start: Boston **Intermediate Goal:** Newark **Goal:** Austin	**Means to Intermediate Goal:** *Commuter flight*, walk, hitchhike, bike, drive, sail, bus
Solution: Take commuter flight to Newark and then catch cheap flight to Austin	

Figure 1–13 *Means-Ends Analysis*

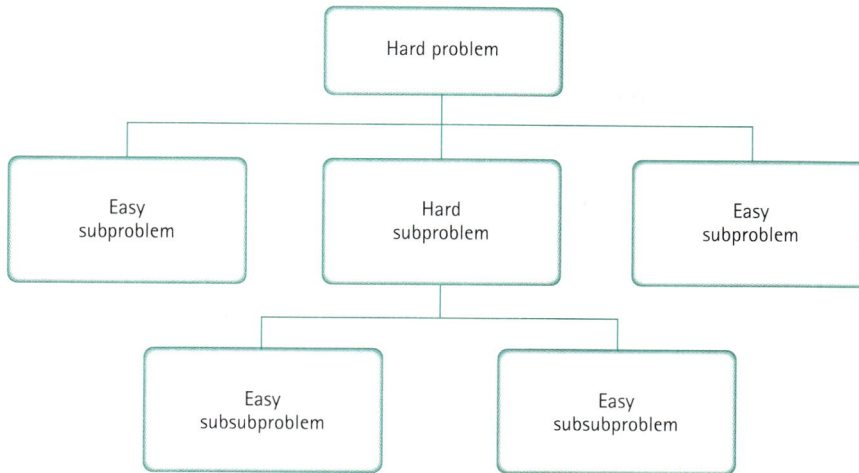

Figure 1–14   *Divide and Conquer*

familiar-things and divide-and-conquer approaches. You look at the big problem and see that it can be divided into smaller problems for which solutions already exist. Solving the big problem is just a matter of putting the existing solutions together, like mortaring together blocks to form a wall (see Figure 1–15).

Merging Solutions

Another way to combine existing solutions is to merge them on a step-by-step basis. For example, to compute the average of a list of values, we must both sum and count

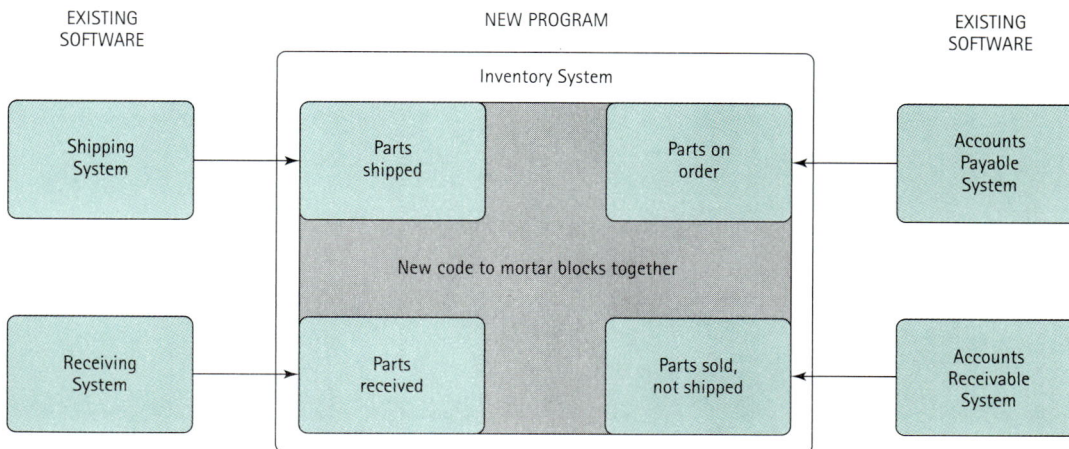

Figure 1–15   *Building-Block Approach*

the values. If we already have separate solutions for summing values and for counting values, we can combine them. But if we first do the summing and then do the counting, we have to read the list twice. We can save steps if we merge these two solutions: Read a value and then add it to the running total and add 1 to our count before going on to the next value. Whenever the solutions to subproblems duplicate steps, think about merging them instead of joining them end-to-end.

Mental Blocks: The Fear of Starting

Writers are all too familiar with the experience of staring at a blank page, not knowing where to begin. Programmers have the same difficulty when they first tackle a big problem. They look at the problem and it seems overwhelming (see Figure 1–16).

Remember that you always have a way to begin solving any problem: Write it down on paper in your own words so that you understand it. Once you paraphrase the problem, you can focus on each of the subparts individually instead of trying to tackle the entire problem at once. This process gives you a clearer picture of the overall problem. It helps you see pieces of the problem that look familiar or that are analogous to other problems you have solved, and it pinpoints areas where something is unclear, where you need more information.

As you write down a problem, you tend to group things together into small, understandable chunks, which may be natural places to split the problem up—to divide and conquer. Your description of the problem may collect all of the information about data

Figure 1–16
Mental Block

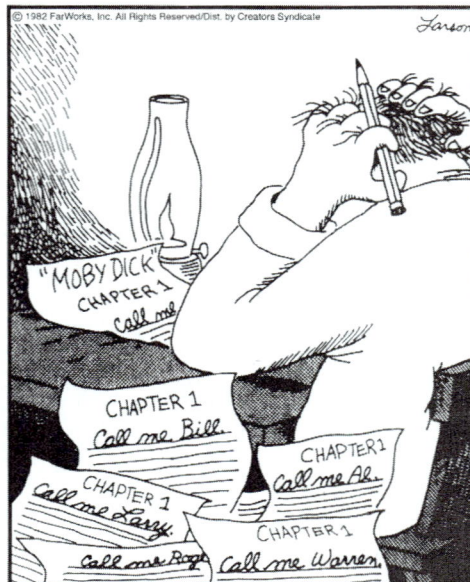

THE FAR SIDE®   By GARY LARSON

and results into one place for easy reference. Then you can see the beginning and ending states necessary for means-ends analysis.

Most mental blocks are caused by not really understanding the problem. Rewriting the problem in your own words is a good way to focus on the subparts of the problem, one at a time, and to understand what is required for a solution.

Algorithmic Problem Solving

Coming up with a step-by-step procedure for solving a particular problem is not always a cut-and-dried process. In fact, it is usually a trial-and-error process requiring several attempts and refinements. We test each attempt to see if it really solves the problem. If it does, fine. If it doesn't, we try again. Solving any nontrivial problem typically requires a combination of the techniques we've described.

Remember that the computer can only do certain things (see p. 13). Your primary concern, then, is how to make the computer transform, manipulate, calculate, or process the input data to produce the desired output. If you keep in mind the allowable instructions in your programming language, you won't design an algorithm that is difficult or impossible to code.

In the case study that follows, we develop a program to determine whether a year is a leap year. It typifies the thought processes involved in writing an algorithm and coding it as a program, and it shows you what a complete C++ program looks like.

Problem–Solving Case Study

Leap Year Algorithm

PROBLEM You need to write a set of instructions that can be used to determine whether a year is a leap year. The instructions must be very clear because they will be used by a class of fourth graders who have just learned about multiplication and division. They plan to use the instructions as part of an assignment to determine if any of their relatives were born in a leap year. To check that the algorithm works correctly, you will code it as a C++ program and test it.

DISCUSSION The rule for determining whether a year is a leap year is that a year must be divisible by four, but not a multiple of 100. When the year is a multiple of 400, it is a leap year anyway. We need to write this set of rules as a series of steps (an algorithm) that can be followed easily by the fourth graders.

First, we break this into major steps using divide and conquer. There are three obvious steps in almost any problem of this type:

1. Get the data.
2. Compute the results.
3. Output the results.

What does it mean to "get the data?" By *get*, we mean *read* or *input* the data. We need one piece of data: a four-digit year. So that the user will know when to enter the value, we must have the computer output a message that indicates when it is ready to accept the value (this is called a *prompting message*, or a *prompt*). Therefore, to have the computer get the data, we have it do these two steps:

> Prompt the user to enter a four-digit year
> Read the year

Next, we check to see if the year that was read can be a leap year (is divisible by four), and then we test whether it is one of the exceptional cases. Our high level algorithm is thus:

Main

> If the year is not divisible by 4,
>   Then the year is not a leap year
>   Otherwise, check for exceptions

Clearly, we need to expand these steps with more detailed instructions, because neither the fourth graders nor the computer know what 'divisible' means. We use means-ends analysis to solve the problem of how to determine if something is divisible by four. Our fourth graders know how to do simple division that results in a quotient and a remainder. So, we can tell them to divide the year by four and if the remainder is zero, then it is divisible by four. Thus, the first line is expanded into the following:

Main revised

> Divide the year by 4
> If the remainder is not 0,
>   then the year is not a leap year
>   otherwise, check for exceptions

Checking for exceptions when the year is divisible by four can be further divided into two parts: checking whether the year is also divisible by 100 and whether it is further divisible by 400. Given how we did the first step, this is easy:

Checking for exceptions

> Divide the year by 100
> If the remainder is 0,
>   then the year is not a leap year
> Divide the year by 400
> If the remainder is 0,
>   then the year is a leap year

These steps are confusing by themselves. When the year is divisible by 400, it also is divisible by 100, so we have one test that says it is a leap year and one that says it is not. What we need to do is to treat the steps as building blocks and combine them. One of the operations that we can use in such situations is also to check when a condition does *not* exist. For example, if the year is divisible by 4 but not by 100, then it must be a leap year. If it is divisible by 100 but not by 400, then it is definitely not a leap year. Thus, the third step (check for exceptions when the year is divisible by 4) expands to the following three tests:

Checking for exceptions revised

> If the year is not divisible by 100,
>   then it is a leap year
> If the year is divisible by 100, but not by 400,
>   then it is not a leap year
> If the year is divisible by 400,
>   then it is a leap year

We can simplify the second test because the first part of it is just the opposite of the first test—we can simply say "otherwise" instead of repeating the test for divisibility by 100. Similarly, the last test is really just the "otherwise" case of the second test. Once we translate each of these simplified tests into steps that the fourth graders know how to perform, we can write the subalgorithm that returns true if the year is a leap year and false otherwise. Let's call this subalgorithm IsLeapYear, and put the year it is to test in parentheses beside the name.

IsLeapYear(year)

> Divide the year by 4
> If the remainder isn't 0,
>   Return false (The year is not a leap year)
>   Otherwise, divide the year by 100 and
> If the remainder isn't 0,
>   Return true (The year is a leap year)
>   Otherwise, divide the year by 400 and
> If the remainder isn't 0
>   Return false (The year is not a leap year)
>   Otherwise, Return true (the year is a leap year)

The only piece left is to write the results. If IsLeapYear returns true, then we write that the year is a leap year; otherwise, we write that it is not a leap year. Now we can write the complete algorithm for this problem.

Main Algorithm

> Prompt the user to enter a four-digit year
> Read the year
> If IsLeapYear(year)
>   Write that the Year is a leap year
> Otherwise
>   Write that the Year is not a leap year

Not only is this algorithm clear, concise, and easy to follow, but once you have finished the next few chapters, you will see that it is easy to translate into a C++ program. We present the program here so that you can compare it to the algorithm. You do not need to know how to read C++ programs to begin to see the similarities. Note that the symbol % is what C++ uses to calculate the remainder, and whatever appears between /* and */ or // and the end of the line is a comment that is ignored by the compiler.

```cpp
//*******************************************************************
// LeapYear program
// This program inputs a year and prints whether the year
// is a leap year or not
//*******************************************************************

#include <iostream>              // Access output stream

using namespace std;

bool IsLeapYear( int );          // Prototype for subalgorithm

int main()
{
    int year;                    // Year to be tested
    cout << "Enter a year AD, for example, 1997."
         << endl;                // Prompt for input
    cin >> year;                 // Read year

    if (IsLeapYear(year))        // Test for leap year
        cout << year << " is a leap year." << endl;
    else
        cout << year << " is not a leap year." << endl;

    return 0;                    // Indicate successful completion
}


//*******************************************************************

bool IsLeapYear( int year )

// IsLeapYear returns true if year is a leap year and
// false otherwise.

{
    if (year % 4 != 0)           // Is year not divisible by 4?
        return false;            // If so, can't be a leap year
    else if (year % 100 != 0)    // Is year not a multiple of 100?
```

```
      return true;              // If so, is a leap year
   else if (year % 400 != 0)    // Is year not a multiple of 400?
      return false;             // If so, then is not a leap year
   else
      return true;              // Is a leap year
}
```

Here is a screen shot of the input and the output.

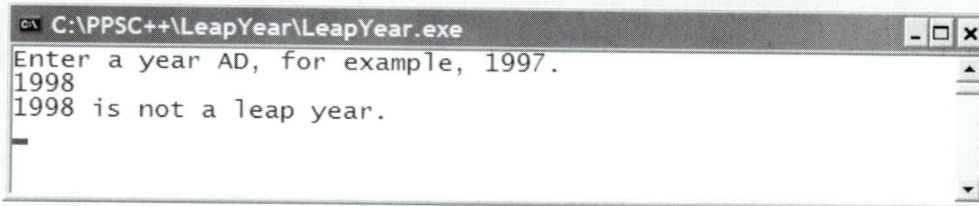

```
C:\PPSC++\LeapYear\LeapYear.exe                          _ □ ✕
Enter a year AD, for example, 1997.
1998
1998 is not a leap year.
```

Summary

We think nothing of turning on the television and sitting down to watch it. It's a communication tool we use to enhance our lives. Computers are becoming as common as televisions, just a normal part of our lives. And like televisions, computers are based on complex principles but are designed for easy use.

Computers are dumb; they must be told what to do. A true computer error is extremely rare (usually due to a component malfunction or an electrical fault). Because we tell the computer what to do, most errors in computer-generated output are really human errors.

Computer programming is the process of planning a sequence of steps for a computer to follow. It involves a problem-solving phase and an implementation phase. After analyzing a problem, we develop and test a general solution (algorithm). This general solution becomes a concrete solution—our program—when we write it in a high-level programming language. The sequence of instructions that makes up our program is then compiled into machine code, the language the computer uses. After correcting any errors ("bugs") that show up during testing, our program is ready to use.

Once we begin to use the program, it enters the maintenance phase. Maintenance involves correcting any errors discovered while the program is being used and changing the program to reflect changes in the user's requirements.

Data and instructions are represented as binary numbers (numbers consisting of just 1s and 0s) in electronic computers. The process of converting data and instructions into a form usable by the computer is called coding.

A programming language reflects the range of operations a computer can perform. The basic control structures in a programming language—sequence, selection, loop, and subprogram—are based on these fundamental operations. In this text, you will learn to write programs in the high-level programming language called C++.

Computers are composed of six basic parts: the memory unit, the arithmetic/logic unit, the control unit, input and output devices, and auxiliary storage devices. The arithmetic/logic unit and control unit together are called the central processing unit. The physical parts of the computer are called hardware. The programs that are executed by the computer are called software.

System software is a set of programs designed to simplify the user/computer interface. It includes the compiler, the operating system, and the editor.

Computing professionals are guided by a set of ethics, as are members of other professions. Among the responsibilities that we have are copying software only with permission, including attribution to other programmers when we make use of their code, guarding the privacy of confidential data, using computer resources only with permission, and carefully engineering our programs so that they work correctly.

We've said that problem solving is an integral part of the programming process. Although you may have little experience programming computers, you have lots of experience solving problems. The key is to stop and think about the strategies you use to solve problems, and then to use those strategies to devise workable algorithms. Among those strategies are asking questions, looking for things that are familiar, solving by analogy, applying means-ends analysis, dividing the problem into subproblems, using existing solutions to small problems to solve a larger problem, merging solutions, and paraphrasing the problem in order to overcome a mental block.

The computer is used widely today in science, engineering, business, government, medicine, consumer goods, and the arts. Learning to program in C++ can help you use this powerful tool effectively.

Quick Check

The Quick Check is intended to help you decide if you've met the goals set forth at the beginning of each chapter. If you understand the material in the chapter, the answer to each question should be fairly obvious. After reading a question, check your response against the answers listed at the end of the Quick Check. If you don't know an answer or don't understand the answer that's provided, turn to the page(s) listed at the end of the question to review the material.

1. What do we call a sequence of instructions that is executed by a computer? (p. 3)
2. How does an algorithm differ from a computer program? (pp. 3–4)
3. How does a programming language differ from a human language? (pp. 5–6)
4. What is the input and output of a compiler? (pp. 10–12)
5. Who invented the C++ programming language? (p. 23)
6. What do we call the combination of the Control Unit and the Arithmetic/Logic Unit? (pp. 15–16)
7. How can you help to keep confidential data private? (p. 25)
8. What are the three phases of the software life cycle? (pp. 3–4)

9. Which of the following tools translates a C++ program into machine language: editor, operating system, compiler, or assembler? (pp. 9–10)
10. What is the general term that we use to refer to the physical components of the computer? (p. 17)
11. When would you use the building-block approach to solve a problem? (pp. 30–31)

Answers

1. A computer program.   2. An algorithm can be written in any language, to be carried out by a person or a processor of any kind. A program is written in a programming language, for execution by a computer.   3. A programming language has a very small vocabulary of words and symbols, and a very precise set of rules that specify the form of valid language constructs (syntax) and the actions that result when a construct is executed by the computer (semantics).   4. The compiler inputs a source program written in a high-level language, and outputs an equivalent program in machine language. Some compilers also output a listing, which is a copy of the source program with error messages inserted.   5. Bjarne Stroustrup at Bell Laboratories.   6. The central processing unit.   7. Use passwords that are difficult to guess, and change them periodically. Encrypt stored data. Ensure that data storage media are kept in a secure area.   8. Problem-solving, implementation, maintenance.   9. Compiler.   10. Hardware.   11. When you see that a problem can be divided into pieces that may correspond to subproblems for which solutions are already known.

Exam Preparation Exercises

1. Match the following terms to their definitions, given below:
   a. Programming
   b. Computer
   c. Algorithm
   d. Computer program
   e. Programming language
   f. Documentation
   g. Information
   h. Data

   i. A programmable device that can store, retrieve, and process data.
   ii. Information in a form a computer can use.
   iii. A sequence of instructions to be performed by a computer.
   iv. A set of rules, symbols, and special words used to construct a computer program.
   v. Planning or scheduling the performance of a task or event.
   vi. Any knowledge that can be communicated.
   vii. The written text and comments that make a program easier for others to understand, use, and modify.
   viii. A step-by-step procedure for solving a problem in a finite amount of time.
2. List the three steps in the problem-solving phase of the software life cycle.

3. List steps in the implementation phase of the software life cycle.

4. If testing uncovers an error, what step in the software life cycle does the programmer return to?

5. Explain why the following series of steps isn't an algorithm, and then rewrite the steps to make a valid algorithm:

    Wake up.
    Go to school.
    Come home.
    Go to sleep.
    Repeat from first step.

6. Match the following terms with their definitions, given below.
    a. Machine language
    b. Assembly language
    c. Assembler
    d. Compiler
    e. Source program
    f. Object program

        i. A program that translates a high-level language into machine code.
        ii. A low-level programming language in which a mnemonic is used to represent each of the instructions for a particular computer.
        iii. The machine language version of a source program.
        iv. A program that translates an assembly language program into machine code.
        v. The language, made up of binary coded instructions, that is used directly by the computer.
        vi. A program written in a high-level programming language.

7. What is the advantage of writing a program in a standardized programming language?

8. What does the control unit do?

9. The editor is a peripheral device. True or false?

10. Memory (RAM) is a peripheral device. True or false?

11. Is it a case of software piracy if you and a friend buy a piece of software together and install it on both of your computers? The license for the software says that it can be registered to just one user.

12. Match the problem-solving strategies to the descriptions following.
    a. Ask questions.
    b. Look for things that are familiar.
    c. Solve by analogy.
    d. Means-ends analysis.
    e. Divide and conquer.
    f. Building-block approach.
    g. Merging solutions.

        i. Break up the problem into more manageable pieces.

ii. Gather more information to help you discover a solution.

iii. Identify aspects of the problem that are similar to a problem in a different domain.

iv. Combine the steps in two or more different algorithms.

v. Identify aspects of the problem that you've solved before.

vi. Join existing problem solutions together.

vii. Look at the input, output, and available operations and find a sequence of operations that transform the input into the output.

Programming Warm-Up Exercises

1. In the following algorithm for making black-and-white photographs, identify the steps that are branches (selection), loops, or references to subalgorithms defined elsewhere.

a. Mix developer according to instructions on package.

b. Pour developer into tray.

c. Mix stop bath according to instructions on package.

d. Pour stop bath into tray.

e. Mix fixer according to instructions on package.

f. Pour fixer into tray.

g. Turn off white lights and turn on safelight.

h. Place negative in enlarger and turn on.

i. Adjust size of image and focus, and then turn off enlarger.

j. Remove one piece of printing paper from paper safe and place in enlarging easel.

k. Turn enlarger on for thirty seconds and then off.

l. Place paper in developer for 1 minute, stop bath for 30 seconds, and fixer for 1 minute.

m. Turn on white lights and inspect the first print, and then turn off white lights.

n1. If first print is too light:

Remove one piece of paper from paper safe, place on easel, and expose for 60 seconds to create a too-dark print. Then place in developer for 1 minute, stop bath for 30 seconds, and fixer for 1 minute.

n2. If first print is too dark:

Remove one piece of paper from paper safe, place on easel, and expose for 15 seconds to create a too-light print. Then place in developer for 1 minute, stop bath for 30 seconds, and fixer for 1 minute.

n3. If first print is about right:

Remove one piece of paper from paper safe, place on easel, and expose for 60 seconds to create a too-dark print. Then place in developer for 1 minute, stop bath for 30 seconds, and fixer for 1 minute. Remove one piece of paper from paper safe, place on easel, and expose for 15 seconds to create a too-light print. Then place in developer for 1 minute, stop bath for 30 seconds, and fixer for 1 minute.

o. Analyze too-light and too-dark prints to estimate base exposure time, and then identify highlights and shadows that require less or more exposure and estimate the necessary time for each area.

p. Remove one piece of paper from paper safe, place on easel, and expose for base exposure time, covering shadow areas for estimated time, and then cover entire print except for highlight areas, which are further exposed as estimated. Then place print in developer for 1 minute, stop bath for 30 seconds, and fixer for 1 minute.

q. Analyze print from step p and adjust estimates of times as appropriate.

r. Repeat steps p and q until a print is obtained with the desired exposure.

s. Document exposure times that result in desired print.

t. Remove one piece of paper from paper safe, place on easel, and expose according to documentation from step s. Then place in developer for 1 minute, stop bath for 30 seconds, and fixer for 4 minutes. Place print in print washer.

u. Repeat step t to create as many prints as needed.

v. Wash all prints for 1 hour.

w. Place prints in print dryer.

2. Write an algorithm for brushing teeth. The instructions must be very simple and exact because the person who will follow them has never done this before, and takes every word literally.

3. Identify the steps in your solution to Exercise 2 that are branches, loops, and references to subalgorithms defined elsewhere.

4. Change the algorithm in Exercise 1 so that 10 properly exposed prints are created each time it is executed.

Case Study Follow-Up

1. Use the algorithm in the leap year case study to decide whether the following years are leap years.

   a. 1900
   b. 2000
   c. 1996
   d. 1998

2. Given the algorithm from the leap year case study with the lines numbered as follows:

   1. Divide the year by 4 and if the remainder isn't 0
   2.   Return false (The year is not a leap year)
   3.   Otherwise, divide the year by 100 and if the remainder isn't 0,
   4.   Return true (The year is a leap year)
   5.   Otherwise, divide the year by 400 and if the remainder isn't 0,
   6.   Return false (The year is not a leap year)
   7.   Otherwise, Return true (the year is a leap year)

Indicate which line of the algorithm tells you whether the date is a leap year in each of the following cases.

a.   1900 Line =
b.   1945 Line =
c.   1600 Line =
d.   1492 Line =
e.   1776 Line =

3. How would you extend the leap year algorithm to tell you also when a year is a millennium year (a multiple of 1000)?
4. Use the leap year algorithm to determine whether you were born in a leap year.
5. Extend the leap year algorithm so that it tells you when the next leap year will be, if the input year is not a leap year.
6. Compare the algorithm for determining the leap year with the C++ program that is shown in the case study. Using the numbering scheme for the algorithm from Question 2, decide which line (or lines) of the algorithm corresponds to which line (or lines) of the program shown here.

Line Number

```
              {
_____          if (year % 4 != 0)
_____              return false;
_____          else if (year % 100 !=  0)
_____              return true;
_____          else if (year % 400 != 0)
_____              return false;
_____          else return true;
              }
```

C++ Syntax and Semantics, and the Program Development Process

Goals

Knowledge Goals

- *To understand how a C++ program is composed of one or more subprograms (functions).*
- *To know what a metalanguage is, and how it is used.*
- *To understand the concept of a data type.*
- *To learn the steps involved in entering and running a program.*

Skill Goals

To be able to:

- *Read syntax templates in order to understand the formal rules governing C++ programs.*
- *Create and recognize legal C++ identifiers.*
- *Declare named constants and variables of type* `char` *and* `string`.
- *Distinguish reserved words in C++ from user-defined identifiers.*
- *Assign values to variables.*
- *Construct simple string expressions made up of constants, variables, and the concatenation operator.*
- *Construct a statement that writes to an output stream.*
- *Determine what is printed by a given output statement.*
- *Use comments to clarify your programs.*
- *Construct simple C++ programs.*

2.1 The Elements of C++ Programs

Programmers develop solutions to problems using a programming language. In this chapter, we start looking at the rules and symbols that make up the C++ programming language. We also review the steps required to create a program and make it work on a computer.

C++ Program Structure

In Chapter 1, we talked about the four basic structures for expressing actions in a programming language: sequence, selection, loop, and subprogram. We said that subprograms allow us to write parts of our program separately and then assemble them into final form. In C++, all subprograms are referred to as **functions**, and a C++ program is a collection of one or more functions.

> **Function** A subprogram in C++.

Each function performs some particular task, and collectively they all cooperate to solve the entire problem.

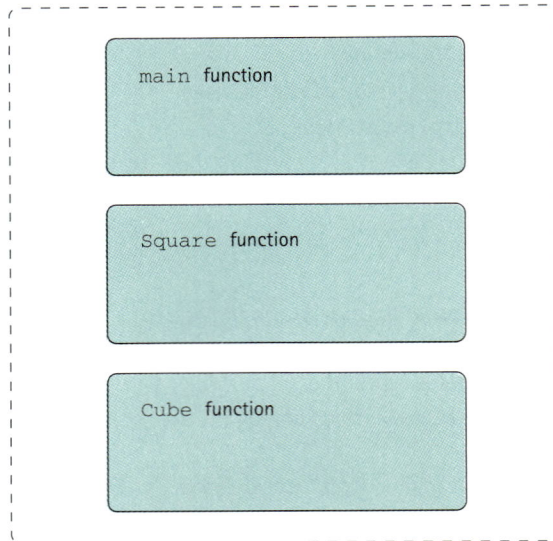

Every C++ program must have a function named `main`. Execution of the program always begins with the `main` function. You can think of `main` as the master and the other functions as the servants. When `main` wants the function `Square` to perform a task, `main` calls (or *invokes*) `Square`. When the `Square` function completes execution of its statements, it obediently returns control to the master, `main`, so the master can continue executing.

Let's look at an example of a C++ program with three functions: `main`, `Square`, and `Cube`. Don't be too concerned with the details in the program—just observe its overall look and structure.

```
#include <iostream>

using namespace std;

int Square( int );
int Cube( int );

int main()
{
    cout << "The square of 27 is " << Square(27) << endl;
    cout << "and the cube of 27 is " << Cube(27) << endl;
    return 0;
}

int Square( int n )
{
    return n * n;
}

int Cube( int n )
{
    return n * n * n;
}
```

In each of the three functions, the left brace ({) and right brace (}) mark the beginning and end of the statements to be executed. Statements appearing between the braces are known as the *body* of the function.

Execution of a program always begins with the first statement of the main function. In our program, the first statement is

```
cout << "The square of 27 is " << Square(27) << endl;
```

This is an output statement that causes information to be printed on the computer's display screen. You will learn how to construct output statements like this later in the chapter. Briefly, this statement prints two items. The first is the message

```
The square of 27 is
```

The second to be printed is the value obtained by calling (invoking) the Square function, with the value 27 as the number to be squared. As the servant, the Square function performs its task of squaring the number and sending the computed result (729) back to its *caller*, the main function. Now main can continue executing by printing the value 729 and proceeding to its next statement.

In a similar fashion, the second statement in main prints the message

```
and the cube of 27 is
```

and then invokes the `Cube` function and prints the result, 19683. The complete output produced by executing this program is, therefore,

```
The square of 27 is 729
and the cube of 27 is 19683
```

Both `Square` and `Cube` are examples of *value-returning functions*. A value-returning function returns a single value to its caller. The word `int` at the beginning of the first line of the `Square` function

```
int Square( int n )
```

states that the function returns an integer value.

Now look at the `main` function again. You'll see that the first line of the function is

```
int main()
```

The word `int` indicates that `main` is a value-returning function that should return an integer value. And it does. After printing the square and cube of 27, `main` executes the statement

```
return 0;
```

to return the value 0 to its caller. But who calls the `main` function? The answer is: the computer's operating system.

When you work with C++ programs, the operating system is considered to be the caller of the `main` function. The operating system expects `main` to return a value when `main` finishes executing. By convention, a return value of 0 means everything went OK. A return value of anything else (typically 1, 2, ...) means something went wrong. Later in this book we look at situations in which you might want to return a value other than 0 from `main`. For the time being, we always conclude the execution of `main` by returning the value 0.

We have looked only briefly at the overall picture of what a C++ program looks like—a collection of one or more functions, including `main`. We have also mentioned what is special about the `main` function—it is a required function, execution begins there, and it returns a value to the operating system. Now it's time to begin looking at the details of the C++ language.

Syntax and Semantics

A programming language is a set of rules, symbols, and special words used to construct a program. There are rules for both **syntax** (grammar) and **semantics** (meaning).

Syntax is a formal set of rules that defines exactly what combinations of letters, numbers, and symbols can be used in a programming language. There is no room for ambiguity in the syntax of a programming language because the computer can't

Syntax The formal rules governing how valid instructions are written in a programming language.

Semantics The set of rules that determines the meaning of instructions written in a programming language.

think; it doesn't "know what we mean." To avoid ambiguity, syntax rules themselves must be written in a very simple, precise, formal language called a **metalanguage**.

> **Metalanguage** A language that is used to write the syntax rules for another language.

Learning to read a metalanguage is like learning to read the notations used in the rules of a sport. Once you understand the notations, you can read the rule book. It's true that many people learn a sport simply by watching others play, but what they learn is usually just enough to allow them to take part in casual games. You could learn C++ by following the examples in this book, but a serious programmer, like a serious athlete, must take the time to read and understand the rules.

Syntax rules are the blueprints we use to build instructions in a program. They allow us to take the elements of a programming language—the basic building blocks of the language—and assemble them into *constructs*, syntactically correct structures. If our program violates any of the rules of the language—by misspelling a crucial word or leaving out an important comma, for instance—the program is said to have *syntax errors* and cannot compile correctly until we fix them.

Theoretical Foundations

Metalanguages

Metalanguage is the word *language* with the prefix *meta-*, which means "beyond" or "more comprehensive." A metalanguage is a language that goes beyond a normal language by allowing us to speak precisely about that language. It is a language for talking about languages. One of the oldest computer-oriented metalanguages is *Backus-Naur Form* (*BNF*), which is named for John Backus and Peter Naur, who developed it in 1960. BNF syntax definitions are written out using letters, numbers, and special symbols. For example, an *identifier* (a name for something in a program) in C++ must be at least one letter or underscore (_), which may or may not be followed by additional letters, underscores, or digits. The BNF definition of an identifier in C++ is as follows.

```
<Identifier> ::= <Nondigit> | <Nondigit> <NondigitOrDigitSequence>
<NondigitOrDigitSequence> ::= <NondigitOrDigit> | <NondigitOrDigit> <NondigitOrDigitSequence>
<NondigitOrDigit> ::= <Nondigit> | <Digit>
<Nondigit> ::= _ | A | B | C | D | E | F | G | H | I | J | K | L | M | N | O | P | Q | R | S | T | U | V | W | X | Y | Z |
               a | b | c | d | e | f | g | h | i | j | k | l | m | n | o | p | q | r | s | t | u | v | w | x | y | z
<Digit> ::= 0 | 1 | 2 | 3 | 4 | 5 | 6 | 7 | 8 | 9
```

(continued) ▼

Metalanguages

Where the symbol ::= is read "is defined as," the symbol | means "or," the symbols < and > are used to enclose words called *nonterminal symbols* (symbols that still need to be defined), and everything else is called a *terminal symbol*.

The first line of the definition reads as follows: "An identifier is defined as either a nondigit or a nondigit followed by a nondigit-or-digit sequence." This line contains nonterminal symbols that must be defined. In the second line, the nonterminal symbol NondigitOrDigitSequence is defined as either a NondigitOrDigit or a NondigitOrDigit followed by another NondigitOrDigitSequence. The self-reference in the definition is a roundabout way of saying that a NondigitOrDigitSequence can be a series of one or more nondigits or digits. The third line defines NondigitOrDigit to be either a Nondigit or a Digit. In the fourth and last lines, we finally encounter terminal symbols, which define Nondigit to be an underscore or any upper- or lowercase letter and Digit as any one of the numeric symbols 0 through 9.

BNF is an extremely simple language, but that simplicity leads to syntax definitions that can be long and difficult to read. An alternative metalanguage, the syntax diagram, is easier to follow. It uses arrows to indicate how symbols can be combined. The syntax diagrams that define an identifier in C++ appear below and on the next page.

To read the diagrams, start at the left and follow the arrows. When you come to a branch, take any one of the branch paths. Symbols in boldface are terminal symbols, and words not in boldface are nonterminal symbols.

The first diagram shows that an identifier consists of a nondigit followed, optionally, by any number of nondigits or digits. The second diagram defines the nonterminal symbol Nondigit to be an underscore or any one of the alphabetic characters. The third diagram defines Digit to be one of the numeric characters. Here, we have eliminated the BNF nonterminal symbols NondigitOrDigit-Sequence and NondigitOrDigit by using arrows in the first syntax diagram to allow a sequence of consecutive nondigits or digits.

Identifier

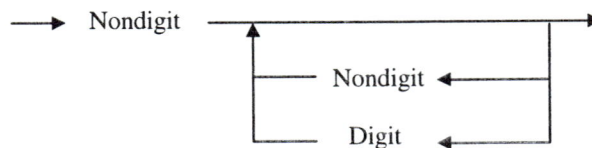

(continued) ▼

Metalanguages

Nondigit

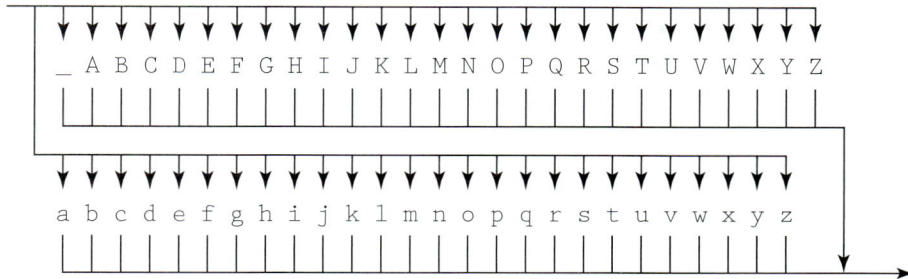

Digit

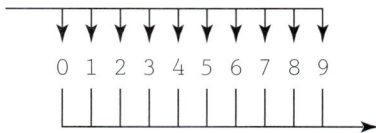

Syntax diagrams are easier to interpret than BNF definitions, but they still can be difficult to read. In this text, we introduce another metalanguage, called a *syntax template*. Syntax templates show at a glance the form a C++ construct takes.

One final note: Metalanguages only show how to write instructions that the compiler can translate. They do not define what those instructions do (their semantics). Formal languages for defining the semantics of a programming language exist, but they are beyond the scope of this text. Throughout this book, we describe the semantics of C++ in English.

Syntax Templates

In this book, we write the syntax rules for C++ using a metalanguage called a *syntax template*. A syntax template is a generic example of the C++ construct being defined. Graphic conventions show which portions are optional and which can be repeated. A boldface word or symbol is a literal word or symbol in the C++ language. A nonbold-face word can be replaced by another template. A curly brace is used to indicate a list of items, from which one item can be chosen.

Let's look at an example. This template defines an identifier in C++:

Identifier

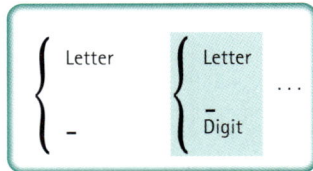

The shading indicates a part of the definition that is optional. The three dots (...) mean that the preceding symbol or shaded block can be repeated. Thus, an identifier in C++ must begin with a letter or underscore and is optionally followed by one or more letters, underscores, or digits.

Remember that a word not in boldface type can be replaced with another template. These are the templates for Letter and Digit:

Letter

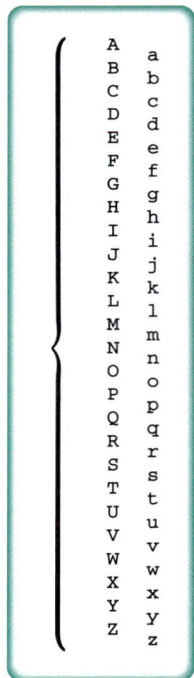

Digit

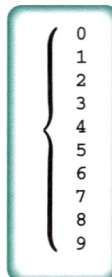

In these templates, the braces again indicate lists of items from which any one item can be chosen. So a letter can be any one of the upper- or lowercase letters, and a digit can be any of the numeric characters 0 through 9.

Now let's look at the syntax template for the C++ `main` function:

MainFunction

```
int main()
{
    Statement
        ⋮
}
```

The `main` function begins with the word `int`, followed by the word `main` and then left and right parentheses. This first line of the function is the *heading*. After the heading, the left brace signals the start of the statements in the function (its body). The shading and the three dots indicate that the function body consists of zero or more statements. (In this diagram we have placed the three dots vertically to suggest that statements usually are arranged vertically, one above the next.) Finally, the right brace indicates the end of the function.

In principle, the syntax template allows the function body to have no statements at all. In practice, however, the body should include a Return statement because the word `int` in the function heading states that `main` returns an integer value. Thus, the shortest C++ program is

```
int main()
{
    return 0;
}
```

As you might guess, this program does absolutely nothing useful when executed!

As we introduce C++ language constructs throughout the book, we use syntax templates to display the proper syntax. At the publisher's Web site, you will find these syntax templates gathered into one central location.*

When you finish this chapter, you should know enough about the syntax and semantics of statements in C++ to write simple programs. But before we can talk about writing statements, we must look at how names are written in C++ and at some of the elements of a program.

---

*The publisher's Web site is www.`problemsolvingcpp`.`jbpub`.`com`

Naming Program Elements: Identifiers

As we noted in our discussion of metalanguages, identifiers are used in C++ to name things—things such as subprograms and places in the computer's memory. Identifiers are made up of letters (A–Z, a–z), digits (0–9), and the underscore character (_), but must begin with a letter or underscore.

> **Identifier** A name associated with a function or data object and used to refer to that function or data object.

Remember that an identifier *must* start with a letter or underscore:

Identifier

```
{ Letter    { Letter  . . .
{ _         { _
            { Digit
```

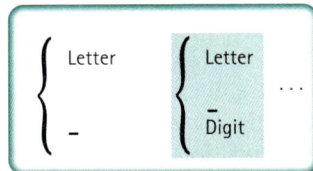

(Identifiers beginning with an underscore have special meanings in some C++ systems, so it is best to begin an identifier with a letter.)

Here are some examples of valid identifiers:

```
sum_of_squares   J9   box_22A   GetData   Bin3D4   count
```

And here are some examples of invalid identifiers and the reasons why they are invalid:

Invalid Identifier	Explanation
40Hours	Identifiers cannot begin with a digit.
Get Data	Blanks are not allowed in identifiers.
box-22	The hyphen (–) is a math symbol (minus) in C++.
cost_in_$	Special symbols such as $ are not allowed.
int	The word int is predefined in the C++ language.

> **Reserved word** A word that has special meaning in C++; it cannot be used as a programmer-defined identifier.

The last identifier in the table, int, is an example of a reserved word. Reserved words are words that have specific uses in C++; you cannot use them as programmer-defined identifiers. Appendix A lists all of the reserved words in C++.

The LeapYear program in Chapter 1 uses the programmer-defined identifiers in the following list. (Most of the other identifiers in the program are C++ reserved words.) Notice that we chose the names to convey how the identifiers are used.

Identifier	How It Is Used
year	Year to be tested
IsLeapYear	Whether year is a leap year

Matters of Style

Using Meaningful, Readable Identifiers

The names we use to refer to things in our programs are totally meaningless to the computer. The computer behaves in the same way whether we call the value 3.14159265 pi or cake, as long as we always call it the same thing. However, it is much easier for somebody to figure out how a program works if the names we choose for elements actually tell something about them. Whenever you have to make up a name for something in a program, try to pick one that is meaningful to a person reading the program.

C++ is a *case-sensitive* language. Uppercase letters are different from lowercase letters. The identifiers

PRINTTOPPORTION   printtopportion   pRiNtToPpOrTiOn   PrintTopPortion

are four distinct names and are not interchangeable in any way. As you can see, the last of these forms is the easiest to read. In this book, we use combinations of uppercase letters, lowercase letters, and underscores in identifiers. We explain our conventions for choosing between uppercase and lowercase as we proceed through this chapter.

Now that we've seen how to write identifiers, we look at some of the things that C++ allows us to name.

Data and Data Types

A computer program operates on data (stored internally in memory, stored externally on disk or tape, or input from a device such as a keyboard, scanner, or electrical sensor)

Data type A specific set of data values, along with a set of operations on those values.

and produces output. In C++, each piece of data must be of a specific **data type**. The data type determines how the data is represented in the computer and the kinds of processing the computer can perform on it.

Some types of data are used so frequently that C++ defines them for us. Examples of these *standard* (or *built-in*) *types* are `int` (for working with integer numbers), `float` (for working with real numbers having decimal points), and `char` (for working with character data).

Additionally, C++ allows programmers to define their own data types—*programmer-defined* (or *user-defined*) *types*. Beginning in Chapter 10, we show you how to define your own data types.

In this chapter, we focus on two data types—one for representing data consisting of a single character, the other for representing strings of characters. In the next chapter, we examine the numeric types (such as `int` and `float`) in detail.

Background Information

Data Storage

Where does a program get the data it needs to operate? Data is stored in the computer's memory. Remember that memory is divided into a large number of separate locations or cells, each of which can hold a piece of data. Each memory location has a unique address to which we refer when we store or retrieve data. We can visualize memory as a set of post office boxes, with the box numbers as the addresses used to designate particular locations.

(continued) ▼

> ### Data Storage
>
> Of course, the actual address of each location in memory is a binary number in a machine language code. In C++ we use identifiers to name memory locations; the compiler then translates them into binary for us. This is one of the advantages of a high-level programming language: It frees us from having to keep track of the numeric addresses of the memory locations in which our data and instructions are stored.

The `char` Data Type   The built-in type `char` describes data consisting of one alphanumeric character—a letter, a digit, or a special symbol:

```
'A'    'a'    '8'    '2'    '+'    '-'    '$'    '?'    '*'    ' '
```

Each machine uses a particular *character set*, the set of alphanumeric characters it can represent. (See Appendix E for some sample character sets.) Notice that each character is enclosed in single quotes (apostrophes). The C++ compiler needs the quotes to differentiate, say, between the character data '8' and the integer value 8 because the two are stored differently inside the machine. Notice also that the blank, ' ', is a valid character.*

You wouldn't want to add the character 'A' to the character 'B' or subtract the character '3' from the character '8', but you might want to compare character values. Each character set has a *collating sequence*, a predefined ordering of all the characters. Although this sequence varies from one character set to another, 'A' always compares less than 'B', 'B' less than 'C', and so forth. And '1' compares less than '2', '2' less than '3', and so on. None of the identifiers in the LeapYear program is of type `char`.

The `string` Data Type   Whereas a value of type `char` is limited to a single character, a *string* is a sequence of characters, such as a word, name, or sentence, enclosed in double quotes. For example, the following are strings in C++:

```
"Problem Solving"    "C++"    "Programming and "    " "    " . "
```

---

*Most programming languages use ASCII (the American Standard Code for Information Interchange) to represent the English alphabet and other symbols. Each ASCII character is stored in a single byte of memory.

A newer character set called Unicode includes the larger alphabets of many international human languages. A single Unicode character occupies two bytes of memory. C++ provides the data type `wchar_t` (for "wide character") to accommodate larger character sets such as Unicode. In C++, the notation L`'something'` denotes a value of type `wchar_t`, where the *something* depends on the particular wide character set being used. We do not examine wide characters any further in this book.

A string must be typed entirely on one line. For example, the string

```
"This string is invalid because it
is typed on more than one line."
```

is not valid because it is split across two lines. In this situation, the C++ compiler issues an error message at the first line. The message may say something like "UNTERMINATED STRING," depending on the particular compiler.

The quotes are not considered to be part of the string but are simply there to distinguish the string from other parts of a C++ program. For example, `"amount"` (in double quotes) is the character string made up of the letters *a, m, o, u, n,* and *t* in that order. On the other hand, `amount` (without the quotes) is an identifier, perhaps the name of a place in memory. The symbols `"12345"` represent a string made up of the characters *1, 2, 3, 4,* and *5* in that order. If we write `12345` without the quotes, it is an integer quantity that can be used in calculations.

A string containing no characters is called the *null string* (or *empty string*). We write the null string using two double quotes with nothing (not even spaces) between them:

```
""
```

The null string is not equivalent to a string of spaces; it is a special string that contains no characters.

To work with string data, this book uses a data type named `string`. This data type is not part of the C++ language (that is, it is not a built-in type). Rather, `string` is a programmer-defined type that is supplied by the C++ *standard library*, a large collection of prewritten functions and data types that any C++ programmer can use. Operations on `string` data include comparing the values of strings, searching a string for a particular character, and joining one string to another. We look at some of these operations later in this chapter and cover additional operations in subsequent chapters. None of the identifiers in the LeapYear program is of type `string`, although string values are used directly in several places in the program.

Naming Elements: Declarations

Identifiers can be used to name both constants and variables. In other words, an identifier can be the name of a memory location whose contents are not allowed to change or it can be the name of a memory location whose contents can change.

> **Declaration** A statement that associates an identifier with a data object, a function, or a data type so that the programmer can refer to that item by name.

How do we tell the computer what an identifier represents? By using a **declaration**, a statement that associates a name (an identifier) with a description of an element in a C++ program (just as a dictionary definition associates a name with a description of the thing being named). In a declaration, we name an identifier and what it represents. For example, the LeapYear program uses the declaration

```
int year;
```

to announce that `year` is the name of a variable whose contents are of type `int`. When we declare a variable, the compiler picks a location in memory to be associated with the identifier. We don't have to know the actual address of the memory location because the computer automatically keeps track of it for us.

Suppose that when we mailed a letter, we only had to put a person's name on it and the post office would look up the address. Of course, everybody in the world would need a different name; otherwise, the post office wouldn't be able to figure out whose address was whose. The same is true in C++. Each identifier can represent just one thing (except under special circumstances, which we talk about in Chapters 7 and 8). Every identifier you use in a program must be different from all others.

Constants and variables are collectively called *data objects*. Both data objects and the actual instructions in a program are stored in various memory locations. You have seen that a group of instructions—a function—can be given a name. A name also can be associated with a programmer-defined data type.

In C++, you must declare every identifier before it is used. This allows the compiler to verify that the use of the identifier is consistent with what it was declared to be. If you declare an identifier to be a constant and later try to change its value, the compiler detects this inconsistency and issues an error message.

There is a different form of declaration statement for each kind of data object, function, or data type in C++. The forms of declarations for variables and constants are introduced here; others are covered in later chapters.

Variables A program operates on data. Data is stored in memory. While a program is executing, different values may be stored in the same memory location at different times. This kind of memory location is called a **variable**, and its content is the *variable value*. The symbolic name that we associate with a memory location is the *variable name* or *variable identifier* (see Figure 2–1). In practice, we often refer to the variable name more briefly as the *variable*.

> **Variable** A location in memory, referenced by an identifier, that contains a data value that can be changed.

Declaring a variable means specifying both its name and its data type. This tells the compiler to associate a name with a memory location whose contents are of a specific

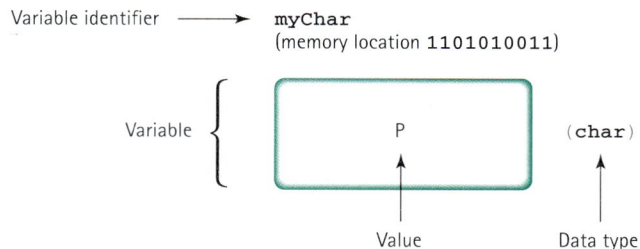

Figure 2–1 *Variable*

type (for example, `char` or `string`). The following statement declares `myChar` to be a variable of type `char`:

```
char myChar;
```

In C++, a variable can contain a data value only of the type specified in its declaration. Because of the above declaration, the variable `myChar` can contain *only* a `char` value. If the C++ compiler comes across an instruction that tries to store a `float` value into `myChar`, it generates extra instructions to convert the `float` value to the proper type. In Chapter 3, we examine how such type conversions take place.

Here's the syntax template for a variable declaration:

VariableDeclaration

DataType Identifier , Identifier . . . ;

where DataType is the name of a data type such as `char` or `string`. Notice that a variable declaration always ends with a semicolon.

From the syntax template, you can see that it is possible to declare several variables in one statement:

```
char letter, middleInitial, ch;
```

Here, all three variables are declared to be `char` variables. Our preference, though, is to declare each variable with a separate statement:

```
char letter;
char middleInitial;
char ch;
```

With this form it is easier, when modifying a program, to add new variables to the list or delete ones you no longer want.

Declaring each variable with a separate statement also allows you to attach comments to the right of each declaration, as shown here:

```
float payRate;    // Employee's pay rate
float hours;      // Hours worked
float wages;      // Wages earned
int   empNum;     // Employee ID number
```

These declarations tell the compiler to reserve memory space for three `float` variables—`payRate`, `hours`, and `wages`—and one `int` variable, `empNum`. The comments explain to someone reading the program what each variable represents.

Now that we've seen how to declare variables in C++, let's look at how to declare constants.

Constants   All single characters (enclosed in single quotes) and strings (enclosed in double quotes) are constants.

```
'A'    '@'    "Howdy boys"    "Please enter an employee number:"
```

In C++ as in mathematics, a constant is something whose value never changes. When we use the actual value of a constant in a program, we are using a **literal value** (or *literal*).

An alternative to the literal constant is the **named constant** (or **symbolic constant**), which is introduced in a declaration statement. A named constant is just another way of representing a literal value. Instead of using the literal value in an instruction, we give it a name in a declaration statement, then use that name in the instruction. For example, we can write an instruction that prints the title of this book using the literal string "Programming and Problem Solving with C++". Or we can declare a named constant called BOOK_TITLE that equals the same string and then use the constant name in the instruction. That is, we can use either

> **Literal value**   Any constant value written in a program.
>
> **Named constant (symbolic constant)**   A location in memory, referenced by an identifier, that contains a data value that cannot be changed.

```
"Programming and Problem Solving with C++"
```

or

```
BOOK_TITLE
```

in the instruction.

Using the literal value of a constant may seem easier than giving it a name and then referring to it by that name. But, in fact, named constants make a program easier to read because they make the meaning of literal constants clearer. Named constants also make it easier to change a program later on.

This is the syntax template for a constant declaration:

ConstantDeclaration

```
const DataType Identifier = LiteralValue;
```

Notice that the reserved word `const` begins the declaration, and an equal sign (=) appears between the identifier and the literal value.

The following are examples of constant declarations:

```
const string STARS = "********";
const char   BLANK = ' ';
const string BOOK_TITLE = "Programming and Problem Solving with C++";
const string MESSAGE = "Error condition";
```

As we have done above, many C++ programmers capitalize the entire identifier of a named constant and separate the English words with an underscore. The idea is to let the reader quickly distinguish between variable names and constant names when they appear in the middle of a program.

It's a good idea to add comments to constant declarations as well as variable declarations. We describe in comments what each constant represents:

```
const float MAX_HOURS = 40.0;    // Maximum normal work hours
const float OVERTIME = 1.5;      // Overtime pay rate factor
```

Matters of Style

Capitalization of Identifiers

Programmers often use capitalization as a quick visual clue to what an identifier represents. Different programmers adopt different conventions for using uppercase letters and lowercase letters. Some people use only lowercase letters, separating the English words in an identifier with the underscore character:

```
pay_rate    emp_num   pay_file
```

The conventions we use in this book are as follows:

- For identifiers representing variables, we begin with a lowercase letter and capitalize each successive English word.

  ```
  lengthInYards    middleInitial    hours
  ```

- Names of programmer-written functions and programmer-defined data types (which we examine later in the book) are capitalized in the same manner as variable names except that they begin with capital letters.

  ```
  CalcPay(payRate, hours, wages)    Cube(27)    MyDataType
  ```

Capitalizing the first letter allows a person reading the program to tell at a glance that an identifier represents a function name or data type rather than a variable. However, we cannot use

(continued) ▼

Capitalization of Identifiers

this capitalization convention everywhere. C++ expects every program to have a function named `main`—all in lowercase letters—so we cannot name it `Main`. Nor can we use `Char` for the built-in data type `char`. C++ reserved words use all lowercase letters, as do most of the identifiers declared in the standard library (such as `string`).

- For identifiers representing named constants, we capitalize every letter and use underscores to separate the English words.

```
BOOK_TITLE     OVERTIME     MAX_LENGTH
```

This convention, widely used by C++ programmers, is an immediate signal that `BOOK_TITLE` is a named constant and not a variable, a function, or a data type.

These conventions are only that—conventions. C++ does not require this particular style of capitalizing identifiers. You may wish to capitalize in a different fashion. But whatever system you use, it is essential that you use a consistent style throughout your program. A person reading your program will be confused or misled if you use a random style of capitalization.

Taking Action: Executable Statements

Up to this point, we've looked at ways of declaring data objects in a program. Now we turn our attention to ways of acting, or performing operations, on data.

Assignment   The value of a variable can be set or changed through an **assignment statement**. For example,

> **Assignment statement**   A statement that stores the value of an expression into a variable.

```
lastName = "Lincoln";
```

assigns the string value "`Lincoln`" to the variable `lastName` (that is, it stores the sequence of characters "Lincoln" into the memory associated with the variable named `lastName`).

Here's the syntax template for an assignment statement:

AssignmentStatement

> Variable = Expression;

> **Expression** An arrangement of identifiers, literals, and operators that can be evaluated to compute a value of a given type.
>
> **Evaluate** To compute a new value by performing a specified set of operations on given values.

The semantics (meaning) of the assignment operator (=) is "store"; the value of the **expression** is *stored* into the variable. Any previous value in the variable is destroyed and replaced by the value of the expression.

Only one variable can be on the left-hand side of an assignment statement. An assignment statement is *not* like a math equation ($x + y = z + 4$); the expression (what is on the right-hand side of the assignment operator) is **evaluated**, and the resulting value is stored into the single variable on the left of the assignment operator. A variable keeps its assigned value until another statement stores a new value into it.

Given the declarations

```
string  firstName;
string  middleName;
string  lastName;
string  title;
char    middleInitial;
char    letter;
```

the following assignment statements are valid:

```
firstName = "Abraham";
middleName = firstName;
middleName = "";
lastName = "Lincoln";
title = "President";
middleInitial = ' ';
letter = middleInitial;
```

However, these assignments are not valid:

Invalid Assignment Statement	Reason
`middleInitial = "A.";`	`middleInitial` is of type `char`; `"A."` is a string.
`letter = firstName;`	`letter` is of type `char`; `firstName` is of type `string`.
`firstName = Thomas;`	Thomas is an undeclared identifier.
`"Edison" = lastName;`	Only a variable can appear to the left of =.
`lastName = ;`	The expression to the right of = is missing.

String Expressions   Although we can't perform arithmetic on strings, the `string` data type provides a special string operation, called *concatenation*, that uses the + operator. The result of concatenating (joining) two strings is a new string containing the characters from both strings. For example, given the statements

```
string bookTitle;
string phrase1;
string phrase2;

phrase1 = "Programming and ";
phrase2 = "Problem Solving";
```

we could write

```
bookTitle = phrase1 + phrase2;
```

This statement retrieves the value of `phrase1` from memory and concatenates the value of `phrase2` to form a new, temporary string containing the characters

```
"Programming and Problem Solving"
```

This temporary string (which is of type `string`) is then assigned to (stored into) book-Title.

The order of the strings in the expression determines how they appear in the resulting string. If we instead write

```
bookTitle = phrase2 + phrase1;
```

then `bookTitle` contains

```
"Problem SolvingProgramming and "
```

Concatenation works with named `string` constants, literal strings, and `char` data as well as with `string` variables. The only restriction is that at least one of the operands of the + operator *must* be a `string` variable or named constant (so you cannot use expressions like `"Hi"` + `"there"` or `'A'` + `'B'`). For example, if we have declared the following constants:

```
const string WORD1 = "rogramming";
const string WORD3 = "Solving";
const string WORD5 = "C++";
```

then we could write the following assignment statement to store the title of this book into the variable `bookTitle`:

```
bookTitle = 'P' + WORD1 + " and Problem " + WORD3 + " with " + WORD5;
```

As a result, `bookTitle` contains the string

```
"Programming and Problem Solving with C++"
```

The preceding example demonstrates how we can combine identifiers, `char` data, and literal strings in a concatenation expression. Of course, if we simply want to assign the complete string to `bookTitle`, we can do so directly:

```
bookTitle = "Programming and Problem Solving with C++";
```

But occasionally we encounter a situation in which we want to add some characters to an existing string value. Suppose that `bookTitle` already contains "`Programming and Problem Solving`" and that we wish to complete the title. We could use a statement of the form

```
bookTitle = bookTitle + " with C++";
```

Such a statement retrieves the value of `bookTitle` from memory, concatenates the string "` with C++`" to form a new string, and then stores the new string back into `bookTitle`. The new string replaces the old value of `bookTitle` (which is destroyed).

Keep in mind that concatenation works only with values of type `string`. Even though an arithmetic plus sign is used for the operation, we cannot concatenate values of numeric data types, such as `int` and `float`, with strings.

If you are using pre–standard C++ (any version of C++ prior to the ISO/ANSI standard) and your standard library does not provide the `string` type, see Section D.1 of Appendix D for a discussion of how to proceed.

Output   Have you ever asked someone, "Do you know what time it is?" only to have the person smile smugly, say, "Yes, I do," and walk away? This situation is like the one that currently exists between you and the computer. You now know enough C++ syntax to tell the computer to assign values to variables and to concatenate strings, but the computer won't give you the results until you tell it to write them out.

In C++ we write out the values of variables and expressions by using a special variable named `cout` (pronounced "see-out") along with the *insertion operator* (`<<`):

```
cout << "Hello";
```

This statement displays the characters `Hello` on the *standard output device*, usually the display screen.

The variable `cout` is predefined in C++ systems to denote an *output stream*. You can think of an output stream as an endless sequence of characters going to an output device. In the case of `cout`, the output stream goes to the standard output device.

The insertion operator `<<` (often pronounced as "put to") takes two operands. Its left-hand operand is a stream expression (in the simplest case, just a stream variable such as `cout`). Its right-hand operand is an expression, which could be as simple as a literal string:

```
cout << "The title is ";
cout << bookTitle + ", 2nd Edition";
```

The insertion operator converts its right-hand operand to a sequence of characters and inserts them into (or, more precisely, appends them to) the output stream. Notice how the << points in the direction the data is going—*from* the expression written on the right *to* the output stream on the left.

You can use the << operator several times in a single output statement. Each occurrence appends the next data item to the output stream. For example, we can write the preceding two output statements as

```
cout << "The title is " << bookTitle + ", 2nd Edition";
```

If `bookTitle` contains "American History", both versions produce the same output:

```
The title is American History, 2nd Edition
```

The output statement has the following form:

OutputStatement

```
cout << Expression << Expression . . . ;
```

The following output statements yield the output shown. These examples assume that the char variable `ch` contains the value '2', the string variable `firstName` contains "Marie", and the string variable `lastName` contains "Curie".

Statement	What Is Printed (□means blank)
`cout << ch;`	2
`cout << "ch = " << ch;`	ch□=□2
`cout << firstName + " " + lastName;`	Marie□Curie
`cout << firstName << lastName;`	MarieCurie
`cout << firstName << ' ' << lastName;`	Marie□Curie
`cout << "ERROR MESSAGE";`	ERROR□MESSAGE
`cout << "Error=" << ch;`	Error=2

An output statement prints literal strings exactly as they appear. To let the computer know that you want to print a literal string—not a named constant or variable— you must remember to use double quotes to enclose the string. If you don't put quotes around a string, you'll probably get an error message (such as "UNDECLARED IDENTI- FIER") from the C++ compiler. If you want to print a string that includes a double quote, you must type a backslash (\) character and a double quote, with no space between them, in the string. For example, to print the characters

```
Al "Butch" Jones
```

the output statement looks like this:

```
cout << "Al \"Butch\" Jones";
```

To conclude this introductory look at C++ output, we should mention how to terminate an output line. Normally, successive output statements cause the output to continue along the same line of the display screen. The sequence

```
cout << "Hi";
cout << "there";
```

writes the following to the screen, all on the same line:

```
Hithere
```

To print the two words on separate lines, we can do this:

```
cout << "Hi" << endl;
cout << "there" << endl;
```

The output from these statements is

```
Hi
there
```

The identifier endl (meaning "end line") is a special C++ feature called a *manipulator*. We discuss manipulators in the next chapter. For now, the important thing to note is that endl lets you finish an output line and go on to the next line whenever you wish.

Beyond Minimalism: Adding Comments to a Program

All you need to create a working program is the correct combination of declarations and executable statements. The compiler ignores comments, but they are of enormous help to anyone who must read the program. Comments can appear anywhere in a program except in the middle of an identifier, a reserved word, or a literal constant.

C++ comments come in two forms. The first is any sequence of characters enclosed by the /* */ pair. The compiler ignores anything within the pair. Here's an example:

```
string idNumber;    /* Identification number of the aircraft */
```

The second, and more common, form begins with two slashes (//) and extends to the end of that line of the program:

```
string idNumber;    // Identification number of the aircraft
```

The compiler ignores anything after the two slashes.

Writing fully commented programs is good programming style. A comment should appear at the beginning of a program to explain what the program does:

```
// This program computes the weight and balance of a Beechcraft
// Starship-1 airplane, given the amount of fuel, number of
// passengers, and weight of luggage in fore and aft storage.
// It assumes that there are two pilots and a standard complement
// of equipment, and that passengers weigh 170 pounds each
```

Another good place for comments is in constant and variable declarations, where the comments explain how each identifier is used. In addition, comments should introduce each major step in a long program and should explain anything that is unusual or difficult to read (for example, a lengthy formula).

It is important to make your comments concise and to arrange them in the program so that they are easy to see and it is clear what they refer to. If comments are too long or crowd the statements in the program, they make the program more difficult to read—just the opposite of what you intended!

2.2 Program Construction

We have looked at basic elements of C++ programs: identifiers, declarations, variables, constants, expressions, statements, and comments. Now let's see how to collect these elements into a program. As you saw earlier, C++ programs are made up of functions, one of which must be named main. A program also can have declarations that lie outside of any function. The syntax template for a program looks like this:

Program

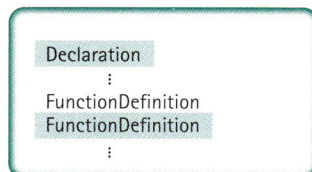

A function definition consists of the function heading and its body, which is delimited by left and right braces:

FunctionDefinition

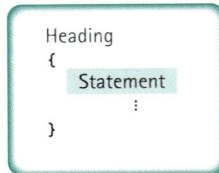

```
Heading
{
    Statement
        ⋮
}
```

Here's an example of a program with just one function, the main function:

```cpp
//*******************************************************************
// PrintName program
// This program prints a name in two different formats
//*******************************************************************
#include <iostream>
#include <string>

using namespace std;

const string FIRST = "Herman";     // Person's first name
const string LAST = "Smith";       // Person's last name
const char   MIDDLE = 'G';         // Person's middle initial

int main()
{
    string firstLast;     // Name in first-last format
    string lastFirst;     // Name in last-first format

    firstLast = FIRST + " " + LAST;
    cout << "Name in first-last format is " << firstLast << endl;

    lastFirst = LAST + ", " + FIRST + ", ";
    cout << "Name in last-first-initial format is ";
    cout << lastFirst << MIDDLE << '.' << endl;


    return 0;
}
```

The program begins with a comment that explains what the program does. Immediately after the comment, the following lines appear:

```
#include <iostream>
#include <string>

using namespace std;
```

The #include lines instruct the C++ system to insert into our program the contents of the files named iostream and string. The first file contains information that C++ needs in order to output values to a stream such as cout. The second file contains information about the programmer-defined data type string. We discuss the purpose of these #include lines and the using statement a little later in the chapter.

Next comes a declaration section in which we define the constants FIRST, LAST, and MIDDLE. Comments explain how each identifier is used. The rest of the program is the function definition for our main function. The first line is the function heading: the reserved word int, the name of the function, and then opening and closing parentheses. (The parentheses inform the compiler that main is the name of a function, not a variable or named constant.) The body of the function includes the declarations of two variables, firstLast and lastFirst, followed by a list of executable statements. The compiler translates these executable statements into machine language instructions. During the execution phase of the program, these are the instructions that are executed.

Our main function finishes by returning 0 as the function value:

```
return 0;
```

Remember that main returns an integer value to the operating system when it completes execution. This integer value is called the *exit status*. On most computer systems, you return an exit status of 0 to indicate successful completion of the program; otherwise, you return a nonzero value.

Notice how we use spacing in the PrintName program to make it easy for someone to read. We use blank lines to separate statements into related groups, and we indent the entire body of the main function. The compiler doesn't require us to format the program this way; we do so only to make it more readable. We have more to say in the next chapter about formatting a program.

Blocks (Compound Statements)

The body of a function is an example of a *block* (or *compound statement*). This is the syntax template for a block:

Block

```
{
    Statement
     ⋮
}
```

A block is just a sequence of zero or more statements enclosed (delimited) by a { } pair. Now we can redefine a function definition as a heading followed by a block:

FunctionDefinition

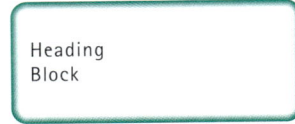

```
Heading
Block
```

In later chapters when we learn how to write functions other than `main`, we define the syntax of Heading in detail. In the case of the `main` function, Heading is simply

```
int main()
```

Here is the syntax template for a statement, limited to the C++ statements discussed in this chapter:

Statement

```
{ NullStatement
  Declaration
  AssignmentStatement
  OutputStatement
  Block
```

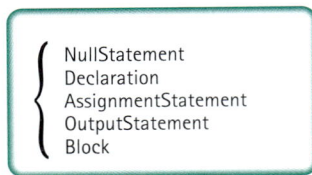

A statement can be empty (the *null statement*). The null statement is just a semicolon (;) and looks like this:

```
;
```

It does absolutely nothing at execution time; execution just proceeds to the next statement. It is not used often.

As the syntax template shows, a statement also can be a declaration, an executable statement, or even a block. The latter means that you can use an entire block wherever a single statement is allowed. In later chapters in which we introduce the syntax for branching and looping structures, this fact is very important.

We use blocks often, especially as parts of other statements. Leaving out a { } pair can dramatically change the meaning as well as the execution of a program. This is why we always indent the statements inside a block—the indentation makes a block easy to spot in a long, complicated program.

Notice in the syntax templates for the block and the statement that there is no mention of semicolons. Yet the PrintName program contains many semicolons. If you look back at the templates for constant declaration, variable declaration, assignment statement, and output statement, you can see that a semicolon is required at the end of each kind of statement. However, the syntax template for the block shows no semicolon after the right brace. The rule for using semicolons in C++, then, is quite simple: Terminate each statement *except* a compound statement (block) with a semicolon.

One more thing about blocks and statements: According to the syntax template for a statement, a declaration is officially considered to be a statement. A declaration, therefore, can appear wherever an executable statement can. In a block, we can mix declarations and executable statements if we wish:

```cpp
{
    char ch;
    ch = 'A';
    cout << ch;
    string str;
    str = "Hello";
    cout << str;
}
```

It's far more common, though, for programmers to group the declarations together before the start of the executable statements:

```cpp
{
    char    ch;
    string str;

    ch = 'A';
    cout << ch;
    str = "Hello";
    cout << str;
}
```

The C++ Preprocessor

Imagine that you are the C++ compiler. You are presented with the following program. You are to check it for syntax errors and, if there are no syntax errors, you are to translate it into machine language code.

```cpp
//***********************************
// This program prints Happy Birthday
//***********************************

int main()
{
    cout << "Happy Birthday" << endl;
    return 0;
}
```

You, the compiler, recognize the identifier `int` as a C++ reserved word and the identifier `main` as the name of a required function. But what about the identifiers `cout` and `endl`? The programmer has not declared them as variables or named constants, and they are not reserved words. You have no choice but to issue an error message and give up.

To fix this program, the first thing we must do is insert a line near the top that says

```
#include <iostream>
```

just as we did in the PrintName program (as well as in the sample program at the beginning of this chapter and the LeapYear program of Chapter 1).

The line says to insert the contents of a file named `iostream` into the program. This file contains declarations of `cout`, `endl`, and other items needed to perform stream input and output. The `#include` line is not handled by the C++ compiler but by a program known as the *preprocessor*.

The preprocessor concept is fundamental to C++. The preprocessor is a program that acts as a filter during the compilation phase. Your source program passes through the preprocessor on its way to the compiler (see Figure 2–2).

A line beginning with a pound sign (#) is not considered to be a C++ language statement (and thus is not terminated by a semicolon). It is called a *preprocessor directive*. The preprocessor expands an `#include` directive by physically inserting the contents of the named file into your source program. A file whose name appears in an `#include` directive is called a *header file*. Header files contain constant, variable, data type, and function declarations needed by a program.

In the directives

```
#include <iostream>
#include <string>
```

the angle brackets < > are required. They tell the preprocessor to look for the files in the standard *include directory*—a location in the computer system that contains all the header files that are related to the C++ standard library. The file `iostream` contains declarations of input/output facilities, and the file `string` contains declarations about the `string` data type. In Chapter 3, we make use of standard header files other than `iostream` and `string`.

In the C language and in pre–standard C++, the standard header files end in the suffix .h (for example, `iostream.h`), where the *h* suggests "header file." In ISO/ANSI C++, the standard header files no longer use the .h suffix.

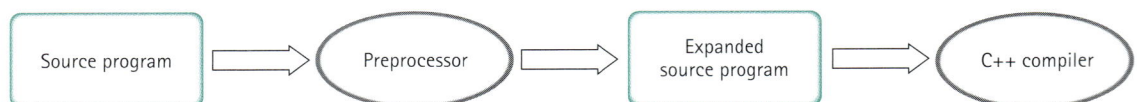

Figure 2–2   *C++ Preprocessor*

An Introduction to Namespaces

In our Happy Birthday program, even if we add the preprocessor directive #include <iostream>, the program will not compile. The compiler *still* doesn't recognize the identifiers cout and endl. The problem is that the header file iostream (and, in fact, every standard header file) declares all of its identifiers to be in a *namespace* called std:

```
namespace std
{
    ⋮   Declarations of variables, data types, and so forth
}
```

An identifier declared within a namespace block can be accessed directly only by statements within that block. To access an identifier that is "hidden" inside a namespace, the programmer has several options. We describe two options here. Chapter 8 describes namespaces in more detail.

The first option is to use a *qualified name* for the identifier. A qualified name consists of the name of the namespace, then the :: operator (the *scope resolution operator*), and then the desired identifier:

```
std::cout
```

With this approach, our program looks like the following:

```
#include <iostream>

int main()
{
    std::cout << "Happy Birthday" << std::endl;
    return 0;
}
```

Notice that both cout and endl must be qualified.

The second option is to use a statement called a *using directive:*

```
using namespace std;
```

When we place this statement near the top of the program before the main function, we make *all* the identifiers in the std namespace accessible to our program without having to qualify them:

```
#include <iostream>

using namespace std;

int main()
{
    cout << "Happy Birthday" << endl;
    return 0;
}
```

This second option is the one we used in the PrintName program and the sample program at the beginning of the chapter. In many of the following chapters, we continue to use this method. However, in Chapter 8 we discuss why it is not advisable to use the method in large programs.

If you are using a pre–standard C++ compiler that does not recognize namespaces and the newer header files (iostream, string, and so forth), you should turn to Section D.2 of Appendix D for a discussion of incompatibilities.

2.3 More About Output

We can control both the horizontal and vertical spacing of our output to make it more appealing (and understandable). Let's look first at vertical spacing.

Creating Blank Lines

We control vertical spacing by using the endl manipulator in an output statement. You have seen that a sequence of output statements continues to write characters across the current line until an endl terminates the line. Here are some examples:

Statements	Output Produced*

```cout << "Hi there, ";```
```cout << "Lois Lane. " << endl;```
```cout << "Have you seen ";```
```cout << "Clark Kent?" << endl;```
	Hi there, Lois Lane.
	
	Have you seen Clark Kent?

```cout << "Hi there, " << endl;```
```cout << "Lois Lane. " << endl;```
```cout << "Have you seen " << endl;```
```cout << "Clark Kent?" << endl;```
	Hi there,
	Lois Lane.
	Have you seen
	Clark Kent?

```cout << "Hi there, " << endl;```
```cout << "Lois Lane. ";```
```cout << "Have you seen " << endl;```
```cout << "Clark Kent?" << endl;```
	Hi there,
	
	Lois Lane. Have you seen
	Clark Kent?

*The output lines are shown next to the output statement that ends each of them. There are no blank lines in the actual output from these statements.

What do you think the following statements print out?

```
cout << "Hi there, " << endl;
cout << endl;
cout << "Lois Lane." << endl;
```

The first output statement causes the words *Hi there,* to be printed; the `endl` causes the screen cursor to go to the next line. The next statement prints nothing but goes on to the next line. The third statement prints the words *Lois Lane.* and terminates the line. The resulting output is the three lines

```
Hi there,

Lois Lane.
```

Whenever you use an `endl` immediately after another `endl`, a blank line is produced. As you might guess, three consecutive uses of `endl` produce two blank lines, four consecutive uses produce three blank lines, and so forth.

Note that we have a great deal of flexibility in how we write an output statement in a C++ program. We could combine the three preceding statements into two statements:

```
cout << "Hi there, " << endl << endl;
cout << "Lois Lane." << endl;
```

In fact, we could do it all in one statement. One possibility is

```
cout << "Hi there, " << endl << endl << "Lois Lane." << endl;
```

Here's another:

```
cout << "Hi there, " << endl << endl
     << "Lois Lane." << endl;
```

The last example shows that you can spread a single C++ statement onto more than one line of the program. The compiler treats the semicolon, not the physical end of a line, as the end of a statement.

Inserting Blanks Within a Line

To control the horizontal spacing of the output, one technique is to send extra blank characters to the output stream. (Remember that the blank character, generated by pressing the spacebar on a keyboard, is a perfectly valid character in C++.)

For example, to produce this output:

```
*   *   *   *   *   *   *   *   *

*   *   *   *   *   *   *   *   *   *

  *   *   *   *   *   *   *   *   *
```

you would use these statements:

```
cout << "  *   *   *   *   *   *   *   *    *" << endl << endl;
cout << "*   *   *   *   *   *   *   *    *" << endl << endl;
cout << "  *   *   *   *   *   *   *    *" << endl;
```

All of the blanks and asterisks are enclosed in double quotes, so they print literally as they are written in the program. The extra `endl` manipulators give you the blank lines between the rows of asterisks.

If you want blanks to be printed, you *must* enclose them in quotes. The statement

```
cout << '*' <<                                        '*';
```

produces the output

```
**
```

Despite all of the blanks we included in the output statement, the asterisks print side by side because the blanks are not enclosed by quotes.

2.4 Program Entry, Correction, and Execution

Once you have a program on paper, you must enter it on the keyboard. In this section, we examine the program entry process in general. You should consult the manual for your specific computer to learn the details.

Entering a Program

The first step in entering a program is to get the computer's attention. With a personal computer, this usually means turning it on if it is not already running. Workstations connected to a network are usually left running all the time. You must *log on* to such a machine to get its attention. This means entering a user name and a password. The password system protects information that you've stored in the computer from being tampered with or destroyed by someone else.

Once the computer is ready to accept your commands, you tell it that you want to enter a program by having it run the editor. The editor is a program that allows you to create and modify programs by entering information into an area of the computer's secondary storage called a **file**.

> **File** A named area in secondary storage that is used to hold a collection of data; the collection of data itself.

A file in a computer system is like a file folder in a filing cabinet. It is a collection of data that has a name associated with it. You usually choose the name for the file when you create it with the editor. From that point on, you refer to the file by the name you've given it.

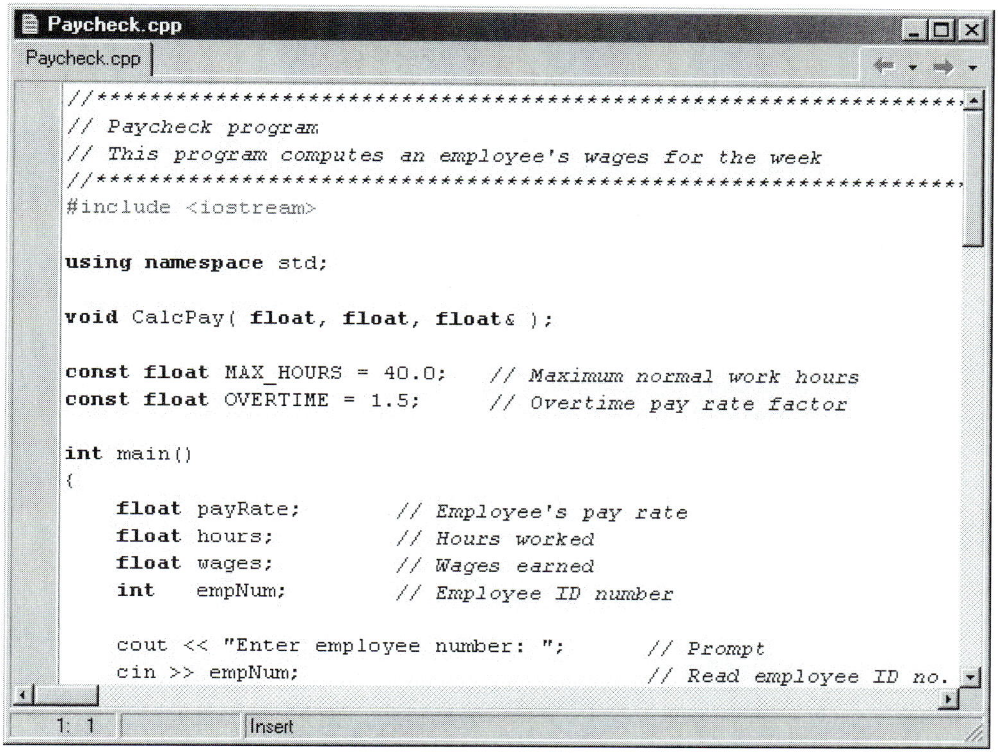

```
Paycheck.cpp                                                    _ □ ✕
Paycheck.cpp                                              ← ▾   → ▾

//***************************************************************
// Paycheck program
// This program computes an employee's wages for the week
//***************************************************************
#include <iostream>

using namespace std;

void CalcPay( float, float, float& );

const float MAX_HOURS = 40.0;     // Maximum normal work hours
const float OVERTIME = 1.5;       // Overtime pay rate factor

int main()
{
    float payRate;        // Employee's pay rate
    float hours;          // Hours worked
    float wages;          // Wages earned
    int   empNum;         // Employee ID number

    cout << "Enter employee number: ";        // Prompt
    cin >> empNum;                             // Read employee ID no.

  1: 1                    Insert
```

Figure 2–3   *Display Screen for an Editor*

There are so many different types of editors, each with different features, that we can't begin to describe them all here. But we can describe some of their general characteristics.

The basic unit of information in an editor is a display screen full of characters. The editor lets you change anything that you see on the screen. When you create a new file, the editor clears the screen to show you that the file is empty. Then you enter your program, using the mouse and keyboard to go back and make corrections as necessary. Figure 2–3 shows an example of an editor's display screen.

Compiling and Running a Program

Once your program is stored in a file, you compile it by issuing a command to run the C++ compiler. The compiler translates the program, then stores the machine language version into a file. The compiler may display a window with messages indicating errors in the program. Some systems let you click on an error message to automatically position the cursor in the editor window at the point where the error was detected.

If the compiler finds errors in your program (syntax errors), you have to determine their cause, go back to the editor and fix them, and then run the compiler again. Once your program compiles without errors, you can run (execute) it.

Some systems automatically run a program when it compiles successfully. On other systems, you have to issue a separate command to run the program. Still other systems require that you specify an extra step called *linking* between compiling and running a program. Whatever series of commands your system uses, the result is the same: Your program is loaded into memory and executed by the computer.

Even though a program runs, it still may have errors in its design. The computer does exactly what you tell it to do, even if that's not what you wanted it to do. If your program doesn't do what it should (a *logic error*), you have to go back to the algorithm and fix it, and then go to the editor and fix the program. Finally, you compile and run the program again. This *debugging* process is repeated until the program does what it is supposed to do (see Figure 2–4).

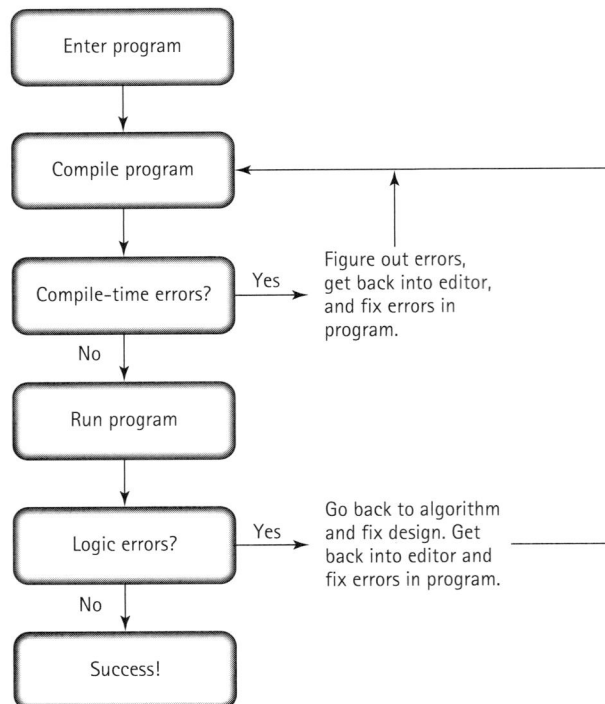

Figure 2–4   *Debugging Process*

Finishing Up

On a workstation, once you finish working on your program you have to *log off* by issuing a command with the mouse or keyboard. This frees up the workstation so that someone else can use it. It also prevents someone from walking up after you leave and tampering with your files.

On a personal computer, when you're done working you save your files and quit the editor. Turning off the power wipes out what's in the computer's memory, but your files are stored safely on disk. It is a wise precaution to periodically back up (make a copy of) your program files onto a removable diskette. When a disk in a computer suffers a hardware failure, it is often impossible to retrieve your files. With a backup copy on a diskette, you can restore your files to the disk once it is repaired.

Be sure to read the manual for your particular system and editor before you enter your first program. Don't panic if you have trouble at first—almost everyone does. It becomes much easier with practice. That's why it's a good idea to first go through the process with a program such as PrintName, where mistakes don't matter—unlike a class programming assignment!

Problem–Solving Case Study

Printing a Chessboard

PROBLEM Your college is hosting a chess tournament, and the people running the tournament want to record the final positions of the pieces in each game on a sheet of paper with a chessboard preprinted on it. Your job is to write a program to preprint these pieces of paper. The chessboard is an eight-by-eight pattern of squares that alternate between black and white, with the upper left square being white. You need to print out squares of light characters (spaces) and dark characters (such as *) in this pattern to form the chessboard.

DISCUSSION You could simply type up a program consisting of a series of output statements with alternating patterns of blanks and asterisks. But the organizers aren't sure exactly what they want the chessboard to look like, and you decide it would be safer to write the program in a manner that allows the design of the chessboard to be modified easily.

It is easy to make a changeable chessboard if the design is built up using string variables. You can begin by defining string constants for rows of characters that make up the black and white areas. Then you can concatenate these to form variables containing the alternating patterns of black and white that are repeated to print a row of chessboard squares. For example, suppose your initial design for the chessboard looks like this:

```
            * * * * * * * *      * * * * * * * *      * * * * * * * *      * * * * * * * *
            * * * * * * * *      * * * * * * * *      * * * * * * * *      * * * * * * * *
            * * * * * * * *      * * * * * * * *      * * * * * * * *      * * * * * * * *
            * * * * * * * *      * * * * * * * *      * * * * * * * *      * * * * * * * *
            * * * * * * * *      * * * * * * * *      * * * * * * * *      * * * * * * * *
* * * * * * * *      * * * * * * * *      * * * * * * * *      * * * * * * * *
* * * * * * * *      * * * * * * * *      * * * * * * * *      * * * * * * * *
* * * * * * * *      * * * * * * * *      * * * * * * * *      * * * * * * * *
* * * * * * * *      * * * * * * * *      * * * * * * * *      * * * * * * * *
* * * * * * * *      * * * * * * * *      * * * * * * * *      * * * * * * * *
            * * * * * * * *      * * * * * * * *      * * * * * * * *      * * * * * * * *
            * * * * * * * *      * * * * * * * *      * * * * * * * *      * * * * * * * *
            * * * * * * * *      * * * * * * * *      * * * * * * * *      * * * * * * * *
            * * * * * * * *      * * * * * * * *      * * * * * * * *      * * * * * * * *
            * * * * * * * *      * * * * * * * *      * * * * * * * *      * * * * * * * *
* * * * * * * *      * * * * * * * *      * * * * * * * *      * * * * * * * *
* * * * * * * *      * * * * * * * *      * * * * * * * *      * * * * * * * *
* * * * * * * *      * * * * * * * *      * * * * * * * *      * * * * * * * *
* * * * * * * *      * * * * * * * *      * * * * * * * *      * * * * * * * *
* * * * * * * *      * * * * * * * *      * * * * * * * *      * * * * * * * *
            * * * * * * * *      * * * * * * * *      * * * * * * * *      * * * * * * * *
            * * * * * * * *      * * * * * * * *      * * * * * * * *      * * * * * * * *
            * * * * * * * *      * * * * * * * *      * * * * * * * *      * * * * * * * *
            * * * * * * * *      * * * * * * * *      * * * * * * * *      * * * * * * * *
            * * * * * * * *      * * * * * * * *      * * * * * * * *      * * * * * * * *
* * * * * * * *      * * * * * * * *      * * * * * * * *      * * * * * * * *
* * * * * * * *      * * * * * * * *      * * * * * * * *      * * * * * * * *
* * * * * * * *      * * * * * * * *      * * * * * * * *      * * * * * * * *
* * * * * * * *      * * * * * * * *      * * * * * * * *      * * * * * * * *
* * * * * * * *      * * * * * * * *      * * * * * * * *      * * * * * * * *
            * * * * * * * *      * * * * * * * *      * * * * * * * *      * * * * * * * *
            * * * * * * * *      * * * * * * * *      * * * * * * * *      * * * * * * * *
            * * * * * * * *      * * * * * * * *      * * * * * * * *      * * * * * * * *
            * * * * * * * *      * * * * * * * *      * * * * * * * *      * * * * * * * *
            * * * * * * * *      * * * * * * * *      * * * * * * * *      * * * * * * * *
* * * * * * * *      * * * * * * * *      * * * * * * * *      * * * * * * * *
* * * * * * * *      * * * * * * * *      * * * * * * * *      * * * * * * * *
* * * * * * * *      * * * * * * * *      * * * * * * * *      * * * * * * * *
* * * * * * * *      * * * * * * * *      * * * * * * * *      * * * * * * * *
* * * * * * * *      * * * * * * * *      * * * * * * * *      * * * * * * * *
```

You can begin by defining constants for WHITE and BLACK that contain eight blanks and eight asterisks respectively, and then concatenate these together into variables that follow the patterns

```
WHITE + BLACK + WHITE + BLACK + WHITE + BLACK + WHITE + BLACK
```

and

```
BLACK + WHITE + BLACK + WHITE + BLACK + WHITE + BLACK + WHITE
```

that can then be printed with cout statements the appropriate number of times in order to create the chessboard.

From this discussion we know that there are two constants and two variables, as summarized in the following tables:

Constants

Name	Value	Function
BLACK	"********"	Characters forming one line of a black square
WHITE	" "	Characters forming one line of a white square

Variables

Name	Data Type	Description
whiteRow	string	A row beginning with a white square
blackRow	string	A row beginning with a black square

If we look carefully at the chessboard, the algorithm jumps out at us. We need to output five whiteRows, five blackRows, five whiteRows, five blackRows, five whiteRows, five blackRows, five whiteRows, and five blackRows. We can summarize this in our algorithm to output the five whiteRows and five blackRows four times.

> Repeat four times
>   Output five whiteRows
>   Output five blackRows

```cpp
//*******************************************************************
// Chessboard program
// This program prints a chessboard pattern that is built up from
// basic strings of white and black characters.
//*******************************************************************

#include <iostream>
#include <string>
using namespace std;

const string BLACK = "********";  // Define a line of a black square
const string WHITE = "        ";  // Define a line of a white square

int main ()
{
    string whiteRow;              // A row beginning with a white square
    string blackRow;              // A row beginning with a black square

    // Create a white-black row by concatenating the basic strings
    whiteRow = WHITE + BLACK + WHITE + BLACK +
               WHITE + BLACK + WHITE + BLACK;
    // Create a black-white row by concatenating the basic strings
    blackRow = BLACK + WHITE + BLACK + WHITE +
               BLACK + WHITE + BLACK + WHITE;

    // Print five white-black rows
    cout << whiteRow << endl;
    cout << whiteRow << endl;
    cout << whiteRow << endl;
    cout << whiteRow << endl;
    cout << whiteRow << endl;

    // Print five black-white rows
    cout << blackRow << endl;
    cout << blackRow << endl;
    cout << blackRow << endl;
    cout << blackRow << endl;
    cout << blackRow << endl;

    // Print five white-black rows
    cout << whiteRow << endl;
    cout << whiteRow << endl;
    cout << whiteRow << endl;
    cout << whiteRow << endl;
    cout << whiteRow << endl;
```

```
   // Print five black-white rows
   cout << blackRow << endl;
   cout << blackRow << endl;
   cout << blackRow << endl;
   cout << blackRow << endl;
   cout << blackRow << endl;

   // Print five white-black rows
   cout << whiteRow << endl;
   cout << whiteRow << endl;
   cout << whiteRow << endl;
   cout << whiteRow << endl;
   cout << whiteRow << endl;

   // Print five black-white rows
   cout << blackRow << endl;
   cout << blackRow << endl;
   cout << blackRow << endl;
   cout << blackRow << endl;
   cout << blackRow << endl;

   // Print five white-black rows
   cout << whiteRow << endl;
   cout << whiteRow << endl;
   cout << whiteRow << endl;
   cout << whiteRow << endl;
   cout << whiteRow << endl;

   // Print five black-white rows
   cout << blackRow << endl;
   cout << blackRow << endl;
   cout << blackRow << endl;
   cout << blackRow << endl;
   cout << blackRow << endl;

   return 0;
}
```

There are eight blocks of five lines that look alike. In Chapter 6, we introduce a looping state-ment that allows us to shorten this program considerably.

After you show the printout from this program to the organizers of the tournament, they sug-gest that the board would look better with the "#" character instead of "*" filling the black squares. You cheerfully agree to make this change because you know that the only difference in the pro-gram is that the value of the constant BLACK becomes "########".

Testing and Debugging

1. Every identifier that isn't a C++ reserved word must be declared. If you use a name that hasn't been declared—either by your own declaration statements or by including a header file—you get an error message.

2. If you try to declare an identifier that is the same as a reserved word in C++, you get an error message from the compiler. See Appendix A for a list of reserved words.

3. C++ is a case-sensitive language. Two identifiers that are capitalized differently are treated as two different identifiers. The word `main` and all C++ reserved words use only lowercase letters.

4. To use identifiers from the standard library, such as `cout` and `string`, you must either (a) give a qualified name such as `std::cout` or (b) put a `using` directive near the top of your program:

   ```
   using namespace std;
   ```

5. Check for mismatched quotes in `char` and string literals. Each `char` literal begins and ends with an apostrophe (single quote). Each string literal begins and ends with a double quote.

6. Be sure to use only the apostrophe (`'`) to enclose `char` literals. Most keyboards also have a reverse apostrophe (`` ` ``), which is easily confused with the apostrophe. If you use the reverse apostrophe, the compiler issues an error message.

7. To use a double quote within a literal string, use the two symbols `\"` in a row. If you use just a double quote, it ends the string, and the compiler then sees the remainder of the string as an error.

8. In an assignment statement, be sure that the identifier to the left of = is a variable and not a named constant.

9. In assigning a value to a `string` variable, the expression to the right of = must be a `string` expression, a literal string, or a `char`.

10. In a concatenation expression, at least one of the two operands of + must be of type `string`. For example, the operands cannot both be literal strings or `char` values.*

11. Make sure your statements end in semicolons (except compound statements, which do not have a semicolon after the right brace).

---

*The invalid concatenation expression `"Hi"` + `"there"` results in a syntax error message such as "INVALID POINTER ADDITION." This can be confusing, especially because the topic of pointers is not covered until much later in this book.

Summary

The syntax (grammar) of the C++ language is defined by a metalanguage. In this text, we use a form of metalanguage called syntax templates. We describe the semantics (meaning) of C++ statements in English.

Identifiers are used in C++ to name things. Some identifiers, called reserved words, have predefined meanings in the language; others are created by the programmer. The identifiers you invent are restricted to those *not* reserved by the C++ language. Reserved words are listed in Appendix A.

Identifiers are associated with memory locations by declarations. A declaration may give a name to a location whose value does not change (a constant) or to one whose value can change (a variable). Every constant and variable has an associated data type. C++ provides many built-in data types, the most common of which are `int`, `float`, and `char`. Additionally, C++ permits programmer-defined types such as the `string` type from the standard library.

The assignment operator is used to change the value of a variable by assigning it the value of an expression. At execution time, the expression is evaluated and the result is stored into the variable. With the `string` type, the plus sign (+) is an operator that concatenates two strings. A string expression can concatenate any number of strings to form a new `string` value.

Program output is accomplished by means of the output stream variable `cout`, along with the insertion operator (<<). Each insertion operation sends output data to the standard output device. When an `endl` manipulator appears instead of a data item, the computer terminates the current output line and goes on to the next line.

Output should be clear, understandable, and neatly arranged. Messages in the output should describe the significance of values. Blank lines (produced by successive uses of the `endl` manipulator) and blank spaces within lines help to organize the output and improve its appearance.

A C++ program is a collection of one or more function definitions (and optionally some declarations outside of any function). One of the functions *must* be named `main`. Execution of a program always begins with the `main` function. Collectively, the functions all cooperate to produce the desired results.

Quick Check

1. What is the name of the one function that every C++ program must have? (p. 46)
2. What is the purpose of a metalanguage? (pp. 49–51)
3. What is a data type? (pp. 55–56)
4. If you discover a logic error in your program, do you go directly to the editor and start changing the code? (pp. 78–80)
5. Use the following syntax template to decide if the string "C++ 4th edition" is a valid "Sentence." (pp. 51–53)

Sentence

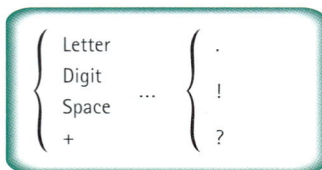

6. Which of the following are valid C++ identifiers? (pp. 54–55)

   Hello   Bob   4th-edition   C++   maximum   all_4_one

7. The only difference between a variable declaration and a constant declaration is that the reserved word `const` precedes the declaration. True or false? (pp. 59–62)

8. The reserved words listed in Appendix A cannot be used as identifiers. True or false? (p. 54)

9. Write a statement to assign the letter "A" to the `char` variable `initial`. (pp. 63–64)

10. What value is stored in the variable `name` by the following statement? (pp. 65–66)

    ```
    name = "Alexander" + " Q. " + "Smith";
    ```

11. Write a statement that sends the value in variable `name` to the stream `cout`. (pp. 66–68)

12. What is printed by the following statement, given the value assigned to `name` in Exercise 10? (pp. 68–69)

    ```
    cout << name << " Jr." << endl;
    ```

13. What are the two ways to write comments in C++? (pp. 68–69)

14. Fill in the blanks in the following statements, which appear at the beginning of a program. (pp. 69–71)

    ```
    #include <_____>
    #include <_____>

    using namespace _____;
    ```

Answers

1. `main`   2. To provide a language for expressing the syntax rules of a programming language. 3. A specific set of values, together with a set of operations that can be applied to those values. 4. No. You go back to the algorithm, correct the general solution to the problem, and then translate the correction into code before you use the editor to change your program.   5. No. According to the template, a Sentence must end in a period, exclamation point, or question mark.   6. `Hello`, `Bob`, `maximum`, and `all_4_one` are the valid C++ identifiers.   7. False. The constant declaration

also assigns a literal value to the identifier. 8. True. Identifiers must differ from reserved words. 9. `initial = 'A';` 10. `Alexander Q. Smith` 11. `cout << name;` 12. The string `Alexander Q. Smith Jr.` is output and then successive output will appear on the next line. 13. Between the delimiters `/*` and `*/`, or following `//` to the end of the line.

14. `#include <iostream>`
    `#include <string>`

    `using namespace std;`

Exam Preparation Exercises

1. Mark the following identifiers as either valid or invalid.

		Valid	Invalid
a.	`theDog`	_____	_____
b.	`all-In-One`	_____	_____
c.	`const`	_____	_____
d.	`recycling`	_____	_____
e.	`DVD_ROM`	_____	_____
f.	`elizabeth_the_2nd`	_____	_____
g.	`2morrow`	_____	_____
h.	`page#`	_____	_____

2. Match the following terms with the definitions given below.
   a. Function
   b. Syntax
   c. Semantics
   d. Metalanguage
   e. Identifier
   f. Data type
   g. Variable
   h. Named constant
   i. Literal
   j. Expression
      i. An identifier referring to a value that can be changed.
      ii. A specific set of values, along with operations that can be applied to those values.
      iii. A value that appears in a program.
      iv. The set of rules that determines the meaning of instructions written in a programming language.
      v. A language that is used to write the rules for another language.
      vi. A subprogram in C++.
      vii. A name that is used to refer to a function or data object.
      viii. An arrangement of identifiers, literals, and operators that can be evaluated.

      ix. The formal rules governing how valid instructions are written in a programming language.

      x. An identifier referring to a value that cannot be changed.

3. A reserved word is a named constant that is predefined in C++. True or false?

4. What is wrong with the following syntax template for a C++ identifier?

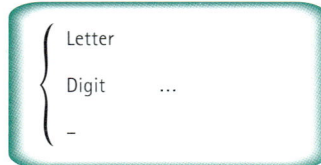

> Letter
>
> Digit   ...
>
> –

5. A `char` literal can be enclosed either in single or double quotes. True or false?

6. The null string represents a string containing no characters. True or false?

7. Concatenation only works with a `char` value when its other operand is a string value. True or false?

8. What is output by the following statement?

```
cout << "Four score and" << endl << "seven years ago"
     << "our fathers" << endl
     << "brought forth on this" << endl
     << "continent a new nation..." << endl
```

9. Given these assignments to string variables:

```
string1 = "Bjarne Stroustrup";
string2 = "C";
string3 = "programming language";
string4 = "++ because it is a successor to the ";
string5 = " named his new ";
```

What is the value of the following expression?

```
string1 + string5 + string3 + " " + string2 + string4 + string2
+ " " + string3 + "."
```

10. How do we insert a double quote into a string?

11. What danger is associated with the use of the /* and */ form of comment, and is avoided by use of the // comment form?

12. What are the limitations associated with the // form of comment?

13. What is the name of the << operator, and how might we pronounce it in reading a line of code that contains it?

14. Can we concatenate `endl` with a string in an expression? Explain.

15. What does the #include preprocessor directive do?

16. If you do not include the line

```
using namespace std;
```

at the start of a program, how must you change the following output statement to work correctly?

```
cout << "Hello everybody!" << endl;
```

17. What is the name of the C++ construct that begins with { and ends with }?
18. How do you write a string that is too long to fit on a single line?
19. Reorder the following lines to make a working program.

```
{
}
#include <iostream>

const string TITLE = "Dr.";
cout << "Hello " + TITLE + " Stroustrup!";
int main()
#include <string>
return 0;
using namespace std;
```

Programming Warm-Up Exercises

1. Write an output statement that prints today's date and then goes to the next line.
2. Write a single output statement that outputs the following three lines:

```
He said, "How is that possible?"
She replied, "Using manipulators."
"Of course!" he exclaimed.
```

3. Write declarations for the following:
   a. A named constant, called ANSWER, of type string with the value "True"
   b. A char variable with the name middleInitial
   c. A string variable with the name courseTitle
   d. A named char constant, called PERCENT, with the value '%'
4. Change the three declarations in the printName program on page 70 so that it prints your name.
5. Given the following declarations:

```
const string PART1 = "Pro";
const string PART2 = "gramming and ";
const string PART3 = "blem Solving with C++";
```

write an output statement that prints the title of this book, using only the cout stream, the stream insertion operator, and the above named constants.

6. Write an expression that results in a string containing the title of this book, using only the concatenation operator and the declarations of Exercise 5.
7. Write C++ output statements to print the following exactly as shown here (a portion of the text found on page iv of this book, relating the action of a weaver's loom to the complexity of human thought). You should write one output statement for each line of text.

```
Yet the web of thought has no such creases
And is more like a weaver's masterpieces;
One step a thousand threads arise,
Hither and thither shoots each shuttle,
The threads flow on unseen and subtle,
Each blow effects a thousand ties.
```

8. Fill in the missing lines in the following program, which outputs:

```
Rev. H.G. Jones
```

 _____
 _____

 _____

```
const string TITLE = "Rev. ";
const char FIRST = 'H';
const char MID 'G';
```

 _____

 _____

```
{
    cout << TITLE << FIRST << DOT << MID << DOT << " Jones";
```

 _____

9. Enter and run the following program. Be sure to type it exactly as it appears here, but substitute your name and the date as indicated.

```
//*****************************************************************
// Program entry and compilation exercise
// Your name goes here
// Today's date goes here
//*****************************************************************

#include <iostream>
#include <string>

using namespace std;

const string STARS35 = "***********************************";
const char    STAR = '*';
const string BLANKS33 = "                                 ";
const string MSG = "Welcome to C++ Programming!";
const string BLANKS3 = "   ";

int main()
```

```
{
    cout << STARS35 << endl << STAR << BLANKS33 << STAR << endl;
    cout << STAR << BLANKS3 << MSG << BLANKS3 << STAR << endl;
    cout << STAR << BLANKS33 << STAR << endl << STARS35 << endl;
}
```

Programming Problems

1. Write a program that prints out your course schedule for a single week. Here's an example of the output for one day:

    ```
    Monday   9:00 Computer Science 101
    Monday  11:00 Physics 201
    Monday   2:00 Dance 153
    ```

    Use named string constants wherever possible to avoid retyping any words or numbers. Be sure to include appropriate comments in your code, choose meaningful identifiers, and use indentation as we do with the programs in this chapter.

2. Write a program that prints out all six permutations of the ordering of the following three lines. Declare a named constant for each line and write an output statement for each permutation. Be sure to include appropriate comments in your code, choose meaningful identifiers, and use indentation as we do with the programs in this chapter.

    ```
    I saw the big brown bear.
    The big brown bear saw me.
    Oh! What a frightening experience!
    ```

3. Write a program that displays a checkerboard pattern made of stars and blanks, as shown below. A checkerboard is eight squares by eight squares. This will be easier if you first declare two named string constants representing the two different row patterns. Be sure to include appropriate comments in your code, choose meaningful identifiers, and use indentation as we do with the programs in this chapter.

    ```
     *   *   *   *
    *   *   *   *
     *   *   *   *
    *   *   *   *
     *   *   *   *
    *   *   *   *
     *   *   *   *
    *   *   *   *
    ```

4. Write a program that prints out business cards for yourself. A card should include your name, address, phone number(s), and email. You also can make up a company name and put that on the card if you wish. To save paper, the

program should print eight cards per page, arranged in two columns of four cards. Thus, to reduce typing, you should declare a named string constant for each line of the card, and then write output statements to print the eight cards using those constants. Be sure to include appropriate comments in your code, choose meaningful identifiers, and use indentation as we do with the programs in this chapter.

Case Study Follow-Up

1. What change would you have to make to the Chessboard program to cause the black squares to be printed with the "%" character instead of "*"?
2. How would you change the Chessboard program to print periods in the white squares instead of blanks?
3. How would the Chessboard program change if you wanted to reverse the colors (that is, make black squares white and vice versa) without changing the constant declarations or the values of `whiteRow` and `blackRow`?
4. Change the Chessboard program so that the squares are 10 characters wide by 8 rows high.
5. The organizers of the chess tournament find it difficult to write in the black squares of the printed chessboard. They want you to change the program so that the black squares have a blank space in their center that is four characters wide and two lines high. (*Hint:* You may have to define another string constant.)
6. How many characters are stored in each of the string variables in the Chessboard program?

Numeric Types, Expressions, and Output

Knowledge Goals

- *To understand implicit type coercion and explicit type conversion.*
- *To recognize and understand the purpose of function arguments.*
- *To learn and use additional operations associated with the* `string` *type.*
- *To learn how to format program statements in a clear and readable fashion.*

Goals

Skill Goals

To be able to:

- *Declare named constants and variables of type* `int` *and* `float`.
- *Construct simple arithmetic expressions.*
- *Evaluate simple arithmetic expressions.*
- *Construct and evaluate expressions that contain multiple arithmetic operations.*
- *Call (invoke) a value-returning function.*
- *Use C++ library functions in expressions.*
- *Call (invoke) a void function (one that does not return a function value).*
- *Use C++ manipulators to format output.*

In Chapter 2, we examined enough C++ syntax to be able to construct simple programs using assignment and output. We focused on the `char` and `string` types and saw how to construct expressions using the concatenation operator. In this chapter we continue to write programs that use assignment and output, but we concentrate on additional built-in data types: `int` and `float`. These numeric types are supported by numerous operators that allow us to construct complex arithmetic expressions. We show how to make expressions even more powerful by using *library functions*— prewritten functions that are part of every C++ system and are available for use by any program.

We also return to the subject of formatting the output. In particular, we consider the special features that C++ provides for formatting numbers in the output. We finish by looking at some additional operations on `string` data.

3.1   Overview of C++ Data Types

The C++ built-in data types are organized into simple types, structured types, and address types (see Figure 3–1). Do not feel overwhelmed by the quantity of data types shown in this figure. Our purpose is simply to give you an overall picture of what is available in C++. This chapter concentrates on the integral and floating types. Details of the other types come later in the book. First we look at the integral types (those used primarily to represent integers), and then we consider the floating types (used to represent real numbers containing decimal points).

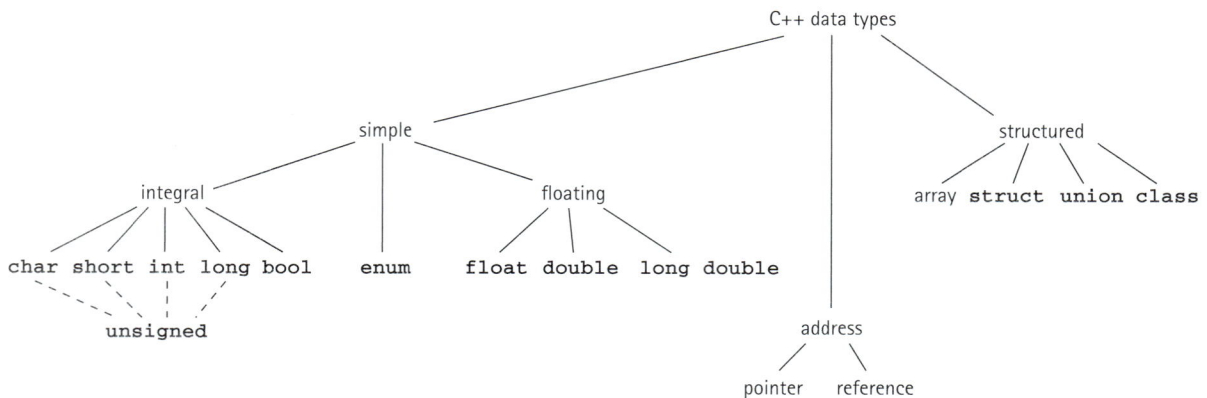

Figure 3–1   *C++ Data Types*

3.2 Numeric Data Types

You already are familiar with the basic concepts of integer and real numbers in math. However, as used on a computer, the corresponding data types have certain limitations, which we now consider.

Integral Types

The data types `char`, `short`, `int`, and `long` are known as integral types (or integer types) because they refer to integer values—whole numbers with no fractional part. (We postpone talking about the remaining integral type, `bool`, until Chapter 5.)

In C++, the simplest form of integer value is a sequence of one or more digits:

```
22   16   1   498   0   4600
```

Commas are not allowed.

In most cases, a minus sign preceding an integer value makes the integer negative:

```
-378   -912
```

The exception is when you explicitly add the reserved word `unsigned` to the data type name:

```
unsigned int
```

An `unsigned` integer value is assumed to be only positive or zero. The `unsigned` types are used primarily in specialized situations. We rarely use `unsigned` in this book.

The data types `char`, `short`, `int`, and `long` are intended to represent different sizes of integers, from smaller (fewer bits) to larger (more bits). The sizes are machine dependent (that is, they may vary from machine to machine). For one particular machine, we might picture the sizes this way:

`char` memory cell

`short` memory cell

`int` memory cell

`long` memory cell

On another machine, the size of an `int` might be the same as the size of a `long`. In general, the more bits there are in the memory cell, the larger the integer value that can be stored.

Although we used the `char` type in Chapter 2 to store character data such as `'A'`, there are reasons why C++ classifies `char` as an integral type. Chapter 10 discusses the reasons.

`int` is by far the most common data type for manipulating integer data. In the LeapYear program of Chapter 1, the identifier, `year`, is of data type `int`. You nearly always use `int` for manipulating integer values, but sometimes you have to use `long` if your program requires values larger than the maximum `int` value. (On some personal computers, the range of `int` values is from `-32768` through `+32767`. More commonly, `int`s range from `-2147483648` through `+2147483647`.) If your program tries to compute a value larger than your machine's maximum value, the result is *integer overflow*. Some machines give you an error message when overflow occurs, but others don't. We talk more about overflow in later chapters.

One caution about integer values in C++: A literal constant beginning with a zero is taken to be an octal (base–8) number instead of a decimal (base–10) number. If you write

```
015
```

the C++ compiler takes this to mean the decimal number 13. If you aren't familiar with the octal number system, don't worry about why an octal 15 is the same as a decimal 13. The important thing to remember is not to start a decimal integer constant with a zero (unless you simply want the number 0, which is the same in both octal and decimal). In Chapter 10, we discuss the various integral types in more detail.

Floating-Point Types

Floating-point types (or floating types), the second major category of simple types in C++, are used to represent real numbers. Floating-point numbers have an integer part and a fractional part, with a decimal point in between. Either the integer part or the fractional part, but not both, may be missing. Here are some examples:

```
18.0    127.54    0.57    4.    193145.8523    .8
```

Starting `0.57` with a zero does not make it an octal number. It is only with integer values that a leading zero indicates an octal number.

Just as the integral types in C++ come in different sizes (`char`, `short`, `int`, and `long`), so do the floating-point types. In increasing order of size, the floating-point types are `float`, `double` (meaning double precision), and `long double`. Again, the exact sizes are machine dependent. Each larger size potentially gives us a wider range of values and more precision (the number of significant digits in the number), but at the expense of more memory space to hold the number.

Floating-point values also can have an exponent, as in scientific notation. (In scientific notation, a number is written as a value multiplied by 10 to some power.) Instead of writing 3.504×10^{12}, in C++ we write `3.504E12`. The E means exponent of base 10. The number preceding the letter `E` doesn't need to include a decimal point. Here are some examples of floating-point numbers in scientific notation:

```
1.74536E-12    3.652442E4    7E20
```

Most programs don't need the `double` and `long double` types. The `float` type usually provides sufficient precision and range of values for floating-point numbers. Most personal computers provide `float` values with a precision of six or seven significant digits and a maximum value of about `3.4E+38`. We use floating-point values to represent money and interest rate in the case study at the end of the chapter.

We talk more about floating-point numbers in Chapter 10. But there is one more thing you should know about them now. Computers cannot always represent floating-point numbers exactly. You learned in Chapter 1 that the computer stores all data in binary (base–2) form. Many floating-point values can only be approximated in the binary number system. Don't be surprised if your program prints out the number 4.8 as 4.7999998. In most cases, slight inaccuracies in the rightmost fractional digits are to be expected and are not the result of programmer error.

3.3 Declarations for Numeric Types

Just as with the types `char` and `string`, we can declare named constants and variables of type `int` and `float`. Such declarations use the same syntax as before, except that the literals and the names of the data types are different.

Named Constant Declarations

In the case of named constant declarations, the literal values in the declarations are numeric instead of being characters in single or double quotes. For example, here are some constant declarations that define values of type `int` and `float`. For comparison, declarations of `char` and `string` values are included.

```
const float  PI = 3.14159;
const float  E = 2.71828;
const int    MAX_SCORE = 100;
const int    MIN_SCORE = -100;
const char   LETTER = 'W';
const string NAME = "Elizabeth";
```

Although character and string literals are put in quotes, literal integers and floating-point numbers are not, because there is no chance of confusing them with identifiers. Why? Because identifiers must start with a letter or underscore, and numbers must start with a digit or sign.

Software Engineering Tip

Using Named Constants Instead of Literals

It's a good idea to use named constants instead of literals. In addition to making your program more readable, named constants can make your program easier to modify. Suppose you wrote a program last year to compute taxes. In several places you used the literal 0.05, which was the sales tax rate at the time. Now the rate has gone up to 0.06. To change your program, you must locate every literal 0.05 and change it to 0.06. And if 0.05 is used for some other reason—to compute deductions, for example—you need to look at each place where it is used, figure out what it is used for, and then decide whether to change it.

The process is much simpler if you use a named constant. Instead of using a literal constant, suppose you had declared a named constant, TAX_RATE, with a value of 0.05. To change your program, you would simply change the declaration, setting TAX_RATE equal to 0.06. This one modification changes all of the tax rate computations without affecting the other places where 0.05 is used.

C++ allows us to declare constants with different names but the same value. If a value has different meanings in different parts of a program, it makes sense to declare and use a constant with an appropriate name for each meaning.

Named constants also are reliable; they protect us from mistakes. If you mistype the name PI as PO, the C++ compiler tells you that the name PO has not been declared. On the other hand, even though we recognize that the number 3.14149 is a mistyped version of pi (3.14159), the number is perfectly acceptable to the compiler. It won't warn us that anything is wrong.

Variable Declarations

We declare numeric variables the same way in which we declare char and string variables, except that we use the names of numeric types. The following are valid variable declarations:

```
int     studentCount;     // Number of students
int     sumOfScores;      // Sum of their scores
float   average;          // Average of the scores
char    grade;            // Student's letter grade
string  stuName;          // Student's name
```

Given the declarations

```
int    num;
int    alpha;
float  rate;
char   ch;
```

the following are appropriate assignment statements:

Variable	Expression
alpha =	2856;
rate =	0.36;
ch =	'B';
num =	alpha;

In each of these assignment statements, the data type of the expression matches the data type of the variable to which it is assigned. Later in the chapter we see what happens if the data types do not match.

3.4 Simple Arithmetic Expressions

Now that we have looked at declaration and assignment, we consider how to calculate with values of numeric types. Calculations are performed with expressions. We first look at simple expressions that involve at most one operator so that we may examine each operator in detail. Then, we move on to compound expressions that combine multiple operations.

Arithmetic Operators

Expressions are made up of constants, variables, and operators. The following are all valid expressions:

```
alpha + 2        rate - 6.0        4 - alpha        rate        alpha * num
```

The operators allowed in an expression depend on the data types of the constants and variables in the expression. The *arithmetic operators* are

+	Unary plus
-	Unary minus
+	Addition
-	Subtraction

```
*           Multiplication
        ⎧   Floating-point division (floating-point result)
/   ⎨
        ⎩   Integer division (no fractional part)
%           Modulus (remainder from integer division)
```

The first two operators are **unary operators**—they take just one operand. The remaining five are **binary operators**, taking two operands. Unary plus and minus are used as follows:

| Unary operator | An operator that has just one operand. |
| Binary operator | An operator that has two operands. |

```
-54    +259.65    -rate
```

Programmers rarely use the unary plus. Without any sign, a numeric constant is assumed to be positive anyway.

You may not be familiar with integer division and modulus (%). Let's look at them more closely. Note that % is used only with integers. When you divide one integer by another, you get an integer quotient and a remainder. Integer division gives only the integer quotient, and % gives only the remainder. (If either operand is negative, the sign of the remainder may vary from one C++ compiler to another.)

$$
\begin{array}{r}
3 \\
2\overline{)6} \\
6 \\
\hline
0
\end{array}
\;\leftarrow 6/2 \qquad\qquad
\begin{array}{r}
3 \\
2\overline{)7} \\
6 \\
\hline
1
\end{array}
\;\leftarrow 7/2
$$

$0 \leftarrow 6 \% 2 \qquad\qquad 1 \leftarrow 7 \% 2$

In contrast, floating-point division yields a floating-point result. The expression

```
7.0 / 2.0
```

yields the value 3.5.

Here are some expressions using arithmetic operators and their values:

Expression	Value
3 + 6	9
3.4 - 6.1	−2.7
2 * 3	6
8 / 2	4
8.0 / 2.0	4.0
8 / 8	1
8 / 9	0
8 / 7	1
8 % 8	0
8 % 9	8
8 % 7	1
0 % 7	0
5 % 2.3	error (both operands must be integers)

Be careful with division and modulus. The expressions `7.0 / 0.0`, `7 / 0`, and `7 % 0` all produce errors. The computer cannot divide by zero.

Because variables are allowed in expressions, the following are valid assignments:

```
alpha = num + 6;
alpha = num / 2;
num = alpha * 2;
num = 6 % alpha;
alpha = alpha + 1;
num = num + alpha;
```

As we saw with assignment statements involving `string` expressions, the same variable can appear on both sides of the assignment operator. In the case of

```
num = num + alpha;
```

the value in `num` and the value in `alpha` are added together, and then the sum of the two values is stored back into `num`, replacing the previous value stored there. This example shows the difference between mathematical equality and assignment. The mathematical equality

$$num = num + alpha$$

is true only when *alpha* equals 0. The assignment statement

```
num = num + alpha;
```

is valid for *any* value of `alpha`.

Here's a simple program that uses arithmetic expressions:

```
//*****************************************************************
// FreezeBoil program
// This program computes the midpoint between
// the freezing and boiling points of water
//*****************************************************************
#include <iostream>

using namespace std;

const float FREEZE_PT = 32.0;    // Freezing point of water
const float BOIL_PT = 212.0;     // Boiling point of water

int main()
{
    float avgTemp;                   // Holds the result of averaging
                                     //    FREEZE_PT and BOIL_PT
```

```
cout << "Water freezes at " << FREEZE_PT << endl;
cout << " and boils at " << BOIL_PT << " degrees." << endl;

avgTemp = FREEZE_PT + BOIL_PT;
avgTemp = avgTemp / 2.0;

cout << "Halfway between is ";
cout << avgTemp << " degrees." << endl;

return 0;
}
```

The program begins with a comment that explains what the program does. Next comes a declaration section where we define the constants FREEZE_PT and BOIL_PT. The body of the main function includes a declaration of the variable avgTemp and then a sequence of executable statements. These statements print a message, add FREEZE_PT and BOIL_PT, divide the sum by 2, and finally print the result.

Increment and Decrement Operators

In addition to the arithmetic operators, C++ provides *increment* and *decrement operators*:

++	Increment
--	Decrement

These are unary operators that take a single variable name as an operand. For integer and floating-point operands, the effect is to add 1 to (or subtract 1 from) the operand. If num currently contains the value 8, the statement

```
num++;
```

causes num to contain 9. You can achieve the same effect by writing the assignment statement

```
num = num + 1;
```

but C++ programmers typically prefer the increment operator. (Recall from Chapter 1 how the C++ language got its name: C++ is an enhanced ["incremented"] version of the C language.)

The ++ and -- operators can be either *prefix* operators

```
++num;
```

or postfix operators

```
num++;
```

Both of these statements behave in exactly the same way; they add 1 to whatever is in num. The choice between the two is a matter of personal preference.

C++ allows the use of ++ and - - in the middle of a larger expression:

```
alpha = num++ * 3;
```

In this case, the postfix form of ++ does *not* give the same result as the prefix form. In Chapter 10, we explain the ++ and - - operators in detail. In the meantime, you should use them only to increment or decrement a variable as a separate, stand-alone statement:

IncrementStatement

{
  Variable ++ ;

  ++ Variable ;
}

DecrementStatement

{
  Variable -- ;

  -- Variable ;
}

3.5 Compound Arithmetic Expressions

The expressions we've used so far have contained at most a single arithmetic operator. We also have been careful not to mix integer and floating-point values in the same expression. Now we look at more complicated expressions—ones that are composed of several operators and ones that contain mixed data types.

Precedence Rules

Arithmetic expressions can be made up of many constants, variables, operators, and parentheses. In what order are the operations performed? For example, in the assignment statement

```
avgTemp = FREEZE_PT + BOIL_PT / 2.0;
```

is FREEZE_PT + BOIL_PT calculated first or is BOIL_PT / 2.0 calculated first?

The basic arithmetic operators (unary +, unary -, + for addition, - for subtraction, * for multiplication, / for division, and % for modulus) are ordered the same way mathematical operators are, according to *precedence rules*:

Highest precedence level:	Unary + Unary -
Middle level:	* / %
Lowest level:	+ -

Because division has higher precedence than addition, the expression in the example above is implicitly parenthesized as

```
FREEZE_PT + (BOIL_PT / 2.0)
```

That is, we first divide `BOIL_PT` by 2.0 and then add `FREEZE_PT` to the result.

You can change the order of evaluation by using parentheses. In the statement

```
avgTemp = (FREEZE_PT + BOIL_PT) / 2.0;
```

`FREEZE_PT` and `BOIL_PT` are added first, and then their sum is divided by 2.0. We evaluate subexpressions in parentheses first and then follow the precedence of the operators.

When an arithmetic expression has several binary operators with the same precedence, their *grouping order* (or *associativity*) is from left to right. The expression

```
int1 - int2 + int3
```

means (`int1` - `int2`) + `int3`, not `int1` - (`int2` + `int3`). As another example, we would use the expression

```
(float1 + float2) / float1 * 3.0
```

to evaluate the expression in parentheses first, then divide the sum by `float1`, and multiply the result by 3.0. Below are some more examples.

Expression	Value
`10 / 2 * 3`	15
`10 % 3 - 4 / 2`	-1
`5.0 * 2.0 / 4.0 * 2.0`	5.0
`5.0 * 2.0 / (4.0 * 2.0)`	1.25
`5.0 + 2.0 / (4.0 * 2.0)`	5.25

In C++, all unary operators (such as unary + and unary -) have right-to-left associativity. Though this fact may seem strange at first, it turns out to be the natural grouping order. For example, - + x means - (+ x) rather than the meaningless (- +) x.

Type Coercion and Type Casting

Integer values and floating-point values are stored differently inside a computer's memory. The pattern of bits that represents the constant 2 does not look at all like the pattern of bits representing the constant 2.0. (In Chapter 10, we examine why floating-point numbers need a special representation inside the computer.) What happens if we mix integer and floating-point values together in an assignment statement or an arithmetic expression? Let's look first at assignment statements.

Assignment Statements If you make the declarations

```
int    someInt;
float someFloat;
```

then `someInt` can hold *only* integer values, and `someFloat` can hold *only* floating-point values. The assignment statement

```
someFloat = 12;
```

may seem to store the integer value 12 into `someFloat`, but this is not true. The computer refuses to store anything other than a `float` value into `someFloat`. The compiler inserts extra machine language instructions that first convert 12 into 12.0 and then store 12.0 into `someFloat`. This implicit (automatic) conversion of a value from one data type to another is known as **type coercion**.

> **Type coercion** The implicit (automatic) conversion of a value from one data type to another.

The statement

```
someInt = 4.8;
```

also causes type coercion. When a floating-point value is assigned to an `int` variable, the fractional part is truncated (cut off). As a result, `someInt` is assigned the value 4.

With both of the assignment statements above, the program would be less confusing for someone to read if we avoided mixing data types:

```
someFloat = 12.0;
someInt = 4;
```

More often, it is not just constants but entire expressions that are involved in type coercion. Both of the assignments

```
someFloat = 3 * someInt + 2;
someInt = 5.2 / someFloat - anotherFloat;
```

lead to type coercion. Storing the result of an `int` expression into a `float` variable generally doesn't cause loss of information; a whole number such as 24 can be represented in floating-point form as 24.0. However, storing the result of a floating-point expression into an `int` variable can cause loss of information because the fractional part is truncated. It is easy to overlook the assignment of a floating-point expression to an `int` variable when we try to discover why our program is producing the wrong answers.

To make our programs as clear (and error free) as possible, we can use explicit **type casting** (or **type conversion**). A C++ *cast operation* consists of a data type name and then, within parentheses, the expression to be converted:

> Type casting   The explicit conversion of a value from one data type to another; also called type conversion.

```
someFloat = float(3 * someInt + 2);
someInt = int(5.2 / someFloat - anotherFloat);
```

Both of the statements

```
someInt = someFloat + 8.2;
someInt = int(someFloat + 8.2);
```

produce identical results. The only difference is in clarity. With the cast operation, it is perfectly clear to the programmer and to others reading the program that the mixing of types is intentional, not an oversight. Countless errors have resulted from unintentional mixing of types.

Note that there is a nice way to round off rather than truncate a floating-point value before storing it into an `int` variable. Here is the way to do it:

```
someInt = int(someFloat + 0.5);
```

With pencil and paper, see for yourself what gets stored into `someInt` when `someFloat` contains 4.7. Now try it again, assuming `someFloat` contains 4.2. (This technique of rounding by adding 0.5 assumes that `someFloat` is a positive number.)

Arithmetic Expressions   So far we have been talking about mixing data types across the assignment operator (=). It's also possible to mix data types within an expression:

```
someInt * someFloat
4.8 + someInt - 3
```

Such expressions are called **mixed type** (or **mixed mode**) **expressions.**

> Mixed type expression   An expression that contains operands of different data types; also called mixed mode expression.

Whenever an integer value and a floating-point value are joined by an operator, implicit type coercion occurs as follows.

1. The integer value is temporarily coerced to a floating-point value.
2. The operation is performed.
3. The result is a floating-point value.

Let's examine how the machine evaluates the expression 4.8 + someInt - 3, where someInt contains the value 2. First, the operands of the + operator have mixed types, so the value of someInt is coerced to 2.0. (This conversion is only temporary; it does not affect the value that is stored in someInt.) The addition takes place, yielding a value of 6.8. Next, the subtraction (-) operator joins a floating-point value (6.8) and an integer value (3). The value 3 is coerced to 3.0, the subtraction takes place, and the result is the floating-point value 3.8.

Just as with assignment statements, you can use explicit type casts within expressions to lessen the risk of errors. Writing expressions such as

```
float(someInt)  *  someFloat
4.8 +  float(someInt  -  3)
```

makes it clear what your intentions are.

Explicit type casts are not only valuable for program clarity, but also are mandatory in some cases for correct programming. Given the declarations

```
int    sum;
int    count;
float  average;
```

suppose that sum and count currently contain 60 and 80, respectively. If sum represents the sum of a group of integer values and count represents the number of values, let's find the average value:

```
average = sum / count;     // Wrong
```

Unfortunately, this statement stores the value 0.0 into average. Here's why. The expression to the right of the assignment operator is not a mixed type expression. Both operands of the / operator are of type int, so integer division is performed. 60 divided by 80 yields the integer value 0. Next, the machine implicitly coerces 0 to the value 0.0 before storing it into average. The way to find the average correctly, as well as clearly, is this:

```
average = float(sum) / float(count);
```

This statement gives us floating-point division instead of integer division. As a result, the value 0.75 is stored into average.

As a final remark about type coercion and type conversion, you may have noticed that we have concentrated only on the int and float types. It is also possible to stir char values, short values, and double values into the pot. The results can be confusing and unexpected. In Chapter 10, we return to the topic with a more detailed discussion. In the meantime, you should avoid mixing values of these types within an expression.

May We Introduce...

Blaise Pascal

One of the great historical figures in the world of computing was the French mathematician and religious philosopher Blaise Pascal (1623–1662), the inventor of one of the earliest known mechanical calculators.

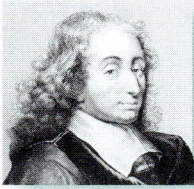

Pascal's father, Etienne, was a noble in the French court, a tax collector, and a mathematician. Pascal's mother died when Pascal was 3 years old. Five years later, the family moved to Paris and Etienne took over the education of the children. Pascal quickly showed a talent for mathematics. When he was only 17, he published a mathematical essay that earned the jealous envy of René Descartes, one of the founders of modern geometry. (Pascal's work actually had been completed before he was 16.) It was based on a theorem, which he called the *hexagrammum mysticum*, or mystic hexagram, that described the inscription of hexagons in conic sections (parabolas, hyperbolas, and ellipses). In addition to the theorem (now called Pascal's theorem), his essay included over 400 corollaries.

When Pascal was about 20, he constructed a mechanical calculator that performed addition and subtraction of eight-digit numbers. That calculator required the user to dial in the numbers to be added or subtracted; then the sum or difference appeared in a set of windows. It is believed that his motivation for building this machine was to aid his father in collecting taxes. The earliest version of the machine does indeed split the numbers into six decimal digits and two fractional digits, as would be used for calculating sums of money. The machine was hailed by his contemporaries as a great advance in mathematics, and Pascal built several more in different forms. It achieved such popularity that many fake, nonfunctional copies were built by others and displayed as novelties. Several of Pascal's calculators still exist in various museums.

Pascal's box, as it is called, was long believed to be the first mechanical calculator. However, in 1950, a letter from Wilhelm Shickard to Johannes Kepler written in 1624 was discovered. This letter described an even more sophisticated calculator built by Shickard 20 years prior to Pascal's box. Unfortunately, the machine was destroyed in a fire and never rebuilt.

During his twenties, Pascal solved several difficult problems related to the cycloid curve, indirectly contributing to the development of differential calculus. Working with Pierre de Fermat, he laid the foundation of the calculus of probabilities and combinatorial analysis. One of the results of this work came to be known as Pascal's triangle, which simplifies the calculation of the coefficients of the expansion of $(x + y)^n$, where n is a positive integer.

Pascal also published a treatise on air pressure and conducted experiments that showed that barometric pressure decreases with altitude, helping to confirm theories that had been proposed by Galileo and Torricelli. His work on fluid dynamics forms a significant part of the foundation of that field. Among the most famous of his contributions is Pascal's law, which states that pressure applied to a fluid in a closed vessel is transmitted uniformly throughout the fluid.

(continued) ▼

Blaise Pascal

When Pascal was 23, his father became ill, and the family was visited by two disciples of Jansenism, a reform movement in the Catholic Church that had begun 6 years earlier. The family converted, and 5 years later one of his sisters entered a convent. Initially, Pascal was not so taken with the new movement, but by the time he was 31, his sister had persuaded him to abandon the world and devote himself to religion.

His religious works are considered no less brilliant than his mathematical and scientific writings. Some consider *Provincial Letters*, his series of 18 essays on various aspects of religion, as the beginning of modern French prose.

Pascal returned briefly to mathematics when he was 35, but a year later his health, which had always been poor, took a turn for the worse. Unable to perform his usual work, he devoted himself to helping the less fortunate. Three years later, he died while staying with his sister, having given his own house to a poor family.

3.6 Function Calls and Library Functions

Value-Returning Functions

At the beginning of Chapter 2, we showed a program consisting of three functions: main, Square, and Cube. Here is a portion of the program:

```
int main()
{
    cout << "The square of 27 is " << Square(27) << endl;
    cout << "and the cube of 27 is " << Cube(27) << endl;
    return 0;
}

int Square( int n )
{
    return n * n;
}

int Cube( int n )
{
    return n * n * n;
}
```

We said that all three functions are value-returning functions. Square returns to its caller a value—the square of the number sent to it. Cube returns a value—the cube of the number sent to it. And main returns to the operating system a value—the program's exit status.

Let's focus for a moment on the `Cube` function. The `main` function contains a statement

```
cout << " and the cube of 27 is " << Cube(27) << endl;
```

In this statement, the master (`main`) causes the servant (`Cube`) to compute the cube of 27 and give the result back to `main`. The sequence of symbols

```
Cube(27)
```

is a **function call** or **function invocation**. The computer temporarily puts the `main` function on hold and starts the `Cube` function running. When `Cube` has finished doing its work, the computer goes back to `main` and picks up where it left off.

> **Function call (function invocation)**   The mechanism that transfers control to a function.

In the above function call, the number 27 is known as an *argument* (or *actual parameter*). Arguments make it possible for the same function to work on many different values. For example, we can write statements like these:

```
cout << Cube(4);
cout << Cube(16);
```

Here's the syntax template for a function call:

FunctionCall

> FunctionName (**ArgumentList**)

> **Argument list**   A mechanism by which functions communicate with each other.

The **argument list** is a way for functions to communicate with each other. Some functions, like `Square` and `Cube`, have a single argument in the argument list. Other functions, like `main`, have no arguments in the list. And some functions have two, three, or more arguments in the argument list, separated by commas.

Value-returning functions are used in expressions in much the same way that variables and constants are. The value computed by a function simply takes its place in the expression. For example, the statement

```
someInt = Cube(2) * 10;
```

stores the value 80 into `someInt`. First the `Cube` function is executed to compute the cube of 2, which is 8. The value 8—now available for use in the rest of the expression—is multiplied by 10. Note that a function call has higher precedence than multiplication, which makes sense if you consider that the function result must be available before the multiplication takes place.

Here are several facts about value-returning functions:

- The function call is used within an expression; it does not appear as a separate statement.
- The function computes a value (*result*) that is then available for use in the expression.
- The function returns exactly one result—no more, no less.

The `Cube` function expects to be given (or *passed*) an argument of type `int`. What happens if the caller passes a `float` argument? The answer is that the compiler applies implicit type coercion. The function call `Cube(6.9)` computes the cube of 6, not 6.9.

Although we have been using literal constants as arguments to `Cube`, the argument could just as easily be a variable or named constant. In fact, the argument to a value-returning function can be any expression of the appropriate type. In the statement

```
alpha = Cube(int1 * int1 + int2 * int2);
```

the expression in the argument list is evaluated first, and only its result is passed to the function. For example, if `int1` contains 3 and `int2` contains 5, the above function call passes 34 as the argument to `Cube`.

An expression in a function's argument list can even include calls to functions. For example, we could use the `Square` function to rewrite the above assignment statement as follows:

```
alpha = Cube(Square(int1) + Square(int2));
```

Library Functions

Certain computations, such as taking square roots or finding the absolute value of a number, are very common in programs. It would be an enormous waste of time if every programmer had to start from scratch and create functions to perform these tasks. To help make the programmer's life easier, every C++ system includes a standard library—a large collection of prewritten functions, data types, and other items that any C++ programmer may use. Here is a very small sample of some standard library functions:

Header File*	Function	Argument Type(s)	Result Type	Result (Value Returned)
`<cstdlib>`	`abs(i)`	`int`	`int`	Absolute value of i
`<cmath>`	`cos(x)`	`float`	`float`	Cosine of x (x is in radians)
`<cmath>`	`fabs(x)`	`float`	`float`	Absolute value of x
`<cstdlib>`	`labs(j)`	`long`	`long`	Absolute value of j
`<cmath>`	`pow(x, y)`	`float`	`float`	x raised to the power y (if x = 0.0, y must be positive; if x ≤ 0.0, y must be a whole number)
`<cmath>`	`sin(x)`	`float`	`float`	Sine of x (x is in radians)
`<cmath>`	`sqrt(x)`	`float`	`float`	Square root of x (x ≥ 0.0)

*The names of these header files are not the same as in pre-standard C++. If you are working with pre-standard C++, see Section D.2 of Appendix D.

Technically, the entries in the table marked `float` should all say `double`. These library functions perform their work using double-precision floating-point values. But because of type coercion, the functions work just as you would like them to when you pass `float` values to them.

Using a library function is easy. First, you place an `#include` directive near the top of your program, specifying the appropriate header file. This directive ensures that the C++ preprocessor inserts declarations into your program that give the compiler some information about the function. Then, whenever you want to use the function, you just make a function call.* Here's an example:

```cpp
#include <iostream>
#include <cmath>        // For sqrt() and fabs()

using namespace std;
   ⋮
float alpha;
float beta;
   ⋮
alpha = sqrt(7.3 + fabs(beta));
```

Remember from Chapter 2 that all identifiers in the standard library are in the namespace `std`. If we omit the `using` directive from the above code, we must use qualified names for the library functions (`std::sqrt`, `std::fabs`, and so forth).

The C++ standard library provides dozens of functions for you to use. Appendix C lists a much larger selection than we have presented here. You should glance briefly at this appendix now, keeping in mind that much of the terminology and C++ language notation will make sense only after you have read further into the book.

Void Functions

In this chapter, the only kind of function that we have looked at is the value-returning function. C++ provides another kind of function as well. For example, the following definition for function `CalcPay` begins with the word `void` instead of a data type like `int` or `float`:

```cpp
void CalcPay( ...  )
{
    ⋮
}
```

---

*Some systems require you to specify a particular compiler option if you use the math functions. For example, with some versions of UNIX, you must add the option `-lm` when compiling your program.

`CalcPay` is an example of a function that doesn't return a function value to its caller. Instead, it just performs some action and then quits. We refer to a function like this as a *non-value-returning function*, a *void-returning function*, or, most briefly, a **void function**. In some programming languages, a void function is known as a **procedure**.

> **Void function (procedure)** A function that does not return a function value to its caller and is invoked as a separate statement.
>
> **Value-returning function** A function that returns a single value to its caller and is invoked from within an expression.

Void functions are invoked differently from **value-returning functions**. With a value-returning function, the function call appears in an expression. With a void function, the function call is a separate, stand-alone statement. In the LeapYear program, `main` calls the `IsLeapYear` function in an expression like this:

```
if (IsLeapYear(year))
```

On the other hand, a call to a void function has the flavor of a command or built-in instruction:

```
DoThis(x, y, z);
DoThat();
```

For the next few chapters, we won't be writing our own functions (except `main`). Instead, we'll be concentrating on how to use existing functions, including functions for performing stream input and output. Some of these functions are value-returning functions; others are void functions. Again, we emphasize the difference in how you invoke these two kinds of functions: A call to a value-returning function occurs in an expression, whereas a call to a void function occurs as a separate statement.

3.7 Formatting the Output

To format a program's output means to control how it appears visually on the screen or on a printer. In Chapter 2, we considered two kinds of output formatting: creating extra blank lines by using the `endl` manipulator and inserting blanks within a line by putting extra blanks into literal strings. In this section, we examine how to format the output values themselves.

Integers and Strings

By default, consecutive integer and string values are output with no spaces between them. If the variables `i`, `j`, and `k` contain the values 15, 2, and 6, respectively, the statement

```
cout << "Results: " << i << j << k;
```

outputs the stream of characters

```
Results: 1526
```

Without spacing between the numbers, this output is difficult to interpret.

To separate the output values, you could print a single blank (as a `char` constant) between the numbers:

```
cout << "Results: " << i << ' ' << j << ' ' << k;
```

This statement produces the output

```
Results: 15 2 6
```

If you want even more spacing between items, you can use literal strings containing blanks, as we discussed in Chapter 2:

```
cout << "Results: " << i << "    " << j << "    " << k;
```

Here, the resulting output is

```
Results: 15     2     6
```

Another way to control the horizontal spacing of the output is to use *manipulators*. For some time now, we have been using the `endl` manipulator to terminate an output line. In C++, a manipulator is a rather curious thing that behaves like a function but travels in the disguise of a data object. Like a function, a manipulator causes some action to occur. But like a data object, a manipulator can appear in the midst of a series of insertion operations:

```
cout << someInt << endl << someFloat;
```

Manipulators are used only in input and output statements.

Here's a revised syntax template for the output statement, showing that not only arithmetic and string expressions but also manipulators are allowed:

OutputStatement

```
cout << ExpressionOrManipulator << ExpressionOrManipulator ... ;
```

The C++ standard library supplies many manipulators, but for now we look at only five of them: `endl`, `setw`, `fixed`, `showpoint`, and `setprecision`. The `endl`, `fixed`, and `showpoint` manipulators come "for free" when we #include the header file `iostream` to perform I/O. The other two manipulators, `setw` and `setprecision`, require that we also #include the header file `iomanip`:

```
#include <iostream>
#include <iomanip>
```

```
using namespace std;
    ⋮
cout << setw(5) << someInt;
```

The manipulator setw—meaning "set width"—lets us control how many character positions the next data item should occupy when it is output. (setw is only for formatting numbers and strings, not char data.) The argument to setw is an integer expression called the *fieldwidth specification*; the group of character positions is called the *field*. The next data item to be output is printed *right-justified* (filled with blanks on the left to fill up the field).

Let's look at an example. Assuming two int variables have been assigned values as follows:

```
ans = 33;
num = 7132;
```

then the following output statements produce the output shown to their right.

Statement	Output (⛶ means blank)

1. `cout << setw(4) << ans`
`<< setw(5) << num`
`<< setw(4) << "Hi";`
	⛶⛶33⛶7132⛶⛶Hi
	  4 5 4

2. `cout << setw(2) << ans`
`<< setw(4) << num`
`<< setw(2) << "Hi";`
	337132Hi
	 2 4 2

3. `cout << setw(6) << ans`
`<< setw(3) << "Hi"`
`<< setw(5) << num;`
	⛶⛶⛶⛶33⛶Hi⛶7132
	    6 3 5

4. `cout << setw(7) << "Hi"` `<< setw(4) << num;`	⛶⛶⛶⛶⛶Hi7132 7 4
5. `cout << setw(1) << ans` `<< setw(5) << num;`	33⛶7132 ↑ 5 Field automatically expands to fit the two-digit value

In (1), each value is specified to occupy enough positions so that there is at least one space separating them. In (2), the values all run together because the fieldwidth specified for each value is just large enough to hold the value. This output obviously is not very readable. It's better to make the fieldwidth larger than the minimum size required so that some space is left between values. In (3), there are extra blanks for readability; in (4), there are not. In (5), the fieldwidth is not large enough for the value in ans, so it automatically expands to make room for all of the digits.

Setting the fieldwidth is a one-time action. It holds only for the very next item to be output. After this output, the fieldwidth resets to 0, meaning "extend the field to exactly as many positions as are needed." In the statement

```
cout << "Hi" << setw(5) << ans << num;
```

the fieldwidth resets to 0 after ans is output. As a result, we get the output

```
Hi    337132
```

Floating-Point Numbers

You can specify a fieldwidth for floating-point values just as for integer values. But you must remember to allow for the decimal point when you specify the number of character positions. The value 4.85 requires four output positions, not three. If x contains the value 4.85, the statement

```
cout << setw(4) << x << endl
     << setw(6) << x << endl
     << setw(3) << x << endl;
```

produces the output

```
4.85
  4.85
4.85
```

In the third line, a fieldwidth of 3 isn't sufficient, so the field automatically expands to accommodate the number.

There are several other issues related to output of floating-point numbers. First, large floating-point values are printed in scientific (E) notation. The value 123456789.5 may print on some systems as

```
1.23457E+08
```

You can use the manipulator named fixed to force all subsequent floating-point output to appear in decimal form rather than scientific notation:

```
cout << fixed << 3.8 * x;
```

Second, if the number is a whole number, C++ doesn't print a decimal point. The value 95.0 prints as

```
95
```

To force decimal points to be displayed in subsequent floating-point output, even for whole numbers, you can use the manipulator `showpoint`:

```
cout << showpoint << floatVar;
```

(If you are using a pre–standard version of C++, the `fixed` and `showpoint` manipulators may not be available. See Section D.3 of Appendix D for an alternative way of achieving the same results.)

Third, you often would like to control the number of *decimal places* (digits to the right of the decimal point) that are displayed. If your program is supposed to print the 5% sales tax on a certain amount, the statement

```
cout << "Tax is $" << price * 0.05;
```

may output

```
Tax is $17.7435
```

Here, you clearly would prefer to display the result to two decimal places. To do so, use the `setprecision` manipulator as follows:

```
cout << fixed << setprecision(2) << "Tax is $" << price * 0.05;
```

Provided that `fixed` has already been specified, the argument to `setprecision` specifies the desired number of decimal places. Unlike `setw`, which applies only to the very next item printed, the value sent to `setprecision` remains in effect for all subsequent output (until you change it with another call to `setprecision`). Here are some examples of using `setprecision` in conjunction with `setw`:

Value of x	Statement	Output (☐ means blank)
	`cout << fixed;`	
310.0	`cout << setw(10)`	
	`     << setprecision(2) << x;`	☐☐☐☐310.00
310.0	`cout << setw(10)`	
	`     << setprecision(5) << x;`	☐310.00000
310.0	`cout << setw(7)`	
	`     << setprecision(5) << x;`	310.00000 (expands to nine positions)
4.827	`cout << setw(6)`	
	`     << setprecision(2) << x;`	☐☐4.83 (last displayed digit is rounded off)
4.827	`cout << setw(6)`	
	`     << setprecision(1) << x;`	☐☐☐4.8 (last displayed digit is rounded off)

Again, the total number of print positions is expanded if the fieldwidth specified by `setw` is too narrow. However, the number of positions for fractional digits is controlled entirely by the argument to `setprecision`.

The following table summarizes the manipulators we have discussed in this section. Manipulators without arguments are available through the header file `iostream`. Those with arguments require the header file `iomanip`.

Header File	Manipulator	Argument Type	Effect
`<iostream>`	`endl`	None	Terminates the current output line
`<iostream>`	`showpoint`	None	Forces display of decimal point in floating-point output
`<iostream>`	`fixed`	None	Suppresses scientific notation in floating-point output
`<iomanip>`	`setw(n)`	int	Sets fieldwidth to n*
`<iomanip>`	`setprecision(n)`	int	Sets floating-point precision to n digits

*`setw` is only for numbers and strings, not `char` data. Also, `setw` applies only to the very next output item, after which the fieldwidth is reset to 0 (meaning "use only as many positions as are needed").

Matters of Style

Program Formatting

As far as the compiler is concerned, C++ statements are *free format*: They can appear anywhere on a line, more than one can appear on a single line, and one statement can span several lines. The compiler only needs blanks (or comments or new lines) to separate important symbols, and it needs semicolons to terminate statements. However, it is extremely important that your programs be readable, both for your sake and for the sake of anyone else who has to examine them.

When you write an outline for an English paper, you follow certain rules of indentation to make it readable. These same kinds of rules can make your programs easier to read. It is much easier to spot a mistake in a neatly formatted program than in a messy one. Thus, you should keep your program neatly formatted while you are working on it. If you've gotten lazy and let your program become messy while making a series of changes, take the time to straighten it up. Often the source of an error becomes obvious during the process of formatting the code.

Take a look at the following program for computing the cost per square foot of a house. Although it compiles and runs correctly, it does not conform to any formatting standards.

```
// HouseCost program
// This program computes the cost per square foot of
    // living space for a house, given the dimensions of
```

(continued) ▼

Program Formatting

```
// the house, the number of stories, the size of the
// nonliving space, and the total cost less land
#include <iostream>
#include <iomanip>// For setw() and setprecision()
using namespace
std;
const float WIDTH = 30.0; // Width of the house
    const float LENGTH = 40.0; // Length of the house
const float STORIES = 2.5; // Number of full stories
const float NON_LIVING_SPACE = 825.0;// Garage, closets, etc.

const float PRICE = 150000.0; // Selling price less land
int main() { float grossFootage;// Total square footage
    float livingFootage;        // Living area
float costPerFoot;      // Cost/foot of living area
   cout << fixed << showpoint;   // Set up floating-pt.
//    output format

grossFootage = LENGTH * WIDTH * STORIES; livingFootage =
grossFootage - NON_LIVING_SPACE; costPerFoot = PRICE /
livingFootage; cout << "Cost per square foot is "
<< setw(6) << setprecision(2) << costPerFoot << endl;
return 0; }
```

Now look at the same program with proper formatting:

```
//*****************************************************************
// HouseCost program
// This program computes the cost per square foot of
// living space for a house, given the dimensions of
// the house, the number of stories, the size of the
// nonliving space, and the total cost less land
//*****************************************************************
#include <iostream>
#include <iomanip>    // For setw() and setprecision()

using namespace std;

const float WIDTH = 30.0;               // Width of the house
const float LENGTH = 40.0;              // Length of the house
const float STORIES = 2.5;              // Number of full stories
const float NON_LIVING_SPACE = 825.0;   // Garage, closets, etc.
const float PRICE = 150000.0;           // Selling price less land

int main()
{
    float grossFootage;         // Total square footage
    float livingFootage;        // Living area
    float costPerFoot;          // Cost/foot of living area
```

(continued) ▼

Program Formatting

```
cout << fixed << showpoint;              // Set up floating-pt.
                                         //   output format

grossFootage = LENGTH * WIDTH * STORIES;
livingFootage = grossFootage - NON_LIVING_SPACE;
costPerFoot = PRICE / livingFootage;

cout << "Cost per square foot is "
     << setw(6) << setprecision(2) << costPerFoot << endl;
return 0;
}
```

Need we say more?

Appendix F talks about programming style. Use it as a guide when you are writing programs.

3.8 Additional string Operations

Now that we have introduced numeric types and function calls, we can take advantage of additional features of the string data type. In this section, we introduce four functions that operate on strings: length, size, find, and substr.

The length and size Functions

The length function, when applied to a string variable, returns an unsigned integer value that equals the number of characters currently in the string. If myName is a string variable, a call to the length function looks like this:

```
myName.length()
```

You specify the name of a string variable (here, myName), then a dot (period), and then the function name and argument list. The length function requires no arguments to be passed to it, but you still must use parentheses to signify an empty argument list. Also, length is a value-returning function, so the function call must appear within an expression:

```
string firstName;
string fullName;
```

```
firstName = "Alexandra";
cout << firstName.length() << endl;        // Prints 9
fullName = firstName + " Jones";
cout << fullName.length() << endl;         // Prints 15
```

Perhaps you are wondering about the syntax in a function call like

```
firstName.length()
```

This expression uses a C++ notation called *dot notation*. There is a dot (period) between the variable name `firstName` and the function name `length`. Certain programmer-defined data types, such as `string`, have functions that are tightly associated with them, and dot notation is required in the function calls. If you forget to use dot notation, writing the function call as

```
length()
```

you get a compile-time error message, something like "UNDECLARED IDENTIFIER." The compiler thinks you are trying to call an ordinary function named `length`, not the `length` function associated with the `string` type. In Chapter 4, we discuss the meaning behind dot notation.

Some people refer to the length of a string as its *size*. To accommodate both terms, the `string` type provides a function named `size`. Both `firstName.size()` and `firstName.length()` return the same value.

We said that the `length` function returns an unsigned integer value. If we want to save the result into a variable `len`, as in

```
len = firstName.length();
```

then what should we declare the data type of `len` to be? To keep us from having to guess whether `unsigned int` or `unsigned long` is correct for the particular compiler we're working with, the `string` type defines a data type `size_type` for us to use:

```
string firstName;
string::size_type len;

firstName = "Alexandra";
len = firstName.length();
```

Notice that we must use the qualified name `string::size_type` (just as we do with identifiers in namespaces) because the definition of `size_type` is otherwise hidden inside the definition of the `string` type.

Before leaving the `length` and `size` functions, we should make a remark about capitalization of identifiers. In the guidelines given in Chapter 2, we said that in this book we begin the names of programmer-defined functions and data types with uppercase letters. We follow this convention when we write our own functions and data types in later chapters. However, we have no control over the capitalization of items supplied by the C++ standard library. Identifiers in the standard library generally use all-lowercase letters.

The find Function

The `find` function searches a string to find the first occurrence of a particular substring and returns an unsigned integer value (of type `string:: size_type`) giving the result of the search. The substring, passed as an argument to the function, can be a literal string or a `string` expression. If `str1` and `str2` are of type `string`, the following are valid function calls:

```
str1.find("the")        str1.find(str2)        str1.find(str2 + "abc")
```

In each case above, `str1` is searched to see if the specified substring can be found within it. If so, the function returns the position in `str1` where the match begins. (Positions are numbered starting at 0, so the first character in a string is in position 0, the second is in position 1, and so on.) For a successful search, the match must be exact, including identical capitalization. If the substring could not be found, the function returns the special value `string::npos`, a named constant meaning "not a position within the string." (`string::npos` is the largest possible value of type `string::size_type`, a number like `4294967295` on many machines. This value is suitable for "not a valid position" because the `string` operations do not let any string become this long.)

Given the code segment

```
string phrase;
string::size_type position;

phrase = "The dog and the cat";
```

the statement

```
position = phrase.find("the");
```

assigns to `position` the value 12, whereas the statement

```
position = phrase.find("rat");
```

assigns to `position` the value `string::npos`, because there was no match.

The argument to the `find` function can also be a `char` value. In this case, `find` searches for the first occurrence of that character within the string and returns its position (or `string::npos`, if the character was not found). For example, the code segment

```
string theString;

theString = "Abracadabra";
cout << theString.find('a');
```

outputs the value 3, which is the position of the first occurrence of a lowercase *a* in theString.

Below are some more examples of calls to the find function, assuming the following code segment has been executed:

```
string str1;
string str2;

str1 = "Programming and Problem Solving";
str2 = "gram";
```

Function Call	Value Returned by Function
str1.find("and")	12
str1.find("Programming")	0
str2.find("and")	string::npos
str1.find("Pro")	0
str1.find("ro" + str2)	1
str1.find("Pr" + str2)	string::npos
str1.find(' ')	11

Notice in the fourth example that there are two copies of the substring "Pro" in str1, but find returns only the position of the first copy. Also notice that the copies can be either separate words or parts of words—find merely tries to match the sequence of characters given in the argument list. The final example demonstrates that the argument can be as simple as a single character, even a single blank.

The substr Function

The substr function returns a particular substring of a string. Assuming myString is of type string, here is a sample function call:

```
myString.substr(5, 20)
```

The first argument is an unsigned integer that specifies a position within the string, and the second is an unsigned integer that specifies the length of the desired substring. The function returns the piece of the string that starts with the specified position and continues for the number of characters given by the second argument. Note that substr doesn't change myString; it returns a new, temporary string value that is a copy of a portion of the string. Following are some examples, assuming the statement

```
myString = "Programming and Problem Solving";
```

has been executed.

Function Call	String Contained in Value Returned by Function
`myString.substr(0, 7)`	`"Program"`
`myString.substr(7, 8)`	`"ming and"`
`myString.substr(10, 0)`	`""`
`myString.substr(24, 40)`	`"Solving"`
`myString.substr(40, 24)`	None. Program terminates with an execution error message.

In the third example, specifying a length of 0 produces the null string as the result. The fourth example shows what happens if the second argument specifies more characters than are present after the starting position: `substr` returns the characters from the starting position to the end of the string. The last example illustrates that the first argument, the position, must not be beyond the end of the string.

Because `substr` returns a value of type `string`, you can use it with the concatenation operator (+) to copy pieces of strings and join them together to form new strings. The `find` and `length` functions can be useful in determining the location and end of a piece of a string to be passed to `substr` as arguments.

Here is a program that uses several of the `string` operations:

```cpp
//****************************************************************
// StringOps program
// This program demonstrates several string operations
//****************************************************************
#include <iostream>
#include <string>     // For string type

using namespace std;

int main()
{
    string fullName;
    string name;
    string::size_type startPos;

    fullName = "Jonathan Alexander Peterson";
    startPos = fullName.find("Peterson");
    name = "Mr. " + fullName.substr(startPos, 8);
    cout << name << endl;
    return 0;
}
```

This program outputs `Mr. Peterson` when it is executed. First it stores a string into the variable `fullName`, and then it uses `find` to locate the start of the name `Peterson` within the string. Next, it builds a new string by concatenating the literal `"Mr. "` with the characters `Peterson`, which are copied from the original string. Last, it prints out the new string. As we see in later chapters, string operations are an important aspect of many computer programs.

The following table summarizes the `string` operations we have looked at in this chapter.

Function Call (s is of type `string`)	Argument Type(s)	Result Type	Result (Value Returned)
`s.length()` `s.size()`	None	`string::size_type`	Number of characters in the string
`s.find(arg)`	`string`, literal string, or `char`	`string::size_type`	Starting position in `s` where `arg` was found; if not found, result is `string::npos`
`s.substr(pos,len)`	`string::size_type`	`string`	Substring of at most `len` characters, starting at position `pos` of `s`. If `len` is too large, it means "to the end" of string `s`. If `pos` is too large, execution of the program is terminated.*

*Technically, if `pos` is too large, the program generates what is called an *out-of-range exception*—a topic we cover in Chapter 17. Unless we write additional program code to deal explicitly with this out-of-range exception, the program simply terminates with a message such as "ABNORMAL PROGRAM TERMINATION."

Software Engineering Tip

Understanding Before Changing

When you are in the middle of getting a program to run and you come across an error, it's tempting to start changing parts of the program to try to make it work. *Don't!* You'll nearly always make things worse. It's essential that you understand what is causing the error and carefully think through the solution. The only thing you should try is running the program with different data to determine the pattern of the unexpected behavior.

There is no magic trick that can automatically fix a program. If the compiler tells you that a semicolon or a right brace is missing, you need to examine the program and determine precisely what the problem is. Perhaps you accidentally typed a colon instead of a semicolon. Or maybe there's an extra left brace.

(continued) ▼

Understanding Before Changing

If the source of a problem isn't immediately obvious, a good rule of thumb is to leave the computer and go somewhere where you can quietly look over a printed copy of the program. Studies show that people who do all of their debugging away from the computer actually get their programs to work in less time *and in the end produce better programs* than those who continue to work on the machine—more proof that there is still no mechanical substitute for human thought.*

*Basili, V. R., and Selby, R. W., "Comparing the Effectiveness of Software Testing Strategies," *IEEE Trans. on Software Engineering* SE-13, no. 12 (1987): 1278–1296.

Problem–Solving Case Study

Mortgage Payment Calculator

PROBLEM Your parents are thinking about refinancing their mortgage, and have asked you to help them with the calculations. Now that you're learning C++, you realize that you can save yourself a lot of calculator button-pressing by writing a program to do the calculations automatically.

DISCUSSION In the case study in Chapter 1, we said that there are often three obvious steps in almost any problem of this type:

1. Get the data.
2. Compute the results.
3. Output the results.

The data we need in this problem are the amount of money to borrow, the number of years for the loan, and the interest rate. From these three values, the monthly payment can be calculated. Although you could solve this problem for your parents using paper and pencil, you might as well write a program to solve it. You can make the data values constants now and later; when you learn how to input values, you can rewrite the program.

After a chat with your parents, you find that they still owe $50,000 on the house and have exactly 7 years worth of payments to go. The latest quote from their credit union is for an interest rate of 5.24 with no closing costs.

Define Constants

Set LOAN_AMOUNT = 50000.00
Set NUMBER_OF_YEARS = 7
Set INTEREST_RATE = 0.0524

You vaguely recall seeing the formula for determining payments, using compound interest, but you can't remember it. You decide to go to the Internet and look it up.

$$\frac{\text{Amount} * (1 + \text{Monthly Interest})^{\text{number of payments}} * \text{Monthly Interest}}{(1 + \text{Monthly Interest})^{\text{number of payments}} - 1}$$

Hmmm. This may actually be easier to do on the computer than on a calculator. Two values taken to the number of payments power looks daunting. Fortunately, the C++ `<cmath>` header file, which we looked at earlier, contains a number of mathematical functions including the power function. Before you actually enter the values in the formula, two intermediate values need to be calculated: monthly interest rate and number of payments.

Calculate Values

Set monthlyInterest to YEARLY_INTEREST divided by 12
Set numberOfPayments to NUMBER_OF_YEARS times 12
Set payment to (LOAN_AMOUNT * pow(monthlyInterest+1,
   numberOfPayments) * monthlyInterest) /
   (pow(monthlyInterest+1, numberOfPayments) – 1)

Now all that is left is to print out the answer in a clear, concise format. Let's use a precision of 2 for the floating point values and a fixed format.

Output Results

Print "For a loan amount of "LOAN_AMOUNT " with an interest rate of "
   YEARLY_INTEREST " and a " NUMBER_OF_YEARS " year mortgage, "
Print "your monthly payments are $" payment "."

From the algorithm we can create tables of constants and variables to help us write the declarations for the program.

Constants

Name	Value	Function
LOAN_AMOUNT	50000.00	Amount of the loan
YEARLY_INTEREST	0.0524	Yearly interest rate
NUMBER_OF_YEARS	7	Number of years

Variables

Name	Data Type	Description
monthlyInterest	float	Monthly interest rate
numberOfPayments	int	Total number of payments
payment	int	Monthly payment

```cpp
//****************************************************************
// Mortgage Payment Calculator program
// This program determines the monthly payments on a mortgage given
// the loan amount, the yearly interest, and the number of years.
//****************************************************************

#include <iostream>                    // Access cout
#include <cmath>                       // Access power function
#include <iomanip>                     // Access manipulators
using namespace std;

const float LOAN_AMOUNT = 50000.00;    // Amount of the loan
const float YEARLY_INTEREST = 0.0524;  // Yearly interest rate
const int NUMBER_OF_YEARS = 7;         // Number of years

int main()
{
    // local variables
    float monthlyInterest;             // Monthly interest rate
    int numberOfPayments;              // Total number of payments
    float payment;                     // Monthly payment

    // Calculate values
    monthlyInterest = YEARLY_INTEREST / 12;
```

```
numberOfPayments = NUMBER_OF_YEARS * 12;
payment = (LOAN_AMOUNT *
          pow(monthlyInterest + 1, numberOfPayments)
          * monthlyInterest)/( pow(monthlyInterest + 1,
          numberOfPayments) - 1 );

// Output results
cout << fixed << setprecision(2) << "For a loan amount of "
     << LOAN_AMOUNT  << " with an interest rate of "
     << YEARLY_INTEREST << " and a " << NUMBER_OF_YEARS
     << " year mortgage, " << endl;
cout << " your monthly payments are $" << payment
     << "." << endl;
return 0;
}
```

Here is a screen shot of the output.

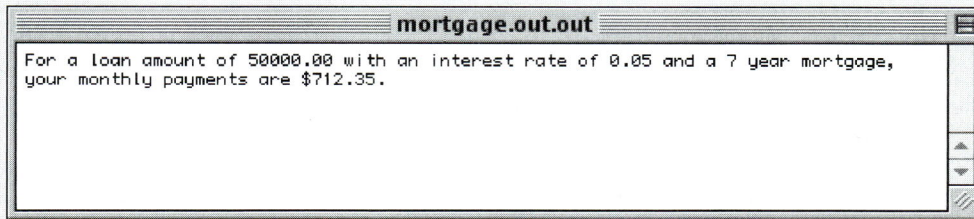

```
mortgage.out.out
For a loan amount of 50000.00 with an interest rate of 0.05 and a 7 year mortgage,
your monthly payments are $712.35.
```

Something looks strange about the output: The interest should be 0.0524, not 0.05. The decision to use a precision of 2 was correct for dollars and cents, but not for interest rates, which are rarely whole percentages. You are asked to make this correction in Case Study Follow-Up Exercise 1.

Testing and Debugging

1. An `int` constant other than 0 should not start with a zero. If it starts with a zero, it is an octal (base–8) number.

2. Watch out for integer division. The expression `47 / 100` yields 0, the integer quotient. This is one of the major sources of wrong output in C++ programs.

3. When using the `/` and `%` operators, remember that division by zero is not allowed.

4. Double-check every expression according to the precedence rules to be sure that the operations are performed in the desired order.

5. Avoid mixing integer and floating-point values in expressions. If you must mix them, consider using explicit type casts to reduce the chance of mistakes.

6. For each assignment statement, check that the expression result has the same data type as the variable to the left of the assignment operator (=). If not, consider using an explicit type cast for clarity and safety. And remember that storing a floating-point value into an `int` variable truncates the fractional part.

7. For every library function you use in your program, be sure to #include the appropriate header file.

8. Examine each call to a library function to see that you have the right number of arguments and that the data types of the arguments are correct.

9. With the `string` type, positions of characters within a string are numbered starting at 0, not 1.

10. If the cause of an error in a program is not obvious, leave the computer and study a printed listing. Change your program only after you understand the source of the error.

Summary

C++ provides several built-in numeric data types, of which the most commonly used are `int` and `float`. The integral types are based on the mathematical integers, but the computer limits the range of integer values that can be represented. The floating-point types are based on the mathematical notion of real numbers. As with integers, the computer limits the range of floating-point numbers that can be represented. Also, it limits the number of digits of precision in floating-point values. We can write literals of type `float` in several forms, including scientific (E) notation.

Much of the computation of a program is performed in arithmetic expressions. Expressions can contain more than one operator. The order in which the operations are performed is determined by precedence rules. In arithmetic expressions, multiplication, division, and modulus are performed first, then addition and subtraction. Multiple binary (two-operand) operations of the same precedence are grouped from left to right. You can use parentheses to override the precedence rules.

Expressions may include function calls. C++ supports two kinds of functions: value-returning functions and void functions. A value-returning function is called by writing its name and argument list as part of an expression. A void function is called by writing its name and argument list as a complete C++ statement.

The C++ standard library is an integral part of every C++ system. The library contains many prewritten data types, functions, and other items that any programmer can use. These items are accessed by using #include directives to the C++ preprocessor, which inserts the appropriate header files into the program.

In output statements, the `setw`, `showpoint`, `fixed`, and `setprecision` manipulators control the appearance of values in the output. These manipulators do not affect the values actually stored in memory, only their appearance when displayed on the output device.

Not only should the output produced by a program be easy to read, but the format of the program itself should be clear and readable. C++ is a free-format language. A consistent style that uses indentation, blank lines, and spaces within lines helps you (and other programmers) understand and work with your programs.

Quick Check

1. What happens to the fractional portion of a floating-point number when it is converted to an integer type? (p. 107)
2. Where do arguments appear, and what is their purpose? (pp. 107–109)
3. What is the value of the following expression, given that the string variable quickCheck contains the string "My friend I shall be pedagogic"? (pp. 122–127)

   ```
   quickCheck.substr(10, 20) + " " + quickCheck.substr(0, 9) + "."
   ```

4. Neatly formatting a program makes it easier to find errors. True or false? (pp. 120–123)
5. How does the declaration of named constants and variables of type int and float differ from declarations of named constants and variables of type string? (pp. 99–101)
6. How would you write an expression that gives the remainder of dividing integer1 by integer2? (pp. 101–104)
7. If integer1 contains 37 and integer2 contains 7, what is the result of the expression in exercise 6? (pp. 101–104)
8. What is the result of the following expression? (pp. 105–106)

   ```
   27 + 8 * 6 - 44 % 5
   ```

9. Write an expression that computes the square root of 17.5. (pp. 111-114)
10. How does a call to a void function differ from a call to a value-returning function? (pp. 114–115)
11. Which stream manipulator would you use to set the output precision for floating-point values? (pp. 115–120)

Answers

1. The fractional part is truncated.   2. They appear in the call to a function, between parentheses, and are used to pass data to or from a function.   3. "I shall be pedagogic My friend."   4. True.
5. The declarations are exactly the same, except that we use the reserved word int or float instead of string, and we assign a numerical value to the constant rather than a string value.
6. integer1 % integer2   7. 37 % 7 = 2   8. 27 + (8 * 6) – (44 % 5) = 27 + 48 – 4 = 71
9. sqrt(17.5)   10. A void function call appears as a separate statement rather than being part of an expression.   11. setprecision

Exam Preparation Exercises

1. The integer and floating types in C++ are considered (simple, address, structured) data types. (Circle one)

2. What are the four integral types in C++? List them in order of size, from smallest to largest.

3. What is the result if the computer tries to calculate a value that is larger than the maximum integer allowed for a given integral type?

4. In a floating-point value, what does it mean when the letter E appears as part of a number?

5. Label each of the following as an integer or floating-point declaration, and whether it is a constant or a variable declaration.

	integer / floating	constant / variable
a. `const int tracksOnDisk = 17;`	_____	_____
b. `float timeOfTrack;`	_____	_____
c. `const float maxTimeOnDisk = 74.0;`	_____	_____
d. `short tracksLeft;`	_____	_____
e. `float timeLeft;`	_____	_____
f. `long samplesInTrack;`	_____	_____
g. `const double sampleRate = 262144.5;`	_____	_____

6. What are the two meanings of the / operator?

7. What is the result of each of the following expressions?
   a. `27 + 8 / 5 - 7`
   b. `27.0 + 8.0 / 5.0 - 7.0`
   c. `25 % 7 + 9.0`
   d. `17++`
   e. `int(15.0 + 12.0 * 2.2 - 3 * 7)`
   f. `23--`
   g. `18 / 1.0`

8. List the following operators in the order of highest precedence to lowest precedence. If a set of operators has the same precedence, write them enclosed in square brackets within the ordered list.

   ```
   *     +     %     /     -     unary -     ()
   ```

9. The increment and decrement operators can either precede or follow their operand. True or false?

10. Match the following terms to the definitions given below.
    a. Unary operator
    b. Binary operator
    c. Type coercion
    d. Type casting
    e. Mixed type expression
    f. Argument list

g. Void function

  i. A computation involving both floating-point and integer values.
  ii. An operator with two operands.
  iii. A function that is called as a separate statement.
  iv. Explicitly changing a value of one type into another.
  v. The values that appear between the parentheses in a function call.
  vi. An operator with just one operand.
  vii. Implicitly changing a value of one type into another.
11. The statement

```
count = count + 1;
```

is equivalent to what C++ operator?
12. How do you write a C++ cast operation?
13. Is `main` a value-returning or a void function?
14. Show precisely what the following statement outputs.

```
cout << setw(6) << showpoint << setprecision(2) << 215.0;
```

15. The prefix and postfix forms of the increment operator (++) always behave the same way. We can use them interchangeably anywhere in C++ code. True or false? Explain your answer.
16. What data type do we use to declare a variable to hold the result of applying the `length` function to a string?
17. Given that the `string` variables `str1` and `str2` contain

```
"you ought to start with logic"
```

and

```
"ou"
```

respectively, what is the result of each of the following expressions?
a. `str1.length()`
b. `str1.find(str2)`
c. `str1.substr(4, 25)`
d. `str1.substr(4, 25).find(str2)`
e. `str1.substr.(str1.find("logic"), 3)`
f. `str1.substr(24, 5).find(str2.substr(0,1))`
g. `str1.find("end")`
18. What does the manipulator `fixed` do?

Programming Warm-Up Exercises

1. Write an expression to convert a time stored in the `int` variables `hours`, `minutes`, and `seconds` into the number of seconds represented by the time. For example, if `hours` contains 2, `minutes` contains 20, and `seconds` contains 12, then the result of your expression should be 8412.

2. Given an int variable days that contains a number of days,
   a. Write an expression that gives the number of whole weeks corresponding to days. For example, if days contains 23, then the number of whole weeks is 3.
   b. Write an expression that gives the number of days remaining after taking the whole weeks out of the value in days. For example, if days contains 23, then the number of days remaining after 3 whole weeks is 2.
3. Given int variables called dollars, quarters, dimes, nickels, and pennies, write an expression that computes the total amount of the money represented in the variables. The result should be an integer value representing the number of pennies in the total.
4. Given the same variables as in Exercise 3, compute the total but store it in a floating-point variable so that the integral part is dollars and the fractional part is cents.
5. Write an assignment statement that adds 3 to the value in int variable count.
6. Write expressions that implement the following formulas.
   a. $3X + Y$
   b. $A^2 + 2B + C$
   c. $\left(\dfrac{A + B}{C - D}\right) \times \left(\dfrac{X}{Y}\right)$
   d. $\dfrac{\left(\dfrac{A^2 + 2B + C}{D}\right)}{XY}$
   e. $\sqrt{|A - B|}$
   f. $X^{-\cos(Y)}$
7. Write a series of assignment statements that find the first three positions of the string "and" in a string variable sentence. The positions should be stored in int variables called first, second, and third. You may declare additional variables if necessary. The contents of sentence should remain unchanged.
8. Write an assignment statement to find the first blank in a string variable called name. Store the result plus one in the int variable startOfMiddle.
9. Write an output statement that prints the value in float variable money in eight spaces on the line, with a leading $ sign, and two digits of decimal precision.
10. Write an output statement that prints the value in double variable distance in fifteen spaces on a line with five digits of decimal precision.
11. If you include the header file climits in a program, the constants INT_MAX and INT_MIN are provided, which give the highest and lowest int values that can be represented. Write the include statement for this file, and an output statement that displays the two values, identified with appropriate labels.
12. Complete the following C++ program. The program should compute and output the Celsius value corresponding to the given Fahrenheit value.

```
//************************************************
// Celsius program
// This program outputs the Celsius temperature
// corresponding to a given Fahrenheit temperature
//************************************************

#include <iostream>

using namespace std;

int main()
{
    const float fahrenheit = 72.0;
```

Programming Problems

1. Write a C++ program that computes and outputs the volume of a cone, given the diameter of its base and its height. The formula for computing the cone's volume is:

$$\frac{1}{3}\pi \times Radius^2 \times Height$$

Be sure to use proper formatting and appropriate comments in your code. The output should be clearly labeled.

2. Write a C++ program that computes the mean and standard deviation of a set of four integer values. The mean is the sum of the four values divided by 4, and the formula for the standard deviation is:

$$s = \sqrt{\frac{\sum_{i=1}^{n}(x_i - \bar{x})^2}{n-1}}$$

Where $n = 4$, x_i refers to each of the four values, and $\bar{x}$ is the mean. Note that although the individual values are integers, the results are floating-point values. Be sure to use proper formatting and appropriate comments in your code. The output should be clearly labeled and neatly formatted.

3. The factorial of a number n (written $n!$) is the number times the factorial of itself minus one. This self-referential definition is easiest to understand through an example. The factorial of 2 is 2 * 1. The factorial of 3 is 3 * 2 * 1. The factorial of 4 is 4 * 3 * 2 * 1, and so on. Factorials grow very large, very quickly. An approximation to the factorial for larger values is given by Stirling's formula, which is:

$$n! = e^{-n}n^n\sqrt{2\pi n}$$

The exp function in the <cmath> header file gives the value of e raised to given power (see Appendix C.5). We've already discussed all of the other functions that are needed to write this formula. Write a C++ program that computes the factorial of 15 both directly and with Stirling's formula, and outputs both results, together with their difference. You will need to use the `double` type for this computation. Be sure to use proper formatting and appropriate comments in your code. The output should be clearly labeled and neatly formatted.

4. The number of permutations of a set of *n* items take *r* at a time is given by the formula:

$$\frac{n!}{r!(n-r)!}$$

Where *n*! is the factorial of *n*. (See Programming Problem 3 for a discussion of ways to compute the factorial.) If there are 18 people in your class and you want to divide the class into programming teams of 3 members, you can compute the number of different teams that can be arranged using the above formula. Write a C++ program that determines the number of potential team arrangements. You will need to use the double type for this computation. Be sure to use proper formatting and appropriate comments in your code. The output should be labeled clearly and formatted neatly.

5. Write a C++ program that takes a string containing a full name, and outputs each part of the name separately. The name should be in the form of first, middle, and last name separated from each other by a single space. For example, if the name string contains

   `"John Jacob Schmidt"`

   then the program would output:

   ```
   First name: John
   Middle name: Jacob
   Last name: Schmidt
   ```

6. Extend Programming Problem 5 to output the length of each name. This problem can be solved using a combination of the string operations presented in this chapter. Be sure to use proper formatting and appropriate comments in your code. The output should be clearly labeled and neatly formatted.

Case Study Follow-Up

1. Change the output statements so that the interest rate prints to 4 decimal places, but the dollar amounts remain at 2 decimal places.
2. The program assumes that the number of years left on the old mortgage is an even multiple of 12. Change the program so that the constant is the number of months left, not the number of years.
3. We usually speak of interest rates as percentages. Rewrite the program so that the interest rate is set as a percentage; that is, 5.24 rather than 0.0524.
4. The calculation of `monthlyInterest + 1` is made twice. Rewrite the program making this calculation only once. In your judgment, which version of the program is better? Justify your answer.

Program Input and the Software Design Process

Knowledge Goals

- *To understand the value of appropriate prompting messages for interactive programs.*
- *To know when noninteractive input/output is appropriate and how it differs from interactive input/output.*
- *To understand the basic principles of object-oriented design.*

Skill Goals

To be able to:

- *Construct input statements to read values into a program.*
- *Determine the contents of variables assigned values by input statements.*
- *Write programs that use data files for input and output.*
- *Apply the functional decomposition methodology to solve a simple problem.*
- *Take a functional decomposition and code it in C++, using self-documenting code.*

A program needs data on which to operate. We have been writing all of the data values in the program itself, in literal and named constants. If this were the only way we could enter data, we would have to rewrite a program each time we wanted to apply it to a different set of values. In this chapter, we look at ways of entering data into a program while it is running.

Once we know how to input data, process the data, and output the results, we can begin to think about designing more complicated programs. We have talked about general problem-solving strategies and writing simple programs. For a simple problem, it's easy to choose a strategy, write the algorithm, and code the program. But as problems become more complex, we have to use a more organized approach. In the second part of this chapter, we look at two general methodologies for developing software: object-oriented design and functional decomposition.

4.1 Getting Data into Programs

One of the biggest advantages of computers is that a program can be used with many different sets of data. To do so, we must keep the data separate from the program until the program is executed. Then instructions in the program copy values from the data set into variables in the program. After storing these values into the variables, the program can perform calculations with them (see Figure 4–1).

The process of placing values from an outside data set into variables in a program is called *input*. In widely used terminology, the computer is said to *read* outside data into the variables. The data for the program can come from an input device or from a file on an auxiliary storage device. We look at file input later in this chapter; here we consider the *standard input device*, the keyboard.

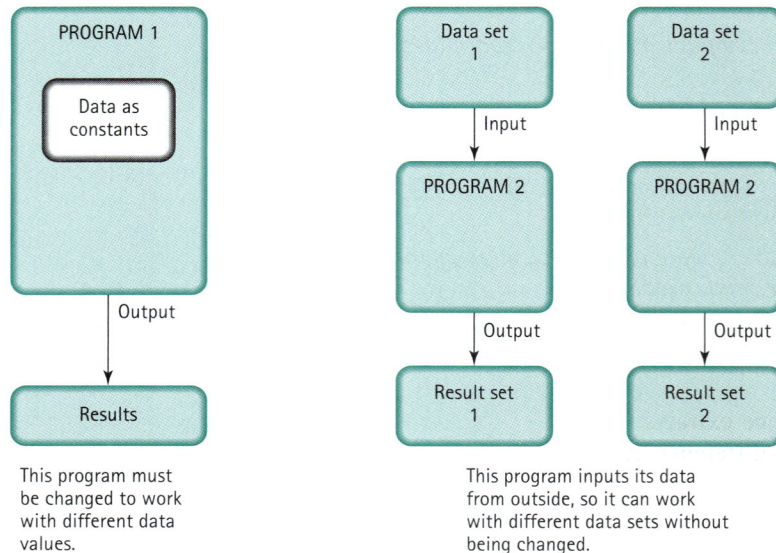

This program must be changed to work with different data values.

This program inputs its data from outside, so it can work with different data sets without being changed.

Figure 4–1 *Separating the Data from the Program*

Input Streams and the Extraction Operator (>>)

The concept of a stream is fundamental to input and output in C++. As we stated in Chapter 3, you can think of an output stream as an endless sequence of characters going from your program to an output device. Likewise, think of an *input stream* as an endless sequence of characters coming into your program from an input device.

To use stream I/O, you must use the preprocessor directive

```
#include <iostream>
```

The header file iostream contains, among other things, the definitions of two data types: istream and ostream. These are data types representing input streams and output streams, respectively. The header file also contains declarations that look like this:

```
istream cin;
ostream cout;
```

The first declaration says that cin (pronounced "see-in") is a variable of type istream. The second says that cout (pronounced "see-out") is a variable of type ostream. Furthermore, cin is associated with the standard input device (the keyboard), and cout is associated with the standard output device (usually the display screen).

As you have already seen, you can output values to cout by using the insertion operator (<<), which is sometimes pronounced "put to":

```
cout << 3 * price;
```

In a similar fashion, you can input data from cin by using the *extraction operator* (>>), sometimes pronounced "get from":

```
cin >> cost;
```

When the computer executes this statement, it inputs the next number you type on the keyboard (425, for example) and stores it into the variable cost.

The extraction operator >> takes two operands. Its left-hand operand is a stream expression (in the simplest case, just the variable cin). Its right-hand operand is a variable into which we store the input data. For the time being, we assume the variable is of a simple type (char, int, float, and so forth). Later in the chapter we discuss the input of string data.

You can use the >> operator several times in a single input statement. Each occurrence extracts (inputs) the next data item from the input stream. For example, there is no difference between the statement

```
cin >> length >> width;
```

and the pair of statements

```
cin >> length;
cin >> width;
```

Using a sequence of extractions in one statement is a convenience for the programmer.

When you are new to C++, you may get the extraction operator (>>) and the insertion operator (<<) reversed. Here is an easy way to remember which one is which: Always begin the statement with either `cin` or `cout`, and use the operator that points in the direction in which the data is going. The statement

```
cout << someInt;
```

sends data from the variable `someInt` *to* the output stream. The statement

```
cin >> someInt;
```

sends data from the input stream *to* the variable `someInt`.

Here's the syntax template for an input statement:

InputStatement

```
cin >> Variable >> Variable  . . . ;
```

Unlike the items specified in an output statement, which can be constants, variables, or complicated expressions, the items specified in an input statement can *only* be variable names. Why? Because an input statement indicates where input data values should be stored. Only variable names refer to memory locations where we can store values while a program is running.

When you enter input data at the keyboard, you must be sure that each data value is appropriate for the data type of the variable in the input statement.

Data Type of Variable in an >> Operation	Valid Input Data
char	A single printable character other than a blank
int	An int literal constant, optionally preceded by a sign
float	An int or float literal constant (possibly in scientific, E, notation), optionally preceded by a sign

Notice that when you input a number into a `float` variable, the input value doesn't have to have a decimal point. The integer value is automatically coerced to a `float` value. Any other mismatches, such as trying to input a `float` value into an `int` variable or a `char` value into a `float` variable, can lead to unexpected and sometimes serious results. Later in this chapter we discuss what might happen.

When looking for the next input value in the stream, the `>>` operator skips any leading *whitespace characters*. Whitespace characters are blanks and certain nonprintable characters such as the character that marks the end of a line. (We talk about this end-of-line character in the next section.) After skipping any whitespace characters, the `>>` operator proceeds to extract the desired data value from the input stream. If this data value is a `char` value, input stops as soon as a single character is input. If the data value is `int` or `float`, input of the number stops at the first character that is inappropriate for the data type, such as a whitespace character. Here are some examples, where i, j, and k are `int` variables, ch is a `char` variable, and x is a `float` variable:

Statement	Data	Contents After Input
1. `cin >> i;`	32	i = 32
2. `cin >> i >> j;`	4 60	i = 4, j = 60
3. `cin >> i >> ch >> x;`	25 A 16.9	i = 25, ch = 'A', x = 16.9
4. `cin >> i >> ch >> x;`	25	
	A	
	16.9	i = 25, ch = 'A', x = 16.9
5. `cin >> i >> ch >> x;`	25A16.9	i = 25, ch = 'A', x = 16.9
6. `cin >> i >> j >> x;`	12 8	i = 12, j = 8
		(Computer waits for a third number)
7. `cin >> i >> x;`	46 32.4 15	i = 46, x = 32.4
		(15 is held for later input)

Examples (1) and (2) are straightforward examples of integer input. Example (3) shows that you do not use quotes around character data values when they are input (quotes around character constants are needed in a program, though, to distinguish them from identifiers). Example (4) demonstrates how the process of skipping whitespace characters includes going on to the next line of input if necessary. Example (5) shows that the first character encountered that is inappropriate for a numeric data type ends the number. Input for the variable i stops at the input character A, after which the A is stored into ch, and then input for x stops at the end of the input line. Example (6) shows that if you are at the keyboard and haven't entered enough values to satisfy the input statement, the computer waits (and waits and waits …) for more data. Example (7) shows that if more values are entered than there are variables in the input statement, the extra values remain waiting in the input stream until they can be read by the next input statement. If there are extra values left when the program ends, the computer disregards them.

The Reading Marker and the Newline Character

To help explain stream input in more detail, we introduce the concept of the *reading marker*. The reading marker works like a bookmark, but instead of marking a place in a book, it keeps track of the point in the input stream where the computer should continue reading. The reading marker indicates the next character waiting to be read. The extraction operator >> leaves the reading marker on the character following the last piece of data that was input.

Each input line has an invisible end-of-line character (the *newline character*) that tells the computer where one line ends and the next begins. To find the next input value, the >> operator crosses line boundaries (newline characters) if it has to.

Where does the newline character come from? What is it? The answer to the first question is easy. When you are working at a keyboard, you generate a newline character yourself each time you hit the Return or Enter key. Your program also generates a newline character when it uses the endl manipulator in an output statement. The endl manipulator outputs a newline, telling the screen cursor to go to the next line. The answer to the second question varies from computer system to computer system. The newline character is a nonprintable control character that the system recognizes as meaning the end of a line, whether it's an input line or an output line.

In a C++ program, you can refer directly to the newline character by using the two symbols \n, a backslash and an n with no space between them. Although \n consists of two symbols, it refers to a single character—the newline character. Just as you can store the letter *A* into a char variable ch like this:

```
ch = 'A';
```

so you can store the newline character into a variable:

```
ch = '\n';
```

You also can put the newline character into a string, just as you can any printable character:

```
cout << "Hello\n";
```

This last statement has exactly the same effect as the statement

```
cout << "Hello" << endl;
```

But back to our discussion of input. Let's look at some examples using the reading marker and the newline character. In the following table, i is an int variable, ch is a char variable, and x is a float variable. The input statements produce the results shown. The part of the input stream printed in color is what has been extracted by input statements. The reading marker, denoted by the shaded block, indicates the next character waiting to be read. The \n denotes the newline character produced by striking the Return or Enter key.

Statements	Contents After Input	Marker Position in the Input Stream
1.		25 A 16.9\n
cin >> i;	i = 25	25 A 16.9\n
cin >> ch;	ch = 'A'	25 A 16.9\n
cin >> x;	x = 16.9	25 A 16.9\n
2.		25\n
		A\n
		16.9\n
cin >> i;	i = 25	25 \n
		A\n
		16.9\n
cin >> ch;	ch = 'A'	25\n
		A\n
		16.9\n
cin >> x;	x = 16.9	25\n
		A\n
		16.9\n
3.		25A16.9\n
cin >> i;	i = 25	25A16.9\n
cin >> ch;	ch = 'A'	25A16.9\n
cin >> x;	x = 16.9	25A16.9\n

Reading Character Data with the get Function

As we have discussed, the >> operator skips any leading whitespace characters (such as blanks and newline characters) while looking for the next data value in the input stream. Suppose that ch1 and ch2 are char variables and the program executes the statement

```
cin >> ch1 >> ch2;
```

If the input stream consists of

```
R 1
```

then the extraction operator stores 'R' into ch1, skips the blank, and stores '1' into ch2. (Note that the char value '1' is not the same as the int value 1. The two are stored completely differently in a computer's memory. The extraction operator interprets the same data in different ways, depending on the data type of the variable that's being filled.)

What if we had wanted to input *three* characters from the input line: the *R*, the blank, and the 1? With the extraction operator, it's not possible. Whitespace characters such as blanks are skipped over.

The `istream` data type provides a second way in which to read character data, in addition to the >> operator. You can use the `get` function, which inputs the very next character in the input stream without skipping any whitespace characters. A function call looks like this:

```
cin.get(someChar);
```

The `get` function is associated with the `istream` data type, and you must use dot notation to make a function call. (Recall that we used dot notation in Chapter 3 to invoke certain functions associated with the `string` type. Later in this chapter we explain the reason for dot notation.) To use the `get` function, you give the name of an `istream` variable (here, `cin`), then a dot (period), and then the function name and argument list. Notice that the call to `get` uses the syntax for calling a void function, not a value-returning function. The function call is a complete statement; it is not part of a larger expression.

The effect of the above function call is to input the next character waiting in the stream—even if it is a whitespace character like a blank—and store it into the variable `someChar`. The argument to the `get` function *must* be a variable, not a constant or arbitrary expression; we must tell the function where we want it to store the input character.

Using the `get` function, we now can input all three characters of the input line

```
R 1
```

We can use three consecutive calls to the `get` function:

```
cin.get(ch1);
cin.get(ch2);
cin.get(ch3);
```

or we can do it this way:

```
cin >> ch1;
cin.get(ch2);
cin >> ch3;
```

The first version is probably a bit clearer for someone to read and understand.

Here are some more examples of character input using both the >> operator and the `get` function. `ch1`, `ch2`, and `ch3` are all `char` variables. As before, \n denotes the newline character.

Statements	Contents After Input	Marker Position in the Input Stream
1.		A B\n CD\n
`cin >> ch1;`	ch1 = 'A'	A▮B\n CD\n
`cin >> ch2;`	ch2 = 'B'	A B▮\n CD\n
`cin >> ch3;`	ch3 = 'C'	A B\n CD▮\n
2.		A B\n CD\n
`cin.get(ch1);`	ch1 = 'A'	A▮B\n CD\n
`cin.get(ch2);`	ch2 = ' '	A B▮\n CD\n
`cin.get(ch3);`	ch3 = 'B'	A B▮\n CD\n
3.		A B\n CD\n
`cin >> ch1;`	ch1 = 'A'	A▮B\n CD\n
`cin >> ch2;`	ch2 = 'B'	A B▮\n CD\n
`cin.get(ch3);`	ch3 = '\n'	A B\n CD▮\n

Theoretical Foundations

More About Functions and Arguments

When your `main` function tells the computer to go off and follow the instructions in another function, `SomeFunc`, the `main` function is *calling* `SomeFunc`. In the call to `SomeFunc`, the arguments in the argument list are *passed* to the function. When `SomeFunc` finishes, the computer *returns* to the `main` function.

With some functions you have seen, like `sqrt` and `abs`, you can pass constants, variables, and arbitrary expressions to the function. The `get` function for reading character data, however, accepts only a variable as an argument. The `get` function stores a value into its argument when it returns, and only variables can have values stored into them while a program is running. Even though `get` is called as a void function—not a value-returning function—it *returns* or *passes back* a value through its argument list. The point to remember is that you can use arguments both to send data into a function and to get results back out.

Skipping Characters with the `ignore` Function

Most of us have a specialized tool lying in a kitchen drawer or in a toolbox. It gathers dust and cobwebs because we almost never use it. But when we suddenly need it, we're glad we have it. The `ignore` function associated with the `istream` type is like this specialized tool. You rarely have occasion to use `ignore`; but when you need it, you're glad it's available.

The `ignore` function is used to skip (read and discard) characters in the input stream. It is a function with two arguments, called like this:

```
cin.ignore(200, '\n');
```

The first argument is an `int` expression; the second, a `char` value. This particular function call tells the computer to skip the next 200 input characters *or* to skip characters until a newline character is read, whichever comes first.

Here are some examples that use a `char` variable `ch` and three `int` variables, `i`, `j`, and `k`:

Statements	Contents After Input	Marker Position in the Input Stream
1.		957 34 1235\n 128 96\n
`cin >> i >> j;`	i = 957, j = 34	957 34 1235\n 128 96\n
`cin.ignore(100, '\n');`		957 34 1235\n 128 96\n
`cin >> k;`	k = 128	957 34 1235\n 128 96\n

2.
`cin >> ch;`
`cin.ignore(100, 'B');`
`cin >> i;`
	ch = 'A'
	
	i = 16
		A 22 B 16 C 19\n
		A 22 B 16 C 19\n
		A 22 B 16 C 19\n
		A 22 B 16 C 19\n

3.
`cin.ignore(2, '\n');`
`cin >> ch;`
	
	ch = 'C'
		ABCDEF\n
		ABCDEF\n
		ABCDEF\n

Example (1) shows the most common use of the `ignore` function, which is to skip the rest of the data on the current input line. Example (2) demonstrates the use of a character other than '\n' as the second argument. We skip over all input characters until a *B* has been found, then read the next input number into `i`. In both (1) and (2), we are focusing on the second argument to the `ignore` function, and we arbitrarily choose any large number, such as 100, for the first argument. In (3), we change our focus and concentrate on the first argument. Our intention is to skip the next two input characters on the current line.

Reading String Data

To input a character string into a `string` variable, we have two options. The first is to use the extraction operator (>>). When reading input characters into a `string` variable, the >> operator skips any leading whitespace characters such as blanks and newlines. It then reads successive characters into the variable, stopping at the first *trailing* whitespace character (which is not consumed, but remains as the first character waiting in the input stream). For example, assume we have the following code:

```
string firstName;
string lastName;

cin >> firstName >> lastName;
```

If the input stream initially looks like this (where ☐ denotes a blank):

```
☐☐Mary☐Smith☐☐☐18
```

then our input statement stores the four characters `Mary` into `firstName`, stores the five characters `Smith` into `lastName`, and leaves the input stream as

```
☐☐☐18
```

Although the >> operator is widely used for string input, it has a potential drawback: it cannot be used to input a string that has blanks within it. (Remember that it stops reading as soon as it encounters a whitespace character.) This fact leads us to the second option for performing string input: the `getline` function. A call to this function looks like this:

```
getline(cin, myString);
```

The function call, which does not use dot notation, requires two arguments. The first is an input stream variable (here, `cin`) and the second is a `string` variable. The `getline` function does not skip leading whitespace characters and continues until it reaches the newline character `'\n'`. That is, `getline` reads and stores an entire input line, embedded blanks and all. Note that with `getline`, the newline character is consumed (but is not stored into the string variable). Given the code segment

```
string inputStr;

getline(cin, inputStr);
```

and the input line

␣␣Mary␣Smith␣␣␣18

the result of the call to `getline` is that all 17 characters on the input line (including blanks) are stored into `inputStr`, and the reading marker is positioned at the beginning of the next input line.

The following table summarizes the differences between the `>>` operator and the `getline` function when reading string data into `string` variables.

Statement	Skips Leading Whitespace?	Stops Reading When?
`cin >> inputStr;`	Yes	When a trailing whitespace character is encountered (which is *not* consumed)
`getline(cin, inputStr);`	No	When '\n' is encountered (which *is* consumed)

4.2 Interactive Input/Output

In Chapter 1, we defined an interactive program as one in which the user communicates directly with the computer. Many of the programs that we write are interactive. There is a certain "etiquette" involved in writing interactive programs that has to do with instructions for the user to follow.

To get data into an interactive program, we begin with *input prompts*, printed messages that explain what the user should enter. Without these messages, the user has no idea what data values to type. In many cases, a program also should print out all of the data values typed in so that the user can verify that they were entered correctly. Printing out the input values is called *echo printing*. Here's a program showing the proper use of prompts:

```
//***************************************************************
// Prompts program
// This program demonstrates the use of input prompts
//***************************************************************
#include <iostream>
#include <iomanip>      // For setprecision()

using namespace std;

int main()
```

```
{
    int    partNumber;
    int    quantity;
    float unitPrice;
    float totalPrice;

    cout << fixed << showpoint              // Set up floating-pt.
         << setprecision(2);                //    output format

    cout << "Enter the part number:" << endl;         // Prompt
    cin >> partNumber;

    cout << "Enter the quantity of this part ordered:" // Prompt
         << endl;
    cin >> quantity;

    cout << "Enter the unit price for this part:"      // Prompt
         << endl;
    cin >> unitPrice;

    totalPrice = quantity * unitPrice;
    cout << "Part " << partNumber                      // Echo print
         << ", quantity " << quantity
         << ", at $ " << unitPrice << " each" << endl;
    cout << "totals $ " << totalPrice << endl;
    return 0;
}
```

Here is the program's output, with the user's input shown in color:

```
Enter the part number:
4671
Enter the quantity of this part ordered:
10
Enter the unit price for this part:
27.25
Part 4671, quantity 10, at $ 27.25 each
totals $ 272.50
```

The amount of information you should put into your prompts depends on who is going to be using a program. If you are writing a program for people who are not famil-iar with computers, your messages should be more detailed. For example, "Type a four-digit part number, then press the key marked Enter." If the program is going to be used frequently by the same people, you might shorten the prompts: "Enter PN" and "Enter

Qty." If the program is for very experienced users, you can prompt for several values at once and have them type all of the values on one input line:

```
Enter PN, Qty, Unit Price:
4176 10 27.25
```

In programs that use large amounts of data, this method saves the user keystrokes and time. However, it also makes it easier for the user to enter values in the wrong order. In such situations, echo printing the data is especially important.

Whether a program should echo print its input or not also depends on how experienced the users are and on the task the program is to perform. If the users are experienced and the prompts are clear, as in the first example, then echo printing is probably not required. If the users are novices or multiple values can be input at once, echo printing should be used. If the program inputs a large quantity of data and the users are experienced, rather than echo print the data, it may be stored in a separate file that can be checked after all of the data is input. We discuss how to store data into a file later in this chapter.

Prompts are not the only way in which programs interact with users. It can be helpful to have a program print out some general instructions at the beginning ("Press Enter after typing each data value. Enter a negative number when done."). When data is not entered in the correct form, a message that indicates the problem should be printed. For users who haven't worked much with computers, it's important that these messages be informative and "friendly." The message

```
ILLEGAL DATA VALUES!!!!!!!
```

is likely to upset an inexperienced user. Moreover, it doesn't offer any constructive information. A much better message would be

```
That is not a valid part number.
Part numbers must be no more than four digits long.
Please reenter the number in its proper form:
```

In Chapter 5, we introduce the statements that allow us to test for erroneous data.

4.3 Noninteractive Input/Output

Although we tend to use examples of interactive I/O in this text, many programs are written using noninteractive I/O. A common example of noninteractive I/O on large computer systems is batch processing (see Chapter 1). Remember that in batch processing, the user and the computer do not interact while the program is running. This method is most effective when a program is going to input or output large amounts of data. An example of batch processing is a program that inputs a file containing semester grades for thousands of students and prints grade reports to be mailed out.

When a program must read in many data values, the usual practice is to prepare them ahead of time, storing them into a disk file. This allows the user to go back and make changes or corrections to the data as necessary before running the program. When a program is designed to print lots of data, the output can be sent directly to a high-speed printer or another disk file. After the program has been run, the user can examine the data at leisure. In the next section, we discuss input and output with disk files.

Programs designed for noninteractive I/O do not print prompting messages for input. It is a good idea, however, to echo print each data value that is read. Echo printing allows the person reading the output to verify that the input values were prepared correctly. Because noninteractive programs tend to print large amounts of data, their output often is in the form of a table—columns with descriptive headings.

Most C++ programs are written for interactive use. But the flexibility of the language allows you to write noninteractive programs as well. The biggest difference is in the input/output requirements. Noninteractive programs are generally more rigid about the organization and format of the input and output data.

4.4   File Input and Output

In everything we've done so far, we've assumed that the input to our programs comes from the keyboard and that the output from our programs goes to the screen. We look now at input/output to and from files.

Files

Earlier we defined a file as a named area in secondary storage that holds a collection of information (for example, the program code we have typed into the editor). The information in a file usually is stored on an auxiliary storage device, such as a disk. Our programs can read data from a file in the same way they read data from the keyboard, and they can write output to a disk file in the same way they write output to the screen.

Why would we want a program to read data from a file instead of the keyboard? If a program is going to read a large quantity of data, it is easier to enter the data into a file with an editor than to enter it while the program is running. With the editor, we can go back and correct mistakes. Also, we do not have to enter the data all at once; we can take a break and come back later. And if we want to rerun the program, having the data stored in a file allows us to do so without retyping the data.

Why would we want the output from a program to be written to a disk file? The contents of a file can be displayed on a screen or printed. This gives us the option of looking at the output over and over again without having to rerun the program. Also, the output stored in a file can be read into another program as input.

Using Files

If we want a program to use file I/O, we have to do four things:

1. Request the preprocessor to include the header file `fstream`.
2. Use declaration statements to declare the file streams we are going to use.
3. Prepare each file for reading or writing by using a function named `open`.
4. Specify the name of the file stream in each input or output statement.

Including the Header File `fstream`   Suppose we want Chapter 3's Mortgage program (p. 130) to read data from a file and to write its output to a file. The first thing we must do is use the preprocessor directive

```
#include <fstream>
```

Through the header file `fstream`, the C++ standard library defines two data types, `ifstream` and `ofstream` (standing for *input file stream* and *output file stream*). Consistent with the general idea of streams in C++, the `ifstream` data type represents a stream of characters coming from an input file, and `ofstream` represents a stream of characters going to an output file.

All of the `istream` operations you have learned about—the extraction operator (`>>`), the `get` function, and the `ignore` function—are also valid for the `ifstream` type. And all of the `ostream` operations, such as the insertion operator (`<<`) and the `endl`, `setw`, and `setprecision` manipulators, apply also to the `ofstream` type. To these basic operations, the `ifstream` and `ofstream` types add some more operations designed specifically for file I/O.

Declaring File Streams   In a program, you declare stream variables the same way that you declare any variable—you specify the data type and then the variable name:

```
int       someInt;
float     someFloat;
ifstream  inFile;
ofstream  outFile;
```

(You don't have to declare the stream variables `cin` and `cout`. The header file `iostream` already does this for you.)

For our Mortgage program, let's name the input and output file streams `inData` and `outData`. We declare them like this:

```
ifstream inData;      // Holds loan amount, interest, and length
ofstream outData;     // Holds input values and monthly payments
```

Note that the `ifstream` type is for input files only, and the `ofstream` type is for output files only. With these data types, you cannot read from and write to the same file.

Opening Files   The third thing we have to do is prepare each file for reading or writing, an act called *opening a file*. Opening a file causes the computer's operating system to perform certain actions that allow us to proceed with file I/O.

In our example, we want to read from the file stream `inData` and write to the file stream `outData`. We open the relevant files by using these statements:

```
inData.open("loan.in");
outData.open("loan.out");
```

Both of these statements are function calls (notice the telltale arguments—the mark of a function). In each function call, the argument is a literal string enclosed by quotes. The first statement is a call to a function named `open`, which is associated with the `ifstream` data type. The second is a call to another function (also named `open`) associated with the `ofstream` data type. As we have seen earlier, we use dot notation (as in `inData.open`) to call certain library functions that are tightly associated with data types.

Exactly what does an `open` function do? First, it associates a stream variable used in your program with a physical file on disk. Our first function call creates a connection between the stream variable `inData` and the actual disk file, named `loan.in`. (Names of file streams must be identifiers; they are variables in your program. But some computer systems do not use this syntax for file names on disk. For example, many systems allow or even require a dot within a file name.) Similarly, the second function call associates the stream variable `outData` with the disk file `loan.out`. Associating a program's name for a file (`outData`) with the actual name for the file (`loan.out`) is much the same as associating a program's name for the standard output device (`cout`) with the actual device (the screen).

The next thing the `open` function does depends on whether the file is an input file or an output file. With an input file, the `open` function sets the file's reading marker to the first piece of data in the file. (Each input file has its own reading marker.)

With an output file, the `open` function checks to see whether the file already exists. If the file doesn't exist, `open` creates a new, empty file for you. If the file already exists, `open` erases the old contents of the file. Then the writing marker is set at the beginning of the empty file (see Figure 4–2). As output proceeds, each successive output operation advances the writing marker to add data to the end of the file.

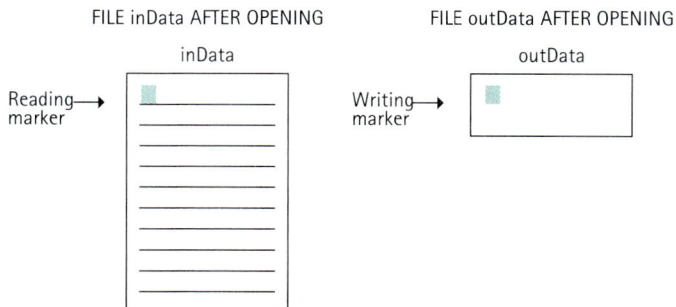

Figure 4–2   *The Effect of Opening a File*

Because the reason for opening files is to *prepare* the files for reading or writing, you must open the files before using any input or output statements that refer to the files. In a program, it's a good idea to open files right away to be sure that the files are prepared before the program attempts any file I/O.

```
    ⋮

int main()
{

    ⋮        } Declarations

    // Open the files

    inData.open("loan.in");
    outData.open("loan.out");
       ⋮

}
```

In addition to the `open` function, the `ifstream` and `ofstream` types have a `close` function associated with each. This function has no arguments and may be used as follows.

```
ifstream inFile;

inFile.open("mydata.dat");    // Open the file
   ⋮                          // Read and process the file data
inFile.close();               // Close the file
   ⋮
```

Closing a file causes the operating system to perform certain wrap-up activities on the disk and to break the connection between the stream variable and the disk file.

Should you always call the `close` function when you're finished reading or writing a file? In some programming languages, it's extremely important that you remember to do so. In C++, however, a file is automatically closed when program control leaves the block (compound statement) in which the stream variable is declared. (Until we get to Chapter 7, this block is the body of the `main` function.) When control leaves this block, a special function associated with each of `ifstream` and `ofstream` called a *destructor* is implicitly executed, and this destructor function closes the file for you. Consequently, you don't often see C++ programs explicitly calling the `close` function. On the other hand, many programmers like to make it a regular habit to call the `close` function explicitly, and you may wish to do so yourself.

Specifying File Streams in Input/Output Statements   There is just one more thing we have to do in order to use files. As we said earlier, all `istream` operations also are valid for the `ifstream` type, and all `ostream` operations are valid for the `ofstream` type. So, to read from or write to a file, all we need to do in our input and output statements is substitute the appropriate file stream variable for `cin` or `cout`. In our Mortgage program, we would use a statement like

```
inData >> loanAmount >> yearlyInterest >> numberOfYears;
```

to instruct the computer to read data from the file `inData`. Similarly, all of the output statements that write to the file `outData` would specify `outData`, not `cout`, as the destination:

```
outData << fixed << setprecision(2) << "For a loan amount of "
        << loanAmount
        << " with an interest rate of " << setprecision(4)
        << yearlyInterest  << " and a "
        << numberOfYears << " year mortgage, " << endl;
outData << fixed << setprecision(2)
        << "your monthly payments are $" << payment
        << "." << endl;
```

What is nice about C++ stream I/O is that we have a uniform syntax for performing I/O operations, regardless of whether we're working with the keyboard and screen, with files, or with other I/O devices.

An Example Program Using Files

The reworked Mortgage program is shown below. Now it reads its input from the file `inData` and writes its output to the file `outData`. Compare this program with the original version on page 130 and notice that named constants have disappeared because the data are now input at execution time. Notice also that to set up the floating-point output format, the `fixed` and `setprecision` manipulators are applied to the `outData` stream variable, not to `cout`.

```
//****************************************************************
// Mortgage Payment Calculator program
// This program determines the monthly payments on a mortgage given
// the loan amount, the yearly interest rate, and the number of
// years.
//****************************************************************

#include <fstream>
#include <cmath>
#include <iomanip>

using namespace std;
```

```cpp
#include <fstream>
#include <cmath>
#include <iomanip>

using namespace std;

int main()
{

    // Input variables
    float loanAmount;
    float yearlyInterest;
    int numberOfYears;
    ofstream outData;
    ifstream inData;

    // Local variables
    float monthlyInterest;
    int numberOfPayments;
    float payment;

    inData.open("loan.in");
    outData.open("loan.out");

    // Read values from the file
    inData >> loanAmount >> yearlyInterest >> numberOfYears;

    // Calculate values
    monthlyInterest = yearlyInterest * 0.01 / 12;
    numberOfPayments = numberOfYears * 12;
    payment = (loanAmount
            * pow(1 + monthlyInterest, numberOfPayments)
            *  monthlyInterest)
            /(pow(1 + monthlyInterest, numberOfPayments) - 1 );

    // Output results
    outData << fixed << setprecision(2) << "For a loan amount of "
            << loanAmount
            << " with an interest rate of " << setprecision(4)
            << yearlyInterest  << " and a "
            << numberOfYears << " year mortgage, " << endl;
    outData << fixed << setprecision(2)
            << "your monthly payments are $" << payment
            << "." << endl;
```

```
    inData.close();
    outData.close();
    return 0;
}
```

Before running the program, you would use the editor to create and save a file `loan.in` to serve as input. The contents of the file might look like this:

```
50000.00 0.05 5
```

In writing the new Mortgage program, what happens if you mistakenly specify `cout` instead of `outData` in one of the output statements? Nothing disastrous; the output of that one statement merely goes to the screen instead of the output file. And what if, by mistake, you specify `cin` instead of `inData` in the input statement? The consequences are not as pleasant. When you run the program, the computer will appear to go dead (to *hang*). Here's the reason: Execution reaches the input statement and the computer waits for you to enter the data from the keyboard. But you don't know that the computer is waiting. There's no message on the screen prompting you for input, and you are assuming (wrongly) that the program is getting its input from a data file. So the computer waits, and you wait, and the computer waits, and you wait. Every programmer at one time or another has had the experience of thinking the computer has hung, when, in fact, it is working just fine, silently waiting for keyboard input.

Run-Time Input of File Names

Until now, our examples of opening a file for input have included code similar to the following:

```
ifstream inFile;

inFile.open("datafile.dat");
  ⋮
```

The `open` function associated with the `ifstream` data type requires an argument that specifies the name of the actual data file on disk. By using a literal string, as in the example above, the file name is fixed at compile time. Therefore, the program works only for this one particular disk file.

We often want to make a program more flexible by allowing the file name to be determined at *run time*. A common technique is to prompt the user for the name of the file, read the user's response into a variable, and pass the variable as an argument to the `open` function. In principle, the following code should accomplish what we want. Unfortunately, the compiler does not allow it.

```
ifstream inFile;
string    fileName;

cout << "Enter the input file name: ";
cin >> fileName;
inFile.open(fileName);                    // Compile-time error
```

The problem is that the open function does not expect an argument of type string. Instead, it expects a *C string*. A C string (so named because it originated in the C language, the forerunner of C++) is a limited form of string whose properties we discuss much later in the book. A literal string, such as "datafile.dat", happens to be a C string and thus is acceptable as an argument to the open function.

To make the above code work correctly, we need to convert a string variable to a C string. The string data type provides a value-returning function named c_str that is applied to a string variable as follows:

```
fileName.c_str()
```

This function returns the C string that is equivalent to the one contained in the fileName variable. (The original string contained in fileName is not changed by the function call.) The primary purpose of the c_str function is to allow programmers to call library functions that expect C strings, not string strings, as arguments.

Using the c_str function, we can code the run-time input of a file name as follows:

```
ifstream inFile;
string    fileName;

cout << "Enter the input file name: ";
cin >> fileName;
inFile.open(fileName.c_str());
```

4.5 Input Failure

When a program inputs data from the keyboard or an input file, things can go wrong. Let's suppose that we're executing a program. It prompts us to enter an integer value, but we absentmindedly type some letters of the alphabet. The input operation fails because of the invalid data. In C++ terminology, the cin stream has entered the *fail state*. Once a stream has entered the fail state, any further I/O operations using that stream are considered to be null operations—that is, they have no effect at all. Unfortunately for us, *the computer does not halt the program or give any error message.* The computer just continues executing the program, silently ignoring each additional attempt to use that stream.

Invalid data is the most common reason for input failure. When your program inputs an `int` value, it is expecting to find only digits in the input stream, possibly preceded by a plus or minus sign. If there is a decimal point somewhere within the digits, does the input operation fail? Not necessarily; it depends on where the reading marker is. Let's look at an example.

Assume that a program has `int` variables `i`, `j`, and `k`, whose contents are currently 10, 20, and 30, respectively. The program now executes the following two statements:

```
cin >> i >> j >> k;
cout << "i: " << i << "   j: " << j << "   k: " << k;
```

If we type these characters for the input data:

```
1234.56 7 89
```

then the program produces this output:

```
i: 1234   j: 20   k: 30
```

Let's see why.

Remember that when reading `int` or `float` data, the extraction operator `>>` stops reading at the first character that is inappropriate for the data type (whitespace or otherwise). In our example, the input operation for `i` succeeds. The computer extracts the first four characters from the input stream and stores the integer value 1234 into `i`. The reading marker is now on the decimal point:

```
1234.56 7 89
```

The next input operation (for `j`) fails; an `int` value cannot begin with a decimal point. The `cin` stream is now in the fail state, and the current value of `j` (20) remains unchanged. The third input operation (for `k`) is ignored, as are all the rest of the statements in our program that read from `cin`.

Another way to make a stream enter the fail state is to try to open an input file that doesn't exist. Suppose that you have a data file on your disk named `myfile.dat`. In your program you have the following statements:

```
ifstream inFile;

inFile.open("myfil.dat");
inFile >> i >> j >> k;
```

In the call to the `open` function, you misspelled the name of your disk file. At run time, the attempt to open the file fails, so the stream `inFile` enters the fail state. The next three input operations (for `i`, `j`, and `k`) are null operations. Without issuing any error message, the program proceeds to use the (unknown) contents of `i`, `j`, and `k` in calculations. The results of these calculations are certain to be puzzling.

The point of this discussion is not to make you nervous about I/O but to make you aware. The Testing and Debugging section at the end of this chapter offers suggestions for avoiding input failure, and Chapters 5 and 6 introduce program statements that let you test the state of a stream.

4.6 Software Design Methodologies

Over the last two chapters and the first part of this one, we have introduced elements of the C++ language that let us input data, perform calculations, and output results. The programs we wrote were short and straightforward because the problems to be solved were simple. We are ready to write programs for more complicated problems, but first we need to step back and look at the overall process of programming.

As you learned in Chapter 1, the programming process consists of a problem-solving phase and an implementation phase. The problem-solving phase includes *analysis* (analyzing and understanding the problem to be solved) and *design* (designing a solution to the problem). Given a complex problem—one that results in a 10,000-line program, for example—it's simply not reasonable to skip the design process and go directly to writing C++ code. What we need is a systematic way of designing a solution to a problem, no matter how complicated the problem is.

In the remainder of this chapter, we describe two important methodologies for designing solutions to more complex problems: *functional decomposition* and *object-oriented design*. These methodologies help you create solutions that can be easily implemented as C++ programs. The resulting programs are readable, understandable, and easy to debug and modify.

> **Object-oriented design** A technique for developing software in which the solution is expressed in terms of objects—self-contained entities composed of data and operations on that data.
>
> **Functional decomposition** A technique for developing software in which the problem is divided into more easily handled subproblems, the solutions of which create a solution to the overall problem.

One software design methodology that is in widespread use is known as **object-oriented design** (OOD). C++ evolved from the C language primarily to facilitate the use of the OOD methodology. In the next two sections, we present the essential concepts of OOD; we expand our treatment of the approach later in the book. OOD is often used in conjunction with the other methodology that we discuss in this chapter, **functional decomposition.**

OOD focuses on entities (*objects*) consisting of data and operations on the data. In OOD, we solve a problem by identifying the components that make up a solution and identifying how those components interact with each other through operations on the data that they contain. The result is a design for a set of objects that can be assembled to form a solution to a problem. In contrast, functional decomposition views the solution to a problem as a task to be accomplished. It focuses on the sequence of operations that are required to complete the task. When the problem requires a sequence of steps that is long or complex, we divide it into subproblems that are easier to solve.

The choice of which methodology we use depends on the problem at hand. For example, a large problem might involve several sequential phases of processing, such as gathering data and verifying its correctness with noninteractive processing, analyzing the data interactively, and printing reports noninteractively at the conclusion of the analysis. This process has a natural functional decomposition. Each of the phases, however, may best be solved by a set of objects that represent the data and the operations that can be applied to it. Some of the individual operations may be sufficiently complex that they require further decomposition, either into a sequence of operations or into another set of objects.

If you look at a problem and see that it is natural to think about it in terms of a collection of component parts, then you should use OOD to solve it. For example, a banking problem may require a `checkingAccount` object with associated operations `OpenAccount`, `WriteCheck`, `MakeDeposit`, and `IsOverdrawn`. The `checkingAccount` object consists of not only data (the account number and current balance, for example) but also these operations, all bound together into one unit.

On the other hand, if you find that it is natural to think of the solution to the problem as a series of steps, then you should use functional decomposition. For example, when computing some statistical measures on a large set of real numbers, it is natural to decompose the problem into a sequence of steps that read a value, perform calculations, and then repeat the sequence. The C++ language and the standard library supply all of the operations that we need, and we simply write a sequence of those operations to solve the problem.

4.7   What Are Objects?

Let's take a closer look at what objects are and how they work before we examine OOD further. We said earlier that an object is a collection of data together with associated operations. Several programming languages, called *object-oriented programming languages*, have been created specifically to support OOD. Examples are C++, Java, Smalltalk, CLOS, Eiffel, and Object-Pascal. In these languages, a *class* is a programmer-defined data type from which objects are created. Although we did not say it at the time, we have been using classes and objects to perform input and output in C++. `cin` is an object of a data type (class) named `istream`, and `cout` is an object of a class `ostream`. As we explained earlier, the header file `iostream` defines the classes `istream` and `ostream` and also declares `cin` and `cout` to be objects of those classes:

```
istream cin;
ostream cout;
```

Similarly, the header file `fstream` defines classes `ifstream` and `ofstream`, from which you can declare your own input file stream and output file stream objects.

Another example you have seen already is `string`—a programmer-defined class from which you create objects by using declarations such as

```
string lastName;
```

In Figure 4–3, we picture the `cin` and `lastName` objects as entities that have a private part and a public part. The private part includes data and functions that the user cannot access and doesn't need to know about in order to use the object. The public part, shown as ovals in the side of the object, represents the object's *interface*. The interface consists of operations that are available to programmers wishing to use the object. In C++, public operations are written as functions and are known as *member functions*. Except for operations using symbols such as `<<` and `>>`, a member function is invoked by giving the name of the class object, then a dot, and then the function name and argument list:

```
cin.ignore(100, '\n');
cin.get(someChar);
cin >> someInt;
len = lastName.length();
pos = lastName.find('A');
```

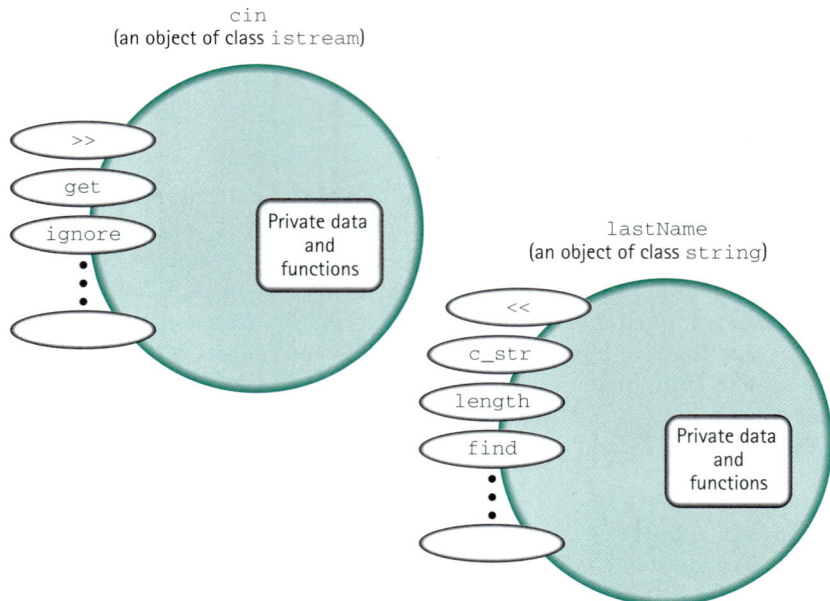

Figure 4–3   *Objects and Their Operations*

4.8   Object-Oriented Design

The first step in OOD is to identify the major objects in the problem, together with their associated operations. The final problem solution is ultimately expressed in terms of these objects and operations.

OOD leads to programs that are collections of objects. Each object is responsible for one part of the entire solution, and the objects communicate by accessing each other's member functions. There are many libraries of prewritten classes, including the C++ standard library, public libraries (called *freeware* or *shareware*), libraries that are sold commercially, and libraries that are developed by companies for their own use. In many cases, it is possible to browse through a library, choose classes you need for a problem, and assemble them to form a substantial portion of your program. Putting existing pieces together in this fashion is an excellent example of the building-block approach we discussed in Chapter 1.

When there isn't a suitable class available in a library, it is necessary to define a new class. We see how this is done in Chapter 11. The design of a new class begins with the specification of its interface. We must decide what operations are needed on the outside of the class to make its objects useful. Once the interface is defined, we can design the implementation of the class, including all of its private members.

One of the goals in designing an interface is to make it flexible so the new class can be used in unforeseen circumstances. For example, we may provide a member function that converts the value of an object into a string, even though we don't need this capability in our program. When the time comes to debug the program, it may be very useful to display values of this type as strings.

Useful features are often absent from an interface, sometimes due to lack of foresight and sometimes for the purpose of simplifying the design. It is quite common to discover a class in a library that is almost right for your purpose but is missing some key feature. OOD addresses this situation with a concept called *inheritance*, which allows you to adapt an existing class to meet your particular needs. You can use inheritance to add features to a class (or restrict the use of existing features) without having to inspect and modify its source code. Inheritance is considered such an integral part of object-oriented programming that a separate term, *object-based programming*, is used to describe programming with objects but not inheritance.

In Chapter 14, we see how to define classes that inherit members from existing classes. Together, OOD, class libraries, and inheritance can dramatically reduce the time and effort required to design, implement, and maintain large software systems.

To summarize the OOD process: We identify the major components of a problem solution and how they interact. We then look in the available libraries for classes that correspond to the components. When we find a class that is almost right, we can use inheritance to adapt it. When we can't find a class that corresponds to a component, we must design a new class. Our design specifies the interface for the class, and we then implement the interface with public and private members as necessary. OOD isn't always used in isolation. Functional decomposition may be used in designing member functions within a class or in coordinating the interactions of objects.

In this section, we have presented only an introduction to OOD. A more complete discussion requires knowledge of topics that we explore in Chapters 5 through 10: flow of control, programmer-written functions, and more about data types. In Chapters 11 through 13, we learn how to write our own classes, and we return to OOD in Chapter 14. Until then, our programs are relatively small, so we use object-based programming and functional decomposition to arrive at our problem solutions.

4.9 Functional Decomposition

The second design technique we use is functional decomposition (it's also called *structured design*, *top-down design*, *stepwise refinement*, and *modular programming*). In functional decomposition, we work from the abstract (a list of the major steps in our solution) to the particular (algorithmic steps that can be translated directly into C++ code). You can also think of this as working from a high-level solution, leaving the details of implementation unspecified, down to a fully detailed solution.

The easiest way to solve a problem is to give it to someone else and say, "Solve this problem." This is the most abstract level of a problem solution: a single-statement solution that encompasses the entire problem without specifying any of the details of implementation. It's at this point that we programmers are called in. Our job is to turn the abstract solution into a concrete solution, a program.

If the solution clearly involves a series of major steps, we break it down (decompose it) into pieces. In the process, we move to a lower level of abstraction—that is, some of the implementation details (but not too many) are now specified. Each of the major steps becomes an independent subproblem that we can work on separately. In a very large project, one person (the *chief architect or team leader*) formulates the subproblems and then gives them to other members of the programming team, saying, "Solve this problem." In the case of a small project, we give the subproblems to ourselves. Then we choose one subproblem at a time to solve. We may break the chosen subproblem into another series of steps that, in turn, become smaller subproblems. Or we may identify components that are naturally represented as objects. The process continues until each subproblem cannot be divided further or has an obvious solution.

Why do we work this way? Why not simply write out all of the details? Because it is much easier to focus on one problem at a time. For example, suppose you are working on part of a program to output certain values and discover that you need a complex formula to calculate an appropriate fieldwidth for printing one of the values. Calculating fieldwidths is not the purpose of this part of the program. If you shift your focus to the calculation, you are likely to forget some detail of the overall output process. What you do is write down an abstract step—"Calculate the fieldwidth required"—and go on with the problem at hand. Once you've written the major steps, you can go back to solving the step that does the calculation.

By subdividing the problem, you create a hierarchical structure called a *tree structure*. Each level of the tree is a complete solution to the problem that is less abstract (more detailed) than the level above it. Figure 4–4 shows a generic solution tree for a problem. Steps that are shaded have enough implementation details to be translated

Top   Abstract

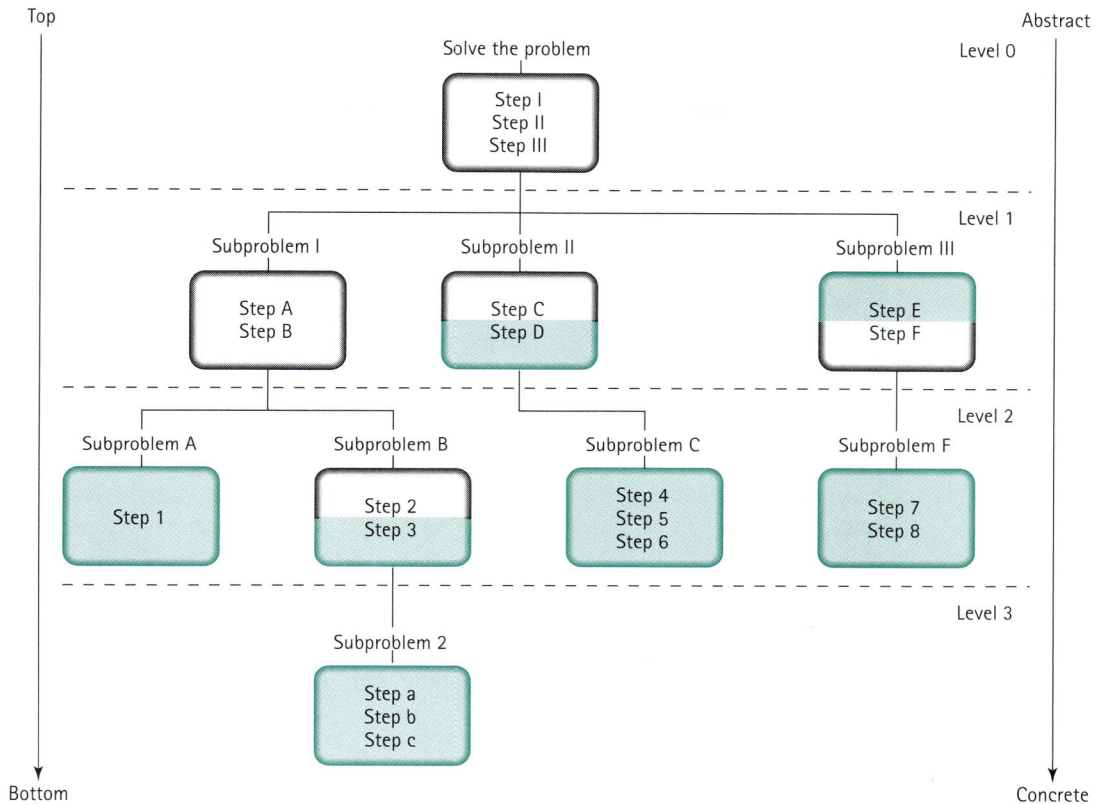

Figure 4–4   *Hierarchical Solution Tree*

directly into C++ statements. These are **concrete steps**. Those that are not shaded are **abstract steps**; they reappear as subproblems in the next level down. Each box in the figure represents a **module**. Modules are the basic building blocks in a functional decomposition. The diagram in Figure 4–4 is also called a *module structure chart*.

    Like OOD, functional decomposition uses the divide-and-conquer approach to problem solving. Both techniques break up large problems into smaller units that are easier to handle. The difference is that in OOD the units are objects, whereas the units in functional decomposition are modules representing algorithms.

Concrete step   A step for which the implementation details are fully specified.

Abstract step   A step for which some implementation details remain unspecified.

Module   A self-contained collection of steps that solves a problem or subproblem; can contain both concrete and abstract steps.

Modules

A module begins life as an abstract step in the next-higher level of the solution tree. It is completed when it solves a given subproblem—that is, when it specifies a series of steps that does the same thing as the higher-level abstract step. At this stage, a module is **functionally equivalent** to the abstract step. (Don't confuse our use of *function* with C++ functions. Here we use the term to refer to the specific role that the module or step plays in an algorithmic solution.)

> **Functional equivalence** A property of a module that performs exactly the same operation as the abstract step it defines. A pair of modules are also functionally equivalent to each other when they perform exactly the same operation.
>
> **Functional cohesion** A property of a module in which all concrete steps are directed toward solving just one problem, and any significant subproblems are written as abstract steps.

In a properly written module, the only steps that directly address the given subproblem are concrete steps; abstract steps are used for significant new subproblems. This is called **functional cohesion.**

The idea behind functional cohesion is that each module should do just one thing and do it well. Functional cohesion is not a well-defined property; there is no quantitative measure of cohesion. It is a product of the human need to organize things into neat chunks that are easy to understand and remember. Knowing which details to make concrete and which to leave abstract is a matter of experience, circumstance, and personal style. For example, you might decide to include a fieldwidth calculation in a printing module if there isn't so much detail in the rest of the module that it becomes confusing. On the other hand, if the calculation is performed several times, it makes sense to write it as a separate module and just refer to it each time you need it.

Writing Cohesive Modules   Here's one approach to writing modules that are cohesive:

1. Think about how you would solve the subproblem by hand.

2. Begin writing down the major steps.

3. If a step is simple enough that you can see how to implement it directly in C++, it is at the concrete level; it doesn't need any further refinement.

4. If you have to think about implementing a step as a series of smaller steps or as several C++ statements, it is still at an abstract level.

5. If you are trying to write a series of steps and start to feel overwhelmed by details, you probably are bypassing one or more levels of abstraction. Stand back and look for pieces that you can write as more abstract steps.

We could call this the "procrastinator's technique." If a step is cumbersome or difficult, put it off to a lower level; don't think about it today, think about it tomorrow. Of course, tomorrow does come, but the whole process can be applied again to the subproblem. A trouble spot often seems much simpler when you can focus on it. And eventually the whole problem is broken up into manageable units.

As you work your way down the solution tree, you make a series of design decisions. If a decision proves awkward or wrong (and many times it does!), you can backtrack (go back up the tree to a higher-level module) and try something else. You don't have to scrap your whole design—only the small part you are working on. There may be many intermediate steps and trial solutions before you reach a final design.

Pseudocode   You'll find it easier to implement a design if you write the steps in pseudocode. *Pseudocode* is a mixture of English statements and C++-like control structures that can be translated easily into C++. (We've been using pseudocode in the algorithms in the Problem-Solving Case Studies.) When a concrete step is written in pseudocode, it should be possible to rewrite it directly as a C++ statement in a program.

Implementing the Design

The product of functional decomposition is a hierarchical solution to a problem with multiple levels of abstraction. Figure 4–5 shows a functional decomposition for the Mortgage program of Chapter 3. This kind of solution forms the basis for the implementation phase of programming.

How do we translate a functional decomposition into a C++ program? If you look closely at Figure 4–5, you can see that the concrete steps (those that are shaded) can be assembled into a complete algorithm for solving the problem. The order in which they are assembled is determined by their position in the tree. We start at the top of the tree, at level 0, with the first step, "Define Constants." Because it is abstract, we must go to the next level, level 1. There we find a series of concrete steps that correspond to this step; this series of steps becomes the first part of our algorithm. Because the conversion process is now concrete, we can go back to level 0 and go on to the next step, "Calculate Values." Because it is abstract, we go to level 1 and find a series of concrete steps that correspond to this step; this series of steps becomes the next part of our algorithm. Returning to level 0, we go on to the next step, "Output Results".

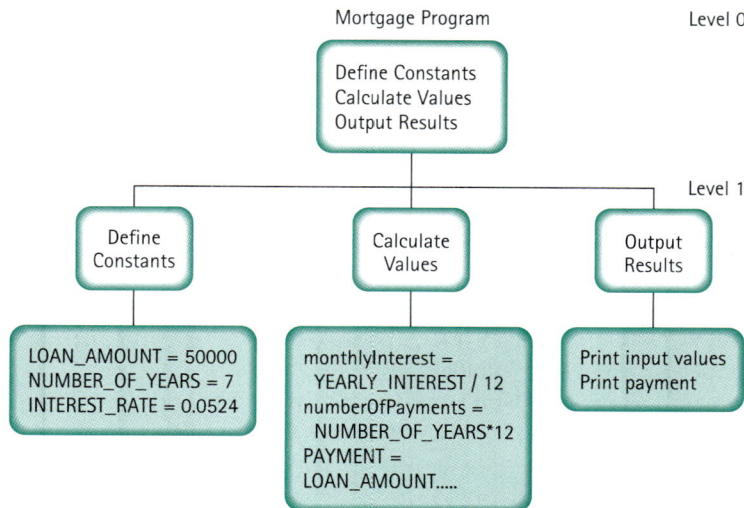

Figure 4–5   *Solution Tree for Mortgage Program*

```
Set LOAN_AMOUNT = 50000.00
Set NUMBER_OF_YEARS = 7
Set INTEREST_RATE = 0.0524
Set monthlyInterest to YEARLY_INTEREST divided by 12
Set numberOfPayments to NUMBER_OF_YEARS times 12
Set payment to (LOAN_AMOUNT *
pow(monthlyInterest+1,numberrOfPayments)
   * monthlyInterest) / (pow(monthlyInterest+1, numberOfPayments) – 1)
Print "For a loan amount of " LOAN_AMOUNT "with an interest rate of "
   YEARLY_INTEREST " and a " NUMBER_OF_YEARS " year mortgage, "
Print "your monthly payments are $" payment "."
```

From this algorithm we can construct a table of the constants and variables required, and then write the declarations and executable statements of the program.

In practice, you write your design not as a tree diagram but as a series of modules grouped by levels of abstraction.

Main   **Level 0**

```
Define Constants
Calculate Values
Output Results
```

Define Constants

```
Set LOAN_AMOUNT = 50000.00
Set NUMBER_OF_YEARS = 7
Set INTEREST_RATE = 0.0524
```

Calculate Values

```
Set monthlyInterest to YEARLY_INTEREST divided by 12
Set numberOfPayments to NUMBER_OF_YEARS times 12
Set payment to (LOAN_AMOUNT * pow(monthlyInterest+1,numberrOfPayments)
   * monthlyInterest) / (pow(monthlyInterest+1, numberOfPayments) – 1)
```

Output Results

> Print "For a loan amount of " LOAN_AMOUNT "with an interest rate of "
>   YEARLY_INTEREST " and a " NUMBER_OF_YEARS " year mortgage, "
> Print "your monthly payments are $" payment "."

If you look at the C++ program for Mortgage, you can see that it closely resembles this solution. The main difference is that we didn't write a "Main module" in Chapter 3. You also can see that the names of the modules have been paraphrased as comments in the code.

The type of implementation that we've introduced here is called *flat* or *inline implementation*. We are flattening the two-dimensional, hierarchical structure of the solution by writing all of the steps as one long sequence. This kind of implementation is adequate when a solution is short and has only a few levels of abstraction. The programs it produces are clear and easy to understand, assuming appropriate comments and good style.

Longer programs, with more levels of abstraction, are difficult to work with as flat implementations. In Chapter 7, you'll see that it is preferable to implement a hierarchical solution by using a *hierarchical implementation*. There we implement many of the modules by writing them as separate C++ functions, and the abstract steps in the design are replaced with calls to those functions.

One of the advantages of implementing modules as functions is that they can be called from different places in a program. For example, if a problem requires that the volume of a cylinder be computed in several places, we could write a single function to perform the calculation and simply call it in each place. This gives us a *semihierarchical implementation*. The implementation does not preserve a pure hierarchy because abstract steps at various levels of the solution tree share one implementation of a module (see Figure 4–6). A shared module actually falls outside the hierarchy because it doesn't really belong at any one level.

Another advantage of implementing modules as functions is that you can pick them up and use them in other programs. Over time, you will build a library of your own functions to complement those that are supplied by the C++ standard library.

We postpone a detailed discussion of hierarchical implementations until Chapter 7. For now, our programs remain short enough for flat implementations to suffice. Chapters 5 and 6 examine topics such as flow of control, preconditions and postconditions, interface design, side effects, and others you'll need in order to develop hierarchical implementations.

From now on, we use the following outline for the functional decompositions in our case studies, and we recommend that you adopt a similar outline in solving your own programming problems:

Problem statement
Input description
Output description

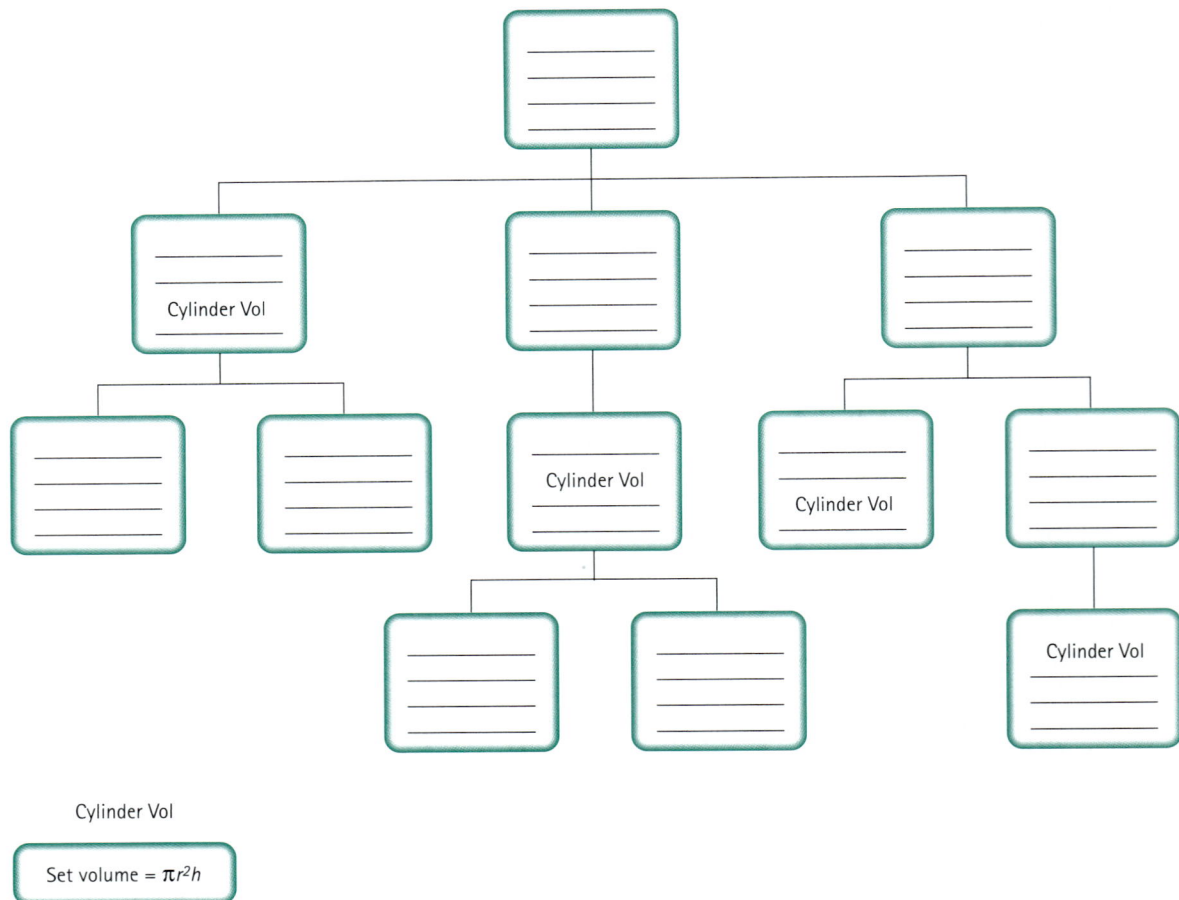

Figure 4–6   *A Semihierarchical Module Structure Chart with a Shared Module*

Discussion
Assumptions (if any)
Main module
Remaining modules by levels
Module structure chart

In some of our case studies, the outline is reorganized, with the input and output descriptions following the discussion. In later chapters, we also expand the outline with additional sections. Don't think of this outline as a rigid prescription—it is more like a list of things to do. We want to be sure to do everything on the list, but the individual circumstances of each problem guide the order in which we do them.

A Perspective on Design

We have looked at two design methodologies, object-oriented design and functional decomposition. Until we learn about additional C++ language features that support OOD, we use functional decomposition (and object-based programming) in the next several chapters to come up with our problem solutions.

An important perspective to keep in mind is that functional decomposition and OOD are not separate, disjoint techniques. OOD decomposes a problem into objects. Objects not only contain data but also have associated operations. The operations on objects require algorithms. Sometimes the algorithms are complicated and must be decomposed into subalgorithms by using functional decomposition. Experienced programmers are familiar with both methodologies and know when to use one or the other, or a combination of the two.

Remember that the problem-solving phase of the programming process takes time. If you spend the bulk of your time analyzing and designing a solution, then coding and implementing the program take relatively little time.

Software Engineering Tip

Documentation

As you create your functional decomposition or object-oriented design, you are developing documentation for your program. *Documentation* includes the written problem specifications, design, development history, and actual code of a program.

Good documentation helps other programmers read and understand a program and is invaluable when software is being debugged and modified (maintained). If you haven't looked at your program for six months and need to change it, you'll be happy that you documented it well. Of course, if someone else has to use and modify your program, documentation is indispensable.

Documentation is both external and internal to the program. External documentation includes the specifications, the development history, and the design documents. Internal documentation includes the program format and self-documenting code—meaningful identifiers and comments. You can use the pseudocode from the design process as comments in your programs.

> **Self-documenting code**   Program code containing meaningful identifiers as well as judiciously used clarifying comments.

This kind of documentation may be sufficient for someone reading or maintaining your programs. However, if a program is going to be used by people who are not programmers, you must provide a user's manual as well.

Be sure to keep documentation up-to-date. Indicate any changes you make in a program in all of the pertinent documentation. Use self-documenting code to make your programs more readable.

Now let's look at a case study that demonstrates functional decomposition.

Problem-Solving Case Study

Display a Name in Multiple Formats

PROBLEM You are beginning to work on a problem that needs to output names in several formats along with the corresponding social security number. As a start, you decide to write a short C++ program that inputs a social security number and a single name and displays it in the different formats so you can be certain that all of your string expressions are correct.

INPUT The social security number and a name in three parts, on file `name.dat`, each separated by one or more white space characters.

OUTPUT The name is to be written in four different formats on file `name.out`:

1. First name, middle name, last name, social security number
2. Last name, first name, middle name, social security number
3. Last name, first name, middle initial, social security number
4. First name, middle initial, last name

DISCUSSION You easily could just type the social security number and the name in the four formats as string literals in the code, but the purpose of this exercise is to develop and test the string expressions that you need for the larger problem. The problem statement doesn't say in which order the parts of the name are entered on the file, but it does say that they are separated by white space. You assume that they are in first name, middle name or initial, and last name order. Because the data are on a file, you don't need to prompt for the values. Once you have the social security number and the name, you just write them out in the various formats.

ASSUMPTION Name is in first, middle, and last order on the file.

Main Module	Level 0

> Open files
> Get social security number
> Get name
> Write data in proper formats
> Close files

Open Files	Level 1

> inData.open("name.dat")
> outData.open("name.out")

The "Get social security number" step can be directly implemented by reading into the string variable. Thus, it doesn't require expansion at Level 1 of our design.

Get Name

Get first name
Get middle name or initial
Get last name

Is there a problem reading the middle name if an initial is in the file rather than a middle name? Not really. You just assume that a middle name is entered and extract the initial from the middle name when you need it for the third and fourth formats. If the initial was entered for the middle name, then the second and third output forms will be the same. What about punctuation in the output? If the last name comes first, it should be followed by a comma, and the middle initial should be followed by a period. Thus, if the initial is entered rather than the middle name, it must be followed by a period. This must be added to the assumptions.

ASSUMPTION Name is in first, middle, and last order, and a period must follow the middle initial if it is entered instead of a middle name.

Write Data in Proper Formats

Write first name, blank, middle name, blank, last name, blank, social
   security number
Write last name, comma, blank first name, blank, middle name, blank,
   social security number
Write last name, comma, blank, first name, blank, middle initial, period,
   blank, social security number
Write first name, blank, middle initial, period, blank, last name

The only thing left to define is the middle initial. We can use the `substr` method to access the first character in the middle name.

Middle Initial   Level 2

Set initial to middleName.substr(0, 1) + period

Close Files

inData.close()
outData.close()

Module Structure Chart

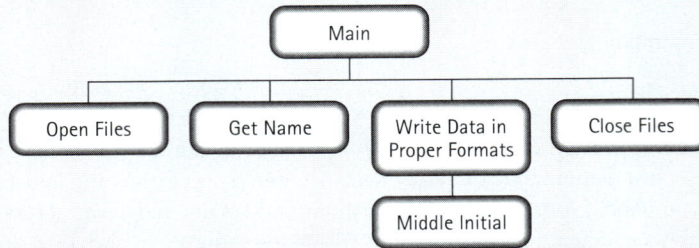

```
                        ┌──────────┐
                        │   Main   │
                        └──────────┘
        ┌────────────────┬──────────┴────────┬────────────────┐
┌───────────────┐ ┌─────────────┐ ┌────────────────┐ ┌───────────────┐
│   Open Files  │ │  Get Name   │ │ Write Data in  │ │  Close Files  │
└───────────────┘ └─────────────┘ │ Proper Formats │ └───────────────┘
                                   └────────────────┘
                                           │
                                  ┌────────────────┐
                                  │ Middle Initial │
                                  └────────────────┘
```

Variables

Name	Data Type	Description
inData	ifstream	Input file
outData	ofstream	Output file
socialNum	string	Social security number
firstName	string	First name
lastName	string	Last name
middleName	string	Middle name
initial	string	Middle initial

```
//*******************************************************************
// Format Names program
// This program reads in a social security number, a first name, a
// middle name or initial, and a last name from file inData.
// The name is written to file outData in three formats:
//     1. First name, middle name, last name, and social security
//     number.
//     2. Last name, first name, middle name, and social
//     security number
//     3. Last name, first name, middle initial, and social security
//     number
//     4. First name, middle initial, last name
//*******************************************************************
```

```cpp
#include <fstream>                        // Access ofstream
#include <string>                         // Access string

using namespace std;

int main()
{
    // Declare and open files
    ifstream inData;
    ofstream outData;
    inData.open("name.dat");
    outData.open("name.out");

    // Declare variables
    string socialNum;                     // Social security number
    string firstName;                     // First name
    string lastName;                      // Last name
    string middleName;                    // Middle name
    string initial;                       // Middle initial

    // Read in data from file inData
    inData >> socialNum >> firstName >> middleName >> lastName;

    // Access middle initial and append a period
    initial = middleName.substr(0, 1) + '.';

    // Output information in required formats
    outData << firstName << ' ' << middleName << ' ' << lastName
            << ' ' << socialNum << endl;
    outData << lastName << ", " << firstName << ' ' << middleName
            << ' ' << socialNum  << endl;
    outData << lastName << ", " << firstName << ' ' << initial
            << ' ' << socialNum  << endl;
    outData << firstName << ' ' << initial << ' ' << lastName;

    // Close files
    inData.close();
    outData.close();
    return 0;
}
```

Here are sample input and output files.

```
name.dat - Notepad
File  Edit  Format  View  Help
333-55-3456 Clara Jones Jacobey
```

```
name.out - Notepad
File  Edit  Format  View  Help
Clara Jones Jacobey 333-55-3456
Jacobey, Clara Jones 333-55-3456
Jacobey, Clara J. 333-55-3456
Clara J. Jacobey
```

Background Information

Programming at Many Scales

To help you put the topics in this book into context, we describe in broad terms the way programming in its many forms is done in "the real world." Obviously, we can't cover every possibility, but we'll try to give you a flavor of the state of the art.

Programming projects range in size from the small scale, in which a student or computer hobbyist writes a short program to try out something new, to large-scale multicompany programming projects involving hundreds of people. Between these two extremes are efforts of many other sizes. There are people who use programming in their professions, even though it isn't their primary job. For example, a scientist might write a special-purpose program to analyze data from a particular experiment.

(continued) ▼

Programming at Many Scales

Even among professional programmers, there are many specialized programming areas. An individual might have a specialty in business data processing, in writing compilers or developing word processors (a specialty known as "tool making"), in research and development support, in graphical display development, in writing entertainment software, or in one of many other areas. However, one person can produce only fairly small programs (a few tens of thousands of lines of code at best). Work of this kind is called *programming in the small*.

A larger application, such as the development of a new operating system, might require hundreds of thousands or even millions of lines of code. Such large-scale projects require teams of programmers, many of them specialists, who must be organized in some manner or they waste valuable time just trying to communicate with one another.

Usually, a hierarchical organization is set up along the lines of the module structure chart. One person, the *chief architect* or *project director*, determines the basic structure of the program and then delegates the responsibility of implementing the major components. These components may be modules produced by a functional decomposition, or they might be classes and objects resulting from an object-oriented design. In smaller projects, the components may be delegated directly to programmers. In larger projects, the components may be given to team leaders, who divide them into subcomponents that are then delegated to individual programmers or groups of programmers. At each stage, the person in charge must have the knowledge and experience necessary to define the next-lower level of the hierarchy and to estimate the resources necessary to implement it. This sort of organization is called *programming in the large*.

Programming languages and software tools can help a great deal in supporting programming in the large. For example, if a programming language lets programmers develop, compile, and test parts of a program independently before they are put together, then it enables several people to work on the program simultaneously. Of course, it is hard to appreciate the complexity of programming in the large when you are writing a small program for a class assignment. However, the experience you gain in this course will be valuable as you begin to develop larger programs.

The following is a classic example of what happens when a large program is developed without careful organization and proper language support. In the 1960s, IBM developed a major new operating system called OS/360, which was one of the first true examples of programming in the large. After the operating system was written, more than 1000 significant errors were found. Despite years of trying to fix these errors, the programmers never did get the number of errors below 1000, and sometimes the "fixes" produced far more errors than they eliminated.

What led to this situation? Hindsight analysis showed that the code was badly organized and that different pieces were so interrelated that nobody could keep it all straight. A seemingly simple change in one part of the code caused several other parts of the system to fail. Eventually, at great expense, an entirely new system was created using better organization and tools.

In those early days of computing, everyone expected occasional errors to occur, and it was still possible to get useful work done with a faulty operating system. Today, however, computers are

(continued) ▼

> ### Programming at Many Scales
>
> used more and more in critical applications such as medical equipment and aircraft control systems, where errors can prove fatal. Many of these applications depend on large-scale programming. If you were stepping onto a modern jetliner right now, you might well pause and wonder, "Just what sort of language and tools did they use when they wrote the programs for this thing?" Fortunately, most large software development efforts today use a combination of good methodology, appropriate language, and extensive organizational tools—an approach known as *software engineering*.

Testing and Debugging

An important part of implementing a program is testing it (checking the results). By now you should realize that there is nothing magical about the computer. It is infallible only if the person writing the instructions and entering the data is infallible. Don't trust it to give you the correct answers until you've verified enough of them by hand to convince yourself that the program is working.

From here on, these Testing and Debugging sections offer tips on how to test your programs and what to do if a program doesn't work the way you expect it to work. But don't wait until you've found a bug to read the Testing and Debugging sections. It's much easier to prevent bugs than to fix them.

When testing programs that input data values from a file, it's possible for input operations to fail. And when input fails in C++, the computer doesn't issue a warning message or terminate the program. The program simply continues executing, ignoring any further input operations on that file. The two most common reasons for input failure are invalid data and the *end-of-file error*.

An end-of-file error occurs when the program has read all of the input data available in the file and needs more data to fill the variables in its input statements. It might be that the data file simply was not prepared properly. Perhaps it contains fewer data items than the program requires. Or perhaps the format of the input data is wrong. Leaving out whitespace between numeric values is guaranteed to cause trouble. For example, we may want a data file to contain three integer values—25, 16, and 42. Look what happens with this data:

```
2516   42
```

and this code:

```
inFile >> i >> j >> k;
```

The first two input operations use up the data in the file, leaving the third with no data to read. The stream `inFile` enters the fail state, so k isn't assigned a new value and the computer quietly continues executing at the next statement in the program.

If the data file is prepared correctly and there is still an end-of-file error, the problem is in the program logic. For some reason, the program is attempting too many input operations. It could be a simple oversight such as specifying too many variables in a particular input statement. It could be a misuse of the `ignore` function, causing values to be skipped inadvertently. Or it could be a serious flaw in the algorithm. You should check all of these possibilities.

The other major source of input failure, invalid data, has several possible causes. The most common is an error in the preparation or entry of the data. Numeric and character data mixed inappropriately in the input can cause the input stream to fail if it is supposed to read a numeric value but the reading marker is positioned at a character that isn't allowed in the number. Another cause is using the wrong variable name (which happens to be of the wrong data type) in an input statement. Declaring a variable to be of the wrong data type is a variation on the problem. Last, leaving out a variable (or including an extra one) in an input statement can cause the reading marker to end up positioned on the wrong type of data.

Another oversight, one that doesn't cause input failure but causes programmer frustration, is to use `cin` or `cout` in an I/O statement when you meant to specify a file stream. If you mistakenly use `cin` instead of an input file stream, the program stops and waits for input from the keyboard. If you mistakenly use `cout` instead of an output file stream, you get unexpected output on the screen.

By giving you a framework that can help you organize and keep track of the details involved in designing and implementing a program, functional decomposition (and, later, object-oriented design) should help you avoid many of these errors in the first place.

In later chapters, you'll see that you can test modules separately. If you make sure that each module works by itself, your program should work when you put all the modules together. Testing modules separately is less work than trying to test an entire program. In a smaller section of code, it's less likely that multiple errors will combine to produce behavior that is difficult to analyze.

Testing and Debugging Hints

1. Input and output statements always begin with the name of a stream object, and the >> and << operators point in the direction in which the data is going. The statement

```
cout << n;
```

sends data *to* the output stream `cout`, and the statement

```
cin >> n;
```

sends data *to* the variable n.

2. When a program inputs from or outputs to a file, be sure each I/O statement from or to the file uses the name of the file stream, not `cin` or `cout`.

3. The `open` function associated with an `ifstream` or `ofstream` object requires a C string as an argument. The argument cannot be a `string` object. At this point in the book, the argument can only be (a) a literal string or (b) the C string returned by the function call `myString.c_str()`, where `myString` is of type `string`.

4. When you open a data file for input, make sure that the argument to the `open` function supplies the correct name of the file as it exists on disk.

5. When reading a character string into a `string` object, the `>>` operator stops at, *but does not consume*, the first trailing whitespace character.

6. Be sure that each input statement specifies the correct number of variables and that each of those variables is of the correct data type.

7. If your input data is mixed (character and numeric values), be sure to deal with intervening blanks.

8. Echo print the input data to verify that each value is where it belongs and is in the proper format. (This is crucial, because an input failure in C++ doesn't produce an error message or terminate the program.)

Summary

Programs operate on data. If data and programs are kept separate, the data is available to use with other programs, and the same program can be run with different sets of input data.

The extraction operator (>>) inputs data from the keyboard or a file, storing the data into the variable specified as its right-hand operand. The extraction operator skips any leading whitespace characters to find the next data value in the input stream. The `get` function does not skip leading whitespace characters; it inputs the very next character and stores it into the `char` variable specified in its argument list. Both the `>>` operator and the `get` function leave the reading marker positioned at the next character to be read. The next input operation begins reading at the point indicated by the marker.

The newline character (denoted by \n in a C++ program) marks the end of a data line. You create a newline character each time you press the Return or Enter key. Your program generates a newline each time you use the `endl` manipulator or explicitly output the \n character. Newline is a control character; it does not print. It controls the movement of the screen cursor or the position of a line on a printer.

Interactive programs prompt the user for each data entry and directly inform the user of results and errors. Designing interactive dialogue is an exercise in the art of communication.

Noninteractive input/output allows data to be prepared before a program is run and allows the program to run again with the same data in the event that a problem crops up during processing.

Data files often are used for noninteractive processing and to permit the output from one program to be used as input to another program. To use these files, you must do four things: (1) include the header file `fstream`, (2) declare the file streams along with your other variable declarations, (3) prepare the files for reading or writing by calling the `open` function, and (4) specify the name of the file stream in each input or output statement that uses it.

Object-oriented design and functional decomposition are methodologies for tackling nontrivial programming problems. Object-oriented design produces a problem solution by focusing on objects and their associated operations. The first step is to identify the major objects in the problem and choose appropriate operations on those objects. An object is an instance of a data type called a class. During object-oriented design, classes can be designed from scratch, obtained from class libraries and used as is, or customized from existing classes by using the technique of inheritance. The result of the design process is a program consisting of self-contained objects that manage their own data and communicate by invoking each other's operations.

Functional decomposition begins with an abstract solution that then is divided into major steps. Each step becomes a subproblem that is analyzed and subdivided further. A concrete step is one that can be translated directly into C++; those steps that need more refining are abstract steps. A module is a collection of concrete and abstract steps that solves a subproblem. Programs can be built out of modules using a flat implementation, a hierarchical implementation, or a semihierarchical implementation.

Careful attention to program design, program formatting, and documentation produces highly structured and readable programs.

Quick Check

1. Why do we need to use prompts for interactive I/O? (pp. 150–152)
2. What conditions would you look for in a problem to decide whether interactive or noninteractive input is appropriate? (pp. 150–152)
3. What is the first step in the object-oriented design process? (pp. 165–166)
4. Write an input statement that reads three integer values into variables a, b, and c. (pp. 141–143)
5. If an input line contains

   ```
   Jones, Walker Thomas
   ```

   what will be the values in the `string` variables `first`, `middle`, and `last` when the following statement is executed? (pp. 149–150)

   ```
   cin >> first >> middle >> last;
   ```

6. After including the header file `fstream`, and declaring a file stream, what is the next step in using a file I/O? (pp. 153–157)
7. What characterizes a concrete step in a functional decomposition design? (pp. 166–167)

8. If you are given a functional decomposition design, how do you implement it? (pp. 169–172)

Answers

1. To tell the user how and when to enter values as input.   2. The amount of data to be input, and whether the data can be prepared for entry before the program is run.   3. To identify the major objects in the problem.   4. `cin >> a >> b >> c;`

5. `first = "Jones,"`
   `middle = "Walker"`
   `last = "Thomas"`

6. Preparing the file for reading or writing with the `open` function.   7. It is a step that can be implemented directly in a programming language.   8. By identifying all of the concrete steps, starting from the top of the tree, and arranging them in the proper order. The sequence of steps is then converted step-by-step into code.

Exam Preparation Exercises

1. The statement

   `cin >> maximum >> minimum;`

   is equivalent to the two statements:

   `cin >> minimum;`
   `cin >> maximum;`

   True or false?

2. What is wrong with each of the following statements?
   a. `cin << score;`
   b. `cout >> maximum;`
   c. `cin >> "Enter data";`
   d. `cin.ignore('Y', 35);`
   e. `getLine(someString, cin);`

3. If input data are entered as follows

   ```
   10   20
   30   40
   50   60
   70   80
   ```

   and the input statements that read it are

   `cin >> a >> b >> c;`
   `cin >> d >> e >> f;`
   `cin >> a >> b;`

   what are the contents of the variables a, b, c, d, e, and f after the statements have executed?

4. If input data are entered as follows:

```
10    20    30    40    50    60
10    20    30    40    50    60
10    20    30    40    50    60
70    80
```

and the input statements that read it are:

```
cin >> a >> b >> c;
cin.ignore(100, '\n');
cin.get(ch1);
cin >> d >> e >> f;
cin.ignore(100, '\n');
cin.ignore(100, '\n');
cin >> a >> b;
```

What are the contents of the variables a, b, c, d, e, and f after the statements have executed?

5. Given the input data

```
January 25, 2005
```

and the input statement

```
cin >> string1 >> string2;
```

a. What is contained in each of the string variables after the statement is executed?
b. Where is the reading marker after the statement is executed?

6. Given the input data

```
January 25, 2005
```

and the input statement

```
getline(cin, string1);
```

a. What is contained in the string variable after the statement is executed?
b. Where is the reading marker after the statement is executed?

7. Given the input data

```
January 25, 2005
```

and the input statement (where the type of each variable is given by its name)

```
cin >> string1 >> int1 >> char1 >> string2;
```

a. What is contained in each of the variables after the statement is executed?
b. Where is the reading marker after the statement is executed?

8. If the reading marker is on the newline character at the end of a line, and you call the get function, what value does it return in its argument?

9. What do the two arguments to the ignore function specify?

10. You are writing a program that inputs a date in the form of mm/dd/yyyy.

    a. Write the output statement to prompt an inexperienced user to enter a date.

    b. Write the output statement to prompt an experienced user to input a date.

11. What are the four steps necessary to use a file for input or output?

12. What are the two file stream data types discussed in this chapter?

13. What is the purpose of the following statements?

```
ifstream inFile;
inFile.open("datafile.dat");
```

14. Correct the following code segment so that it opens the file whose name is entered via the input statement.

```
ifstream inData;
string name;

cout << "Enter the name of the file: ");
cin >> name;
infile.open(name);
```

15. What happens when an input operation is performed on a file that is in the fail state?

16. When you try to open a file that doesn't exist, C++ outputs an error message and terminates execution of the program. True or false?

17. Just opening an input file stream cannot cause it to enter the fail state. True or false?

18. You're writing a program for a rental car company that keeps track of vehicles. What are the major objects in this problem?

19. What C++ construct is used to implement an object?

20. Define the following terms:

    a. Concrete step

    b. Abstract step

    c. Module

    d. Functional equivalence

    e. Functional cohesion

21. What C++ construct do we use to implement modules?

22. Which of the following are member functions of the `istream` class?

    a. `>>`

    b. `ignore`

    c. `get`

    d. `getline`

    e. `cin`

23. The `open` function is a member of both the `ifstream` and the `ofstream` classes. True or false?

Programming Warm-Up Exercises

1. Write a C++ input statement that reads three integer values into variables `int1`, `int2`, and `int3`, in that order.

2. Write a prompting output statement and then an input statement that reads a name into three string variables: `first`, `middle`, and `last`. The name is to be entered in the format: first middle last.

3. Write a prompting output statement and then an input statement that reads a name into a single string variable, `name`. The name is to be entered on one line, in the format: first middle last.

4. Write the statements necessary to prompt for and input three floating point values, and then output their average. For this exercise, assume that the user has no prior experience with computers and thus needs very detailed instructions. To help avoid errors, the user should enter each value separately.

5. Write the statements necessary to prompt for and input three floating point values, and then output their average. For this exercise, assume that the user has plenty of experience with computers and thus needs minimal instructions. The user should enter all three values on one line.

6. Write the declarations and input statements necessary to read each of the following sets of data values into variables of the appropriate types. You choose the names of the variables. In some cases, there are punctuation marks or special symbols that must be skipped.

   a. `100 A 98.6`
   b. `February 23 March 19`
   c. `19, 25, 103.876`
   d. `A a B b`
   e. `$56.45`

7. Write a single input statement that reads the following lines of data into the variables `streetNum`, `street1`, `street2`, `town`, `state`, and `zip`.

   782 Maple Avenue
   Blithe, CO 56103

8. Write the statements necessary to prepare a file called `"temperatures.dat"` for reading as an `ifstream` called `temps`.

9. The file `"temperatures.dat"` contains a list of six temperatures, arranged one per line. Assuming that the file has already been prepared for reading, as described in Exercise 8, write the statements to read in the data from the file and print out the average temperature. You will also need to declare the necessary `float` variables to accomplish this task.

10. Fill in the blanks in the following program:

```
#include <iostream>
#include _____

using namespace std;

_____ inData;
_____ outData;
const float PI = 3.14159265;
float radius;
```

```
float circumference;
float area;

int main()
{
    _____("indata.dat");
    _____("outdata.dat");
    _____ >> radius;
    circumference = radius * 2 * PI;
    area = radius * radius * PI;
    cout << "For the first circle, the circumference is "
         << circumference << " and the area is " << area << endl;
    _____ << radius << " " << circumference << " " << area
         << endl;
    _____ >> radius;
    circumference = radius * 2 * PI;
    area = radius * radius * PI;
    cout << "For the second circle, the circumference is "
         << circumference << " and the area is " << area << endl;
    _____ << radius << " " << circumference << " " << area
         << endl;
    return 0;
}
```

11. Modify the program in Exercise 10 so that it allows the user to enter the name of the output file instead of having the program use `"outdata.dat"`.
12. The file stream `inFile` contains two integer values. Write an input statement that will cause it to enter the fail state.
13. Write a code segment that prompts the user for a file name, reads the file name into a `string` called `filename`, and then opens the file stream `userFile` using the supplied name.
14. Use functional decomposition to write an algorithm for writing and mailing a business letter.
15. What are the objects in the problem described in Exercise 14?

Programming Problems

1. Write an interactive C++ program that inputs a name from the user in the format of:

   ```
   last, first middle
   ```

   The program then should output the name in the format of:

   ```
   first middle last
   ```

The program will have to use string operations to remove the comma from the end of the last name. Be sure to use proper formatting and appropriate comments in your code. The input should have an appropriate prompt, and the output should be labeled clearly and formatted neatly.

2. Write an interactive C++ program that inputs a series of 12 temperatures from the user. It should write out on file `"tempdata.dat"` each temperature and the difference between the current temperature and the one preceding it. The difference is not output for the first temperature that is input. At the end of the program, the average temperature should be displayed for the user via `cout`. For example, given the following input data:

```
34.5 38.6 42.4 46.8 51.3 63.1 60.2 55.9 60.3 56.7 50.3 42.2
```

File `tempdata.dat` would contain:

```
34.5
38.6    4.1
42.4    3.8
46.8    4.4
51.3    4.5
63.1   11.8
60.2   -2.9
55.9   -4.3
60.3    4.4
56.7   -3.6
50.3   -6.4
42.2   -8.1
```

Be sure to use proper formatting and appropriate comments in your code. The input should have appropriate prompts, and the output should be labeled clearly and formatted neatly.

3. Write an interactive C++ program that computes and outputs the mean and standard deviation of a set of four integer values that are input by the user. (If you did Programming Problem 2 in Chapter 3, then you can reuse much of that code here.) The mean is the sum of the four values divided by 4, and the formula for the standard deviation is

$$
s = \sqrt{\frac{\sum_{i=1}^{n}(x_i - \bar{x})^2}{n-1}}
$$

where $n = 4$, x_i refers to each of the four values, and $\bar{x}$ is the mean. Note that although the individual values are integers, the results are floating-point values. Be sure to use proper formatting and appropriate comments in your code. Provide appropriate prompts to the user. The output should be labeled clearly and formatted neatly.

4. Write a C++ program that reads data from a file whose name is input by the user, and that outputs the first word following each of the first three commas in the file. For example, if the file contains the text of this problem, then the program would output:

```
and
if
then
```

Assume that a comma appears within at least every 200 characters in the file. Be sure to use proper formatting and appropriate comments in your code. Provide appropriate prompts to the user. The output should be labeled clearly and formatted neatly.

5. Write a C++ program that allows the user to enter the percentage of the moon's face that appears illuminated, and that outputs the surface area of that portion of the moon. The formula for the surface area of a segment of a sphere is

$$S = 2R^2\theta$$

where R is the radius of the sphere (the moon's radius is 1738.3 km), and θ is the angle of the wedge in radians. There are 2π radians in a circle, so the hemisphere of the moon that we see accounts for at most π radians. Thus, if the user enters 100% (full moon), the angle of the wedge is π and the formula can be evaluated as follows.

$S = 2 \times 1738.3^2 \times 3.14159 = 18985818.672$ square kilometers

If the user enters 50% (first or last quarter), then the angle of the wedge is $\pi \times 0.5$, and so on. Be sure to use proper formatting and appropriate comments in your code. Provide appropriate prompts to the user. The output should be labeled clearly and formatted neatly (limit the decimal precision to three places as in the example above).

Case Study Follow-Up

1. Replace Clara Jones Jacobey's information with your own name as input to the Format Names program.
2. Change this program so that the social security number is written on a line by itself with the various name formats indented five spaces on the next four lines.
3. Change the program so that the name of the input file is read from the keyboard.
4. Change the program so that the names of both the input file and the output file are read from the keyboard.
5. In Chapter 3, the Case Study was a mortgage payment calculator where the data were stored as constants. Rewrite that program so that the information is input from the keyboard.

Conditions, Logical Expressions, and Selection Control Structures

Goals

Knowledge Goals

- To understand how the Boolean operators work.
- To understand the flow of control in a branching statement.
- To understand the flow of control in a nested branching statement.
- To know what preconditions and postconditions are.

Skill Goals

To be able to:

- Construct a simple logical (Boolean) expression to evaluate a given condition.
- Construct a complex logical expression to evaluate a given condition.
- Construct an If-Then-Else statement to perform a specific task.
- Construct an If-Then statement to perform a specific task.
- Construct a set of nested If statements to perform a specific task.
- Trace the execution of a C++ program.
- Test and debug a C++ program.

So far, the statements in our programs have been executed in their physical order. The first statement is executed, then the second, and so on until all of the statements have been executed. But what if we want the computer to execute the statements in some other order? Suppose we want to check the validity of input data and then perform a calculation *or* print an error message, not both. To do so, we must be able to ask a question and then, based on the answer, choose one or another course of action.

The If statement allows us to execute statements in an order that is different from their physical order. We can ask a question with it and do one thing if the answer is yes (true) or another if the answer is no (false). In the first part of this chapter, we deal with asking questions; in the second part, we deal with the If statement itself.

5.1 Flow of Control

The order in which statements are executed in a program is called the **flow of control**. In a sense, the computer is under the control of one statement at a time. When a statement has been executed, control is turned over to the next statement (like a baton being passed in a relay race).

Flow of control is normally sequential (see Figure 5-1). That is, when one statement is finished executing, control passes to the next statement in the program. When we want the flow of control to be nonsequential, we use **control structures**, special statements that transfer control to a statement other than the one that physically comes next. Control structures

> **Flow of control** The order in which the computer executes statements in a program.
>
> **Control structure** A statement used to alter the normally sequential flow of control.

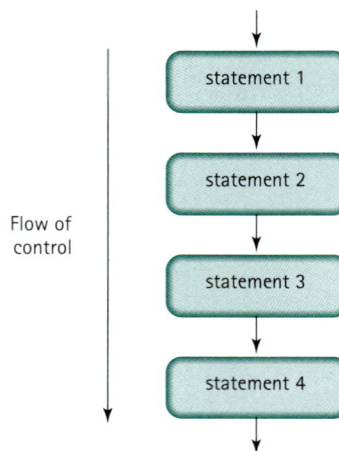

Flow of control

statement 1

statement 2

statement 3

statement 4

Figure 5-1 *Sequential Control*

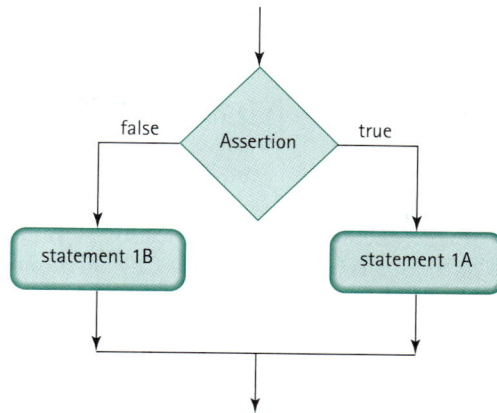

Figure 5–2   *Selection (Branching) Control Structure*

are so important that we focus on them in the remainder of this chapter and in the next four chapters.

Selection

We use a selection (or branching) control structure when we want the computer to choose between alternative actions. We make an assertion, a claim that is either true or false. If the assertion is true, the computer executes one statement. If it is false, it executes another (see Figure 5–2). The computer's ability to solve practical problems is a product of its ability to make decisions and execute different sequences of instructions.

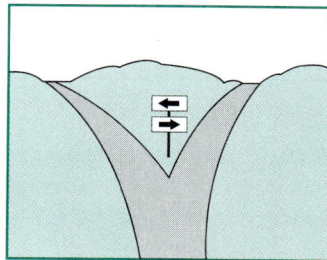

The LeapYear program in Chapter 1 shows the selection process at work. The computer must decide whether a year is a leap year. It does this by testing the assertion that the year is not divisible by 4. If the assertion is true, the computer follows the instructions to return false, indicating that the year is not a leap year. If the assertion is false, the computer goes on to check the exceptions to the general rule. Before we examine selection control structures in C++, let's look closely at how we get the computer to make decisions.

5.2 Conditions and Logical Expressions

To ask a question in C++, we don't phrase it as a question; we state it as an assertion. If the assertion we make is true, the answer to the question is yes. If the statement is not true, the answer to the question is no. For example, if we want to ask, "Are we having spinach for dinner tonight?" we would say, "We are having spinach for dinner tonight." If the assertion is true, the answer to the question is yes. If not, the answer is no.

So, asking questions in C++ means making an assertion that is either true or false. The computer *evaluates* the assertion, checking it against some internal condition (the values stored in certain variables, for instance) to see whether it is true or false.

The `bool` Data Type

In C++, the `bool` data type is a built-in type consisting of just two values, the constants `true` and `false`. The reserved word `bool` is short for Boolean (pronounced 'BOOL-e-un).* Boolean data is used for testing conditions in a program so that the computer can make decisions (with a selection control structure).

We declare variables of type `bool` the same way we declare variables of other types, that is, by writing the name of the data type and then an identifier:

```
bool dataOK;      // True if the input data is valid
bool done;        // True if the process is done
bool taxable;     // True if the item has sales tax
```

Each variable of type `bool` can contain one of two values: `true` or `false`. It's important to understand right from the beginning that `true` and `false` are not variable names and they are not strings. They are special constants in C++ and, in fact, are reserved words.

Background Information

Before the `bool` Type

The C language does not have a `bool` data type, and prior to the ISO/ANSI C++ language standard, neither did C++. In C and pre–standard C++, the value 0 represents *false*, and any nonzero value represents *true*. In these languages, it is customary to use the `int` type to represent Boolean data:

```
int dataOK;
   ⋮
dataOK = 1;    // Store "true" into dataOK
   ⋮
dataOK = 0;    // Store "false" into dataOK
```

(continued) ▼

---

*The word *Boolean* is a tribute to George Boole, a nineteenth-century English mathematician who described a system of logic using variables with just two values, True and False. (See the May We Introduce box on page 203.)

Before the `bool` Type

To make the code more self-documenting, many C and pre–standard C++ programmers prefer to define their own Boolean data type by using a *Typedef statement*. This statement allows you to introduce a new name for an existing data type:

```
typedef int bool;
```

All this statement does is tell the compiler to substitute the word `int` for every occurrence of the word `bool` in the rest of the program. Thus, when the compiler encounters a statement such as

```
bool dataOK;
```

it translates the statement into

```
int dataOK;
```

With the Typedef statement and declarations of two named constants, `true` and `false`, the code at the beginning of this discussion becomes the following:

```
typedef int bool;
const int true = 1;
const int false = 0;
    ⋮
bool dataOK;
    ⋮
dataOK = true;
    ⋮
dataOK = false;
```

With standard C++, none of this is necessary because `bool` is a built-in type. If you are working with pre–standard C++, see Section D.4 of Appendix D for more information about defining your own `bool` type so that you can work with the programs in this book.

Logical Expressions

In programming languages, assertions take the form of *logical expressions* (also called *Boolean expressions*). Just as an arithmetic expression is made up of numeric values and operations, a logical expression is made up of logical values and operations. Every logical expression has one of two values: true or false.

Here are some examples of logical expressions:

- A Boolean variable or constant
- An expression followed by a relational operator followed by an expression
- A logical expression followed by a logical operator followed by a logical expression

Let's look at each of these in detail.

Boolean Variables and Constants   As we have seen, a Boolean variable is a variable declared to be of type `bool`, and it can contain either the value `true` or the value `false`. For example, if `dataOK` is a Boolean variable, then

```
dataOK = true;
```

is a valid assignment statement.

Relational Operators   Another way of assigning a value to a Boolean variable is to set it equal to the result of comparing two expressions with a *relational operator*. Relational operators test a relationship between two values.

Let's look at an example. In the following program fragment, `lessThan` is a Boolean variable and `i` and `j` are `int` variables:

```
cin >> i >> j;
lessThan = (i < j);   // Compare i and j with the "less than"
                      // relational operator, and assign the
                      // truth value to lessThan
```

By comparing two values, we assert that a relationship (like "less than") exists between them. If the relationship does exist, the assertion is true; if not, it is false. These are the relationships we can test for in C++:

Operator	Relationship Tested
==	Equal to
!=	Not equal to
>	Greater than
<	Less than
>=	Greater than or equal to
<=	Less than or equal to

An expression followed by a relational operator followed by an expression is called a *relational expression*. The result of a relational expression is of type `bool`. For example, if `x` is 5 and `y` is 10, the following expressions all have the value `true`:

```
x != y
y > x
x < y
y >= x
x <= y
```

If `x` is the character 'M' and `y` is 'R', the values of the expressions are still `true` because the relational operator <, used with letters, means "comes before in the alphabet," or, more properly, "comes before in the collating sequence of the character set." For example, in the widely used ASCII character set, all of the uppercase letters are in alphabetical order, as are the lowercase letters, but all of the uppercase letters come before the lowercase letters. So

```
'M' < 'R'
```

and

```
'm' < 'r'
```

have the value `true`, but

```
'm' < 'R'
```

has the value `false`.

Of course, we have to be careful about the data types of things we compare. The safest approach is to always compare `ints` with `ints`, `floats` with `floats`, `chars` with `chars`, and so on. If you mix data types in a comparison, implicit type coercion takes place just as in arithmetic expressions. If an `int` value and a `float` value are compared, the computer temporarily coerces the `int` value to its `float` equivalent before making the comparison. As with arithmetic expressions, it's wise to use explicit type casting to make your intentions known:

```
someFloat >= float(someInt)
```

If you compare a `bool` value with a numeric value (probably by mistake), the value `false` is temporarily coerced to the number 0, and `true` is coerced to 1. Therefore, if `boolVar` is a `bool` variable, the expression

```
boolVar < 5
```

yields `true` because 0 and 1 both are less than 5.

Until you learn more about the `char` type in Chapter 10, be careful to compare `char` values only with other `char` values. For example, the comparisons

```
'0' < '9'
```

and

```
0 < 9
```

are appropriate, but

```
'0' < 9
```

generates an implicit type coercion and a result that probably isn't what you expect.

We can use relational operators not only to compare variables or constants, but also to compare the values of arithmetic expressions. In the following table, we compare the results of adding 3 to x and multiplying y by 10 for different values of x and y.

Value of x	Value of y	Expression	Result
12	2	x + 3 <= y * 10	true
20	2	x + 3 <= y * 10	false
7	1	x + 3 != y * 10	false
17	2	x + 3 == y * 10	true
100	5	x + 3 > y * 10	true

Caution: It's easy to confuse the assignment operator (=) and the == relational operator. These two operators have very different effects in a program. Some people pronounce the relational operator as "equals-equals" to remind themselves of the difference.

Comparing Strings Recall from Chapter 4 that string is a class—a programmer-defined type from which you declare variables that are more commonly called objects. Contained within each string object is a character string. The string class is designed such that you can compare these strings using the relational operators. Syntactically, the operands of a relational operator can either be two string objects, as in

```
myString < yourString
```

or a string object and a C string:

```
myString >= "Johnson"
```

However, the operands cannot both be C strings.

Comparison of strings follows the collating sequence of the machine's character set (ASCII, for instance). When the computer tests a relationship between two strings, it begins with the first character of each, compares them according to the collating sequence, and if they are the same repeats the comparison with the next character in each string. The character-by-character test proceeds until either a mismatch is found or the final characters have been compared and are equal. If all their characters are equal, then the two strings are equal. If a mismatch is found, then the string with the character that comes before the other is the "lesser" string.

For example, given the statements

```
string word1;
string word2;

word1 = "Tremendous";
word2 = "Small";
```

the relational expressions in the following table have the indicated values.

Expression	Value	Reason
word1 == word2	false	They are unequal in the first character.
word1 > word2	true	'T' comes after 'S' in the collating sequence.
word1 < "Tremble"	false	Fifth characters don't match, and 'b' comes before 'e'.
word2 == "Small"	true	They are equal.
"cat" < "dog"	Unpredictable	The operands cannot both be C strings.*

*The expression is syntactically legal in C++ but results in a *pointer* comparison, not a string comparison. Pointers are not discussed until Chapter 15.

In most cases, the ordering of strings corresponds to alphabetical ordering. But when strings have mixed-case letters, we can get nonalphabetical results. For example, in a phone book we expect to see Macauley before MacPherson, but the ASCII collating sequence places all uppercase letters before the lowercase letters, so the string "MacPherson" compares as less than "Macauley". To compare strings for strict alphabetical ordering, all the characters must be in the same case. In a later chapter we show an algorithm for changing the case of a string.

If two strings with different lengths are compared and the comparison is equal up to the end of the shorter string, then the shorter string compares as less than the longer string. For example, if word2 contains "Small", the expression

```
word2 < "Smaller"
```

yields true, because the strings are equal up to their fifth character position (the end of the string on the left), and the string on the right is longer.

Logical Operators   In mathematics, the *logical* (or *Boolean*) *operators* AND, OR, and NOT take logical expressions as operands. C++ uses special symbols for the logical operators: && (for AND), || (for OR), and ! (for NOT). By combining relational operators with logical operators, we can make more complex assertions. For example, suppose we want to determine whether a final score is greater than 90 *and* a midterm score is greater than 70. In C++, we would write the expression this way:

```
finalScore > 90 && midtermScore > 70
```

The AND operation (&&) requires both relationships to be true in order for the overall result to be true. If either or both of the relationships are false, the entire result is false.

The OR operation (||) takes two logical expressions and combines them. If *either* or *both* are true, the result is true. Both values must be false for the result to be false. Now we can determine whether the midterm grade is an A *or* the final grade is an A. If either the midterm grade or the final grade equals A, the assertion is true. In C++, we write the expression like this:

```
midtermGrade == 'A' || finalGrade == 'A'
```

The && and || operators always appear between two expressions; they are binary (two-operand) operators. The NOT operator (!) is a unary (one-operand) operator. It precedes a single logical expression and gives its opposite as the result. If (grade == 'A') is false, then !(grade == 'A') is true. NOT gives us a convenient way of reversing the meaning of an assertion. For example,

```
!(hours > 40)
```

is the equivalent of

```
hours <= 40
```

In some contexts, the first form is clearer; in others, the second makes more sense.

The following pairs of expressions are equivalent:

Expression	Equivalent Expression
!(a == b)	a != b
!(a == b || a == c)	a != b && a != c
!(a == b && c > d)	a != b || c <= d

Take a close look at these expressions to be sure you understand why they are equivalent. Try evaluating them with some values for a, b, c, and d. Notice the pattern: The expression on the left is just the one to its right with ! added and the relational and logical operators reversed (for example, == instead of != and || instead of &&). Remember this pattern. It allows you to rewrite expressions in the simplest form.*

Logical operators can be applied to the results of comparisons. They also can be applied directly to variables of type bool. For example, instead of writing

```
isElector = (age >= 18 && district == 23);
```

to assign a value to the Boolean variable isElector, we could use two intermediate Boolean variables, isVoter and isConstituent:

```
isVoter = (age >= 18);
isConstituent = (district == 23);
isElector = isVoter && isConstituent;
```

---

*In Boolean algebra, the pattern is formalized by a theorem called *DeMorgan's law*.

The two tables below summarize the results of applying && and || to a pair of logical expressions (represented here by Boolean variables x and y).

Value of x	Value of y	Value of x && y
true	true	true
true	false	false
false	true	false
false	false	false

Value of x	Value of y	Value of x || y
true	true	true
true	false	true
false	true	true
false	false	false

The following table summarizes the results of applying the ! operator to a logical expression (represented by Boolean variable x).

Value of x	Value of !x
true	false
false	true

Technically, the C++ operators !, &&, and || are not required to have logical expressions as operands. Their operands can be of any simple data type, even floating-point types. If an operand is not of type bool, its value is temporarily coerced to type bool as follows: A 0 value is coerced to false, and any nonzero value is coerced to true. As an example, you sometimes encounter C++ code that looks like this:

```
float height;
bool  badData;
   ⋮
cin >> height;
badData = !height;
```

The assignment statement says to set badData to true if the coerced value of height is false. That is, the statement really is saying, "Set badData to true if height equals

0.0." Although this assignment statement works correctly according to the C++ language, many programmers find the following statement to be more readable:

```
badData = (height == 0.0);
```

Throughout this text we apply the logical operators *only* to logical expressions, not to arithmetic expressions.

Caution: It's easy to confuse the logical operators && and || with two other C++ operators, & and |. We don't discuss the & and | operators here, but we'll tell you that they are used for manipulating individual bits within a memory cell—a role quite different from that of the logical operators. If you accidentally use & instead of &&, or | instead of ||, you won't get an error message from the compiler, but your program probably will compute wrong answers. Some programmers pronounce && as "and-and" and || as "or-or" to avoid making mistakes.

Short-Circuit Evaluation Consider the logical expression

```
i == 1 && j > 2
```

Some programming languages use *full evaluation* of logical expressions. With full evaluation, the computer first evaluates both subexpressions (both i == 1 and j > 2) before applying the && operator to produce the final result.

In contrast, C++ uses short-circuit (or conditional) evaluation of logical expressions. Evaluation proceeds from left to right, and the computer stops evaluating subexpressions as soon as possible—that is, as soon as it knows the truth value of the entire expression. How can the computer know if a lengthy logical expression yields true or false if it doesn't examine all the subexpressions? Let's look first at the AND operation.

> Short-circuit (conditional) evaluation Evaluation of a logical expression in left-to-right order with evaluation stopping as soon as the final truth value can be determined.

An AND operation yields the value true only if both of its operands are true. In the expression above, suppose that the value of i happens to be 95. The first subexpression yields false, so it isn't necessary even to look at the second subexpression. The computer stops evaluation and produces the final result of false.

With the OR operation, the left-to-right evaluation stops as soon as a subexpression yielding true is found. Remember that an OR produces a result of true if either one or both of its operands are true. Given this expression:

```
c <= d || e == f
```

if the first subexpression is true, evaluation stops and the entire result is true. The computer doesn't waste time with an unnecessary evaluation of the second subexpression.

May We Introduce

George Boole

Boolean algebra is named for its inventor, English mathematician George Boole, born in 1815. His father, a tradesman, began teaching him mathematics at an early age. But Boole initially was more interested in classical literature, languages, and religion—interests he maintained throughout his life. By the time he was 20, he had taught himself French, German, and Italian. He was well versed in the writings of Aristotle, Spinoza, Cicero, and Dante, and wrote several philosophical papers himself.

At 16, to help support his family, he took a position as a teaching assistant in a private school. His work there and a second teaching job left him little time to study. A few years later, he opened a school and began to learn higher mathematics on his own. In spite of his lack of formal training, his first scholarly paper was published in the *Cambridge Mathematical Journal* when he was just 24. Boole went on to publish over 50 papers and several major works before he died in 1864, at the peak of his career.

Boole's *The Mathematical Analysis of Logic* was published in 1847. It would eventually form the basis for the development of digital computers. In the book, Boole set forth the formal axioms of logic (much like the axioms of geometry) on which the field of symbolic logic is built.

Boole drew on the symbols and operations of algebra in creating his system of logic. He associated the value 1 with the universal set (the set representing everything in the universe) and the value 0 with the empty set, and restricted his system to these two quantities. He then defined operations that are analogous to subtraction, addition, and multiplication. Variables in the system have symbolic values. For example, if a Boolean variable P represents the set of all plants, then the expression $1 - P$ refers to the set of all things that are not plants. We can simplify the expression by using $-P$ to mean "*not* plants." ($0 - P$ is simply 0 because we can't remove elements from the empty set.) The subtraction operator in Boole's system corresponds to the ! (NOT) operator in C++. In a C++ program, we might set the value of the Boolean variable `plant` to `true` when the name of a plant is entered, whereas `!plant` is `true` when the name of anything else is input.

The expression $0 + P$ is the same as P. However, $0 + P + F$, where F is the set of all foods, is the set of all things that are either plants or foods. So the addition operator in Boole's algebra is the same as the C++ `||` (OR) operator.

The analogy can be carried to multiplication: $0 \times P$ is 0, and $1 \times P$ is P. But what is $P \times F$? It is the set of things that are both plants and foods. In Boole's system, the multiplication operator is the same as the `&&` (AND) operator.

In 1854, Boole published *An Investigation of the Laws of Thought, on Which Are Founded the Mathematical Theories of Logic and Probabilities*. In the book, he described theorems built on his axioms of logic and extended the algebra to show how probabilities could be computed in a logical system. Five years later, Boole published *Treatise on Differential Equations*, then *Treatise on the Calculus of Finite Differences*. The latter is one of the cornerstones of numerical analysis, which deals with the

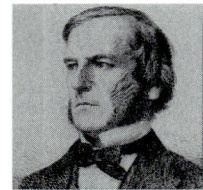

(continued) ▼

George Boole

accuracy of computations. (In Chapter 10, we examine the important role numerical analysis plays in computer programming.)

Boole received little recognition and few honors for his work. Given the importance of Boolean algebra in modern technology, it is hard to believe that his system of logic was not taken seriously until the early twentieth century. George Boole was truly one of the founders of computer science.

Precedence of Operators

In Chapter 3, we discussed the rules of precedence, the rules that govern the evaluation of complex arithmetic expressions. C++'s rules of precedence also govern relational and logical operators. Here's a list showing the order of precedence for the arithmetic, relational, and logical operators (with the assignment operator thrown in as well):

```
!    Unary +   Unary -          Highest precedence
*    /    %
+    -
<    <=    >    >=
==    !=
&&
||
=                               Lowest precedence
```

Operators on the same line in the list have the same precedence. If an expression contains several operators with the same precedence, most of the operators group (or *associate*) from left to right. For example, the expression

```
a / b * c
```

means (a / b) * c, not a / (b * c). However, the unary operators (!, unary +, unary -) group from right to left. Although you'd never have occasion to use this expression:

```
!!badData
```

the meaning of it is !(!badData) rather than the meaningless (!!)badData. Appendix B, "Precedence of Operators," lists the order of precedence for all operators in C++. In skimming the appendix, you can see that a few of the operators associate from right to left (for the same reason we just described for the ! operator).

Parentheses are used to override the order of evaluation in an expression. If you're not sure whether parentheses are necessary, use them anyway. The compiler disregards unnecessary parentheses. So if they clarify an expression, use them. Some programmers like to include extra parentheses when assigning a relational expression to a Boolean variable:

```
dataInvalid = (inputVal == 0);
```

The parentheses are not needed; the assignment operator has the lowest precedence of all the operators we've just listed. So we could write the statement as

```
dataInvalid = inputVal == 0;
```

but some people find the parenthesized version more readable.

One final comment about parentheses: C++, like other programming languages, requires that parentheses always be used in pairs. Whenever you write a complicated expression, take a minute to go through and pair up all of the opening parentheses with their closing counterparts.

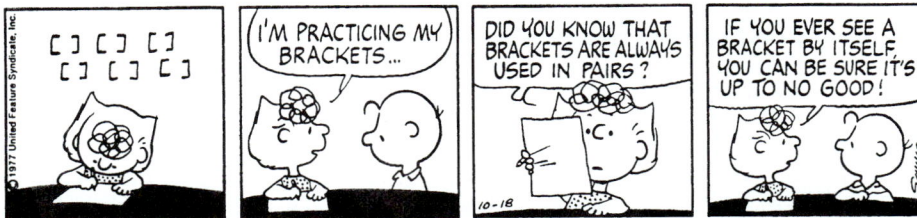

PEANUTS © UFS. Reprinted by permission.

Software Engineering Tip

Changing English Statements into Logical Expressions

In most cases, you can write a logical expression directly from an English statement or mathematical term in an algorithm. But you have to watch out for some tricky situations. Remember our sample logical expression:

```
midtermGrade == 'A' || finalGrade == 'A'
```

In English, you would be tempted to write this expression: "Midterm grade or final grade equals A." In C++, you can't write the expression as you would in English. That is,

```
midtermGrade || finalGrade == 'A'
```

(continued) ▼

Changing English Statements into Logical Expressions

won't work because the || operator is connecting a char value (midtermGrade) and a logical expression (finalGrade == 'A'). The two operands of || should be logical expressions. (Note that this expression is wrong in terms of logic, but it isn't "wrong" to the C++ compiler. Recall that the || operator may legally connect two expressions of any data type, so this example won't generate a syntax error message. The program will run, but it won't work the way you intended.)

A variation of this mistake is to express the English assertion "*i* equals either 3 or 4" as

```
i == 3 || 4
```

Again, the syntax is correct but the semantics are not. This expression always evaluates to true. The first subexpression, i == 3, may be true or false. But the second subexpression, 4, is nonzero and therefore is coerced to the value true. Thus, the || operation causes the entire expression to be true. We repeat: Use the || operator (and the && operator) only to connect two logical expressions. Here's what we want:

```
i == 3 || i == 4
```

In math books, you might see a notation like this:

$$12 < y < 24$$

which means "*y* is between 12 and 24." This expression is legal in C++ but gives an unexpected result. First, the relation 12 < y is evaluated, giving the result true or false. The computer then coerces this result to 1 or 0 in order to compare it with the number 24. Because both 1 and 0 are less than 24, the result is always true. To write this expression correctly in C++, you must use the && operator as follows:

```
12 < y && y < 24
```

Relational Operators with Floating-Point Types

So far, we've talked only about comparing int, char, and string values. Here we look at float values.

Do not compare floating-point numbers for equality. Because small errors in the rightmost decimal places are likely to arise when calculations are performed on floating-point numbers, two float values rarely are exactly equal. For example, consider the following code that uses two float variables named oneThird and x:

```
oneThird = 1.0 / 3.0;
x = oneThird + oneThird + oneThird;
```

We would expect x to contain the value 1.0, but it probably doesn't. The first assignment statement stores an *approximation* of 1/3 into oneThird, perhaps 0.333333. The second statement stores a value like 0.999999 into x. If we now ask the computer to compare x with 1.0, the comparison yields false.

Instead of testing floating-point numbers for equality, we test for *near* equality. To do so, we compute the difference between the two numbers and test to see if the result is less than some maximum allowable difference. For example, we often use comparisons like this:

```
fabs(r - s) < 0.00001
```

where fabs is the floating-point absolute value function from the C++ standard library. The expression fabs(r - s) computes the absolute value of the difference between two float variables r and s. If the difference is less than 0.00001, the two numbers are close enough to call them equal. We discuss this problem with floating-point accuracy in more detail in Chapter 10.

5.3 The If Statement

Now that we've seen how to write logical expressions, let's use them to alter the normal flow of control in a program. The *If statement* is the fundamental control structure that allows branches in the flow of control. With it, we can ask a question and choose a course of action: *If* a certain condition exists, *then* perform one action, *else* perform a different action.

At run time, the computer performs just one of the two actions, depending on the result of the condition being tested. Yet we must include the code for *both* actions in the program. Why? Because, depending on the circumstances, the computer can choose to execute *either* of them. The If statement gives us a way of including both actions in a program and gives the computer a way of deciding which action to take.

The If-Then-Else Form

In C++, the If statement comes in two forms: the *If-Then-Else* form and the *If-Then* form. Let's look first at the If-Then-Else. Here is its syntax template:

IfStatement (the If–Then–Else form)

```
if   ( Expression )
       Statement1A
else
       Statement1B
```

The expression in parentheses can be of any simple data type. Almost without exception, this will be a logical (Boolean) expression; if not, its value is implicitly coerced to

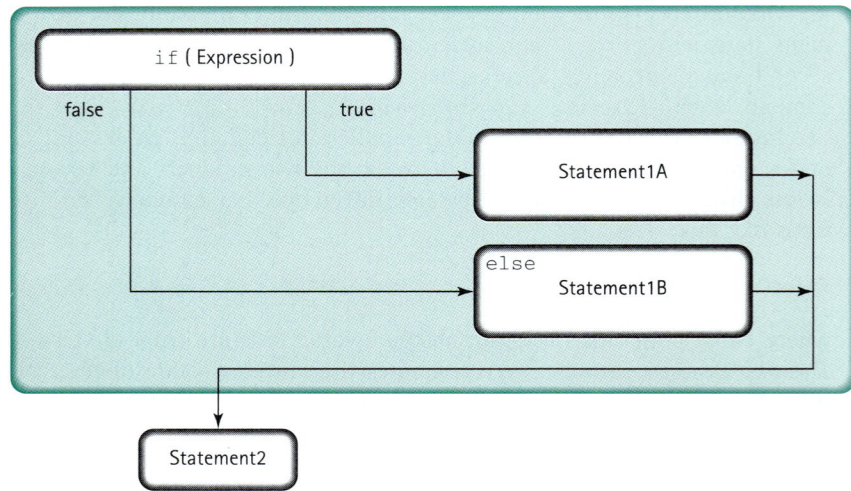

Figure 5–3   *If-Then-Else Flow of Control*

type `bool`. At run time, the computer evaluates the expression. If the value is `true`, the computer executes Statement1A. If the value of the expression is `false`, Statement1B is executed. Statement1A often is called the *then-clause;* Statement1B, the *else-clause.* Figure 5–3 illustrates the flow of control of the If-Then-Else. In the figure, Statement2 is the next statement in the program after the entire If statement.

Notice that a C++ If statement uses the reserved words `if` and `else` but does not include the word *then.* Still, we use the term *If-Then-Else* because it corresponds to how we say things in English: "*If* something is true, *then* do this, *else* do that."

The code fragment below shows how to write an If statement in a program. Observe the indentation of the then-clause and the else-clause, which makes the statement easier to read. And notice the placement of the statement following the If statement.

```
if (hours <= 40.0)
    pay = rate * hours;
else
    pay = rate * (40.0 + (hours - 40.0) * 1.5);
cout << pay;
```

In terms of instructions to the computer, the above code fragment says, "If `hours` is less than or equal to 40.0, compute the regular pay and then go on to execute the output statement. But if `hours` is greater than 40, compute the regular pay and the overtime pay, and then go on to execute the output statement." Figure 5–4 shows the flow of control of this If statement.

If-Then-Else often is used to check the validity of input. For example, before we ask the computer to divide by a data value, we should be sure that the value is not zero.

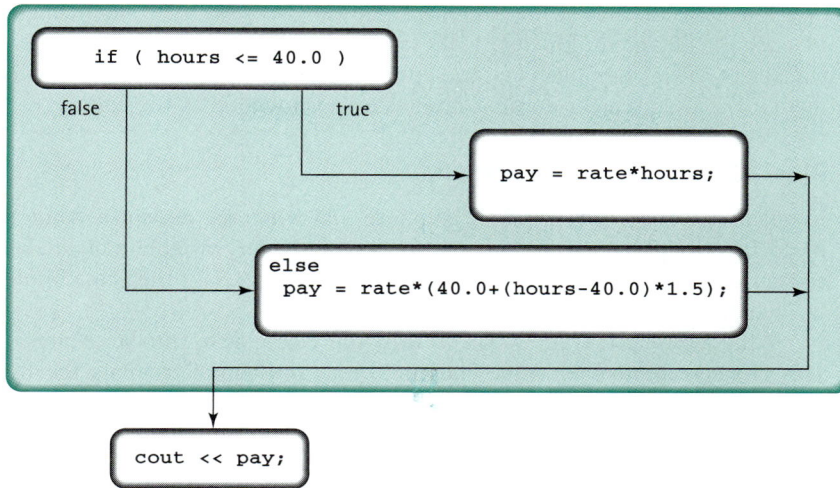

Figure 5–4   *Flow of Control for Calculating Pay*

(Even computers can't divide something by zero. If you try, most computers halt the execution of your program.) If the divisor is zero, our program should print out an error message. Here's the code:

```
if (divisor != 0)
    result = dividend / divisor;
else
    cout << "Division by zero is not allowed." << endl;
```

As another example of an If-Then-Else, suppose we want to determine where in a string variable the first occurrence (if any) of the letter *A* is located. Recall from Chapter 3 that the string class has a member function named find, which returns the position where the item was found (or the named constant string::npos if the item wasn't found). The following code outputs the result of the search:

```
string myString;
string::size_type pos;
        ⋮
pos = myString.find('A');
if (pos == string::npos)
    cout << "No 'A' was found" << endl;
else
    cout << "An 'A' was found in position " << pos << endl;
```

Before we look any further at If statements, take another look at the syntax template for the If-Then-Else. According to the template, there is no semicolon at the end of an If statement. In all of the program fragments above—the worker's pay, division-by-zero, and string search examples—there seems to be a semicolon at the end of each If statement. However, the semicolons belong to the statements in the else-clauses in those examples; assignment statements end in semicolons, as do output statements. The If statement doesn't have its own semicolon at the end.

Blocks (Compound Statements)

In our division-by-zero example, suppose that when the divisor is equal to zero we want to do *two* things: print the error message *and* set the variable named `result` equal to a special value like 9999. We would need two statements in the same branch, but the syntax template seems to limit us to one.

What we really want to do is turn the else-clause into a *sequence* of statements. This is easy. Remember from Chapter 2 that the compiler treats the block (compound statement)

```
{
    ⋮
}
```

like a single statement. If you put a { } pair around the sequence of statements you want in a branch of the If statement, the sequence of statements becomes a single block. For example:

```
if (divisor != 0)
    result = dividend / divisor;
else
{
    cout << "Division by zero is not allowed." << endl;
    result = 9999;
}
```

If the value of `divisor` is 0, the computer both prints the error message and sets the value of `result` to 9999 before continuing with whatever statement follows the If statement.

Blocks can be used in both branches of an If-Then-Else. For example:

```
if (divisor != 0)
{
    result = dividend / divisor;
    cout << "Division performed." << endl;
}
else
{
    cout << "Division by zero is not allowed." << endl;
    result = 9999;
}
```

When you use blocks in an If statement, there's a rule of C++ syntax to remember: *Never use a semicolon after the right brace of a block*. Semicolons are used only to terminate simple statements such as assignment statements, input statements, and output statements. If you look at the examples above, you won't see a semicolon after the right brace that signals the end of each block.

Matters of Style

Braces and Blocks

C++ programmers use different styles when it comes to locating the left brace of a block. The style we use puts the left and right braces directly below the words `if` and `else`, each brace on its own line:

```
if (n >= 2)
{
    alpha = 5;
    beta = 8;
}
else
{
    alpha = 23;
    beta = 12;
}
```

Another popular style is to place the left braces at the end of the `if` line and the `else` line; the right braces still line up directly below the words `if` and `else`. This way of formatting the If statement originated with programmers using the C language, the predecessor of C++.

```
if (n >= 2) {
    alpha = 5;
    beta = 8;
}
else {
    alpha = 23;
    beta = 12;
}
```

It makes no difference to the C++ compiler which style you use (and there are other styles as well). It's a matter of personal preference. Whichever style you use, though, you should always use the same style throughout a program. Inconsistency can confuse the person reading your program and give the impression of carelessness.

The If-Then Form

Sometimes you run into a situation where you want to say, "*If* a certain condition exists, *then* perform some action; otherwise, don't do anything." In other words, you want the computer to skip a sequence of instructions if a certain condition isn't met. You could do this by leaving the `else` branch empty, using only the null statement:

```
if (a <= b)
    c = 20;
else
    ;
```

Better yet, you can simply leave off the `else` part. The resulting statement is the If-Then form of the If statement. This is its syntax template:

IfStatement (the If-Then form)

```
if    ( Expression )
         Statement
```

Here's an example of an If-Then. Notice the indentation and the placement of the statement that follows the If-Then.

```
if (age < 18)
    cout << "Not an eligible ";
cout << "voter." << endl;
```

This statement means that if `age` is less than 18, first print "Not an eligible " and then print "voter." If `age` is not less than 18, skip the first output statement and go directly to print "voter." Figure 5–5 shows the flow of control for an If-Then.

Like the two branches in an If-Then-Else, the one branch in an If-Then can be a block. For example, let's say you are writing a program to compute income taxes. One of the lines on the tax form reads "Subtract line 23 from line 17 and enter result on line 24; if result is less than zero, enter zero and check box 24A." You can use an If-Then to do this in C++:

```
result = line17 - line23;
if (result < 0.0)
{
    cout << "Check box 24A" << endl;
    result = 0.0;
}
line24 = result;
```

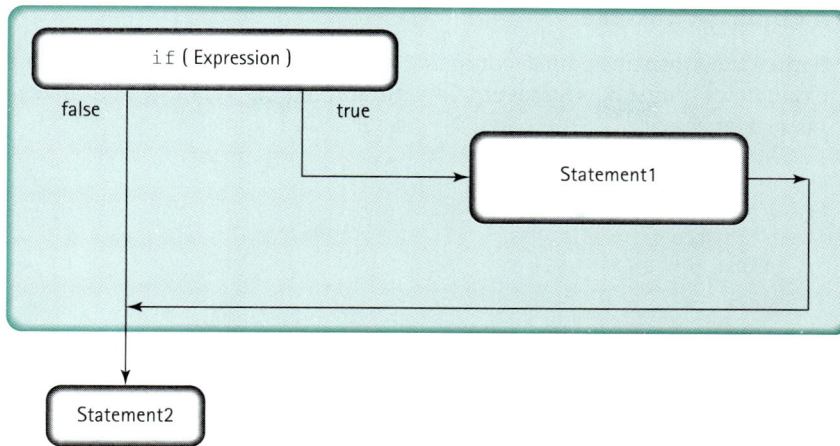

Figure 5–5   *If-Then Flow of Control*

This code does exactly what the tax form says it should. It computes the result of sub-tracting line 23 from line 17. Then it looks to see if `result` is less than 0. If it is, the fragment prints a message telling the user to check box 24A and then sets `result` to 0. Finally, the calculated result (or 0, if the result is less than 0) is stored into a variable named `line24`.

What happens if we leave out the left and right braces in the code fragment above? Let's look at it:

```
result = line17 - line23;                    // Incorrect version
if (result < 0.0)
    cout << "Check box 24A" << endl;
    result = 0.0;
line24 = result;
```

Despite the way we have indented the code, the compiler takes the then-clause to be a single statement—the output statement. If `result` is less than 0, the computer executes the output statement, then sets `result` to 0, and then stores `result` into `line24`. So far, so good. But if `result` is initially greater than or equal to 0, the computer skips the then-clause and proceeds to the statement following the If statement—the assignment statement that sets `result` to 0. The unhappy outcome is that `result` ends up as 0 no matter what its initial value was! The moral here is not to rely on indentation alone; you can't fool the compiler. If you want a compound statement for a then- or else-clause, you must include the left and right braces.

A Common Mistake

Earlier we warned against confusing the = operator and the == operator. Here is an example of a mistake that every C++ programmer is guaranteed to make at least once in his or her career:

```
cin >> n;
if (n = 3)                          // Wrong
    cout << "n equals 3";
else
    cout << "n doesn't equal 3";
```

This code segment *always* prints out

```
n equals 3
```

no matter what was input for n.

Here is the reason: We've used the wrong operator in the If test. The expression n = 3 is not a logical expression; it's called an *assignment expression*. (If an assignment is written as a separate statement ending with a semicolon, it's an assignment *statement*.) An assignment expression has a *value* (above, it's 3) and a *side effect* (storing 3 into n). In the If statement of our example, the computer finds the value of the tested expression to be 3. Because 3 is a nonzero value and thus is coerced to true, the then-clause is executed, no matter what the value of n is. Worse yet, the side effect of the assignment expression is to store 3 into n, destroying what was there.

Our intention is not to focus on assignment expressions; we discuss their use later in the book. What's important now is that you see the effect of using = when you meant to use ==. The program compiles correctly but runs incorrectly. When debugging a faulty program, always look at your If statements to see whether you've made this particular mistake.

5.4 Nested If Statements

There are no restrictions on what the statements in an If can be. Therefore, an If within an If is OK. In fact, an If within an If within an If is legal. The only limitation here is that people cannot follow a structure that is too involved, and readability is one of the marks of a good program.

When we place an If within an If, we are creating a *nested control structure*. Control structures nest much like mixing bowls do, with smaller ones tucked inside larger ones. Here's an example, written in pseudocode:

```
┌─────────────────────────────────────┐
│ IF today is Saturday or Sunday   ◄─── Outer If
│   ┌─────────────────────────────┐
│   │ IF it is raining         ◄─── Inner (nested) If
│   │   Sleep late
│   │ ELSE
│   │   Get up and go outside
│   └─────────────────────────────┘
│ ELSE
│   Go to work
└─────────────────────────────────────┘
```

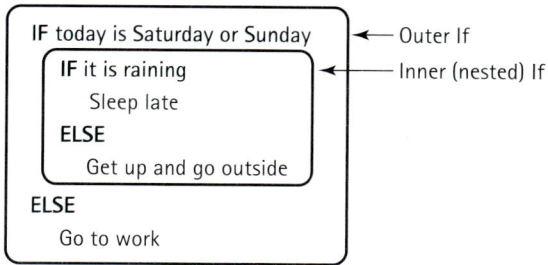

In general, any problem that involves a *multiway branch* (more than two alternative courses of action) can be coded using nested If statements. For example, to print out the name of a month given its number, we could use a sequence of If statements (unnested):

```
if (month == 1)
    cout << "January";
if (month == 2)
    cout << "February";
if (month == 3)
    cout << "March";
    ⋮
if (month == 12)
    cout << "December";
```

But the equivalent nested If structure,

```
if (month == 1)
    cout << "January";
else
    if (month == 2)              // Nested If
        cout << "February";
    else
        if (month == 3)              // Nested If
            cout << "March";
        else
            if (month == 4)              // Nested If
                ⋮
```

is more efficient because it makes fewer comparisons. The first version—the sequence of independent If statements—always tests every condition (all 12 of them), even if the first one is satisfied. In contrast, the nested If solution skips all remaining comparisons after one alternative has been selected. As fast as modern computers are, many applications require so much computation that inefficient algorithms can waste hours of computer time. Always be on the lookout for ways to make your programs more efficient, as long as doing so doesn't make them difficult for other programmers to understand. It's usually better to sacrifice a little efficiency for the sake of readability.

In the last example, notice how the indentation of the then- and else-clauses causes the statements to move continually to the right. Instead, we can use a special indentation style with deeply nested If-Then-Else statements to indicate that the complex structure is just choosing one of a set of alternatives. This general multiway branch is known as an *If-Then-Else-If* control structure:

```cpp
if (month == 1)
    cout << "January";
else if (month == 2)          // Nested If
    cout << "February";
else if (month == 3)          // Nested If
    cout << "March";
else if (month == 4)          // Nested If
    ⋮
else
    cout << "December";
```

This style prevents the indentation from marching continuously to the right. But, more important, it visually conveys the idea that we are using a 12-way branch based on the variable `month`.

It's important to note one difference between the sequence of If statements and the nested If: More than one alternative can be taken by the sequence of Ifs, but the nested If can select only one. To see why this is important, consider the analogy of filling out a questionnaire. Some questions are like a sequence of If statements, asking you to circle all the items in a list that apply to you (such as all your hobbies). Other questions ask you to circle only one item in a list (your age group, for example) and are thus like a nested If structure. Both kinds of questions occur in programming problems. Being able to recognize which type of question is being asked permits you to immediately select the appropriate control structure.

Another particularly helpful use of the nested If is when you want to select from a series of consecutive ranges of values. For example, suppose that we want to print out an appropriate activity for the outdoor temperature, given the following table.

Activity	Temperature
Swimming	Temperature > 85
Tennis	$70 <$ temperature ≤ 85
Golf	$32 <$ temperature ≤ 70
Skiing	$0 <$ temperature ≤ 32
Dancing	Temperature ≤ 0

At first glance, you may be tempted to write a separate If statement for each range of temperatures. On closer examination, however, it is clear that these If conditions are interdependent. That is, if one of the statements is executed, none of the others should be executed. We really are selecting one alternative from a set of possibilities—just the sort of situation in which we can use a nested If structure as a multiway branch. The only difference between this problem and our earlier example of printing the month name from its number is that we must check ranges of numbers in the If expressions of the branches.

When the ranges are consecutive, we can take advantage of that fact to make our code more efficient. We arrange the branches in consecutive order by range. Then, if a particular branch has been reached, we know that the preceding ranges have been eliminated from consideration. Thus, the If expressions must compare the temperature to only the lowest value of each range. Look at the following Activity program.

```cpp
//***************************************************************
// Activity program
// This program outputs an appropriate activity
// for a given temperature
//***************************************************************
#include <iostream>

using namespace std;

int main()
{
    int temperature;     // The outside temperature

    // Read and echo temperature

    cout << "Enter the outside temperature:" << endl;
    cin >> temperature;
    cout << "The current temperature is " << temperature << endl;

    // Print activity

    cout << "The recommended activity is ";
    if (temperature > 85)
        cout << "swimming." << endl;
    else if (temperature > 70)
        cout << "tennis." << endl;
    else if (temperature > 32)
        cout << "golf." << endl;
    else if (temperature > 0)
        cout << "skiing." << endl;
```

```
    else
        cout << "dancing." << endl;

    return 0;
}
```

To see how the If-Then-Else-If structure in this program works, consider the branch that tests for `temperature` greater than 70. If it has been reached, we know that `temperature` must be less than or equal to 85 because that condition causes this particular `else` branch to be taken. Thus, we only need to test whether `temperature` is above the bottom of this range (> 70). If that test fails, then we enter the next else-clause knowing that `temperature` must be less than or equal to 70. Each successive branch checks the bottom of its range until we reach the final `else`, which takes care of all the remaining possibilities.

Note that if the ranges aren't consecutive, then we must test the data value against both the highest and lowest value of each range. We still use an If-Then-Else-If because that is the best structure for selecting a single branch from multiple possibilities, and we may arrange the ranges in consecutive order to make them easier for a human reader to follow. But there is no way to reduce the number of comparisons when there are gaps between the ranges.

The Dangling `else`

When If statements are nested, you may find yourself confused about the `if-else` pairings. That is, to which `if` does an `else` belong? For example, suppose that if a student's average is below 60, we want to print "Failing"; if it is at least 60 but less than 70, we want to print "Passing but marginal"; and if it is 70 or greater, we don't want to print anything.

We code this information with an If-Then-Else nested within an If-Then:

```
if (average < 70.0)
    if (average < 60.0)
        cout << "Failing";
    else
        cout << "Passing but marginal";
```

How do we know to which `if` the `else` belongs? Here is the rule that the C++ compiler follows: In the absence of braces, an `else` is always paired with the closest preceding `if` that doesn't already have an `else` paired with it. We indented the code to reflect this pairing.

Suppose we write the fragment like this:

```
if (average >= 60.0)        // Incorrect version
    if (average < 70.0)
        cout << "Passing but marginal";
else
    cout << "Failing";
```

Here we want the `else` branch attached to the outer If statement, not the inner, so we indent the code as you see it. But indentation does not affect the execution of the code. Even though the `else` aligns with the first `if`, the compiler pairs it with the second `if`. An `else` that follows a nested If-Then is called a *dangling else*. It doesn't logically belong with the nested If but is attached to it by the compiler.

To attach the `else` to the first `if`, not the second, you can turn the outer then-clause into a block:

```
if (average >= 60.0)         // Correct version
{
    if (average < 70.0)
        cout << "Passing but marginal";
}
else
    cout << "Failing";
```

The { } pair indicates that the inner If statement is complete, so the `else` must belong to the outer `if`.

5.5 Testing the State of an I/O Stream

In Chapter 4, we talked about the concept of input and output streams in C++. We introduced the classes `istream`, `ostream`, `ifstream`, and `ofstream`. We said that any of the following can cause an input stream to enter the fail state:

- Invalid input data
- An attempt to read beyond the end of a file
- An attempt to open a nonexistent file for input

C++ provides a way to check whether a stream is in the fail state. In a logical expression, you simply use the name of the stream object (such as `cin`) as if it were a Boolean variable:

```
if (cin)
    ⋮


if ( !inFile )
    ⋮
```

When you do this, you are said to be **testing the state of the stream**. The result of the test is either `true` (meaning the last I/O operation on that stream succeeded) or `false` (meaning the last I/O operation failed).

> **Testing the state of a stream** The act of using a C++ stream object in a logical expression as if it were a Boolean variable; the result is `true` if the last I/O operation on that stream succeeded, and `false` otherwise.

Conceptually, you want to think of a stream object in a logical expression as being a Boolean variable with a value `true` (the stream state is OK) or `false` (the state isn't OK).

Notice in the second If statement above that we typed spaces around the expression `!inFile`. The spaces are not required by C++ but are there for readability. Without the spaces, it is harder to see the exclamation mark:

```
if (!inFile)
```

In an If statement, the way you phrase the logical expression depends on what you want the then-clause to do. The statement

```
if (inFile)
    ⋮
```

executes the then-clause if the last I/O operation on `inFile` succeeded. The statement

```
if ( !inFile )
    ⋮
```

executes the then-clause if `inFile` is in the fail state. (And remember that once a stream is in the fail state, it remains so. Any further I/O operations on that stream are null operations.)

Here's an example that shows how to check whether an input file was opened successfully:

```
//************************************************************
// StreamState program
// This program demonstrates testing the state of a stream
//************************************************************
#include <iostream>
#include <fstream>      // For file I/O

using namespace std;

int main()
{
    int        height;
    int        width;
    ifstream inFile;

    inFile.open("measures.dat");        // Attempt to open input file
    if ( !inFile )                      // Was it opened?
    {
        cout << "Can't open the input file.";   // No--print message
        return 1;                                // Terminate program
    }
    inFile >> height >> width;
```

```
    cout << "For a height of " << height << endl
        << "and a width of " << width << endl
        << "the area is " << height * width << endl;
    return 0;
}
```

In this program, we begin by attempting to open the disk file `measures.dat` for input. Immediately, we check to see whether the attempt succeeded. If it was successful, the value of the expression `!inFile` in the If statement is `false` and the then-clause is skipped. The program proceeds to read data from the file and then perform a computation. It concludes by executing the statement

```
return 0;
```

With this statement, the `main` function returns control to the computer's operating system. Recall that the function value returned by `main` is known as the exit status. The value 0 signifies normal completion of the program. Any other value (typically 1, 2, 3, …) means that something went wrong.

Let's trace through the program again, assuming we weren't able to open the input file. Upon return from the `open` function, the stream `inFile` is in the fail state. In the If statement, the value of the expression `!inFile` is `true`. Thus, the then-clause is executed. The program prints an error message to the user and then terminates, returning an exit status of 1 to inform the operating system of an abnormal termination of the program. (Our choice of the value 1 for the exit status is purely arbitrary. System programmers sometimes use several different values in a program to signal different reasons for program termination. But most people just use the value 1.)

Whenever you open a data file for input, be sure to test the stream state before proceeding. If you forget to, and the computer cannot open the file, your program quietly continues executing and ignores any input operations on the file.

Problem–Solving Case Study

BMI Calculator

PROBLEM A great deal has been said about how overweight much of the American population is today. You can't pick up a magazine that doesn't have an article on the health problems caused by obesity. Rather than looking at a chart that shows the average weight for a particular height, a measure called the Body Mass Index (BMI), which computes a ratio of your weight and height, has become a popular tool to determine an appropriate weight. The formula for non-metric values is:

$$BMI = weight * 703 / height^2$$

BMI correlates with body fat, which can be used to determine if a weight is unhealthy for a certain height. Although the discussion of the BMI in the media is fairly recent, the formula was developed by Adolphe Quetelet, a nineteenth century Belgian statistician. Do a search of the Internet for "body mass index" and you will find more than a million hits. In these references, the formula remains the same but the interpretation of the result varies, depending upon age and sex. Here is the most commonly used generic interpretation:

BMI	Interpretation
< 20	Underweight
20–25	Normal
26–30	Overweight
over 30	Obese

Write a program that calculates the BMI given a weight and height and prints out an appropriate message.

INPUT The problem statement says that the formula is for non-metric values. This means that the weight should be in pounds and the height should be in inches. Thus, the input should be two `float` values: weight and height.

OUTPUT
Prompts for the input values
A message based on the BMI

DISCUSSION To calculate the BMI, you read in the weight and height and plug them into the formula. If you square the height, you must include `<cmath>` to access the `pow` function. It is more efficient to just multiply height by itself.

BMI = weight * 703 / (height * height)

If you were calculating this by hand, you would probably notice if the weight or height were negative and question it. If the semantics of your data imply that the values should be nonnegative, then your program should test to be sure that they are. The program should test each value and use a Boolean variable to report the results. Here is the main module for this algorithm.

Main	Level 0

```
Get Data
Test data
IF data are OK
    Calculate BMI
    Print message indicating status
ELSE
    Print "Invalid data; weight and height must be positive."
```

Which of these steps require(s) expansion? *Get data*, *Test data*, and *Print message indicating status* all require multiple statements in order to solve their particular subproblem. On the other hand, we can translate *Print "Invalid Data: ..."* directly into a C++ output statement. What about the step *CalculateBMI*? We can write it as a single C++ statement, but there's another level of detail that we must fill in—the actual formula to be used. Because the formula is at a lower level of detail than the rest of the main module, we choose to expand *CalculateBMI* as a level 1 module.

Get Data   **Level 1**

> Prompt for weight
> Read weight
> Prompt for height
> Read height

Test Data

> IF weight < 0 OR height < 0
>   Set dataAreOK to false
> ELSE
>   Set dataAreOK to true

Calculate BMI

> Set bodyMassIndex to weight * 703 / (height * height)

Print Message Indicating Status

The problem doesn't say exactly what the message should be, other than reporting the status. Why not jazz up the output a little by printing an appropriate message along with the status.

Status	Message
Underweight	Have a milk shake.
Normal	Have a glass of milk.
Overweight	Have a glass of iced tea.
Obese	See your doctor.

```
Print "Your body mass index is ", bodyMassIndex,  '.'
Print "Interpretation and instructions."
IF bodyMassIndex <20
    Print "Underweight: Have a milk shake."
ELSE IF bodyMassIndex <= 25
    Print "Normal: Have a glass of milk."
ELSE IF bodyMassIndex <= 30
    Print "Overweight: Have a glass of iced tea."
ELSE
    Print "Obese: See your doctor."
```

Module Structure Chart

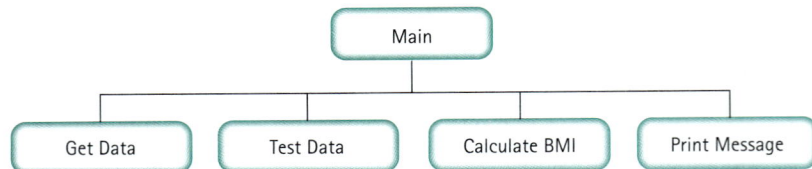

Constants

Name	Value	Function
BMI_CONSTANT	703	Formula constant

Variables

Name	Data Type	Description
weight	float	Weight in pounds
height	float	Height in inches
bodyMassIndex	float	Body mass index
dataAreOK	bool	Reports if data are ok

```
//*************************************************************************
// BMI Program
// This program calculates the body mass index (BMI) given a weight
// in pounds and a height in inches and prints a health message
```

```cpp
// based on the BMI. Input in English measures.
//*********************************************************************

#include <iostream>

using namespace std;

int main()
{
    const int BMI_CONSTANT = 703;         // Constant in non-metric formula
    float weight;                          // Weight in weight
    float height;                          // Height in height
    float bodyMassIndex;                   // Appropriate BMI
    bool dataAreOK;                        // True if data are non-negative

    // Prompt for and input weight and height
    cout << "Enter your weight in pounds. " << endl;
    cin >> weight;
    cout << "Enter your height in inches. " << endl;
    cin >> height;

    // Test Data
    if (weight < 0 || height < 0)
        dataAreOK = false;
    else
        dataAreOK = true;

    if ( dataAreOK)
    {
        // Calculate body mass index

        bodyMassIndex = weight * BMI_CONSTANT / (height * height);

        // Print message indicating status

        cout << "Your body mass index is " << bodyMassIndex
            << ". " << endl;
        cout << "Interpretation and instructions. " << endl;
        if (bodyMassIndex < 20)
            cout << "Underweight: Have a milk shake." << endl;
        else if (bodyMassIndex <= 25)
            cout << "Normal: Have a glass of milk."  << endl;
        else if (bodyMassIndex <=  30)
```

```
            cout << "Overweight: Have a glass of iced tea."  << endl;
        else
            cout << "Obese: See your doctor." << endl;
    }
    else
        cout << "Invalid data; weight and height must be positive."
            << endl;
    return 0;
}
```

Here are screen shots with both good and bad data.

```
C:\PPSC++\BMI\BMI.exe                                              _ □ ×
Enter your weight in pounds.
124
Enter your height in inches.
63.5
Your body mass index is 21.6187.
Interpretation and instructions.
Normal: Have a glass of milk.
```

```
C:\PPSC++\BMI\BMI.exe                                              _ □ ×
Enter your weight in pounds.
-124
Enter your height in inches.
63.5
Invalid data; weight and height must be positive.
```

In this program, we use a nested If structure that is easy to understand although somewhat inefficient. We assign a value to `dataAreOK` in one statement before testing it in the next. We could reduce the code by writing:

```
dataAreOK = !(weight < 0 || height < 0);
```

Using DeMorgan's law, we also could write this statement as:

```
dataAreOK = (weight >= 0 && height >= 0);
```

In fact, we could reduce the code even more by eliminating the variable `dataAreOK` and using:

```
if (weight => 0 && height >= 0)
    :
```

in place of

```
if (dataAreOK)
    :
```

To convince yourself that these three variations work, try them by hand with some test data. If all of these statements do the same thing, how do you choose which one to use? If your goal is efficiency, the final variation—the compound condition in the main If statement—is best. If you are trying to express as clearly as possible what your code is doing, the longer form shown in the program may be best. The other variations lie somewhere in between. (However, some people would find the compound condition in the main If statement to be not only the most efficient, but also the clearest to understand.) There are no absolute rules to follow here, but the general guideline is to strive for clarity, even if you must sacrifice a little efficiency.

Testing and Debugging

In Chapter 1, we discussed the problem-solving and implementation phases of computer programming. Testing is an integral part of both phases. Here, we test both phases of the process used to develop the BMI program. Testing in the problem-solving phase is done after the solution is developed but before it is implemented. In the implementation phase, we test after the algorithm is translated into a program, and again after the program has compiled successfully. The compilation itself constitutes another stage of testing that is performed automatically.

Testing in the Problem-Solving Phase: The Algorithm Walk-Through

Determining Preconditions and Postconditions   To test during the problem-solving phase, we do a *walk-through* of the algorithm. For each module in the functional decomposition, we establish an assertion called a precondition and another called a postcondition. A **precondition** is an assertion that must be true before a module is executed in order for the module to execute correctly. A **postcondition** is an assertion that should be true after the module has executed, if it has done its job correctly. To test a module, we "walk through" the algorithmic steps to confirm that they produce the required postcondition, given the stated precondition.

> **Precondition** An assertion that must be true before a module begins executing.
>
> **Postcondition** An assertion that should be true after a module has executed.

Our algorithm has five modules: the main module, Get Data, Test Data, Calculate BMI, and Print Message Indicating Status. Usually there is no precondition for a main module. Our main module's postcondition is that it outputs the correct results, given the correct input. More specifically, the postcondition for the main module is:

- The computer has input two real values into `weight` and `height`.

- If the input is invalid, an error message has been printed; otherwise, the body mass index has been calculated and an appropriate message has been printed based on the result.

Because Get Data is the first module executed in the algorithm and because it does not assume anything about the contents of the variables it is about to manipulate, it has no precondition. Its postcondition is that it has input two real values into `weight` and `height`.

The precondition for module Test Data is that `weight` and `height` have been assigned meaningful values. Its postcondition is that `dataAreOK` contains `true` if the values in `weight` and `height` are nonnegative; otherwise, `dataAreOK` contains `false`.

The precondition for module Calculate BMI is that `weight` and `height` contain meaningful values. Its postcondition is that the variable named `bodyMassIndex` contains the evaluation of the BMI formula (weight * 703 / (height * height)).

The precondition for module Print Message Indicating Status is that `bodyMassIndex` contains the result of evaluating the BMI formula. Its postcondition is that appropriate documentation and the value in `bodyMassIndex` have been printed, along with the messages: "Underweight: Have a milk shake." if the BMI value is less than 20; "Normal: Have a glass of milk." if the value is less than or equal to 26; "Overweight: Have a glass of ice tea." if the value is less than or equal to 30; and "Obese: See your doctor." if the value is greater than 30.

Below the module preconditions and postconditions are summarized in tabular form. In the table, we use *AND* with its usual meaning in an assertion—the logical AND operation. Also, a phrase like "`someVariable` is assigned" is an abbreviated way of asserting that `someVariable` has already been assigned a meaningful value.

Module	Precondition	Postcondition
Main	—	Two float values have been input AND if the input is valid, the BMI formula is calculated and the value is printed with an appropriate message; otherwise, an error message has been printed.
Get Data	—	`weight` and `height` have been input
Test Data	`weight` and `height` are assigned values	`dataAreOK` contains `true` if `weight` and `height` are nonnegative; otherwise, `dataAreOK` contains `false`.
Calculate BMI	`weight` and `height` are assigned values	`bodyMassIndex` contains the evaluation of the BMI formula.
Print Message Indicating Status	`bodyMassIndex` contains the evaluation of the BMI formula	The value of `bodyMassIndex` has been printed, along with a message interpreting the value.

Performing the Algorithm Walk-Through   Now that we've established the preconditions and postconditions, we walk through the main module. At this point, we are concerned only with the steps in the main module, so for now we assume that each lower-level module executes correctly. At each step, we must determine the current conditions. If the step is a reference to another module, we must verify that the precondition of that module is met by the current conditions.

We begin with the first statement in the main module. Get Data does not have a precondition, and we assume that Get Data satisfies its postcondition that it correctly inputs two real values into `weight` and `height`.

The precondition for module Test Data is that `weight` and `height` are assigned values. This must be the case if Get Data's postcondition is true. Again, because we are concerned only with the step at level 0, we assume that Test Data satisfies its postcondition that `dataAreOK` contains `true` or `false`, depending on the input values.

Next, the If statement checks to see if `dataAreOK` is `true`. If it is, the algorithm performs the then-clause. Assuming that Calculate BMI correctly evaluates the BMI formula and that Print Message Indicating Status prints the result and the appropriate message (remember, we're assuming that the lower-level modules are correct for now), then the If statement's then-clause is correct. If the value in `dataAreOK` is `false`, the algorithm performs the else-clause and prints an error message.

We now have verified that the main (level 0) module is correct, assuming the level 1 modules are correct. The next step is to examine each module at level 1 and answer this question: If the level 2 modules (if any) are assumed to be correct, does this level 1 module do what it is supposed to do? We simply repeat the walk-through process for each module, starting with its particular precondition. In this example, there are no level 2 modules, so the level 1 modules must be complete.

Get Data correctly reads in two values—`weight` and `height`—thereby satisfying its postcondition. (The next refinement is to code this instruction in C++. Whether it is coded correctly or not is *not* an issue in this phase; we deal with the code when we perform testing in the implementation phase.)

Test Data checks to see if both variables contain nonnegative values. The If condition correctly uses OR operators to combine the relational expressions so that if either of them are `true`, the then-clause is executed. It thus assigns `false` to `dataAreOK` if either of the numbers are negative; otherwise, it assigns `true`. The module therefore satisfies its postcondition.

Calculate BMI evaluates the BMI formula: weight * 703 / (height * height). The required postcondition therefore is true. But what if the value of height is 0? Oh, dear! We checked that the inputs are nonnegative, but forgot that height is used as a divisor and thus cannot be 0. We'll need to fix this problem before we release this program for general use.

Print Message Indicating Status outputs the value in `bodyMassIndex` with appropriate documentation. It then compares the result to the standards and prints the appropriate interpretation. "Underweight: Have a milk shake." is printed if the value is less than 20, "Normal: Have a glass of milk." if the value is less than or equal to 26, "Overweight: Have a glass of ice tea." if the value is less than or equal to 30, and "Obese: See your doctor." if the value is greater than 30. Thus, the module satisfies its postcondition.

Once we've completed the algorithm walk-through, we have to correct any discrepancies and repeat the process. When we know that the modules do what they are supposed to do, we start translating the algorithm into our programming language.

A standard postcondition for any program is that the user has been notified of invalid data. You should *validate* every input value for which any restrictions apply. A data-validation If statement tests an input value and outputs an error message if the value is not acceptable. (We validated the data when we tested for negative scores in the BMI program.) The best place to validate data is immediately after it is input. To satisfy the data-validation postcondition, the algorithm also should test the input values to ensure that they aren't too large or too small.

B.C.   **by johnny hart**

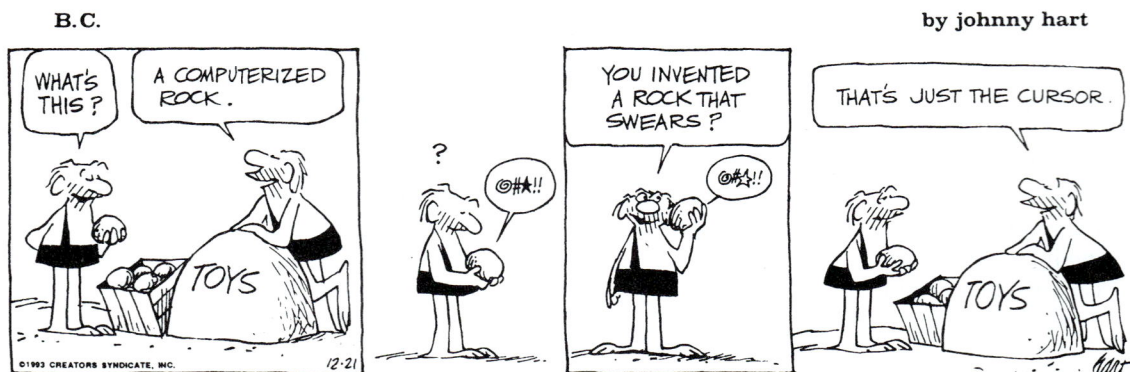

By permission of Johnny Hart and Creators Syndicate, Inc.

Testing in the Implementation Phase

Now that we've talked about testing in the problem-solving phase, we turn to testing in the implementation phase. In this phase, you need to test at several points.

Code Walk-Through   After the code is written, you should go over it line by line to be sure that you've faithfully reproduced the algorithm—a process known as a *code walk-through*. In a team programming situation, you ask other team members to walk through the algorithm and code with you, to double-check the design and code.

Execution Trace   You also should take some actual values and hand-calculate what the output should be by doing an *execution trace* (or *hand trace*). When the program is executed, you can use these same values as input and check the results.

The computer is a very literal device—it does exactly what we tell it to do, which may or may not be what we want it to do. We try to make sure that a program does what we want by tracing the execution of the statements.

We use a nonsense program below to demonstrate the technique. We keep track of the values of the program variables on the right-hand side. Variables with undefined values are indicated with a dash. When a variable is assigned a value, that value is listed in the appropriate column.

Statement	Value of		
	a	b	c
`const int x = 5;`			
`int main()`			
`{`			
`    int a, b, c;`	—	—	—
`    b = 1;`	—	1	—
`    c = x + b;`	—	1	6
`    a = x + 4;`	9	1	6
`    a = c;`	6	1	6
`    b = c;`	6	6	6
`    a = a + b + c;`	18	6	6
`    c = c % x;`	18	6	1
`    c = c * a;`	18	6	18
`    a = a % b;`	0	6	18
`    cout << a << b << c;`	0	6	18
`    return 0;`	0	6	18
`}`			

Now that you've seen how the technique works, let's apply it to the BMI program. We list only the executable statement portion here. The input values are 124 and 63.5.

The then-clause of the first If statement is not executed for these input data, so we do not fill in any of the variable columns to its right. The then-clause of the second If statement is executed, and thus, the else-clause is not. The else-clause of the third If statement is executed, which is another If statement. The then-clause is executed here, leaving the rest of the code unexecuted. We always create columns for all of the variables, even if we know that some will stay empty. Why? Because it's possible that later we'll encounter an erroneous reference to an empty variable; having a column for the variable reminds us to check for just such an error.

Statement	weight	height	BMI	dataIsOK
`cout << "Enter your weight in pounds. " << endl;`	—	—	—	—
`cin >> weight;`	124	—	—	—
`cout << "Enter your height in inches. " << endl;`	124	—	—	—
`cin >> height;`	124	63.5	—	—
`if (weight < 0 || height < 0)`	124	63.5	—	—
`    dataAreOK = false;`				
`else`				
`    dataAreOK = true;`	124	63.5	—	true
`if ( dataAreOK)`	124	63.5	—	true
`{`				
`    bodyMassIndex = weight * BMI_CONSTANT /`				
`        (height * height);`	124	63.5	21.087	true
`    cout << "Your body mass index is "`				
`        << bodyMassIndex << ". " << endl;`	124	63.5	21.087	true
`    cout << "Interpretation and instructions. "`				
`        << endl;`	124	63.5	21.087	true
`    if (bodyMassIndex < 20)`	124	63.5	21.087	true
`        cout <<"Underweight: Have a milk shake."`				
`            << endl;`				
`    else if (bodyMassIndex <= 25)`	124	63.5	21.087	true
`        cout << "Normal: Have a glass of milk."`				
`            << endl;`	124	63.5	21.087	true
`    else if (bodyMassIndex <= 30)`				
`        cout <<`				
`            "Overweight: Have a glass of ice tea."`				
`                << endl;`				
`    else`				
`        cout << "Obese: See your doctor."`				
`            << endl;`				
`}`				
`else`				
`    cout << "Invalid data; weight "`				
`        << "and height must be positive."`				
`        << endl;`				
`return 0;`	124	63.5	21.087	true

When a program contains branches, it's a good idea to retrace its execution with different input data so that each branch is traced at least once. In the next section, we describe how to develop data sets that test each of a program's branches.

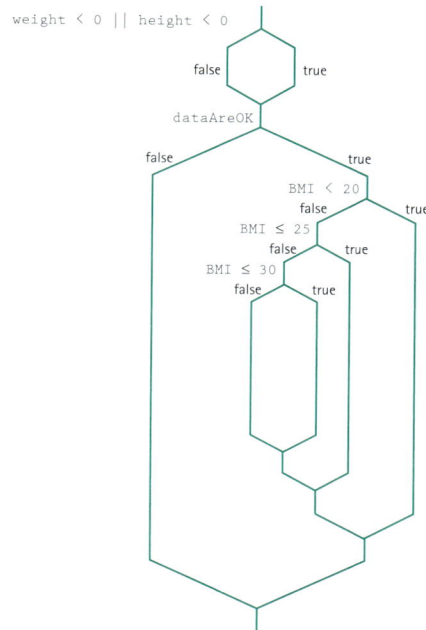

Figure 5–6   *Branching Structure for BMI Program*

Testing Selection Control Structures   To test a program with branches, we need to execute each branch at least once and verify the results. For example, in the BMI program there are five If-Then-Else statements (see Figure 5–6). We need a series of data sets to test the different branches. For example, the following sets of input values for `weight` and `height` cause all of the branches to be executed:

Data Set	Weight in Pounds	Height in Inches	Status
1	110.0	67.5	Underweight
2	120.0	63.0	Normal
3	145.0	62.0	Overweight
4	176.6	60.0	Obese
5	-100	65.0	Error message

Figure 5–7 shows the flow of control through the branching structure of the BMI program for each of these data sets. Every branch in the program is executed at least once through this series of test runs; eliminating any of the test data sets would leave at least one branch untested. This series of data sets provides what is called *minimum complete coverage* of the program's branching structure. Whenever you test a program with branches in it, you should design a series of tests that covers all of the branches. It may

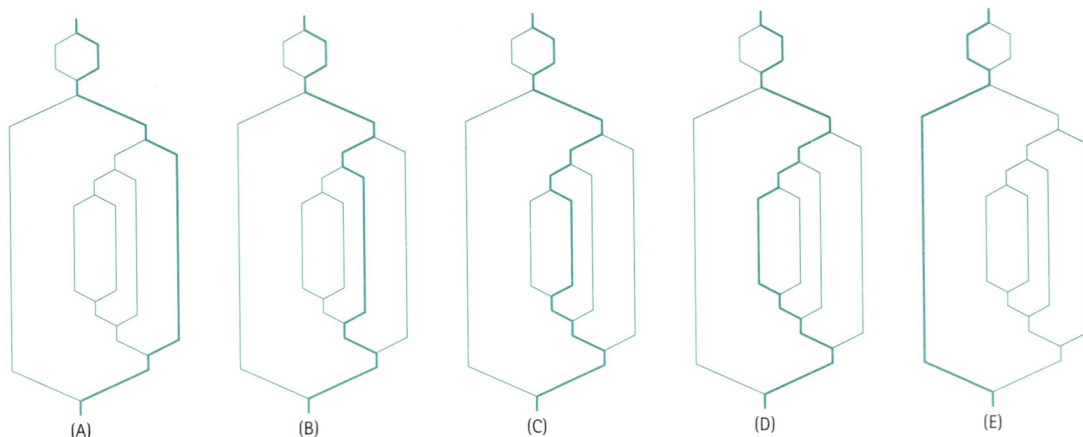

Figure 5-7   *Flow of Control Through BMI Program for Each of Five Data Sets*

help to draw diagrams like those in Figure 5–7 so that you can see which branches are being executed.

Because an action in one branch of a program often affects processing in a later branch, it is critical to test as many *combinations of branches*, or paths, through a program as possible. By doing so, we can be sure that there are no interdependencies that could cause problems. Of course, some combinations of branches may be impossible to follow. For example, if the else is taken in the first branch of the BMI program, the else in the second branch cannot be taken. Shouldn't we try all possible paths? Yes, in theory we should. However, the number of paths in even a small program can be very large.

The approach to testing that we've used here is called *code coverage* because the test data are designed by looking at the code of the program. Code coverage also is called *white box* (or *clear box*) *testing* because we are allowed to see the program code while designing the tests. Another approach to testing, *data coverage*, attempts to test as many allowable data values as possible without regard to the program code. Because we need not see the code in this form of testing, it also is called *black box testing*—we would design the same set of tests even if the code were hidden in a black box.

Complete data coverage is as impractical as complete code coverage for many programs. For example, if a program has four int input values, there are approximately $(2 * \text{INT\_MAX})^4$ possible inputs. (INT_MAX and INT_MIN are constants declared in the header file climits. They represent the largest and smallest possible int values, respectively, on your particular computer and C++ compiler.)

Often, testing is a combination of these two strategies. Instead of trying every possible data value (data coverage), we examine the code (code coverage) and look for ranges of values for which processing is identical. Then we test the values at the boundaries and, sometimes, a value in the middle of each range. For example, a simple condition such as

```
alpha < 0
```

divides the integers into two ranges:

1. `INT_MIN through -1`
2. `0 through INT_MAX`

Thus, we should test the four values `INT_MIN`, −1, 0, and `INT_MAX`. A compound condition such as

```
alpha >= 0 && alpha <= 100
```

divides the integers into three ranges:

1. `INT_MIN through -1`
2. `0 through 100`
3. `101 through INT_MAX`

Thus, we have six values to test. In addition, to verify that the relational operators are correct, we should test for values of 1 (> 0) and 99 (< 100).

Conditional branches are only one factor in developing a testing strategy. We consider more of these factors in later chapters.

The Test Plan

We've discussed strategies and techniques for testing programs, but how do you approach the testing of a specific program? You do it by designing and implementing a test plan—a document that specifies the test cases that should be tried, the reason for each test case, and the expected output. Implementing a test plan involves running the program using the data specified by the test cases in the plan and checking and recording the results.

> **Test plan** A document that specifies how a program is to be tested.
>
> **Test plan implementation** Using the test cases specified in a test plan to verify that a program outputs the predicted results.

The test plan should be developed together with the functional decomposition. As you create each module, write out its precondition and postcondition and note the test data required to verify them. Consider code coverage and data coverage to see if you've left out tests for any aspects of the program (if you've forgotten something, it probably also indicates that a precondition or postcondition is incomplete).

The following table shows a partial test plan for the BMI program. It has six test cases. The first four cases test the different paths through the program for valid data. Two more test cases check that each of the weight and height are validated appropriately by separately entering an invalid score for each.

We should test the program on the end cases; that is, where the BMI is exactly 20, 25, and 30. Because the BMI is calculated and not input, it is difficult to come up with the appropriate input values. The Case Study Follow-Up Exercises asks you to look at this problem, complete this test plan, and implement it.

Test Plan for BMI Program

Reason for Test Case	Input Values	Expected Output	Observed Output
Underweight case	110, 67.5	Your body mass index is 16.9723. Interpretation and instructions. Underweight: Have a milk shake.	
Normal case	120, 63	Your body mass index is 21.2547. Interpretation and instructions. Normal: Have a glass of milk.	
Overweight case	145, 62	Your body mass index is 26.518. Interpretation and instructions. Overweight: Have a glass of ice tea.	
Obese case	176.6, 60	Your body mass index is 34.4861. Interpretation and instructions. Obese: See your doctor.	
Negative weight	-120, 63	Invalid data; weight and height must be positive.	
Negative height	120, -63	Invalid data; weight and height must be positive.	

Implementing a test plan does not guarantee that a program is completely correct. It means only that a careful, systematic test of the program has not demonstrated any bugs. The situation shown in Figure 5–8 is analogous to trying to test a program without a plan—depending only on luck, you may completely miss the fact that a program contains numerous errors. Developing and implementing a written test plan, on the other hand, casts a wide net that is much more likely to find errors.

Tests Performed Automatically During Compilation and Execution

Once a program is coded and test data has been prepared, it is ready for compiling. The compiler has two responsibilities: to report any errors and (if there are no errors) to translate the program into object code.

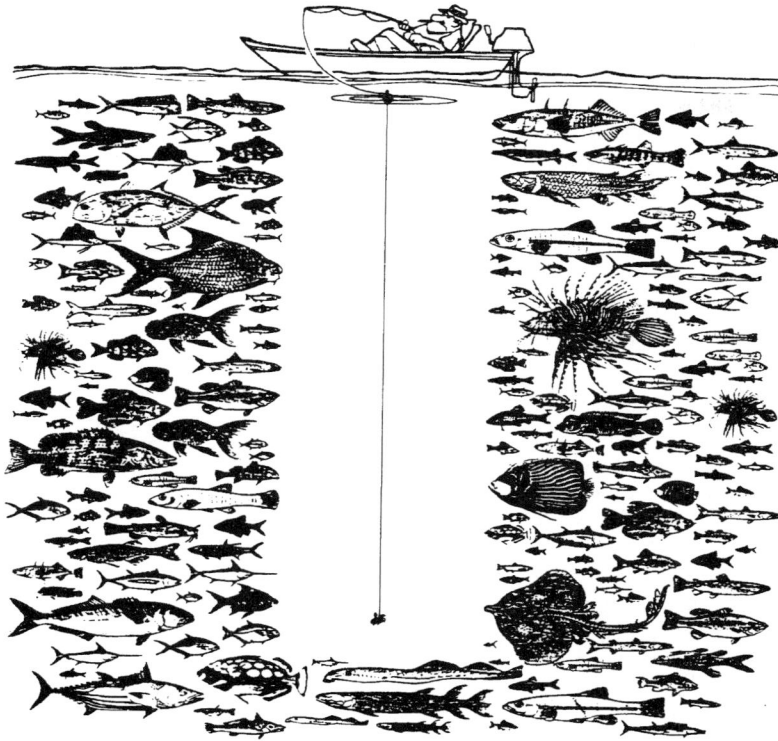

Reprinted by
permission of
Jeff Griffin.

Figure 5–8   *When You Test a Program Without a Plan, You Never Know What You Might Be Missing*

Errors can be syntactic or semantic. The compiler finds syntactic errors. For example, the compiler warns you when reserved words are misspelled, identifiers are undeclared, semicolons are missing, and operand types are mismatched. But it won't find all of your typing errors. If you type > instead of < , you won't get an error message; instead, you get erroneous results when you test the program. It's up to you to design a test plan and carefully check the code to detect errors of this type.

Semantic errors (also called *logic errors*) are mistakes that give you the wrong answer. They are more difficult to locate than syntactic errors and usually surface when a program is executing. C++ detects only the most obvious semantic errors—those that result in an invalid operation (dividing by zero, for example). Although semantic errors sometimes are caused by typing errors, they are more often a product of a faulty algorithm design. The lack of checking whether height is 0 that we found in the algorithm walk-through for the BMI problem is a typical semantic error.

By walking through the algorithm and the code, tracing the execution of the program, and developing a thorough test strategy, you should be able to avoid, or at least quickly locate, semantic errors in your programs.

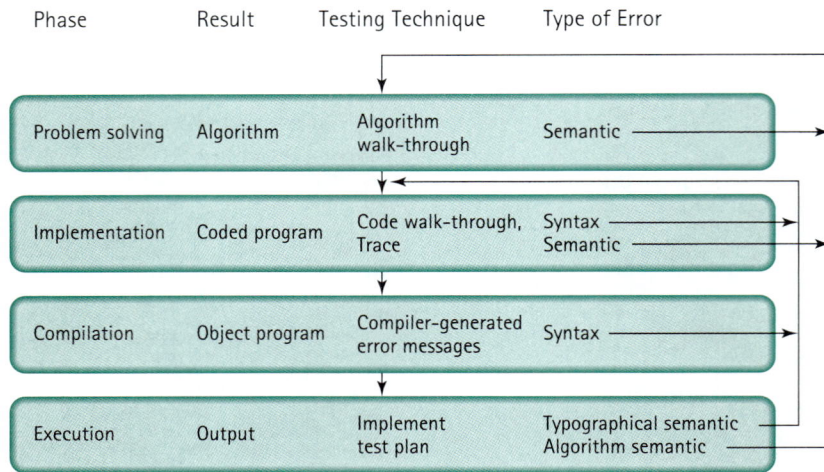

Phase	Result	Testing Technique	Type of Error
Problem solving	Algorithm	Algorithm walk-through	Semantic
Implementation	Coded program	Code walk-through, Trace	Syntax Semantic
Compilation	Object program	Compiler-generated error messages	Syntax
Execution	Output	Implement test plan	Typographical semantic Algorithm semantic

Figure 5–9   *Testing Process*

Figure 5–9 illustrates the testing process we've been discussing. The figure shows where syntax and semantic errors occur and in which phase they can be corrected.

Testing and Debugging Hints

1. C++ has three pairs of operators that are similar in appearance but very different in effect: == and =, && and &, and || and |. Double-check all of your logical expressions to be sure you're using the "equals-equals," "and-and," and "or-or" operators.

2. If you use extra parentheses for clarity, be sure that the opening and closing parentheses match up. To verify that parentheses are properly paired, start with the innermost pair and draw a line connecting them. Do the same for the others, working your way out to the outermost pair. For example,

```
if ( ( (total/scores) > 50)   &&   ( (total/(scores - 1) ) < 100) )
```

Here is a quick way to tell whether you have an equal number of opening and closing parentheses. The scheme uses a single number (the "magic number"), whose value initially is 0. Scan the expression from left to right. At each opening parenthesis, add 1 to the magic number; at each closing parenthesis, subtract 1. At the final closing parenthesis, the magic number should be 0. For example,

```
if (((total/scores) > 50) && ((total/(scores - 1)) < 100))
   0   123              2    1    23      4          32     10
```

3. Don't use =< to mean "less than or equal to"; only the symbol <= works. Likewise, => is invalid for "greater than or equal to"; you must use >= for this operation.

4. In an If statement, remember to use a { } pair if the then-clause or else-clause is a sequence of statements. And be sure not to put a semicolon after the right brace.

5. Echo print all input data. By doing so, you know that your input values are what they are supposed to be.

6. Test for bad data. If a data value must be positive, use an If statement to test the value. If the value is negative or 0, an error message should be printed; otherwise, processing should continue. For example, the following code segment tests whether three test scores are less than 0 or greater than 100.

```
dataOK = true;
if (test1 < 0 || test2 < 0 || test3 < 0)
{
    cout << "Invalid Data:  Score(s) less than zero." << endl;
    dataOK = false;
}
if (test1 > 100 || test2 > 100 || test3 > 100)
{
    cout << "Invalid Data:  Score(s) greater than 100." << endl;
    dataOK = false;
}
```

These If statements test the limits of reasonable scores, and the rest of the program continues only if the data values are reasonable.

7. Take some sample values and try them by hand as we did for the BMI program. (There's more on this method in Chapter 6.)

8. If your program reads data from an input file, it should verify that the file was opened successfully. Immediately after the call to the open function, an If statement should test the state of the file stream.

9. If your program produces an answer that does not agree with a value you've calculated by hand, try these suggestions:

a. Redo your arithmetic.

b. Recheck your input data.

c. Carefully go over the section of code that does the calculation. If you're in doubt about the order in which the operations are performed, insert clarifying parentheses.

d. Check for integer overflow. The value of an int variable may have exceeded INT_MAX in the middle of a calculation. Some systems give an error message when this happens, but most do not.

e. Check the conditions in branching statements to be sure that the correct branch is taken under all circumstances.

Summary

Using logical expressions is a way of asking questions while a program is running. The program evaluates each logical expression, producing the value `true` if the expression is true or the value `false` if the expression is not true.

The If statement allows you to take different paths through a program based on the value of a logical expression. The If-Then-Else is used to choose between two courses of action; the If-Then is used to choose whether or not to take a particular course of action. The branches of an If-Then or If-Then-Else can be any statement, simple or compound. They can even be other If statements.

The algorithm walk-through requires us to define a precondition and a postcondition for each module in an algorithm. Then we need to verify that those assertions are true at the beginning and end of each module. By testing our design in the problem-solving phase, we can eliminate errors that can be more difficult to detect in the implementation phase.

An execution trace is a way of finding program errors once we've entered the implementation phase. It's a good idea to trace a program before you run it, so that you have some sample results against which to check the program's output. A written test plan is an essential part of any program development effort.

Quick Check

1. What are the two values that are the basis for Boolean logic? (p. 194)
2. What does a branch allow the computer to do? (pp. 194–195)
3. What purpose does a nested branch serve? (pp. 192–193)
4. What does a precondition of a module tell us? (pp. 227–228)
5. Write a Boolean expression that is true when the value of the variable `temperature` is greater than 32. (pp. 196–198)
6. Write a Boolean expression that is true when the value of variable `temperature` is in the range of 33 to 211 degrees, and the `bool` variable `fahrenheit` is true. (pp. 199–202)
7. Write an If-Then-Else statement that uses the test from question 5 to output either "`Above freezing.`" or "`Freezing or below.`" (pp. 207–208)
8. Write an If-Then statement that outputs "In range." when the Boolean expression in question 6 is true. (pp. 212–214)
9. Write nested If statements to print messages indicating whether a temperature is below freezing, freezing, above freezing but not boiling, or boiling and above. (pp. 214–218)
10. When tracing a program by hand we write out a table. What do we put in the columns of the table, and what do the rows represent? (pp. 230–233)
11. If a program never seems to take one branch of an If statement, how would you go about debugging it? (pp. 233–235)

Answers

1. True and false.   2. It allows the computer to choose between alternative courses of action, depending on a test of certain conditions.   3. It allows the computer to select among any number of alternative courses of action.   4. A precondition tells us precisely what conditions must exist upon entry to a module for the module to be able to execute correctly.   5. `temperature > 32`
6. `temperature > 32 && temperature < 212 && fahrenheit`
7.
```
if (temperature > 32)
        cout << "Above freezing.";
   else
        cout << "Freezing or below.";
```
8.
```
if (temperature > 32 && temperature < 212 && fahrenheit)
        cout << "In range.";
```
9.
```
if (temperature < 32)
        cout << "Below freezing.";
   else if (temperature == 32)
        cout << "Freezing.";
   else if (temperature < 212)
        cout << "Above freezing and below boiling.";
   else
        cout << "Boiling and above.";
```
10. The columns are the values of the variables, and the rows correspond to the result of executing each statement during the trace.   11. Try different inputs to be sure that there is a problem, then check that the conditional test is written correctly. Working backward from there, check to see that each variable in the test is correctly assigned a value. Verify that all of the preconditions of each related module are satisfied before it executes.

Exam Preparation Exercises

1. Define the term "flow of control."
2. The values `true` and `false` are keywords in C++. True or false?
3. The "equals or greater" operator in C++ is written =>. True or false?
4. Why is it that `'A' < 'B'` and `'a' < 'b'` are both `true`, but `'a' < 'B'` is `false`?
5. If `int1` has the value 12, `int2` has the value 18, and `int3` has the value 21, what is the result of each of the following Boolean expressions?
   a. `int1 < int2 && int2 < int3`
   b. `int1 < int3 || int3 < int2`
   c. `int1 <= int2 - 6`
   d. `int2 <= int1 + 5 || int3 >= int2 + 5`
   e. `!(int1 < 30)`
   f. `!(int2 == int1 && int3 == int1)`
   g. `!(int1 > 25) && !(int2 < 17)`
6. If `string1` has the value `"miniscule"`, `string2` has the value `"minimum"`, and `string3` has the value `"miniature"`, what is the result of each of the following expressions?
   a. `string1 > string2`

b. `string1 > string2 && string2 > string3`

c. `string1.substr(0, 4) == string2.substr(0, 4)`

d. `string1 > "maximum"`

e. `string3.substr(0, 4) == "mini" || string1 == string2`

f. `string3.length() > string1.length() && string1 > string3`

g. `!((string1.substr(8, 1) == string3.substr(8, 1)) && string1.length() == 9)`

7. Why won't the following expression result in a division-by-zero error when `someInt` has the value 0?

```
someInt != 0 && 5/someInt > 10
```

8. The `bool` operators have lower precedence than the arithmetic operators, with the exception of the `!` operator, which has the same precedence as unary minus. True or false?

9. We enclose the logical expression in an If statement in parentheses only to make the code more readable. C++ doesn't require the parentheses. True or false?

10. What does the following If statement do when the value in `someInt` is 77?

```
if (someInt <= 44) || (someInt - 37 < 40)
    cout << "The data is within range.";
else
    cout << "The data doesn't make sense.";
```

11. What does the following If statement do when the value in `string1` is `"The"`?

```
if (string1.length() == 3 && string1.substr(0, 1) = "T")
    cout << "The word may be \"The\"";
else
{
    string1 = "The";
    cout << "The word is now \"The\"";
}
```

12. What does the following If statement do when the value in `float1` is `3.15`?

```
if (fabs(float1 - 3.14) < 0.00000001)
{
    cout << "The area of the circle of radius 6.0 is
            approximately:"
        << endl;
    cout << 6.0 * 6.0 * float1;
}
```

13. Why does the following If statement always output `"false"` regardless of the value in `someInt`?

```
if (someInt = 0)
    cout << "true";
else
    cout << "false";
```

14. What is output by the following code segment when `score` has the value 85?

```
if (score < 50)
    cout << "Failing";
else if (score < 60)
    cout << "Below average";
else if (score < 70)
    cout << "Average";
else if (score < 80)
    cout << "Above average";
else if (score < 90)
    cout << "Very good";
else if (score < 100)
    cout << "Excellent";
```

15. What is output by the following code segment when `score` has the value 85?

```
if (score < 50)
    cout << "Failing";
if (score < 60)
    cout << "Below average";
if (score < 70)
    cout << "Average";
if (score < 80)
    cout << "Above average";
if (score < 90)
    cout << "Very good";
if (score < 100)
    cout << "Excellent";
```

16. How do you fix a nested If statement that has a dangling else?
17. How would you write a Boolean expression in an If statement if you want the statement's Then branch to execute when file `inData` is in the fail state?
18. Is there any limit to how deeply we can nest If statements?

Programming Warm-Up Exercises

1. Write a Boolean expression that is true when the `bool` variable `moon` has the value "`blue`" or the value "`Blue`".
2. Write a Boolean expression that is true when both `inFile1` and `inFile2` are in the fail state.
3. Write a branching statement that reads into a string variable called `someString`, from a file called `inFile` if the file is not in the fail state.
4. Write a branching statement that tests whether one date comes before another. The dates are stored as integers representing the month, day, and year. The variables for the two dates are thus called `month1`, `day1`, `year1`, `month2`, `day2`, and

year2. The statement should output an appropriate message depending on the outcome of the test. For example:

```
12/21/01 comes before 1/27/05
```

or

```
7/14/04 does not come before 7/14/04
```

5. Change the branching statement that you wrote for Exercise 4 so that when the first date doesn't come before the second, it sets the first date equal to the second date in addition to printing the message.

6. Write a Boolean expression that is `true` when either of the `bool` variables `bool1` or `bool2` is `true`, but is `false` whenever both of them are `true` or neither of them is `true`.

7. Write a branching statement that tests whether `score` is in the range of 0 to 100, and outputs an error message if it is not within that range.

8. Change the branching statement that you wrote for Exercise 7 so that when `score` is in the proper range, it adds `score` to a running total variable called `scoreTotal`, and increments a counter called `scoreCount`.

9. Write a code segment that reads an `int` value from each of two files, `infile1` and `infile2`, and if neither file is in the fail state, it writes the lesser value of the two to a file called `outfile`, and reads another value from the file that had the lesser value. If either of the files is in the fail state, then the value from the one that is not in the fail state is written to `outfile`. If both files are in the fail state, then an error message is output to `cout`. The `int` values can be input into variables `value1` and `value2`.

10. Change the following series of If-Then statements into a nested If-Else-If structure.

```
if (score > 100)
    cout << "Duffer.";
if (score <= 100 && score > 80)
    cout << "Weekend regular.";
if (score <= 80 && score > 72)
    cout << "Competitive player.";
if (score <= 72 && score > 68)
    cout << "Turn pro!";
if (score <= 68)
    cout << "Time to go on tour!";
```

11. Write an If structure that outputs the least of three values, `count1`, `count2`, and `count3`. If there is more than one variable with the lowest value, then output the value as many times as it is found in those variables.

12. The following program segment is not supposed to print anything, yet it outputs the first error message, `"Error in maximum: 100"`. What's wrong, and how would you correct it? Why doesn't it output both error messages?

```
maximum = 75;
minimum = 25;
if (maximum = 100)
    cout << "Error in maximum: " << maximum << endl;
if (minimum = 0)
    cout << "Error in minimum: " << minimum << endl;
```

13. Write an If statement that takes the square root of the variable `area` only when its value is nonnegative. Otherwise the statement should set `area` equal to its absolute value and then take the square root of the new value. The result should be assigned to the variable `root`.

14. Write a test plan for the following branching structure.

```
cout << "The water is a ";
if (temp >= 212)
    cout << "gas.";
else if (temp > 32)
    cout << "liquid.";
else
    cout << "solid.";
```

15. Write a test plan for the following branching structure. (Note that the test for leap year given here does not include the special rules for century years.)

```
if (month == 2 && day > 28)
    if (year%4 != 0)
        cout << "Date error. Not a leap year."
    else
        if (day > 29)
            cout << "Date error. Improper day for February."
```

Programming Problems

1. Use functional decomposition to write a C++ program that inputs a letter and outputs the corresponding International Civil Aviation Organization alphabet word (these are the words that pilots use when they need to spell something out over a noisy radio channel). The alphabet is as follows:

A Alpha
B Bravo
C Charlie
D Delta
E Echo
F Foxtrot
G Golf
H Hotel

I   India
J   Juliet
K   Kilo
L   Lima
M   Mike
N   November
O   Oscar
P   Papa
Q   Quebec
R   Romeo
S   Sierra
T   Tango
U   Uniform
V   Victor
W   Whiskey
X   X-ray
Y   Yankee
Z   Zulu

Be sure to use proper formatting and appropriate comments in your code. Provide appropriate prompts to the user. The output should be labeled clearly and formatted neatly.

2. Use functional decomposition to write a C++ program that asks the user to enter their weight and the name of a planet. The program then outputs how much the user would weigh on that planet. The following table gives the factor by which the weight must be multiplied for each planet. The program should output an error message if the user doesn't type a correct planet name. The prompt and the error message should make it clear to the user how a planet name must be entered. Be sure to use proper formatting and appropriate comments in your code. The output should be clearly labeled and neatly formatted.

Mercury   0.4155
Venus   0.8975
Earth   1.0
Moon   0.166
Mars   0.3507
Jupiter   2.5374
Saturn   1.0677
Uranus   0.8947
Neptune   1.1794
Pluto   0.0899

3. Use functional decomposition to write a C++ program that takes a number in the range of 1 to 12 as input, and outputs the corresponding month of the year, where 1 is January, and so on. The program should output an error message if the number entered is not in the required range. The prompt and the error mes-

sage should make it clear to the user how a month number must be entered. Be sure to use proper formatting and appropriate comments in your code. The output should be labeled clearly and formatted neatly.

4. Use functional decomposition to write a C++ program that takes a number in the range of 0 to 6 and a second number in the range of 1 to 366 as input. The first number represents the day of the week on which the year begins, where 0 is Sunday, and so on. The second number indicates the day of the year. The program then outputs the name of the day of the week corresponding to the day of the year. The number of the day of the week can be computed as follows:

(start day + day of year − 1) % 7

The program should output an error message if the numbers entered are not in the required ranges. The prompt and the error message should make it clear to the user how the numbers must be entered. Be sure to use proper formatting and appropriate comments in your code. The output should be labeled clearly and formatted neatly.

5. Use functional decomposition to write a C++ program that takes a number in the range of 1 to 365 as input. The number represents the day of the year. The program then outputs the name of the month (assume the year is not a leap year). You can do this by comparing the day of the year to the number of days in the year that precede the start of each month. For example, 59 days precede March, which has 31 days. So if the day of the year is in the range of 60 through 91, then your program would output March. The program should output an error message if the number entered is not in the required range. The prompt and the error message should make it clear to the user how the number must be entered. Be sure to use proper formatting and appropriate comments in your code. The output should be labeled clearly and formatted neatly.

6. Use functional decomposition to write a C++ program that takes as input three numbers representing the number of pins knocked down by a bowler in three throws. The rules of bowling are that if the first throw is a strike (all ten pins knocked down), then the score is equal to those 10 points plus the number knocked down in the next two throws. The maximum score (three strikes) is thus thirty. If the first throw knocks down fewer than ten pins, but the second throw knocks down the remainder of the ten pins (a spare), then the score is those 10 points plus the number of pins knocked down on the third throw. If the first two throws fail to knock down all of the pins (a blow), then the score is just the total number of pins knocked down in the first two throws. Your program should output the computed score, and also should check for erroneous input. For example, a throw may be in the range of 0 through 10 pins, and the total of the first two throws must be less than or equal to 10, except when the first throw is a strike. Be sure to use proper formatting and appropriate comments in your code. The output should be labeled clearly and formatted neatly, and the error messages should be informative.

7. Use functional decomposition to write a C++ program that computes a dance competition score. There are four judges who mark the dancers in the range of 0

to 10, and the overall score is the average of the three highest scores (the lowest score is excluded). Your program should output an error message, instead of the average, if any of the scores are not in the correct range. Be sure to use proper formatting and appropriate comments in your code. The output should be labeled clearly and formatted neatly, and the error message should indicate clearly which score was invalid.

8. Use functional decomposition to write a C++ program that determines the median of three input numbers. The median is the middle number when the three are arranged in order. However, the user can input the values in any order, so your program must determine which value is between the other two. For example, if the user enters:

```
41.52 27.18 96.03
```

then the program would output:

```
The median of 41.52, 27.18, and 96.03 is 41.52.
```

Once you have the three-number case working, extend the program to handle five numbers. Be sure to use proper formatting and appropriate comments in your code. The output should be labeled clearly and formatted neatly.

Case Study Follow-Up

1. How might you go about choosing values for weight and height so that the BMI values of 20, 25, and 30 might be tested?
2. Change the program so that the BMI is rounded. Choose appropriate cases to test the end conditions. Implement your test plan.
3. Rewrite this program to take metric values for weight and height. Go on the Internet to find the correct formula.
4. Change the original program so that the height is entered in feet and inches. Prompt for and enter them separately.
5. A negative input value for weight or height was considered an error condition in the BMI program. Are there other values for weight or height that should be considered error conditions? Explain.

Looping

Goals

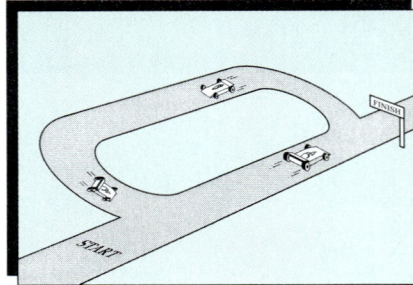

In Chapter 5, we said that the flow of control in a program can differ from the physical order of the statements. The *physical order* is the order in which the statements appear in a program; the order in which we want the statements to be executed is called the *logical order*.

The If statement is one way of making the logical order different from the physical order. Looping control structures are another. A **loop** executes the same statement (simple or compound) over and over, as long as a condition or set of conditions is satisfied.

> **Loop** A control structure that causes a statement or group of statements to be executed repeatedly.

In this chapter, we discuss different kinds of loops and how they are constructed using the While statement. We also discuss *nested loops* (loops that contain other loops) and introduce a notation for comparing the amount of work done by different algorithms.

6.1 The While Statement

The While statement, like the If statement, tests a condition. Here is the syntax template for the While statement:

WhileStatement

```
while ( Expression )
    Statement
```

and this is an example of one:

```
while (inputVal != 25)
    cin >> inputVal;
```

The While statement is a looping control structure. The statement to be executed each time through the loop is called the *body* of the loop. In the example above, the body of the loop is the input statement that reads in a value for `inputVal`. This While statement says to execute the body repeatedly as long as the input value does not equal 25. The While statement is completed (hence, the loop stops) when `inputVal` equals 25. The effect of this loop, then, is to consume and ignore all the values in the input stream until the number 25 is read.

Just like the condition in an If statement, the condition in a While statement can be an expression of any simple data type. Nearly always, it is a logical (Boolean) expression; if not, its value is implicitly coerced to type `bool` (recall that a zero value is coerced to `false`, and any nonzero value is coerced to `true`). The While statement says, "If the value of the expression is `true`, execute the body and then go back and test the expression again. If the expression's value is `false`, skip the body." The loop body is thus executed over and over as long as the expression is `true` when it is tested. When the expression is `false`, the program skips the body and execution continues at the statement immediately following the loop. Of course, if the expression is `false` to begin with, the body is not even executed. Figure 6–1 shows the flow of control of the While statement, where Statement1 is the body of the loop and Statement2 is the statement following the loop.

The body of a loop can be a compound statement (block), which allows us to execute any group of statements repeatedly. Most often we use While loops in the following form:

```
while (Expression)
{
    ⋮
}
```

In this structure, if the expression is `true`, the entire sequence of statements in the block is executed, and then the expression is checked again. If it is still `true`, the statements are executed again. The cycle continues until the expression becomes `false`.

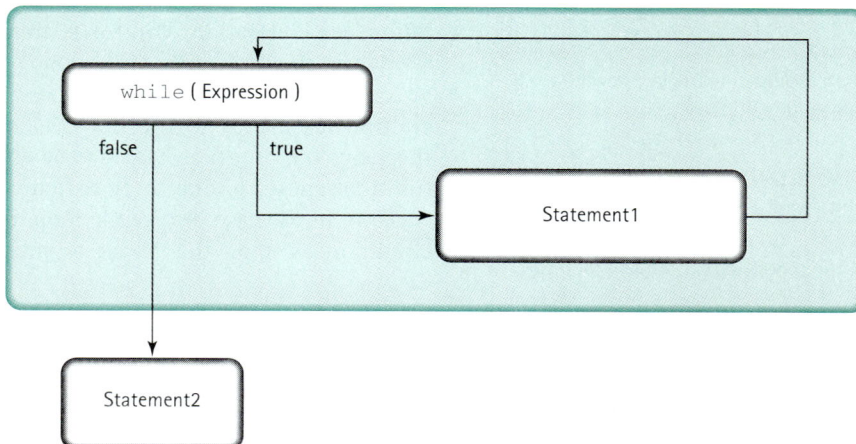

Figure 6–1   *While Statement Flow of Control*

IF-THEN STATEMENT

WHILE STATEMENT

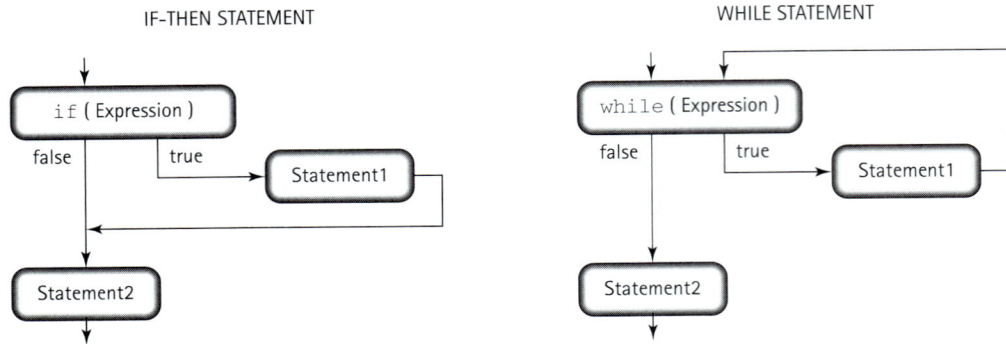

Figure 6–2 *A Comparison of If and While*

Although in some ways the If and While statements are alike, there are fundamental differences between them (see Figure 6–2). In the If structure, Statement1 is either skipped or executed exactly once. In the While structure, Statement1 can be skipped, executed once, or executed over and over. The If is used to *choose* a course of action; the While is used to *repeat* a course of action.

6.2 Phases of Loop Execution

The body of a loop is executed in several phases:

- The moment that the flow of control reaches the first statement inside the loop body is the **loop entry**.
- Each time the body of a loop is executed, a pass is made through the loop. This pass is called an **iteration**.
- Before each iteration, control is transferred to the **loop test** at the beginning of the loop.
- When the last iteration is complete and the flow of control has passed to the first statement following the loop, the program has **exited the loop**. The condition that causes a loop to be exited is the **termination condition**. In the case of a While loop, the termination condition is that the While expression becomes `false`.

Loop entry   The point at which the flow of control reaches the first statement inside a loop.

Iteration   An individual pass through, or repetition of, the body of a loop.

Loop test   The point at which the While expression is evaluated and the decision is made either to begin a new iteration or skip to the statement immediately following the loop.

Loop exit   The point at which the repetition of the loop body ends and control passes to the first statement following the loop.

Termination condition   The condition that causes a loop to be exited.

Notice that the loop exit occurs only at one point: when the loop test is performed. Even though the termination condition may become satisfied midway through the execution of the loop, the current iteration is completed before the computer checks the While expression again.

The concept of looping is fundamental to programming. In this chapter, we spend some time looking at typical kinds of loops and ways of implementing them with the While statement. These looping situations come up again and again when you are analyzing problems and designing algorithms.

6.3 Loops Using the While Statement

In solving problems, you will come across two major types of loops: **count-controlled loops**, which repeat a specified number of times, and **event-controlled loops**, which repeat until something happens within the loop.

If you are making an angel food cake and the recipe reads "Beat the mixture 300 strokes," you are executing a count-controlled loop. If you are making a pie crust and the recipe reads "Cut with a pastry blender until the mixture resembles coarse meal," you are executing an event-controlled loop; you don't know ahead of time the exact number of loop iterations.

> **Count-controlled loop** A loop that executes a specified number of times.
>
> **Event-controlled loop** A loop that terminates when something happens inside the loop body to signal that the loop should be exited.

Count-Controlled Loops

A count-controlled loop uses a variable we call the *loop control variable* in the loop test. Before we enter a count-controlled loop, we have to *initialize* (set the initial value of) the loop control variable and then test it. Then, as part of each iteration of the loop, we must *increment* (increase by 1) the loop control variable. Here's an example in a program that repeatedly outputs "Hello!" on the screen:

```
//****************************************************************
// Hello program
// This program demonstrates a count-controlled loop
//****************************************************************
#include <iostream>

using namespace std;

int main()
{
    int loopCount;      // Loop control variable

    loopCount = 1;                       // Initialization
    while (loopCount <= 10)              // Test
    {
        cout << "Hello!" << endl;
        loopCount = loopCount + 1;       // Incrementation
```

```
    }
    return 0;
}
```

In the Hello program, loopCount is the loop control variable. It is set to 1 before loop entry. The While statement tests the expression

```
loopCount <= 10
```

and executes the loop body as long as the expression is true. Inside the loop body, the main action we want to be repeated is the output statement. The last statement in the loop body increments loopCount by adding 1 to it.

Look at the statement in which we increment the loop control variable. Notice its form:

```
variable = variable + 1;
```

This statement adds 1 to the current value of the variable, and the result replaces the old value. Variables that are used this way are called *counters*. In the Hello program, loop-Count is incremented with each iteration of the loop—we use it to count the iterations. The loop control variable of a count-controlled loop is always a counter.

We've encountered another way of incrementing a variable in C++. The incremen-tation operator (++) increments the variable that is its operand. The statement

```
loopCount++;
```

has precisely the same effect as the assignment statement

```
loopCount = loopCount + 1;
```

From here on, we typically use the ++ operator, as do most C++ programmers.

When designing loops, it is the programmer's responsibility to see that the condi-tion to be tested is set correctly (initialized) before the While statement begins. The pro-grammer also must make sure that the condition changes within the loop so that it eventually becomes false; otherwise, the loop is never exited.

```
loopCount = 1;                    ←Variable loopCount must be initialized
while (loopCount <= 10)
{
        ⋮
    loopCount++;                  ←loopCount must be incremented
}
```

A loop that never exits is called an *infinite loop* because, in theory, the loop executes forever. In the code above, omitting the incrementation of `loopCount` at the bottom of the loop leads to an infinite loop; the While expression is always `true` because the value of `loopCount` is forever 1. If your program goes on running for much longer than you expect it to, chances are that you've created an infinite loop. You may have to issue an operating system command to stop the program.

How many times does the loop in our Hello program execute—9 or 10? To determine this, we have to look at the initial value of the loop control variable and then at the test to see what its final value is. Here we've initialized `loopCount` to 1, and the test indicates that the loop body is executed for each value of `loopCount` up through 10. If `loopCount` starts out at 1 and runs up to 10, the loop body is executed 10 times. If we want the loop to execute 11 times, we have to either initialize `loopCount` to 0 or change the test to

```
loopCount <= 11
```

Event-Controlled Loops

There are several kinds of event-controlled loops: sentinel-controlled, end-of-file-controlled, and flag-controlled. In all of these loops, the termination condition depends on some event occurring while the loop body is executing.

Sentinel-Controlled Loops   Loops often are used to read in and process long lists of data. Each time the loop body is executed, a new piece of data is read and processed. Often a special data value, called a *sentinel* or *trailer value*, is used to signal the program that there is no more data to be processed. Looping continues as long as the data value read is *not* the sentinel; the loop stops when the program recognizes the sentinel. In other words, reading the sentinel value is the event that controls the looping process.

A sentinel value must be something that never shows up in the normal input to a program. For example, if a program reads calendar dates, we could use February 31 as a sentinel value:

```
// This code is incorrect:

while (  !(month == 2 && day == 31) )
{
    cin >> month >> day;              // Get a date
       ⋮                              // Process it
}
```

There is a problem in the loop in the example above. The values of `month` and `day` are not defined before the first pass through the loop. Somehow we have to initialize these variables. We could assign them arbitrary values, but then we would run the risk that the first values input are the sentinel values, which would then be processed as data. Also, it's inefficient to initialize variables with values that are never used.

We can solve the problem by reading the first set of data values *before* entering the loop. This is called a *priming read*. (The idea is similar to priming a pump by pouring a bucket of water into the mechanism before starting it.) Let's add the priming read to the loop:

```
// This is still incorrect:

cin >> month >> day;                    // Get a date--priming read
while ( !(month == 2 && day == 31) )
{
    cin >> month >> day;                // Get a date
        :                               // Process it
}
```

With the priming read, if the first values input are the sentinel values, then the loop correctly does not process them. We've solved one problem, but now there is a problem when the first values input are valid data. Notice that the first thing the program does inside the loop is to get a date, destroying the values obtained by the priming read. Thus, the first date in the data list is never processed. Given the priming read, the *first* thing that the loop body should do is process the data that's already been read. But then at what point do we read the next data set? We do this *last* in the loop. In this way, the While condition is applied to the next data set before it gets processed. Here's how it looks:

```
// This version is correct:

cin >> month >> day;                    // Get a date--priming read
while ( !(month == 2 && day == 31) )
{
        :                               // Process it
    cin >> month >> day;                // Get the next date
}
```

This segment works fine. The first data set is read in; if it is not the sentinel, it gets processed. At the end of the loop, the next data set is read in, and we go back to the beginning of the loop. If the new data set is not the sentinel, it gets processed just like the first. When the sentinel value is read, the While expression becomes `false` and the loop exits (*without* processing the sentinel).

Many times the problem dictates the value of the sentinel. For example, if the problem does not allow data values of 0, then the sentinel value should be 0. Sometimes a combination of values is invalid. The combination of February and 31 as a date is such a case. Sometimes a range of values (negative numbers, for example) is the sentinel. And when you process `char` data one line of input at a time, the newline character (`'\n'`) often serves as the sentinel. Here's a program that reads and prints all of the characters from one line of an input file:

```
//*****************************************************************
// EchoLine program
// This program reads and echoes the characters from one line
// of an input file
//*****************************************************************
#include <iostream>
#include <fstream>                          // For file I/O

using namespace std;

int main()
{
    char      inChar;                       // An input character
    ifstream  inFile;                       // Data file

    inFile.open("text.dat");                // Attempt to open input file
    if ( !inFile )                          // Was it opened?
    {
        cout << "Can't open the input file.";  // No--print message
        return 1;                           // Terminate program
    }

    inFile.get(inChar);                     // Get first character
    while (inChar != '\n')
    {
        cout << inChar;                     // Echo it
        inFile.get(inChar);                 // Get next character
    }
    cout << endl;
    return 0;
}
```

(Notice that for this particular task we use the get function, not the >> operator, to input a character. Remember that the >> operator skips whitespace characters—including blanks and newlines—to find the next data value in the input stream. In this program, we want to input *every* character, even a blank and especially the newline character.)

When you are choosing a value to use as a sentinel, what happens if there aren't any invalid data values? Then you may have to input an extra value in each iteration, a value whose only purpose is to signal the end of the data. For example, look at this code segment:

```
cin >> dataValue >> sentinel;          // Get first data value
while (sentinel == 1)
{
        ⋮                              // Process it
    cin >> dataValue >> sentinel;      // Get next data value
}
```

The second value on each line of the following data set is used to indicate whether or not there is more data. In this data set, when the sentinel value is 0, there is no more data; when it is 1, there is more data.

Data values	Sentinel values
10	1
0	1
-5	1
8	1
-1	1
47	0

What happens if you forget to enter the sentinel value? In an interactive program, the loop executes again, prompting for input. At that point, you can enter the sentinel value, but your program logic may be wrong if you already entered what you thought was the sentinel value. If the input to the program is from a file, once all the data has been read from the file, the loop body is executed again. However, there isn't any data left—because the computer has reached the end of the file—so the file stream enters the fail state. In the next section, we describe a way to use the end-of-file situation as an alternative to using a sentinel.

Before we go on, we mention an issue that is related not to the design of loops but to C++ language usage. In Chapter 5, we talked about the common mistake of using the assignment operator (=) instead of the relational operator (==) in an If condition. This same mistake can happen when you write While statements. See what happens when we use the wrong operator in the previous example:

```
cin >> dataValue >> sentinel;
while (sentinel = 1)                    // Whoops
{
    ⋮
    cin >> dataValue >> sentinel;
}
```

This mistake creates an infinite loop. The While expression is now an assignment expression, not a relational expression. The expression's value is 1 (interpreted in the loop test as true because it's nonzero), and its side effect is to store the value 1 into sentinel, replacing the value that was just input into the variable. Because the While expression is always true, the loop never stops.

End-of-File-Controlled Loops   You already have learned that an input stream (such as cin or an input file stream) goes into the fail state (a) if it encounters unacceptable input data, (b) if the program tries to open a nonexistent input file, or (c) if the program tries to read past the end of an input file. Let's look at the third of these three possibilities.

After a program has read the last piece of data from an input file, the computer is at the end of the file (EOF, for short). At this moment, the stream state is all right. But if we try to input even one more data value, the stream goes into the fail state. We can use this fact to our advantage. To write a loop that inputs an unknown number of data items, we can use the failure of the input stream as a form of sentinel.

In Chapter 5, we described how to test the state of an I/O stream. In a logical expression, we use the name of the stream as though it were a Boolean variable:

```
if (inFile)
    ⋮
```

In a test like this, the result is `true` if the most recent I/O operation succeeded, or `false` if it failed. In a While statement, testing the state of a stream works the same way. Suppose we have a data file containing integer values. If `inData` is the name of the file stream in our program, here's a loop that reads and echoes all of the data values in the file:

```
inData >> intVal;               // Get first value
while (inData)                  // While the input succeeded ...
{
    cout << intVal << endl;     // Echo it
    inData >> intVal;           // Get next value
}
```

Let's trace this code, assuming there are three values in the file: 10, 20, and 30. The priming read inputs the value 10. The While condition is `true` because the input succeeded. Therefore, the computer executes the loop body. First the body prints out the value 10, and then it inputs the second data value, 20. Looping back to the loop test, the expression `inData` is `true` because the input succeeded. The body executes again, printing the value 20 and reading the value 30 from the file. Looping back to the test, the expression is `true`. Even though we are at the end of the file, the stream state is still OK—the previous input operation succeeded. The body executes a third time, printing the value 30 and executing the input statement. This time, the input statement fails; we're trying to read beyond the end of the file. The stream `inData` enters the fail state. Looping back to the loop test, the value of the expression is `false` and we exit the loop.

When we write EOF-controlled loops like the one above, we are expecting that the end of the file is the reason for stream failure. But keep in mind that *any* input error causes stream failure. The above loop terminates, for example, if input fails because of invalid characters in the input data. This fact emphasizes again the importance of echo printing. It helps us verify that all the data was read correctly before the EOF was encountered.

EOF-controlled loops are similar to sentinel-controlled loops in that the program doesn't know in advance how many data items are to be input. In the case of sentinel-controlled loops, the program reads until it encounters the sentinel value. With EOF-controlled loops, it reads until it reaches the end of the file.

Is it possible to use an EOF-controlled loop when we read from the standard input device (via the `cin` stream) instead of a data file? On many systems, yes. With the UNIX operating system, you can type Ctrl-D (that is, you hold down the Ctrl key and tap the D key) to signify end-of-file during interactive input. With the MS-DOS operating system and the CodeWarrior IDE, the end-of-file keystrokes are Ctrl-Z (or sometimes Ctrl-D). Other systems use similar keystrokes. Here's a program segment that tests for EOF on the `cin` stream in UNIX:

```
cout << "Enter an integer (or Ctrl-D to quit): ";
cin >> someInt;
while (cin)
{
    cout << someInt << " doubled is " << 2 * someInt << endl;
    cout << "Next number (or Ctrl-D to quit): ";
    cin >> someInt;
}
```

Flag-Controlled Loops   A *flag* is a Boolean variable that is used to control the logical flow of a program. We can set a Boolean variable to `true` before a While loop; then, when we want to stop executing the loop, we reset it to `false`. That is, we can use the Boolean variable to record whether or not the event that controls the process has occurred. For example, the following code segment reads and sums values until the input value is negative. (`nonNegative` is the Boolean flag; all of the other variables are of type `int`.)

```
sum = 0;
nonNegative = true;              // Initialize flag
while (nonNegative)
{
    cin >> number;
    if (number < 0)              // Test input value
        nonNegative = false;     // Set flag if event occurred
    else
        sum = sum + number;
}
```

Notice that we can code sentinel-controlled loops with flags. In fact, this code uses a negative value as a sentinel.

You do not have to initialize flags to `true`; you can initialize them to `false`. If you do, you must use the NOT operator (`!`) in the While expression and reset the flag to `true` when the event occurs. Compare the code segment above with the one below; both perform the same task. (Assume that `negative` is a Boolean variable.)

```
sum = 0;
negative = false;                 // Initialize flag
while ( !negative )
{
    cin >> number;
    if (number < 0)               // Test input value
        negative = true;          // Set flag if event occurred
    else
        sum = sum + number;
}
```

Looping Subtasks

We have been looking at ways to use loops to affect the flow of control in programs. But looping by itself does nothing. The loop body must perform a task in order for the loop to accomplish something. In this section, we look at three tasks—counting, summing, and keeping track of a previous value—that often are used in loops.

Counting   A common task in a loop is to keep track of the number of times the loop has been executed. For example, the following program fragment reads and counts input characters until it comes to a period. (inChar is of type char; count is of type int.) The loop in this example has a counter variable, but the loop is not a count-controlled loop because the variable is not being used as a loop control variable.

```
count = 0;                        // Initialize counter
cin.get(inChar);                  // Read the first character
while (inChar != '.')
{
    count++;                      // Increment counter
    cin.get(inChar);              // Get the next character
}
```

The loop continues until a period is read. After the loop is finished, count contains one less than the number of characters read. That is, it counts the number of characters up to, but not including, the sentinel value (the period). Notice that if a period is the first character, the loop body is not entered and count contains a 0, as it should. We use a priming read here because the loop is sentinel-controlled.

The counter variable in this example is called an **iteration counter** because its value equals the number of iterations through the loop.

> **Iteration counter**   A counter variable that is incremented with each iteration of a loop.

According to our definition, the loop control variable of a count-controlled loop is an iteration counter. However, as you've just seen, not all iteration counters are loop control variables.

Summing Another common looping task is to sum a set of data values. Notice in the following example that the summing operation is written the same way, regardless of how the loop is controlled.

```
sum = 0;                            // Initialize the sum
count = 1;
while (count <= 10)
{
    cin >> number;                  // Input a value
    sum = sum + number;             // Add the value to sum
    count++;
}
```

We initialize sum to 0 before the loop starts so that the first time the loop body executes, the statement

```
sum = sum + number;
```

adds the current value of sum (0) to number to form the new value of sum. After the entire code fragment has executed, sum contains the total of the ten values read, count contains 11, and number contains the last value read.

Here count is being incremented in each iteration. For each new value of count, there is a new value for number. Does this mean we could decrement count by 1 and inspect the previous value of number? No. Once a new value has been read into number, the previous value is gone forever unless we've saved it in another variable. You'll see how to do that in the next section.

Let's look at another example. We want to count and sum the first ten odd numbers in a data set. We need to test each number to see if it is even or odd. (We can use the modulus operator to find out. If number % 2 equals 1, number is odd; otherwise, it's even.) If the input value is even, we do nothing. If it is odd, we increment the counter and add the value to our sum. We use a flag to control the loop because this is not a normal count-controlled loop. In the following code segment, all variables are of type int except the Boolean flag, lessThanTen.

```
count = 0;                          // Initialize event counter
sum = 0;                            // Initialize sum
lessThanTen = true;                 // Initialize loop control flag
while (lessThanTen)
{
    cin >> number;                  // Get the next value
    if (number % 2 == 1)            // Is the value odd?
    {
        count++;                    // Yes--Increment counter
        sum = sum + number;         // Add value to sum
        lessThanTen = (count < 10); // Update loop control flag
    }
}
```

In this example, there is no relationship between the value of the counter variable and the number of times the loop is executed. We could have written the While expression this way:

```
while (count < 10)
```

but this might mislead a reader into thinking that the loop is count-controlled in the normal way. So, instead, we control the loop with the flag `lessThanTen` to emphasize that `count` is incremented only when an odd number is read. The counter in this example is an **event counter**; it is initialized to 0 and incremented only when a certain event occurs. The counter in the previous example was an *iteration counter;* it was initialized to 1 and incremented during each iteration of the loop.

> **Event counter**   A variable that is incremented each time a particular event occurs.

Keeping Track of a Previous Value   Sometimes we want to remember the previous value of a variable. Suppose we want to write a program that counts the number of not-equal operators (!=) in a file that contains a C++ program. We can do so by simply counting the number of times an exclamation mark (!) followed by an equal sign (=) appears in the input. One way in which to do this is to read the input file one character at a time, keeping track of the two most recent characters, the current value and the previous value. In each iteration of the loop, a new current value is read and the old current value becomes the previous value. When EOF is reached, the loop is finished. Here's a program that counts not-equal operators in this way:

```cpp
//******************************************************************
// NotEqualCount program
// This program counts the occurrences of "!=" in a data file
//******************************************************************
#include <iostream>
#include <fstream>              // For file I/O

using namespace std;

int main()
{
    int      count;            // Number of != operators
    char     prevChar;         // Last character read
    char     currChar;         // Character read in this loop iteration
    ifstream inFile;           // Data file

    inFile.open("myfile.dat");          // Attempt to open input file
    if ( !inFile )                      // Was it opened?
    {
        cout << "** Can't open input file **"   // No--print message
```

```
                      << endl;
            return 1;               // Terminate program
        }
        count = 0;                  // Initialize counter
        inFile.get(prevChar);       // Initialize previous value
        inFile.get(currChar);       // Initialize current value
        while (inFile)              // While previous input succeeded ...
        {
            if (currChar == '=' && // Test for event
                prevChar == '!')
                count++;            // Increment counter
            prevChar = currChar;    // Replace previous value
                                    //    with current value
            inFile.get(currChar);   // Get next value
        }
        cout << count << " != operators were found." << endl;
        return 0;
}
```

Study this loop carefully. It's going to come in handy. There are many problems in which you must keep track of the last value read in addition to the current value.

6.4 How to Design Loops

It's one thing to understand how a loop works when you look at it and something else again to design a loop that solves a given problem. In this section, we look at how to design loops. We can divide the design process into two tasks: designing the control flow and designing the processing that takes place in the loop. We can in turn break each task into three phases: the task itself, initialization, and update. It's also important to specify the state of the program when it exits the loop, because a loop that leaves variables and files in a mess is not well designed.

There are seven different points to consider in designing a loop:

1. What is the condition that ends the loop?
2. How should the condition be initialized?
3. How should the condition be updated?
4. What is the process being repeated?
5. How should the process be initialized?
6. How should the process be updated?
7. What is the state of the program on exiting the loop?

We use these questions as a checklist. The first three help us design the parts of the loop that control its execution. The next three help us design the processing within the loop. The last question reminds us to make sure that the loop exits in an appropriate manner.

Designing the Flow of Control

The most important step in loop design is deciding what should make the loop stop. If the termination condition isn't well thought out, there's the potential for infinite loops and other mistakes. So here is our first question:

- What is the condition that ends the loop?

This question usually can be answered through a close examination of the problem statement. The following table lists some examples.

Key Phrase in Problem Statement	Termination Condition
"Sum 365 temperatures"	The loop ends when a counter reaches 365 (count-controlled loop).
"Process all the data in the file"	The loop ends when EOF occurs (EOF-controlled loop).
"Process until ten odd integers have been read"	The loop ends when ten odd numbers have been input (event counter).
"The end of the data is indicated by a negative test score"	The loop ends when a negative input value is encountered (sentinel-controlled loop).

Now we need statements that make sure the loop gets started correctly and statements that allow the loop to reach the termination condition. So we have to ask the next two questions:

- How should the condition be initialized?
- How should the condition be updated?

The answers to these questions depend on the type of termination condition.

Count-Controlled Loops   If the loop is count-controlled, we initialize the condition by giving the loop control variable an initial value. For count-controlled loops in which the loop control variable is also an iteration counter, the initial value is usually 1. If the process requires the counter to run through a specific range of values, the initial value should be the lowest value in that range.

The condition is updated by increasing the value of the counter by 1 for each iteration. (Occasionally, you may come across a problem that requires a counter to count from some value *down* to a lower value. In this case, the initial value is the greater value, and the counter is decremented by 1 for each iteration.) So, for count-controlled loops that use an iteration counter, these are the answers to the questions:

- Initialize the iteration counter to 1.
- Increment the iteration counter at the end of each iteration.

If the loop is controlled by a variable that is counting an event within the loop, the control variable usually is initialized to 0 and is incremented each time the event occurs. For count-controlled loops that use an event counter, these are the answers to the questions:

- Initialize the event counter to 0.
- Increment the event counter each time the event occurs.

Sentinel-Controlled Loops   In sentinel-controlled loops, a priming read may be the only initialization necessary. If the source of input is a file rather than the keyboard, it also may be necessary to open the file in preparation for reading. To update the condition, a new value is read at the end of each iteration. So, for sentinel-controlled loops, we answer our questions this way:

- Open the file, if necessary, and input a value before entering the loop (priming read).
- Input a new value for processing at the end of each iteration.

EOF-Controlled Loops   EOF-controlled loops require the same initialization as sentinel-controlled loops. You must open the file, if necessary, and perform a priming read. Updating the loop condition happens implicitly; the stream state is updated to reflect success or failure every time a value is input. However, if the loop doesn't read any data, it can never reach EOF, so updating the loop condition means the loop must keep reading data.

Flag-Controlled Loops   In flag-controlled loops, the Boolean flag variable must be initialized to `true` or `false` and then updated when the condition changes.

- Initialize the flag variable to `true` or `false`, as appropriate.
- Update the flag variable as soon as the condition changes.

In a flag-controlled loop, the flag variable essentially remains unchanged until it is time for the loop to end. Then the code detects some condition within the process being repeated that changes the value of the flag (through an assignment statement). Because the update depends on what the process does, at times we have to design the process before we can decide how to update the condition.

Designing the Process Within the Loop

Once we've determined the looping structure itself, we can fill in the details of the process. In designing the process, we first must decide what we want a single iteration to do. Assume for a moment that the process is going to execute only once. What tasks must the process perform?

- What is the process being repeated?

To answer this question, we have to take another look at the problem statement. The definition of the problem may require the process to sum up data values or to keep a count of data values that satisfy some test. For example:

Count the number of integers in the file howMany.

This statement tells us that the process to be repeated is a counting operation.

Here's another example:

Read a stock price for each business day in a week and compute the average price.

In this case, part of the process involves reading a data value. We have to conclude from our knowledge of how an average is computed that the process also involves summing the data values.

In addition to counting and summing, another common loop process is reading data, performing a calculation, and writing out the result. Many other operations can appear in looping processes. We've mentioned only the simplest here; we look at some other processes later on.

After we've determined the operations to be performed if the process is executed only once, we design the parts of the process that are necessary for it to be repeated correctly. We often have to add some steps to take into account the fact that the loop executes more than once. This part of the design typically involves initializing certain variables before the loop and then reinitializing or updating them before each subsequent iteration.

- How should the process be initialized?
- How should the process be updated?

For example, if the process within a loop requires that several different counts and sums be performed, each must have its own statements to initialize variables, increment counting variables, or add values to sums. Just deal with each counting or summing operation by itself—that is, first write the initialization statement, and then write the incrementing or summing statement. After you've done this for one operation, you go on to the next.

The Loop Exit

When the termination condition occurs and the flow of control passes to the statement following the loop, the variables used in the loop still contain values. And if the cin stream has been used, the reading marker has been left at some position in the stream. Or maybe an output file has new contents. If these variables or files are used later in the program, the loop must leave them in an appropriate state. So, the final step in designing a loop is answering this question:

- What is the state of the program on exiting the loop?

Now we have to consider the consequences of our design and double-check its validity. For example, suppose we've used an event counter and that later processing depends on the number of events. It's important to be sure (with an algorithm walk-through) that the value left in the counter is the exact number of events—that it is not off by 1.

Look at this code segment:

```
commaCount = 1;                    // This code is incorrect
cin.get(inChar);
while (inChar != '\n')
{
    if (inChar == ',')
        commaCount++;
    cin.get(inChar);
}
cout << commaCount << endl;
```

This loop reads characters from an input line and counts the number of commas on the line. However, when the loop terminates, commaCount equals the actual number of commas plus 1 because the loop initializes the event counter to 1 before any events take place. By determining the state of commaCount at loop exit, we've detected a flaw in the initialization. commaCount should be initialized to 0.

Designing correct loops depends as much on experience as it does on the application of design methodology. At this point, you may want to read through the Problem-Solving Case Study at the end of the chapter to see how the loop design process is applied to a real problem.

6.5 Nested Logic

In Chapter 5, we described nested If statements. It's also possible to nest While statements. Both While and If statements contain statements and are, themselves, statements. So the body of a While statement or the branch of an If statement can contain other While and If statements. By nesting, we can create complex control structures.

Suppose we want to extend our code for counting commas on one line, repeating it for all the lines in a file. We put an EOF-controlled loop around it:

```
cin.get(inChar);                   // Initialize outer loop
while (cin)                        // Outer loop test
{
    commaCount = 0;                // Initialize inner loop
                                   //   (Priming read is taken care of
                                   //     by outer loop's priming read)
    while (inChar != '\n')         // Inner loop test
    {
        if (inChar == ',')
            commaCount++;
```

```
        cin.get(inChar);            // Update inner termination condition
    }
    cout << commaCount << endl;
    cin.get(inChar);                // Update outer termination condition
}
```

In this code, notice that we have omitted the priming read for the inner loop. The priming read for the outer loop has already "primed the pump." It would be a mistake to include another priming read just before the inner loop; the character read by the outer priming read would be destroyed before we could test it.

Let's examine the general pattern of a simple nested loop. The dots represent places where the processing and update may take place in the outer loop.

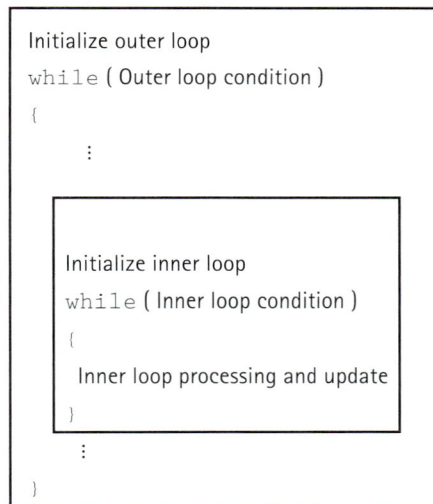

```
Initialize outer loop
while ( Outer loop condition )
{
          ⋮

      Initialize inner loop
      while ( Inner loop condition )
      {
        Inner loop processing and update
      }

          ⋮
}
```

Notice that each loop has its own initialization, test, and update. It's possible for an outer loop to do no processing other than to execute the inner loop repeatedly. On the other hand, the inner loop might be just a small part of the processing done by the outer loop; there could be many statements preceding or following the inner loop.

Let's look at another example. For nested count-controlled loops, the pattern looks like this (where outCount is the counter for the outer loop, inCount is the counter for the inner loop, and limit1 and limit2 are the number of times each loop should be executed):

```
outCount = 1;                       // Initialize outer loop counter
while (outCount <= limit1)
{
    ⋮
    inCount = 1;                    // Initialize inner loop counter
    while (inCount <= limit2)
```

```
{
    ⋮
    inCount++;                    // Increment inner loop counter
}
    ⋮
    outCount++;                   // Increment outer loop counter
}
```

Here, both the inner and outer loops are count-controlled loops, but the pattern can be used with any combination of loops.

The following program fragment shows a count-controlled loop nested within an EOF-controlled loop. The outer loop inputs an integer value telling how many asterisks to print out across a row of the screen. (We use the numbers to the right of the code to trace the execution of the program.)

```
cin >> starCount;                              1
while (cin)                                     2
{
    loopCount = 1;                             3
    while (loopCount <= starCount)             4
    {
        cout << '*';                           5
        loopCount++;                           6
    }
    cout << endl;                              7
    cin >> starCount;                          8
}
cout << "Goodbye" << endl;                     9
```

To see how this code works, let's trace its execution with these data values (<EOF> denotes the end-of-file keystrokes pressed by the user):

```
3
1
<EOF>
```

We'll keep track of the variables starCount and loopCount, as well as the logical expressions. To do this, we've numbered each line (except those containing only a left or right brace). As we trace the program, we indicate the first execution of line 3 by 3.1, the second by 3.2, and so on. Each loop iteration is enclosed by a large brace, and true and false are abbreviated as T and F (see Table 6–1).

Table 6–1   Code trace

| Statement | Variables | | Logical Expressions | | Output |
	starCount	loopCount	cin	loopCount <= starCount	
1.1	3	—	—	—	—
2.1	3	—	T	—	—
3.1	3	1	—	—	—
4.1	3	1	—	T	—
5.1	3	1	—	—	*
6.1	3	2	—	—	—
4.2	3	2	—	T	—
5.2	3	2	—	—	*
6.2	3	3	—	—	—
4.3	3	3	—	T	—
5.3	3	3	—	—	*
6.3	3	4	—	—	—
4.4	3	4	—	F	—
7.1	3	4	—	—	\n (newline)
8.1	1	4	—	—	—
2.2	1	4	T	—	—
3.2	1	1	—	—	—
4.5	1	1	—	T	—
5.4	1	1	—	—	*
6.4	1	2	—	—	—
4.6	1	2	—	F	—
7.2	1	2	—	—	\n (newline)
8.2	1	2	—	—	—
(null operation)					
2.3	1	2	F	—	—
9.1	1	2	—	—	Goodbye

Here's a sample run of the program. The user's input is in color. Again, the symbol <EOF> denotes the end-of-file keystrokes pressed by the user (the symbol would not appear on the screen).

```
3
* * *
1
*
<EOF>
Goodbye
```

Because `starCount` and `loopCount` are variables, their values remain the same until they are explicitly changed, as indicated by the repeating values in Table 6–1. The values of the logical expressions `cin` and `loopCount <= starCount` exist only when the test is made. We indicate this fact with dashes in those columns at all other times.

Designing Nested Loops

To design a nested loop, we begin with the outer loop. The process being repeated includes the nested loop as one of its steps. Because that step is more complex than a single statement, our functional decomposition methodology tells us to make it a separate module. We can come back to it later and design the nested loop just as we would any other loop.

For example, here's the design process for the preceding code segment:

1. *What is the condition that ends the loop?* EOF is reached in the input.

2. *How should the condition be initialized?* A priming read should be performed before the loop starts.

3. *How should the condition be updated?* An input statement should occur at the end of each iteration.

4. *What is the process being repeated?* Using the value of the current input integer, the code should print that many asterisks across one output line.

5. *How should the process be initialized?* No initialization is necessary.

6. *How should the process be updated?* A sequence of asterisks is output and then a newline character is output. There are no counter variables or sums to update.

7. *What is the state of the program on exiting the loop?* The `cin` stream is in the fail state (because the program tried to read past EOF), `starCount` contains the last integer read from the input stream, and the rows of asterisks have been printed along with a concluding message.

From the answers to these questions, we can write this much of the algorithm:

```
Read starCount
WHILE NOT EOF
    Print starCount asterisks
    Output newline
    Read starCount
Print "Goodbye"
```

After designing the outer loop, it's obvious that the process in its body (printing a sequence of asterisks) is a complex step that requires us to design an inner loop. So we repeat the methodology for the corresponding lower-level module:

1. *What is the condition that ends the loop?* An iteration counter exceeds the value of `starCount`.

2. *How should the condition be initialized?* The iteration counter should be initialized to 1.

3. *How should the condition be updated?* The iteration counter is incremented at the end of each iteration.

4. *What is the process being repeated?* The code should print a single asterisk on the standard output device.

5. *How should the process be initialized?* No initialization is needed.

6. *How should the process be updated?* No update is needed.

7. *What is the state of the program on exiting the loop?* A single row of asterisks has been printed, the writing marker is at the end of the current output line, and `loopCount` contains a value one greater than the current value of `starCount`.

Now we can write the algorithm:

```
Read starCount
WHILE NOT EOF
    Set loopCount = 1
    WHILE loopCount <= starCount
        Print '*'
        Increment loopCount
    Output newline
    Read starCount
Print "Goodbye"
```

Of course, nested loops themselves can contain nested loops (called *doubly nested loops*), which can contain nested loops (*triply nested loops*), and so on. You can use this design process for any number of levels of nesting. The trick is to defer details by using the functional decomposition methodology—that is, focus on the outermost loop first and treat each new level of nested loop as a module within the loop that contains it.

It's also possible for the process within a loop to include more than one loop. For example, here's an algorithm that reads and prints people's names from a file, omitting the middle name in the output:

> Read and print first name (ends with a comma)
> WHILE NOT EOF
>   Read and discard characters from middle name (ends with a comma)
>   Read and print last name (ends at newline)
>   Output newline
>   Read and print first name (ends with a comma)

The steps for reading the first name, middle name, and last name require us to design three separate loops. All of these loops are sentinel-controlled.

This kind of complex control structure would be difficult to read if written out in full. There are simply too many variables, conditions, and steps to remember at one time. In the next two chapters, we examine the control structure that allows us to break programs down into more manageable chunks—the subprogram.

Theoretical Foundations

Analysis of Algorithms

If you were given the choice of cleaning a room with a toothbrush or a broom, you probably would choose the broom. Using a broom sounds like less work than using a toothbrush. True, if the room were in a dollhouse, it might be easier to use the toothbrush, but in general a broom is the faster way to clean. If you were given the choice of adding numbers together with a pencil and paper or a calculator, you would probably choose the calculator because it is usually less work. If you were given the choice of walking or driving to a meeting, you would probably choose to drive; it sounds like less work.

What do these examples have in common? What do they have to do with computer science? In each of the situations mentioned, one of the choices seems to involve significantly less work. Precisely measuring the amount of work is difficult in each case because there are unknowns. How large is the room? How many numbers are there? How far away is the meeting? In each case, the unknown information is related to the size of the problem. If the problem is especially small (for example, adding 2 plus 2), our original estimate of which approach to take (using the calculator) might be wrong. However, our intuition is usually correct, because most problems are reasonably large.

In computer science, we need a way of measuring the amount of work done by an algorithm relative to the size of a problem, because there is usually more than one algorithm that solves any

(continued) ▼

Analysis of Algorithms

given problem. We often must choose the most efficient algorithm—the algorithm that does the least work for a problem of a given size.

The amount of work involved in executing an algorithm relative to the size of the problem is called the complexity of the algorithm. We would like to be able to look at an algorithm and determine its complexity. Then we could take two algorithms that perform the same task and determine which completes the task faster (requires less work).

> **Complexity**   A measure of the effort expended by the computer in performing a computation, relative to the size of the computation.

How do we measure the amount of work required to execute an algorithm? We use the total number of *steps* executed as a measure of work. One statement, such as an assignment, may require only one step; another, such as a loop, may require many steps. We define a step as any operation roughly equivalent in complexity to a comparison, an I/O operation, or an assignment.

Given an algorithm with just a sequence of simple statements (no branches or loops), the number of steps performed is directly related to the number of statements. When we introduce branches, however, we make it possible to skip some statements in the algorithm. Branches allow us to subtract steps without physically removing them from the algorithm because only one branch is executed at a time. But because we usually want to express work in terms of the worst-case scenario, we use the number of steps in the longest branch.

Now consider the effect of a loop. If a loop repeats a sequence of 15 simple statements 10 times, it performs 150 steps. Loops allow us to multiply the work done in an algorithm without physically adding statements.

Now that we have a measure for the work done in an algorithm, we can compare algorithms. For example, if algorithm A always executes 3124 steps and algorithm B always does the same task in 1321 steps, then we can say that algorithm B is more efficient—that is, it takes fewer steps to accomplish the same task.

If an algorithm, from run to run, always takes the same number of steps or fewer, we say that it executes in an amount of time bounded by a constant. Such algorithms are referred to as having *constant-time* complexity. Be careful: Constant time doesn't mean small; it means that the amount of work done does not exceed some amount from one run to another.

If a loop executes a fixed number of times, the work done is greater than the physical number of statements but still is constant. What happens if the number of loop iterations can change from one run to the next? Suppose a data file contains N data values to be processed in a loop. If the loop reads and processes one value during each iteration, then the loop executes N iterations. The amount of work done thus depends on a variable, the number of data values. The variable N determines the size of the problem in this example.

If we have a loop that executes N times, the number of steps to be executed is some factor times N. The factor is the number of steps performed within a single iteration of the loop.

(continued) ▼

Analysis of Algorithms

Specifically, the work done by an algorithm with a data-dependent loop is given by the expression

$$\overbrace{S_1 \times N}^{\text{Steps performed by the loop}} + \underbrace{S_0}_{\substack{\text{Steps performed} \\ \text{outside the loop}}}$$

where S_1 is the number of steps in the loop body (a constant for a given simple loop), N is the number of iterations (a variable representing the size of the problem), and S_0 is the number of steps outside the loop. Mathematicians call expressions of this form *linear*; hence, algorithms such as this are said to have *linear-time* complexity. Notice that if N grows very large, the term $S_1 \times N$ dominates the execution time. That is, S_0 becomes an insignificant part of the total execution time. For example, if S_0 and S_1 are each 20 steps, and N is 1,000,000, then the total number of steps is 20,000,020. The 20 steps contributed by S_0 are a tiny fraction of the total.

What about a data-dependent loop that contains a nested loop? The number of steps in the inner loop, S_2, and the number of iterations performed by the inner loop, L, must be multiplied by the number of iterations in the outer loop:

$$\overbrace{(S_2 \times L \times N)}^{\substack{\text{Steps performed} \\ \text{by the nested loop}}} + \overbrace{(S_1 \times N)}^{\substack{\text{Steps performed} \\ \text{by the outer loop}}} + \overbrace{S_0}^{\substack{\text{Steps performed outside} \\ \text{the outer loop}}}$$

By itself, the inner loop performs $S_2 \times L$ steps, but because it is repeated N times by the outer loop, it accounts for a total of $S_2 \times L \times N$ steps. If L is a constant, then the algorithm still executes in linear time.

Now, suppose that for each of the N outer loop iterations, the inner loop performs N steps ($L = N$). Here the formula for the total steps is

$$(S_2 \times N \times N) + (S_1 \times N) + S_0$$

(continued) ▼

Analysis of Algorithms

or

$$\left(S_2 \times N^2\right) + \left(S_1 \times N\right) + S_0$$

Because N^2 grows much faster than N (for large values of N), the inner loop term ($S_2 \times N^2$) accounts for the majority of steps executed and of the work done. The corresponding execution time is thus essentially proportional to N^2. Mathematicians call this type of formula *quadratic*. If we have a doubly nested loop in which each loop depends on N, then the expression is

$$\left(S_3 \times N^3\right) + \left(S_2 \times N^2\right) + \left(S_1 \times N\right) + S_0$$

and the work and time are proportional to N^3 whenever N is reasonably large. Such a formula is called *cubic*.

The following table shows the number of steps required for each increase in the exponent of N, where N is a size factor for the problem, such as the number of input values.

N	N^0 (Constant)	N^1 (Linear)	N^2 (Quadratic)	N^3 (Cubic)
1	1	1	1	1
10	1	10	100	1,000
100	1	100	10,000	1,000,000
1,000	1	1,000	1,000,000	1,000,000,000
10,000	1	10,000	100,000,000	1,000,000,000,000
100,000	1	100,000	10,000,000,000	1,000,000,000,000,000

As you can see, each time the exponent increases by 1, the number of steps is multiplied by an additional order of magnitude (factor of 10). That is, if N is made 10 times greater, the work involved in an N^2 algorithm increases by a factor of 100, and the work involved in an N^3 algorithm increases by a factor of 1000. To put this in more concrete terms, an algorithm with a doubly nested loop in which each loop depends on the number of data values takes 1000 steps for 10 input values and 1 quadrillion steps for 100,000 values. On a computer that executes 1 billion instructions per second, the latter case would take about 12 days to run.

The table also shows that the steps outside of the innermost loop account for an insignificant portion of the total number of steps as N gets bigger. Because the innermost loop dominates the

(continued) ▼

Analysis of Algorithms

total time, we classify the complexity of an algorithm according to the highest order of N that appears in its complexity expression, called the *order of magnitude*, or simply the *order*, of that expression. So we talk about algorithms having "order N squared complexity" (or cubed or so on) or we describe them with what is called *Big-O notation*. We express the complexity by putting the highest-order term in parentheses with a capital O in front. For example, $O(1)$ is constant time, $O(N)$ is linear time, $O(N^2)$ is quadratic time, and $O(N^3)$ is cubic time.

Determining the complexities of different algorithms allows us to compare the work they require without having to program and execute them. For example, if you had an $O(N^2)$ algorithm and a linear algorithm that performed the same task, you probably would choose the linear algorithm. We say *probably* because an $O(N^2)$ algorithm actually may execute fewer steps than an $O(N)$ algorithm for small values of N. Remember that if the size factor N is small, the constants and lower-order terms in the complexity expression may be significant.

Let's look at an example. Suppose that algorithm A is $O(N^2)$ and that algorithm B is $O(N)$. For large values of N, we would normally choose algorithm B because it requires less work than A. But suppose that in algorithm B, $S_0 = 1000$ and $S_1 = 1000$. If $N = 1$, then algorithm B takes 2000 steps to execute. Now suppose that for algorithm A, $S_0 = 10$, $S_1 = 10$, and $S_2 = 10$. If $N = 1$, then algorithm A takes only 30 steps. Here is a table that compares the number of steps taken by these two algorithms for different values of N.

N	Algorithm A	Algorithm B
1	30	2,000
2	70	3,000
3	130	4,000
10	1,110	11,000
20	4,210	21,000
30	9,310	31,000
50	25,510	51,000
100	101,010	101,000
1,000	10,010,010	1,001,000
10,000	1,000,100,010	10,001,000

From this table we can see that the $O(N^2)$ algorithm A is actually faster than the $O(N)$ algorithm B, up to the point that N equals 100. Beyond that point, algorithm B becomes more efficient. Thus, if we know that N is always less than 100 in a particular problem, we would choose algorithm A. For example, if the size factor N is the number of test scores on an exam and the class size is limited to

(continued) ▼

> ### Analysis of Algorithms
>
> 30 students, algorithm A would be more efficient. On the other hand, if N is the number of scores at a university with 25,000 students, we would choose algorithm B.
>
> Constant, linear, quadratic, and cubic expressions are all examples of *polynomial* expressions. Algorithms whose complexity is characterized by such expressions are therefore said to execute in *polynomial time* and form a broad class of algorithms that encompasses everything we've discussed so far.
>
> In addition to polynomial-time algorithms, we encounter a logarithmic-time algorithm in Chapter 13. There are also factorial ($O(N!)$), exponential ($O(N^N)$), and hyperexponential ($O(N^{N^N})$) classes of algorithms, which can require vast amounts of time to execute and are beyond the scope of this book. For now, the important point to remember is that different algorithms that solve the same problem can vary significantly in the amount of work they do.

Problem–Solving Case Study

Recording Studio Design

PROBLEM   You've gone to work for a consulting firm that specializes in converting existing rooms into recording studios. They have asked you to write a program that inputs a set of loudness measurements for a room and prints out basic statistics. The measurements are made by playing a series of 12 different tones, and recording the readings from a sound level meter onto a file. The meter readings range from 50 to 126 decibels (a measure of loudness). Your program, however, is to output the measurements relative to the first tone—that is, to show how much each individual reading differs from the first. After all the data have been read, the program is to print out the highest and lowest readings.

INPUT   Twelve real numbers, representing the meter readings, on file "acoustic.dat".

OUTPUT   The 12 input values (echo print) and their values relative to the first reading. At the end of the program, the actual value, relative value, and sequence number of both the highest reading and the lowest.

DISCUSSION   This is easy to do by hand. We simply scan the list, subtracting the first value from each value in the list. As we scan the list, we also keep track of which value from the list is the highest and which is the lowest.

How do we translate this process into an algorithm? Let's take a closer look at what we are doing. To find the largest number in a list, we compare the first and second numbers and remember the larger one. Then, we compare that number with the third one, remembering the larger number. We repeat the process for all of the numbers, and the one we remember at the end is the largest. We use the same process to find the smallest number, only we remember the smaller number instead of the larger one. Consider a sample data set:

Reading Number	Actual Reading	Relative Reading
1	86.0	0.0
2	86.5	0.5
3	88.0	2.0
4	83.5	−2.5
5	88.3	2.3
6	89.6	3.6
7	80.1	−5.9
8	84.0	−2.0
9	86.7	0.7
10	79.3	−6.7
11	74.0	−12.0
12	73.5	−12.5

The maximum reading was number 6 at 89.6 decibels. The lowest was reading 12 at 73.5 decibels.

"Scan the list" in our by-hand algorithm translates into a loop. Now that we understand the process, let's design the looping algorithm using our checklist.

1. *What is the condition that ends the loop?* Because there are exactly 12 values in a set of readings, we use a counter to control the loop. When it exceeds 12, the loop exits.

2. *How should the condition be initialized?* The first value will be input before the loop, because it is a special case — it is the value that is subtracted from all the other values to get their relative values. Also, its relative value is automatically 0.0. Thus, the first iteration of the loop gets the second value, so the counter will start at 2.

3. *How should the condition be updated?* The counter should be incremented at the end of each iteration.

4. *What is the process being repeated?* The process reads a value, echo prints it, subtracts the first value from the new value, prints the result, and checks to see if the new value should replace the current high or low value.

5. *How should the process be initialized?* The first number must be read in. Its relative value is automatically printed as 0.0. It is the initial high and low, and it also is saved as the base reading. The sequence number for both the high and low values will be set to 1 and their relative values will be 0.0.

6. *How should the process be updated?* In each iteration, a new current reading is input. If the current reading is greater than high, it replaces the current high. If current is lower than the current low, then it becomes the new low. We also must save the reading number of the highest and lowest values, and their relative values.

7. *What is the state of the program on exiting the loop?* Twelve readings have been input and echo printed together with twelve relative values. The loop control variable equals 13. high contains the greatest value read, highNumber the number of that value, and highRelative the relative value for that reading; low contains the lowest value, lowNumber holds the number of that reading, and lowRelative has the corresponding relative value.

ASSUMPTIONS   At least 12 real numbers will be input, and all will be within the proper range.

Main Module	Level 0

```
Initialize process
Initialize loop ending condition
WHILE readingNumber < =12 DO
     Update process
     Update ending condition
Print high and low readings
Close file
```

Initialize Process	Level 1

```
Open input file
If not opened ok
     Write error message
     Return 1
Print heading for output
Get baseValue
Print readingNumber 1, baseValue, relativeValue 0.0
Set high to baseValue
Set highNumber to 1
Set highRelative to 0.0
Set low to baseValue
Set low Number to 1
Set lowRelative to 0.0
```

Initialize Loop Ending Condition

```
Set readingNumber to 2
```

Update Process

Get current
Set relative to current – baseValue
Print readingNumber, current, relative
Check for new high
Check for new low

Update Loop Ending Condition

Increment readingNumber

Print High and Low Readings

Print 'Highest reading number is ', highNumber
Print 'Highest reading is ', high
Print 'Highest relative value is ', highRelative
Print 'Lowest reading number is ', lowNumber
Print 'Lowest reading is ', low
Print 'Lowest relative value is ', lowRelative

Check for New High   Level 2

IF current > high
    Set high to current
    Set highNumber to readingNumber
    Set highRelative to relative

Check for New Low

IF current < low
    Set low to current
    Set lowNumber to readingNumber
    Set lowRelative to relative

MODULE STRUCTURE CHART

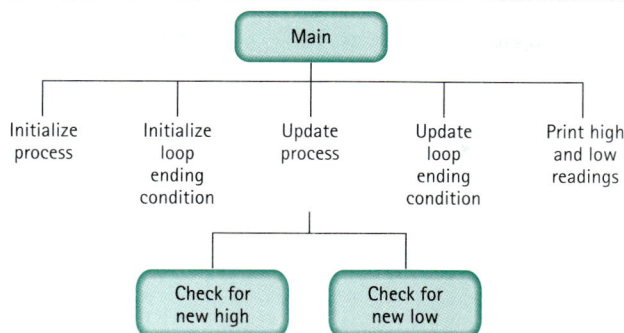

```
//*****************************************************************
// Acoustic Program
// This program inputs 12 sound-level readings, taken in a room
// at different frequencies.  The first reading is used as a
// base value.  For each reading, a value relative to the base is
// calculated and printed.  The program ends by printing the
// highest reading and the lowest reading.
//*****************************************************************

#include <iostream>
#include <fstream>
#include <iomanip>

using namespace std;

int main()
{
    // Declare variables
    float baseValue;         // First reading
    float current;           // Input during each iteration
    float relative;          // Current minus base value
    float high;              // Highest value input
    float highRelative;      // High minus base value
    float low;               // Lowest value input
    float lowRelative;       // Low minus base value
    int highNumber;          // Sequence number of high
    int lowNumber;           // Sequence number of lowest
    int readingNumber;       // Sequence number of current reading

    // Declare and open input file
    ifstream inData;                      // Input file of readings
    inData.open("acoustic.dat");
```

```cpp
    if ( !inData )                          // Did input file open correctly?
    {   // no
        cout << "Can't open input file." << endl;
        return 1;                           // Terminate program
    }

    // Initialize variables and output
    readingNumber = 1;
    relative = 0.0;
    cout << setw(14) << "Reading Number" << setw(15)
         << "Actual Reading << setw(18) << "Relative Reading"
         << endl;

    inData >> baseValue;                    // Input base value

    // Write first line of output
    cout << fixed << showpoint << setprecision(2) << setw(7)
         << readingNumber << setw(19) << baseValue << setw(15)
         << relative << endl;

    // Initialize process
    high = baseValue;
    highNumber = 1;
    highRelative = 0.0;
    low = baseValue;
    lowNumber = 1;
    lowRelative = 0.0;
    readingNumber = 2;                      // Initialize loop ending

    while (readingNumber <= 12)
    {
        inData >> current;                  // Input new reading
        relative = current - baseValue;     // Calculate new relative
        cout << setw(7) << readingNumber << setw(19) << current
             << setw(15) << relative << endl;

        if (current > high)                 // Check for new high
        {
            high = current;
            highNumber = readingNumber;
            highRelative = relative;
        }

      if (current < low)                    // Check for new low
      {
          low = current;
          lowNumber = readingNumber;
```

```
          lowRelative = relative;
     }
   readingNumber++;          // Increment reading number


}


// Print high and low readings
cout << endl;
cout << "Highest reading number is " << highNumber << endl;
cout << "Highest reading is "  << high << endl;
cout << "Highest relative value is " << highRelative << endl;
cout << endl;
cout << "Lowest reading number is " << lowNumber << endl;
cout << "Lowest reading is " << low << endl;
cout << "Lowest relative value is " << lowRelative << endl;

inData.close();
return 0;
}
```

Here is a screen shot of the output.

```
C:\PPSC++\Acoustic\Acoustic.exe                                 - □ ×
Reading Number Actual Reading   Relative Reading
       1               86.00           0.00
       2               86.50           0.50
       3               88.00           2.00
       4               83.50          -2.50
       5               88.30           2.30
       6               89.60           3.60
       7               80.10          -5.90
       8               84.00          -2.00
       9               86.70           0.70
      10               79.30          -6.70
      11               74.00         -12.00
      12               73.50         -12.50

Highest reading number is 6
Highest reading is 89.60
Highest relative value is 3.60

Lowest reading number is 12
Lowest reading is 73.50
Lowest relative value is -12.50
```

Now that you have written the program, you call the president of the consulting firm and fax her the results. After studying the results, she is silent for a moment and says "Oh. Right." "I'm sorry," she says, "but I told you to keep track of the wrong value. We're not interested in the lowest value, but in the lowest *dip in the readings*. You see, the last value is almost always the lowest because it's the lowest tone, and we know that most rooms respond poorly to bass notes. There's nothing we can do about that. But the lowest dip in the readings often occurs with a higher tone and that's usually a sign of a problem that we can fix. Can you change the program to output the lowest dip?" You confirm that a dip is a reading followed by a higher reading.

Now you have to figure out how to recognize a dip in the readings. You draw some graphs with random squiggles on them and pick out the lowest dips by hand. Then you make up some data sets that would generate the graphs. You find that a dip is usually a series of decreasing values followed by increasing values. But it also can be just a series of equal values followed by greater values. The bottom of a dip is merely the lowest value before values start increasing. You know how to keep track of a lowest value, but how do you tell if it is followed by a greater value?

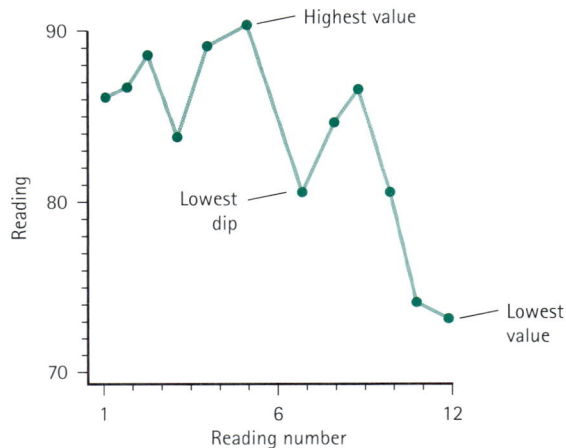

The answer is that you check it after the next value is input. That is, when you read in a new value, you check to see if the preceding value was lower. If it was, then you check to see if it was the lowest value input so far. You've seen the algorithm for keeping track of a previous value, and now you just have to add it to the program.

Now we can return to the checklist and see what must change. The control of the loop stays the same, only the process changes. Thus, we can skip the first three questions.

4. *What is the process being repeated?* It is the same as before, except where we check for the lowest value. Instead, we first check whether the preceding value is less than the current value. If it is, then we check to see if preceding should replace the lowest value so far. In replacing the lowest value, we must assign readingNumber minus one to lowNumber, because the dip occurred with the previous reading. We also could keep track of the previous value of readingNumber, but it is easier to calculate it.

5. *How should the process be initialized?* The change here is that we must initialize preceding. We can set it equal to the first value. We also have to initialize the precedingRelative value to 0.0.

6. *How should the process be updated?* We add steps to set preceding equal to current at the end of the loop, and to saveRelative in precedingRelative for use in the next iteration.

7. *What is the state of the program on exiting the loop?* At this point, preceding holds the last value input and precedingRelative holds the last relative value computed; low holds the value of the lowest dip, lowNumber contains the reading number of the lowest dip, and lowRelative is the difference between the lowest dip and the first value.

Now let's look at the modules that have changed. We'll use italics to indicate the steps that are different:

Initialize Process   Level 1

Open input file
If not opened ok
    Write error message
    Return 1
Print heading for output
Get baseValue
Print readingNumber 1, baseValue, relativeValue 0.0
Set preceding to baseValue
Set precedingRelative to 0.0
Set high to baseValue
Set highNumber to 1
Set highRelative to 0.0
Set low to baseValue
Set lowNumber to 1
Set lowRelative to 0.0

Update Process

Prompt for current
Get current
Set relative to current – baseValue
Print readingNumber, current, relative
Check for new high
Check for new low
Set preceding to current
Set precedingRelative to relative

Print High and Low Readings

Print 'Highest reading number is ', highNumber
Print 'Highest reading is ', high
Print 'Highest relative value is ', highRelative
Print 'Lowest dip is number ', lowNumber
Print 'Lowest dip reading is ', low
Print 'Lowest relative dip is ', lowRelative

Check for New Low

> *IF current > preceding*
>   *IF preceding < low*
>   *Set low to preceding*
>   *Set lowNumber to readingNumber – 1*
>   *Set lowRelative to precedingRelative*

Here's the new version of the program.

```
//*************************************************************
// Acoustic Program
// This program inputs 12 sound-level readings, taken in a room
// at different frequencies.  The first reading is used as a base
// value.  For each reading, a value relative to the base is
// calculated and printed.  The program ends by printing the
// lowest dip in the readings, where a dip is defined as a reading
// followed by a higher reading
//*************************************************************

#include <iostream>
#include <fstream>
#include <iomanip>

using namespace std;

int main()
{
    // Declare variables
    float baseValue;          // First reading
    float preceding;          // Reading preceding current
    float precedingRelative;  // Relative preceding current
    float current;            // Input during each iteration
    float relative;           // Current minus base value
    float high;               // Highest value input
    float highRelative;       // High minus base value
    float low;                // Lowest dip in the readings
    float lowRelative;        // Relative value of low
    int highNumber;           // Sequence number of high
    int lowNumber;            // Sequence number of lowest dip
    int readingNumber;        // Sequence number of current reading

    // Declare and open input file
    ifstream inData;                      // Input file of readings
    inData.open("acoustic.dat");
```

```cpp
if ( !inData )                      // Did input file open correctly?
{    // no
    cout << "Can't open input file." << endl;
    return 1;                        // Terminate program
}

// Initialize variables and output
cout << setw(14) << "Reading Number" << setw(15)
     << "Actual Reading" << setw(18) << "Relative Reading"
     << endl;
inData >> baseValue;
preceding = baseValue;
precedingRelative = 0.0;
highNumber = 1;
lowNumber = 1;
high = baseValue;
low = baseValue;
highRelative = 0.0;
lowRelative = 0.0;
readingNumber = 1;
relative = 0.0;

// Write first line of output
cout << fixed << showpoint << setprecision(2) << setw(7)
     << readingNumber << setw(19)
     << baseValue << setw(15) << relative << endl;

readingNumber = 2;                       // Initialize loop end
while (readingNumber <= 12)
{
    inData >> current;                   // Input new reading
    relative = current - baseValue;      // Calculate new relative
    cout << setw(7) << readingNumber << setw(19) << current
         << setw(15) << relative << endl;

    if (current > high)                  // Check for new high
    {
        high = current;
        highNumber = readingNumber;
        highRelative = relative;
    }

    if (current > preceding)             // Check for new low
    {
        if (preceding < low)
        {
```

```
                    low = preceding;
                    lowNumber = readingNumber - 1;
                    lowRelative = precedingRelative;
                }
            }
        preceding = current;
        precedingRelative = relative;
        readingNumber++;
    }

    // Print high and low readings
    cout << endl;
    cout << "Highest reading number is " << highNumber << endl;
    cout << "Highest reading is "  << high << endl;
    cout << "Highest relative value is " << highRelative << endl;
    cout << endl;
    cout << "Lowest dip is number " << lowNumber << endl;
    cout << "Lowest dip reading is " << low << endl;
    cout << "Lowest relative dip is " << lowRelative << endl;

    inData.close();
    return 0;
}
```

Here is the output screen.

```
C:\PPSC++\Acoustic\Acoustic.exe                                    _ □ ×
Reading Number Actual Reading   Relative Reading
         1             86.00              0.00
         2             86.50              0.50
         3             88.00              2.00
         4             83.50             -2.50
         5             88.30              2.30
         6             89.60              3.60
         7             80.10             -5.90
         8             84.00             -2.00
         9             86.70              0.70
        10             79.30             -6.70
        11             74.00            -12.00
        12             73.50            -12.50

Highest reading number is 6
Highest reading is 89.60
Highest relative value is 3.60

Lowest dip is number 7
Lowest dip reading is 80.10
Lowest relative dip is -5.90
```

Testing and Debugging

Loop-Testing Strategy

Even if a loop has been properly designed and verified, it is still important to test it rigorously because the chance of an error creeping in during the implementation phase is always present. Because loops allow us to input many data sets in one run, and because each iteration may be affected by preceding ones, the test data for a looping program is usually more extensive than for a program with just sequential or branching statements. To test a loop thoroughly, we must check for the proper execution of both a single iteration and multiple iterations.

Remember that a loop has seven parts (corresponding to the seven questions in our checklist). A test strategy must test each part. Although all seven parts aren't implemented separately in every loop, the checklist reminds us that some loop operations serve multiple purposes, each of which should be tested. For example, the incrementing statement in a count-controlled loop may be updating both the process and the ending condition, so it's important to verify that it performs both actions properly with respect to the rest of the loop.

To test a loop, we try to devise data sets that could cause the variables to go out of range or leave the files in improper states that violate either the loop postcondition (an assertion that must be true immediately after loop exit) or the postcondition of the module containing the loop.

It's also good practice to test a loop for four special cases: (1) when the loop is skipped entirely, (2) when the loop body is executed just once, (3) when the loop executes some normal number of times, and (4) when the loop fails to exit.

Statements following a loop often depend on its processing. If a loop can be skipped, those statements may not execute correctly. If it's possible to execute a single iteration of a loop, the results can show whether the body performs correctly in the absence of the effects of previous iterations, which can be very helpful when you're trying to isolate the source of an error. Obviously, it's important to test a loop under normal conditions, with a wide variety of inputs. If possible, you should test the loop with real data in addition to mock data sets. Count-controlled loops should be tested to be sure they execute exactly the right number of times. And finally, if there is any chance that a loop might never exit, your test data should try to make that happen.

Testing a program can be as challenging as writing it. To test a program, you need to step back, take a fresh look at what you've written, and then attack it in every way possible to make it fail. This isn't always easy to do, but it's necessary if your programs are going to be reliable. (A *reliable program* is one that works consistently and without errors regardless of whether the input data is valid or invalid.)

Test Plans Involving Loops

In Chapter 5, we introduced formal test plans and discussed the testing of branches. Those guidelines still apply to programs with loops, but here we provide some additional guidelines that are specific to loops.

Unfortunately, when a loop is embedded in a larger program, it sometimes is difficult to control and observe the conditions under which the loop executes using test data and output alone. In some cases we must use indirect tests. For example, if a loop reads floating-point values from a file and prints their average without echo printing them, you cannot tell directly that the loop processes all the data—if the data values in the file are all the same, then the average appears correct as long as even one of them is processed. You must construct the input file so that the average is a unique value that can be arrived at only by processing all the data.

To simplify our testing of such loops, we would like to observe the values of the variables associated with the loop at the start of each iteration. How can we observe the values of variables while a program is running? Two common techniques are the use of the system's *debugger* program and the use of extra output statements designed solely for debugging purposes. We discuss these techniques in the next section, Testing and Debugging Hints.

Now let's look at some test cases that are specific to the different types of loops that we've seen in this chapter.

Count-Controlled Loops When a loop is count-controlled, you should include a test case that specifies the output for all the iterations. It may help to add an extra column to the test plan that lists the iteration number. If the loop reads data and outputs a result, then each input value should produce a different output to make it easier to spot errors. For example, in a loop that is supposed to read and print 100 data values, it is easier to tell that the loop executes the correct number of iterations when the values are 1, 2, 3, ..., 100 than if they are all the same.

If the program inputs the iteration count for the loop, you need to test the cases in which an invalid count, such as a negative number, is input (an error message should be output and the loop should be skipped), a count of 0 is input (the loop should be skipped), a count of 1 is input (the loop should execute once), and some typical number of iterations is input (the loop should execute the specified number of times).

Event-Controlled Loops In an event-controlled loop, you should test the situation in which the event occurs before the loop, in the first iteration, and in a typical number of iterations. For example, if the event is that EOF occurs, then try an empty file, a file with one data set, and another with several data sets. If your testing involves reading from test files, you should attach printed copies of the files to the test plan and identify each in some way so that the plan can refer to them. It also helps to identify where each iteration begins in the Input and Expected Output columns of the test plan.

When the event is the input of a sentinel value, you need the following test cases: the sentinel is the only data set, the sentinel follows one data set, and the sentinel follows a typical number of data sets. Given that sentinel-controlled loops involve a priming read, it is especially important to verify that the first and last data sets are processed properly.

Testing and Debugging Hints

1. Plan your test data carefully to test all sections of a program.

2. Beware of infinite loops, in which the expression in the While statement never becomes `false`. The symptom: the program doesn't stop. If you are on a system that monitors the execution time of a program, you may see a message such as "TIME LIMIT EXCEEDED."

    If you have created an infinite loop, check your logic and the syntax of your loops. Be sure there's no semicolon immediately after the right parenthesis of the While condition:

    ```
    while (Expression);          // Wrong
       Statement
    ```

    This semicolon causes an infinite loop in most cases; the compiler thinks the loop body is the null statement (the do-nothing statement composed only of a semicolon). In a count-controlled loop, make sure the loop control variable is incremented within the loop. In a flag-controlled loop, make sure the flag eventually changes.

    And, as always, watch for the = versus == problem in While conditions as well as in If conditions. The line

    ```
    while (someVar = 5)          // Wrong (should be ==)
    ```

    produces an infinite loop. The value of the assignment (not relational) expression is always 5, which is interpreted as `true`.

3. Check the loop termination condition carefully and be sure that something in the loop causes it to be met. Watch closely for values that cause one iteration too many or too few (the "off-by-1" syndrome).

4. Remember to use the `get` function rather than the `>>` operator in loops that are controlled by detection of a newline character.

5. Perform an algorithm walk-through to verify that all of the appropriate preconditions and postconditions occur in the right places.

6. Trace the execution of the loop by hand with a code walk-through. Simulate the first few passes and the last few passes very carefully to see how the loop really behaves.

7. Use a *debugger* if your system provides one. A debugger is a program that runs your program in "slow motion," allowing you to execute one instruction at a time and to examine the contents of variables as they change. If you haven't already done so, check to see if a debugger is available on your system.

8. If all else fails, use *debug output statements*—output statements inserted into a program to help debug it. They output messages that indicate the flow of execution in the program or report the values of variables at certain points in the program.

For example, if you want to know the value of variable `beta` at a certain point in a program, you could insert this statement:

```
cout << "beta = " << beta << endl;
```

If this output statement is in a loop, you will get as many values of `beta` output as there are iterations of the body of the loop.

After you have debugged your program, you can remove the debug output statements or just precede them with `//` so that they'll be treated as comments. (This practice is referred to as *commenting out* a piece of code.) You can remove the double slashes if you need to use the statements again.

9. An ounce of prevention is worth a pound of debugging. Use the checklist questions to design your loop correctly at the outset. It may seem like extra work, but it pays off in the long run.

Summary

The While statement is a looping construct that allows the program to repeat a statement as long as the value of an expression is `true`. When the value of the expression becomes `false`, the body of the loop is skipped and execution continues with the first statement following the loop.

With the While statement, you can construct several types of loops that you will use again and again. These types of loops fall into two categories: count-controlled loops and event-controlled loops.

In a count-controlled loop, the loop body is repeated a specified number of times. You initialize a counter variable right before the While statement. This variable is the loop control variable. The control variable is tested against the limit in the While expression. The last statement in the loop body increments the control variable.

Event-controlled loops continue executing until something inside the body signals that the looping process should stop. Event-controlled loops include those that test for a sentinel value in the data, for end-of-file, or for a change in a flag variable.

Sentinel-controlled loops are input loops that use a special data value as a signal to stop reading. EOF-controlled loops are loops that continue to input (and process) data values until there is no more data. To implement them with a While statement, you must test the state of the input stream by using the name of the stream object as if it were a Boolean variable. The test yields `false` when there are no more data values. A flag is a variable that is set in one part of the program and tested in another. In a flag-controlled loop, you must set the flag before the loop begins, test it in the While expression, and change it somewhere in the body of the loop.

Counting is a looping operation that keeps track of how many times a loop is repeated or how many times some event occurs. This count can be used in computations or to control the loop. A counter is a variable that is used for counting. It may be the loop control variable in a count-controlled loop, an iteration counter in a counting loop, or an event counter that counts the number of times a particular condition occurs in a loop.

Summing is a looping operation that keeps a running total of certain values. It is like counting in that the variable that holds the sum is initialized outside the loop. The summing operation, however, adds up unknown values; the counting operation adds a constant (1) to the counter each time.

When you design a loop, there are seven points to consider: how the termination condition is initialized, tested, and updated; how the process in the loop is initialized, performed, and updated; and the state of the program upon exiting the loop. By answering the checklist questions, you can bring each of these points into focus.

To design a nested loop structure, begin with the outermost loop. When you get to where the inner loop must appear, make it a separate module and come back to its design later.

The process of testing a loop is based on the answers to the checklist questions and the patterns the loop might encounter (for example, executing a single iteration, multiple iterations, an infinite number of iterations, or no iterations at all).

Quick Check

1. What are the four phases of loop execution? (pp. 252–253)
2. How is a flag-controlled loop like an event-controlled loop, and how are they different? (pp. 255–261)
3. Does averaging a set of values that are input by a loop involve summing, counting, or both? (pp. 261–264)
4. What type of loop would you use to read a file of drivers' license numbers until a specific number is input? (pp. 264–266)
5. Write a While statement that exits when the int variable count is greater than 10, or the Boolean flag found is true. (pp. 253–258)
6. Write the initialization and update portions of the loop in Exercise 5. The variable found becomes true when the int variable inData contains zero. The count starts at one and is incremented in each iteration. (pp. 264–266)
7. Add a test for end-of-file on cin to the loop in Exercise 6, and add statements to the loop that perform a priming read and an updating read of inData from cin. (pp. 258–260)
8. Add initialization and update operations to the loop in Exercise 7 that cause it to count the occurrences of the value 1 that are input to variable inData, and to sum all of the values read into inData. (pp. 261–263)
9. How would you extend the loop from Exercise 8 so that it would be repeated in its entirety five times? (pp. 268–274)
10. How would you test a looping program that reads hourly temperatures from a file and outputs the daily average? (pp. 291–292)

Answers

1. Entry, iteration, test, exit. **2.** They both exit when an event occurs. But the event-controlled loop tests for the event at the start of each iteration, while the flag-controlled loop checks for the event in the middle of the iteration, setting a flag to be tested at the start of the next iteration. **3.** Both. **4.** An event-controlled loop. (The events would be the input of the number, or reaching end-of-file). **5.** `while (count <= 10 && !found)`

6.
```
count = 1;
found = false;
while (count <= 10 && !found)
{
    count++;
    found = inData == 0;
}
```

7.
```
count = 1;
found = false;
cin >> inData;
while (count <= 10 && !found && cin)
{
    count++;
    found = inData == 0;
    cin >> inData;
}
```

8.
```
onesCount = 0;
sum = 0;
count = 1;
found = false;
cin >> inData;
while (count <= 10 && !found && cin)
{
    if (inData == 1)
        onesCount++;
    sum = sum + inData;
    count++;
    found = inData == 0;
    cin >> inData;
}
```

9. Nest it within a counting loop that counts from 1 to 5. **10.** Run the program with an empty file, a file with 24 input values, a file with fewer than 24 input values, and a file with more than 24 input values. Test the program with 24 input values all the same, and with 24 values that differ so that omitting any of them results in an average that's different from the average of all 24.

Exam Preparation Exercises

1. The While statement exits when the termination condition becomes true. True or false?
2. The body of the While statement is always executed at least once. True or false?
3. Using a block as the body of the While statement enables us to place any number of statements within a loop. True or false?

4. Match the following list of terms with the definitions given below.
   a. Loop entry.
   b. Iteration.
   c. Loop test.
   d. Loop exit.
   e. Termination condition.
   f. Count-controlled loop.
   g. Event-controlled loop.
   h. Iteration counter.
   i. Event counter.
      i. A loop that executes a specified number of times.
      ii. When the flow of control reaches the first statement inside a loop.
      iii. A variable that is incremented each time a particular condition is encountered.
      iv. When the decision is made whether to begin a new iteration or to exit.
      v. A loop that exits when a specific condition is encountered.
      vi. The condition that causes the loop to exit.
      vii. A variable that is incremented with each iteration of a loop.
      viii. When control passes to the statement following the loop.
      ix. An individual pass through a loop.

5. How many times does the following loop execute, and what is its output?

```
count = 1;
while (count <= 12)
{
    cout << count << endl;
    count++;
}
```

6. How many times does the following loop execute, and what is its output?

```
count = 0;
while (count <= 11)
{
    cout << count << ", ";
    count++;
}
```

7. How many times does the following loop execute, and what is its output?

```
count = 1;
while (count < 13)
{
    cout << "$" << count << ".00" << endl;
    count++;
}
```

8. What does the following nested loop structure output?

```
count = 1;
while (count <= 11)
{
    innerCount = 1
    while (innerCount <= (12 - count) / 2)
    {
        cout << " ";
        innerCount++;
    }
    innerCount = 1;
    while (innerCount <= count)
    {
        cout << "@";
        innerCount++;
    }
    cout << endl;
    count++;
}
```

9. What does the following nested loop structure output?

```
count = 1;
while (count <= 10)
{
    innerCount = 1;
    while (innerCount <= 10)
    {
        cout << setw(5) << count * innercount;
        innerCount++;
    }
    cout << endl;
    count++;
}
```

10. The following loop is supposed to sum all of the input values on file `indata`. What's wrong with it? Change the code so that it works correctly.

```
sum = 0;
indata >> number;
while (indata)
{
    indata >> number;
    sum = sum + number;
}
```

11. What sentinel value would you choose for a program that reads names as strings?

12. The following code segment is supposed to write out the odd numbers from 1 to 19. What does it actually output? Change the code to work correctly.

```
number = 1;
while (number < 10)
{
    number++;
    cout << number * 2 - 1 << " ";
}
```

13. Priming reads aren't necessary when a loop is controlled by a sentinel value. True or false?

14. What are the seven questions that must be answered in order to design a loop?

15. The following code segment is supposed to output the average of the five numbers on each input line, for all of the lines in the file. Instead, it simply outputs the sum of all of the numbers in the file. What's wrong with the code segment? Change the code to work correctly.

```
sum = 0;
while (indata)
{
    count = 1;
    while (count <= 5 && indata)
    {
        cin >> number;
        sum = sum + number;
    }
    cout << sum / count << endl;
}
```

Programming Warm-Up Exercises

1. Write a code segment using a While loop that outputs the numbers from –10 to 10.

2. Write a code segment using a While loop that sums the integers, counting up from 1, and stops when the sum is greater than 10,000, printing out the integer that was most recently added to the sum.

3. Write a looping code segment that inputs up to 20 integer scores from file indata, and outputs their average. If the file contains fewer than 20 scores, the segment should still output the correct average. If the file contains more than 20 scores, the additional numbers should be ignored. Be sure to consider what happens if the file is empty.

4. Write a code segment that reads lines of text from file chapter6, and outputs the number of lines in the file that contain the string "code segment".

5. Write a code segment that reads a string from `cin`. The string should be one of, "Yes", "No", "yes", or "no". If it is not, the user should be prompted to input an appropriate response, and the process should repeat. Once a valid response is received, the `bool` variable `yes` should be assigned `true` if the response is "Yes" or "yes" and `false` if the response is "No" or "no".

6. Write a code segment that prints the days of a month in calendar format. The day of the week on which the month begins is represented by an `int` variable `startDay`. When `startDay` is zero, the month begins on a Sunday. The `int` variable `days` contains the number of days in the month. Print a heading with the days of the week as the first line of output. The day numbers should neatly align under these column headings.

7. We could extend the code from Exercise 6 to print a calendar for a year by nesting it within a loop that repeats the code twelve times.
   a. What formula would you use to compute the new start day for the next month?
   b. What additional information would you need to print the calendar for each month?

8. Write a code segment that reads all of the characters on file `textData`, and then outputs the percentage of the characters that are the letter "z".

9. Change the code segment in Exercise 8 so that it stops reading either at the end of the file or after 10,000 characters have been input.

10. Write a code segment that outputs the Fibonacci numbers that are less than 30,000. Each Fibonacci number is the sum of its two predecessors. The first two Fibonacci numbers are 1 and 1. Thus, the sequence begins with:

    1, 1, 2, 3, 5, 8, 13, 21, 34, ...

    Output each number on a separate line.

11. Modify the code segment in Exercise 10 so that it also outputs the position of the Fibonacci number in the sequence. For example:

1	1
2	1
3	2
4	3
5	5
6	8
7	13

12. Write a code segment that inputs an integer from `cin`, and then outputs a row of that many stars on `cout`.

13. How did you answer the checklist questions for Exercise 12?

14. Change the code segment for Exercise 12 to read a series of numbers from file `indata`, and print a row of stars on `cout` for each number read. (You can think of this as printing a bar graph of a data file.)

15. What test data would you use to test the code segment in Exercise 14?

Programming Problems

1. Design and write a C++ program that inputs a series of 24 hourly temperatures from a file, and outputs a bar chart (using stars) of the temperatures for the day. The temperature should be printed to the left of the corresponding bar, and there should be a heading that gives the scale of the chart. The range of temperatures should be from −30 to 120. Because it is hard to display 150 characters on the screen, you should have each star represent a range of 3 degrees. That way, the bars will be at most 50 characters wide. Here is a partial example, showing the heading, the output for a negative temperature, and the output for various positive temperatures. Note how the temperatures are rounded to the appropriate number of stars.

```
Temperatures for 24 hours:
     -30           0          30          60          90         120
 -20        *******|
   0               |
   1               |
   2               |*
   3               |*
   4               |*
   5               |**
  10               |***
  50               |*****************
 100               |******************************
```

Use meaningful variable names, proper indentation, and appropriate comments. Thoroughly test the program using your own data sets.

2. The standard deviation of a set of data values gives us a sense of the dispersion of values within their range. For example, a set of test scores with a small standard deviation indicates that most people's scores were very close to the average score. Some instructors thus use the standard deviation as a way of determining the range of values to assign a particular grade.

Design and write a C++ program that reads a set of scores from the file scores.dat, and outputs their mean and standard deviation on cout. The formula for the standard deviation is

$$ s = \sqrt{\frac{n \sum\limits_{i=1}^{n} x_i^2 - \left(\sum\limits_{i=1}^{n} x_i \right)^2}{n(n-1)}} $$

where n is the number of values and x_i represents the individual values. Thus, to compute the standard deviation, you must sum the squares of the individual values, and also square the sum of the values. All of this reading and summing can be done with a single loop, after which the mean and standard deviation of the scores are computed. Be sure to properly label the output. Use meaningful variable names, proper indentation, and appropriate comments. Thoroughly test the program using your own data sets.

3. You are burning some music CDs for a party. You've arranged a list of songs in the order in which you want to play them. However, you would like to maximize your use of space on the CD, which holds 80 minutes of music. So, you want to figure out the total time for a group of songs and see how well they fit. Write a design and a C++ program to help you do this. The data are on file `songs.dat`. The time is entered as seconds. For example, if a song takes 7 minutes and 42 seconds to play, the data entered for that song would be

462

After all the data has been read, the application should print a message indicating the time remaining on the CD.

The output should be in the form of a table with columns and headings written on a file. For example,

Song Number	Song Time Minutes	Seconds	Total Time Minutes	Seconds
1	5	10	5	10
2	7	42	12	52
5	4	19	17	11
3	4	33	21	44
4	10	27	32	11
6	8	55	41	6
7	5	0	46	6

There are 33 minutes and 54 seconds of space left on the 80 minute CD.

Note that the output converts the input from seconds to minutes and seconds. Use meaningful variable names, proper indentation, and appropriate comments. Thoroughly test the program using your own data sets.

4. A palindrome is a phrase that reads the same both forwards and backwards. Write a C++ program that reads a line from `cin`, prints its characters in reverse order on `cout`, and then pronounces judgment on whether the input line is a palindrome. For example, here are two sample runs of the program:

```
Enter string: able was I ere I saw elba
able was I ere I saw elba

is a palindrome.


Enter string: madam I'm adam
mada m'I madam

is not a palindrome
```

Hint: use the substr function within a loop to extract and print the characters one-by-one from the string, starting at the end of the string, and at the same time, extract the corresponding character starting at the beginning of the string to compare with it.

Use a prompting message, meaningful variable names, proper indentation, and appropriate comments. Thoroughly test the program using your own data sets.

5. You're working for a company that's building an email list from files of mail messages. They would like you to write a program that reads a file called `mail.dat`, and that outputs every string containing the @ sign to file `addresses.dat`. For the purpose of this project, a string is defined as it is by the C++ stream reader—a contiguous sequence of non-whitespace characters. Given the data:

```
From:   sharon@marzipan.edu
Date: Wed, 13 Aug 2003 17:12:33 EDT
Subject: Re: hi
To:   john@meringue.com

John,

Dave's email is dave_smith@icing.org.

ttyl,

sharon
```

Then the program would output on file `addresses.dat`:

```
sharon@marzipan.edu
john@meringue.com
dave_smith@icing.org.
```

Use meaningful variable names, proper indentation, and appropriate comments. Thoroughly test the program using your own data sets.

Case Study Follow-Up

1. The first version of program Acoustic remembers the reading number of the highest reading. If there are multiple readings with the same value, it remembers only the first one. Change the program so that it remembers the last of these values instead. Hint: you only need to add one character to the program.
2. The second version of program Acoustic keeps track of the lowest dip in the readings. If there are two dips that are equal, it remembers the first one. Change the program so that it remembers the last one.
3. Does the loop in program Acoustic use a priming read?

4. What type of loop, event-controlled or count-controlled, is used in program Acoustic?

5. The problem states that the readings are on a file. They equally could well have been entered from the keyboard. Change the revised program so that the values are entered in real time.

6. How might you determine whether it is better to enter data from a file or from the keyboard?

7. Discuss how you might go about devising a test plan for program Acoustic.

Functions

Knowledge Goals

- *To know how functions can be used to reflect the structure of a functional decomposition.*
- *To understand the difference between value and reference parameters.*
- *To know how to use arguments and parameters.*

Skill Goals

To be able to:

- *Write a module of your own design as a void function.*
- *Design the parameter list for each module of a functional decomposition.*
- *Code a program using functions.*
- *Define and use local variables correctly.*
- *Write a program that uses multiple calls to a single function.*

Goals

You have been using C++ functions since we introduced standard library routines such as `sqrt` and `abs` in Chapter 3. By now, you should be quite comfortable with the idea of calling these subprograms to perform a task. So far, we have not considered how the programmer can create his or her own functions other than `main`. That is the topic of this chapter and the next.

You might wonder why we waited until now to look at user-defined subprograms. The reason, and the major purpose for using subprograms, is that we write our own value-returning functions and void functions to help organize and simplify larger programs. Until now, our programs have been relatively small and simple, so we didn't need to write subprograms. Now that we've covered the basic control structures, we are ready to introduce subprograms so that we can begin writing larger and more complex programs.

7.1 Functional Decomposition with Void Functions

As a brief refresher, let's review the two kinds of subprograms with which the C++ language works: value-returning functions and void functions. A value-returning function receives some data through its argument list, computes a single function value, and returns this function value to the calling code. The caller invokes (calls) a value-returning function by using its name and argument list in an expression:

```
y = 3.8 * sqrt(x);
```

In contrast, a void function (*procedure*, in some languages) does not return a function value. Nor is it called from within an expression. Instead, the function call appears as a complete, stand-alone statement. An example is the `get` function associated with the `istream` and `ifstream` classes:

```
cin.get(inputChar);
```

In this chapter, we concentrate exclusively on creating our own void functions. In Chapter 8, we examine how to write value-returning functions.

From the early chapters on, you have been designing your programs as collections of modules. Many of these modules are naturally implemented as *user-defined void functions*. We now look at how to turn the modules in your algorithms into user-defined void functions.

When to Use Functions

In general, you can code any module as a function, although some are so simple that this really is unnecessary. In designing a program, then, we frequently need to decide which modules should be implemented as functions. The decision should be based on whether the overall program is easier to understand as a result. Other factors can affect this decision, but for now this is the simplest heuristic (strategy) to use.

If a module is a single line only, it is usually best to write it directly in the program. Turning it into a function only complicates the overall program, which defeats the purpose of using subprograms. On the other hand, if a module is many lines long, it is easier to understand the program if the module is turned into a function.

Keep in mind that whether you choose to code a module as a function or not affects only the readability of the program and may make it more or less convenient to change the program later. Your choice does not affect the correct functioning of the program.

Writing Modules as Void Functions

It is quite simple to turn a module into a void function in C++. Basically, a void function looks like the `main` function except that the function heading uses `void` rather than `int` as the data type of the function. Additionally, the body of a void function does not contain a statement like

```
return 0;
```

as does `main`. A void function does not return a function value to its caller.

Let's look at a program using void functions. A friend of yours is returning from a long trip, and you want to write a program that prints the following message:

```
* * * * * * * * * * * * * * *
* * * * * * * * * * * * * * *
  Welcome  Home!
* * * * * * * * * * * * * * *
* * * * * * * * * * * * * * *
* * * * * * * * * * * * * * *
* * * * * * * * * * * * * * *
```

Here is a design for the program.

Main	Level 0
Print two lines of asterisks Print "Welcome Home!" Print four lines of asterisks	

| Print 2 Lines | Level 1 |

```
Print "***************"
Print "***************"
```

| Print 4 Lines |

```
Print "***************"
Print "***************"
Print "***************"
Print "***************"
```

If we write the two first-level modules as void functions, the `main` function is simply

```
int main()
{
    Print2Lines();
    cout << "Welcome Home!" << endl;
    Print4Lines();
    return 0;
}
```

Notice how similar this code is to the main module of our functional decomposition. It contains two function calls—one to a function named `Print2Lines` and another to a function named `Print4Lines`. Both of these functions have empty argument lists.

The following code should look familiar to you, but look carefully at the function heading.

```
void Print2Lines()                          // Function heading
{
    cout << "***************" << endl;
    cout << "***************" << endl;
}
```

This segment is a *function definition*. A function definition is the code that extends from the function heading to the end of the block that is the body of the function. The function heading begins with the word `void`, signaling the compiler that this is not a value-returning function. The body of the function executes some ordinary statements and does *not* finish with a `return` statement to return a function value.

Now look again at the function heading. Just like any other identifier in C++, the name of a function cannot include blanks, even though our paper-and-pencil module names do. Following the function name is an empty argument list—that is, there is nothing between the parentheses. Later we see what goes inside the parentheses if a function uses arguments. Now let's put `main` and the other two functions together to form a complete program.

```cpp
//******************************************************************
// Welcome program
// This program prints a "Welcome Home" message
//******************************************************************
#include <iostream>

using namespace std;

void Print2Lines();                       // Function prototypes
void Print4Lines();

int main()
{
    Print2Lines();                        // Function call
    cout << " Welcome Home!" << endl;
    Print4Lines();                        // Function call
    return 0;
}

//******************************************************************

void Print2Lines()                        // Function heading

// This function prints two lines of asterisks

{
    cout << "***************" << endl;
    cout << "***************" << endl;
}

//******************************************************************

void Print4Lines()                        // Function heading

// This function prints four lines of asterisks

{
    cout << "***************" << endl;
    cout << "***************" << endl;
    cout << "***************" << endl;
    cout << "***************" << endl;
}
```

C++ function definitions can appear in any order. We could have chosen to place the `main` function last instead of first, but C++ programmers typically put `main` first and any supporting functions after it.

In the Welcome program, the two statements just before the `main` function are called *function prototypes*. These declarations are necessary because of the C++ rule requiring you to declare an identifier before you can use it. Our `main` function uses the identifiers `Print2Lines` and `Print4Lines`, but the definitions of those functions don't appear until later. We must supply the function prototypes to inform the compiler in advance that `Print2Lines` and `Print4Lines` are the names of functions, that they do not return function values, and that they have no arguments. We say more about function prototypes later in the chapter.

Because the Welcome program is so simple to begin with, it may seem more complicated with its modules written as functions. However, it is clear that it much more closely resembles our functional decomposition. This is especially true of the `main` function. If you handed this code to someone, the person could look at the `main` function (which, as we said, usually appears first) and tell you immediately what the program does—it prints two lines of something, prints "Welcome Home!", and prints four lines of something. If you asked the person to be more specific, he or she could then look up the details in the other function definitions. The person is able to begin with a top-level view of the program and then study the lower-level modules as necessary, without having to read the entire program or look at a module structure chart. As our programs grow to include many modules nested several levels deep, the ability to read a program in the same manner as a functional decomposition aids greatly in the development and debugging process.

May We Introduce

Charles Babbage

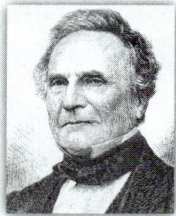

The British mathematician Charles Babbage (1791–1871) is generally credited with designing the world's first computer. Unlike today's electronic computers, however, Babbage's machine was mechanical. It was made of gears and levers, the predominant technology of the 1820s and 1830s.

Babbage actually designed two different machines. The first, called the Difference Engine, was to be used in computing mathematical tables. For example, the Difference Engine could produce a table of squares:

x	x^2
1	1
2	4
3	9
4	16
⋮	⋮

(continued) ▼

Charles Babbage

It was essentially a complex calculator that could not be programmed. Babbage's Difference Engine was designed to improve the accuracy of the computation of tables, not the speed. At that time, all tables were produced by hand, a tedious and error-prone job. Because much of science and engineering depended on accurate table information, an error could have serious consequences. Even though the Difference Engine could perform the calculations only a little faster than a human could, it did so without error. In fact, one of its most important features was that it would stamp its output directly onto copper plates, which could then be placed into a printing press, thereby avoiding even typographical errors.

By 1833, the project to build the Difference Engine had run into financial trouble. The engineer whom Babbage had hired to do the construction was dishonest and had drawn the project out as long as possible so as to extract more money from Babbage's sponsors in the British government. Eventually the sponsors became tired of waiting for the machine and withdrew their support. At about the same time, Babbage lost interest in the project because he had developed the idea for a much more powerful machine, which he called the Analytical Engine—a truly programmable computer.

The idea for the Analytical Engine came to Babbage as he toured Europe to survey the best technology of the time in preparation for constructing the Difference Engine. One of the technologies that he saw was the Jacquard automatic loom, in which a series of paper cards with punched holes was fed through the machine to produce a woven cloth pattern. The pattern of holes constituted a program for the loom and made it possible to weave patterns of arbitrary complexity automatically. In fact, its inventor even had a detailed portrait of himself woven by one of his machines.

Babbage realized that this sort of device could be used to control the operation of a computing machine. Instead of calculating just one type of formula, such a machine could be programmed to perform arbitrarily complex computations, including the manipulation of algebraic symbols. As his associate, Ada Lovelace (the world's first computer programmer), elegantly put it, "We may say most aptly that the Analytical Engine weaves algebraical patterns." It is clear that Babbage and Lovelace fully understood the power of a programmable computer and even contemplated the notion that someday such machines could achieve artificial thought.

Unfortunately, Babbage never completed construction of either of his machines. Some historians believe that he never finished them because the technology of the period could not support such complex machinery. But most feel that Babbage's failure was his own doing. He was both brilliant and somewhat eccentric (it is known that he was afraid of Italian organ grinders, for example). As a consequence, he had a tendency to abandon projects in midstream so that he could concentrate on newer and better ideas. He always believed that his new approaches would enable him to complete a machine in less time than his old ideas would.

(continued) ▼

Charles Babbage

When he died, Babbage had many pieces of computing machines and partial drawings of designs, but none of the plans were complete enough to produce a single working computer. After his death, his ideas were dismissed and his inventions ignored. Only after modern computers were developed did historians recognize the true importance of his contributions. Babbage recognized the potential of the computer an entire century before one was fully developed. Today, we can only imagine how different the world would be if he had succeeded in constructing his Analytical Engine.

7.2 An Overview of User-Defined Functions

Now that we've seen an example of how a program is written with functions, let's look briefly and informally at some of the more important points of function construction and use.

Flow of Control in Function Calls

We said that C++ function definitions can be arranged in any order, although `main` usually appears first. During compilation, the functions are translated in the order in which they physically appear. When the program is executed, however, control begins at the first statement in the `main` function, and the program proceeds in logical sequence. When a function call is encountered, logical control is passed to the first statement in that function's body. The statements in the function are executed in logical order. After the last one is executed, control returns to the point immediately following the function call. Because function calls alter the logical order of execution, functions are considered control structures. Figure 7–1 illustrates this physical versus logical ordering of functions. In the figure, functions A, B, and C are written in the physical order A, B, C but are executed in the order C, B, A.

In the Welcome program, execution begins with the first executable statement in the `main` function (the call to `Print2Lines`). When `Print2Lines` is called, control passes to its first statement and subsequent statements in its body. After the last statement in `Print2Lines` has executed, control returns to the `main` function at the point following the call (the output statement that prints "Welcome Home!").

Function Parameters

Looking at the Welcome program, you can see that `Print2Lines` and `Print4Lines` are very similar functions. They differ only in the number of lines that they print. Do we really need two different functions in this program? Maybe we should write only one

```
int main()                              Module Structure Chart
{
      •
      •
      •
    C();
    B();
    A();
    return 0;
}

void A()
{
      •
      •
      •
}
void B()
{
      •
      •
      •
}
void C()
{
      •
      •
      •
}
```

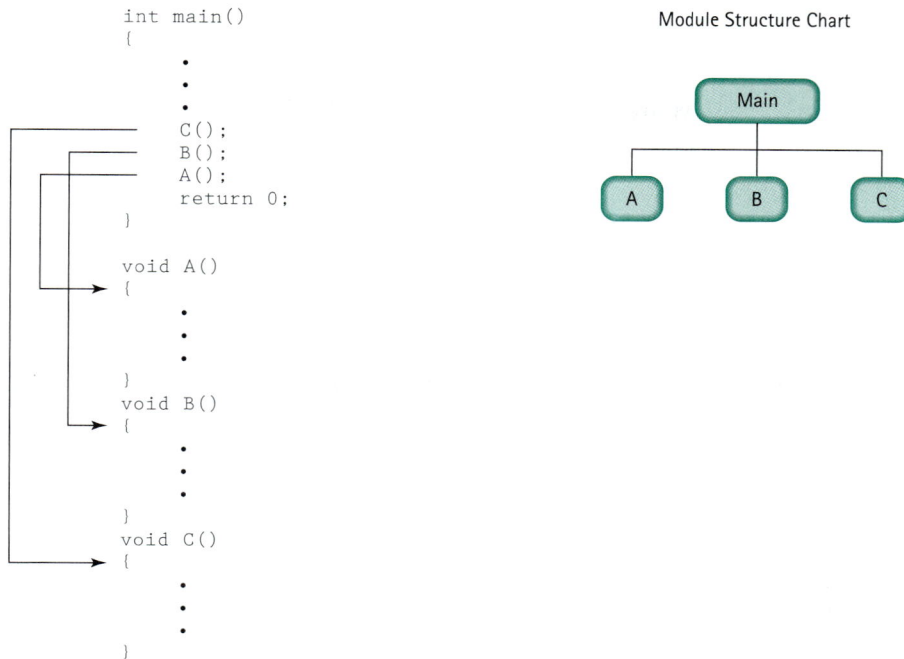

Figure 7–1   *Physical Versus Logical Order of Functions*

function that prints *any* number of lines, where the "any number of lines" is passed as an argument by the caller (main). Here is a second version of the program, which uses only one function to do the printing. We call it NewWelcome.

```cpp
//****************************************************************
// NewWelcome program
// This program prints a "Welcome Home" message
//****************************************************************
#include <iostream>

using namespace std;

void PrintLines( int );                       // Function prototype

int main()
{
    PrintLines(2);
    cout << " Welcome Home!" << endl;
    PrintLines(4);
    return 0;
}
```

```
//************************************************************************

void PrintLines( int numLines )

// This function prints lines of asterisks, where
// numLines specifies how many lines to print

{
    int count;        // Loop control variable

    count = 1;
    while (count <= numLines)
    {
        cout << "***************" << endl;
        count++;
    }
}
```

In the function heading of PrintLines, you see some code between the parentheses that looks like a variable declaration. This is a *parameter declaration*. As you learned in earlier chapters, arguments represent a way for two functions to communicate with each other. Arguments enable the calling function to input (pass) values to another function to use in its processing and—in some cases—to allow the called function to output (return) results to the caller. The items listed in the call to a function are the **arguments**. The variables declared in the function heading are the **parameters**. (Some programmers use the pair of terms *actual argument* and *formal argument* instead of *argument* and *parameter*. Others use the term *actual parameter* in place of *argument*, and *formal parameter* in place of *parameter*.) Notice that the main function in the code above is a *parameterless* function.

Argument   A variable or expression listed in a call to a function; also called *actual argument* or *actual parameter*.

Parameter   A variable declared in a function heading; also called *formal argument* or *formal parameter*.

In the NewWelcome program, the arguments in the two function calls are the constants 2 and 4, and the parameter in the PrintLines function is named numLines. The main function first calls PrintLines with an argument of 2. When control is turned over to PrintLines, the parameter numLines is initialized to 2. Within PrintLines, the count-controlled loop executes twice and the function returns. The second time PrintLines is called, the parameter numLines is initialized to the value of the argument, 4. The loop executes four times, after which the function returns.

Although there is no benefit in doing so, we could write the main function this way:

```
int main()
{
    int lineCount;
```

```
        lineCount = 2;
        PrintLines(lineCount);
        cout << " Welcome Home!" << endl;
        lineCount = 4;
        PrintLines(lineCount);
        return 0;
}
```

In this version, the argument in each call to PrintLines is a variable rather than a constant. Each time main calls PrintLines, a copy of the argument's value is passed to the function to initialize the parameter numLines. This version shows that when you pass a variable as an argument, the argument and the parameter can have different names.

The NewWelcome program brings up a second major reason for using functions—namely, a function can be called from many places in the main function (or from other functions). Use of multiple calls can save a great deal of effort in coding many problem solutions. If a task must be done in more than one place in a program, we can avoid repetitive coding by writing it as a function and then calling it wherever we need it.

If more than one argument is passed to a function, the arguments and parameters are matched by their relative positions in the two lists. For example, if you want PrintLines to print lines consisting of any selected character, not only asterisks, you might rewrite the function so that its heading is

```
void PrintLines( int  numLines,
                 char whichChar )
```

and a call to the function might look like this:

```
PrintLines(3, '#');
```

The first argument, 3, is matched with numLines because numLines is the first parameter. Likewise, the second argument, '#', is matched with the second parameter, whichChar.

7.3 Syntax and Semantics of Void Functions

Function Call (Invocation)

To call (or invoke) a void function, we use its name as a statement, with the arguments in parentheses following the name. A **function call** in a program results in the execution of the

Function call (to a void function) A statement that transfers control to a void function. In C++, this statement is the name of the function, followed by a list of arguments.

body of the called function. This is the syntax template of a function call to a void function:

FunctionCall (to a void function)

FunctionName (ArgumentList);

According to the syntax template for a function call, the argument list is optional. A function is not required to have arguments. However, as the syntax template also shows, the parentheses are required even if the argument list is empty.

If there are two or more arguments in the argument list, you must separate them with commas. Here is the syntax template for ArgumentList:

ArgumentList

Expression , Expression . . .

When a function call is executed, the arguments are passed to the parameters according to their positions, left to right, and control is then transferred to the first executable statement in the function body. When the last statement in the function has executed, control returns to the point from which the function was called.

Function Declarations and Definitions

In C++, you must declare every identifier before it can be used. In the case of functions, a function's declaration must physically precede any function call.

A function declaration announces to the compiler the name of the function, the data type of the function's return value (either `void` or a data type like `int` or `float`), and the data types of the parameters it uses. The NewWelcome program shows a total of three function declarations. The first declaration (the statement labeled "Function prototype") does not include the body of the function. The remaining two declarations—for `main` and `PrintLines`—include bodies for the functions.

Function prototype   A function declaration without the body of the function.

Function definition   A function declaration that includes the body of the function.

In C++ terminology, a function declaration that omits the body is called a **function prototype**, and a declaration that does include the body is a **function definition**. We can use a Venn diagram to picture the fact that all definitions are declarations, but not all declarations are definitions:

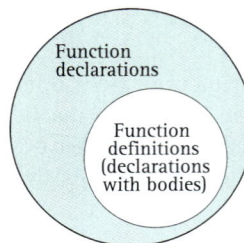

Function declarations

Function definitions (declarations with bodies)

Whether we are talking about functions or variables, the general idea in C++ is that a declaration becomes a definition if it also allocates memory space for the item. (There are exceptions to this rule of thumb, but we don't concern ourselves with them now.) For example, a function prototype is merely a declaration—that is, it specifies the properties of a function: its name, its data type, and the data types of its parameters. But a function definition does more; it causes the compiler to allocate memory for the instructions in the body of the function. (Technically, all of the variable declarations we've used so far have been variable *definitions* as well as declarations—they allocate memory for the variable. In Chapter 8, we see examples of variable declarations that aren't variable definitions.)

The rule throughout C++ is that you can declare an item as many times as you wish, but you can define it only once. In the NewWelcome program, we could include many function prototypes for `PrintLines` (though we'd have no reason to), but only one function definition is allowed.

Function Prototypes   We have said that the definition of the `main` function usually appears first in a program, followed by the definitions of all other functions. To satisfy the requirement that identifiers be declared before they are used, C++ programmers typically place all function prototypes near the top of the program, before the definition of `main`.

A function prototype (known as a *forward declaration* in some languages) specifies in advance the data type of the function value to be returned (or the word `void`) and the data types of the parameters. A prototype for a void function has the following form:

FunctionPrototype (for a void function)

> **void** FunctionName (ParameterList);

As you can see in the syntax template, no body is included for the function, and a semicolon terminates the declaration. The parameter list is optional, to allow for parameterless functions. If the parameter list is present, it has the following form:

ParameterList (in a function prototype)

> Datatype **&** VariableName , DataType **&** VariableName . . .

The ampersand (&) attached to the name of a data type is optional and has a special significance that we cover later in the chapter.

In a function prototype, the parameter list must specify the data types of the parameters, but their names are optional. You could write either

```
void DoSomething( int, float );
```

or

```
void DoSomething( int velocity, float angle );
```

Sometimes it's useful for documentation purposes to supply names for the parameters, but the compiler ignores them.

Function Definitions   You learned in Chapter 2 that a function definition consists of two parts: the function heading and the function body, which is syntactically a block (compound statement). Here's the syntax template for a function definition, specifically, for a void function:

FunctionDefinition (for a void function)

```
void FunctionName ( ParameterList )
{
      Statement
        ⋮

}
```

Notice that the function heading does *not* end in a semicolon the way a function prototype does. It is a common syntax error to put a semicolon at the end of the line.

The syntax of the parameter list differs slightly from that of a function prototype in that you *must* specify the names of all the parameters. Also, it's our style preference (but not a language requirement) to declare each parameter on a separate line:

ParameterList (in a function definition)

```
Datatype & VariableName ,
Datatype & VariableName
  ⋮
```

Local Variables

Because a function body is a block, any function—not only the `main` function—can include variable declarations within its body. These variables are called **local variables** because they are accessible only within the block in which they are declared. As far as the calling code is concerned, they don't exist. If you tried to print the contents of a local variable from another function, a compile-time error such as "UNDECLARED IDENTIFIER" would occur. You

Local variable   A variable declared within a block and not accessible outside of that block.

saw an example of a local variable in the NewWelcome program—the `count` variable declared within the `PrintLines` function.

In contrast to local variables, variables declared outside of all the functions in a program are called *global variables*. We return to the topic of global variables in Chapter 8.

Local variables occupy memory space only while the function is executing. At the moment the function is called, memory space is created for its local variables. When the function returns, its local variables are destroyed.* Therefore, every time the function is called, its local variables start out with their values undefined. Because every call to a function is independent of every other call to that same function, you must initialize the local variables within the function itself. And because local variables are destroyed when the function returns, you cannot use them to store values between calls to the function.

The following code segment illustrates each of the parts of the function declaration and calling mechanism that we have discussed.

```cpp
#include <iostream>

using namespace std;

void TryThis( int, int, float );        // Function prototype

int main()                              // Function definition
{
    int    int1;                        // Variables local to main
    int    int2;
    float  someFloat;
    ⋮
    TryThis(int1, int2, someFloat);     // Function call with three
                                        //    arguments
    ⋮
}

void TryThis( int    param1,            // Function definition with
              int    param2,            //    three parameters
              float  param3 )
{
    int    i;                           // Variables local to TryThis
    float  x;
    ⋮
}
```

---

*We'll see an exception to this rule in the next chapter.

The Return Statement

The `main` function uses the statement

```
return 0;
```

to return the value 0 (or 1 or some other value) to its caller, the operating system. Every value-returning function must return its function value this way.

A void function does not return a function value. Control returns from the function when it "falls off" the end of the body—that is, after the final statement has executed. As you saw in the NewWelcome program, the `PrintLines` function simply prints some lines of asterisks and then returns.

Alternatively, there is a second form of the Return statement. It looks like this:

```
return;
```

This statement is valid *only* for void functions. It can appear anywhere in the body of the function; it causes control to exit the function immediately and return to the caller. Here's an example:

```
void SomeFunc( int n )
{
    if (n > 50)
    {
        cout << "The value is out of range.";
        return;
    }
    n = 412 * n;
    cout << n;
}
```

In this (nonsense) example, there are two ways for control to exit the function. At function entry, the value of n is tested. If it is greater than 50, the function prints a message and returns immediately without executing any more statements. If n is less than or equal to 50, the If statement's then-clause is skipped and control proceeds to the assignment statement. After the last statement, control returns to the caller.

Another way of writing the above function is to use an If-Then-Else structure:

```
void SomeFunc( int n )
{
    if (n > 50)
        cout << "The value is out of range.";
    else
    {
        n = 412 * n;
        cout << n;
    }
}
```

If you asked different programmers about these two versions of the function, you would get differing opinions. Some prefer the first version, saying that it is most straightforward to use Return statements whenever it logically makes sense to do so. Others insist on the *single-entry, single-exit* approach in the second version. With this philosophy, control enters a function at one point only (the first executable statement) and exits at one point only (the end of the body). They argue that multiple exits from a function make the program logic hard to follow and difficult to debug. Other programmers take a position somewhere between these two philosophies, allowing occasional use of the Return statement when the logic is clear. Our advice is to use `return` sparingly; overuse can lead to confusing code.

Matters of Style

Naming Void Functions

When you choose a name for a void function, keep in mind how calls to it will look. A call is written as a statement; therefore, it should sound like a command or an instruction to the computer. For this reason, it is a good idea to choose a name that is an imperative verb or has an imperative verb as part of it. (In English, an imperative verb is one representing a command: *Listen! Look! Do something!*) For example, the statement

```
Lines(3);
```

has no verb to suggest that it's a command. Adding the verb *Print* makes the name sound like an action:

```
PrintLines(3);
```

When you are picking a name for a void function, write down sample calls with different names until you come up with one that sounds like a command to the computer.

Header Files

From the very beginning, we have been using #include directives that request the C++ preprocessor to insert the contents of header files into our programs:

```
#include <iostream>
#include <cmath>       // For sqrt() and fabs()
#include <fstream>     // For file I/O
#include <climits>     // For INT_MAX and INT_MIN
```

Exactly what do these header files contain?

It turns out that there is nothing magical about header files. Their contents are nothing more than a series of C++ declarations. There are declarations of items such as named constants (INT_MAX, INT_MIN), classes (istream, ostream, string), and objects (cin, cout). But most of the items in a header file are function prototypes.

Suppose that your program needs to use the library function sqrt in a statement like this:

```
y = sqrt(x);
```

Every identifier must be declared before it can be used. If you forget to #include the header file cmath, the compiler gives you an "UNDECLARED IDENTIFIER" error message. The file cmath contains function prototypes for sqrt and other math-oriented library functions. With this header file included in your program, the compiler not only knows that the identifier sqrt is the name of a function but it also can verify that your function call is correct with respect to the number of arguments and their data types.

Header files save you the trouble of writing all of the library function prototypes yourself at the beginning of your program. With just one line—the #include directive—you cause the preprocessor to go out and find the header file and insert the prototypes into your program. In later chapters, we see how to create our own header files that contain declarations specific to our programs.

7.4 Parameters

When a function is executed, it uses the arguments given to it in the function call. How is this done? The answer to this question depends on the nature of the parameters. C++ supports two kinds of parameters: **value parameters** and **reference parameters**. With a value parameter, which is declared without an ampersand (&) at the end of the data type name, the function receives a copy of the argument's value. With a reference parameter, which is declared by adding an ampersand to the data type name, the function receives the location (memory address) of the caller's argument. Before we examine in detail the difference between these two kinds of parameters, let's look at an example of a function heading with a mixture of reference and value parameter declarations.

> **Value parameter** A parameter that receives a copy of the value of the corresponding argument.
>
> **Reference parameter** A parameter that receives the location (memory address) of the caller's argument.

```
void Example( int&  param1,      // A reference parameter
              int   param2,      // A value parameter
              float param3 )     // Another value parameter
```

With simple data types—int, char, float, and so on—a value parameter is the default (assumed) kind of parameter. In other words, if you don't do anything special (add an ampersand), a parameter is assumed to be a value parameter. To specify a reference parameter, you have to go out of your way to do something extra (attach an ampersand).

Let's look at both kinds of parameters, starting with value parameters.

Value Parameters

In the NewWelcome program, the `PrintLines` function heading is

```
void PrintLines( int numLines )
```

The parameter `numLines` is a value parameter because its data type name doesn't end in &. If the function is called using an argument `lineCount`,

```
PrintLines(lineCount);
```

then the parameter `numLines` receives a copy of the value of `lineCount`. At this moment, there are two copies of the data—one in the argument `lineCount` and one in the parameter `numLines`. If a statement inside the `PrintLines` function were to change the value of `numLines`, this change would not affect the argument `lineCount` (remember, there are two copies of the data). Using value parameters thus helps us avoid unintentional changes to arguments.

Because value parameters are passed copies of their arguments, anything that has a value may be passed to a value parameter. This includes constants, variables, and even arbitrarily complicated expressions. (The expression is simply evaluated and a copy of the result is sent to the corresponding value parameter.) For the `PrintLines` function, the following function calls are all valid:

```
PrintLines(3);
PrintLines(lineCount);
PrintLines(2 * abs(10 - someInt));
```

There must be the same number of arguments in a function call as there are parameters in the function heading.* Also, each argument should have the same data type as the parameter in the same position. Notice how each parameter in the following example is matched to the argument in the same position (the data type of each argument below is what you would assume from its name):

Function heading: `void ShowMatch(float num1, int num2, char letter)`

Function call: `ShowMatch(floatVariable, intVariable, charVariable);`

---

*This statement is not the whole truth. C++ has a special language feature—*default parameters*—that lets you call a function with fewer arguments than parameters. We do not cover default parameters in this book.

If the matched items are not of the same data type, implicit type coercion takes place. For example, if a parameter is of type int, an argument that is a float expression is coerced to an int value before it is passed to the function. As usual in C++, you can avoid unintended type coercion by using an explicit type cast or, better yet, by not mixing data types at all.

As we have stressed, a value parameter receives a copy of the argument, and therefore the caller's argument cannot be accessed directly or changed. When a function returns, the contents of its value parameters are destroyed, along with the contents of its local variables. The difference between value parameters and local variables is that the values of local variables are undefined when a function starts to execute, whereas value parameters are automatically initialized to the values of the corresponding arguments.

Because the contents of value parameters are destroyed when the function returns, they cannot be used to return information to the calling code. What if we *do* want to return information by modifying the caller's arguments? We must use the second kind of parameter available in C++: reference parameters. Let's look at these now.

Reference Parameters

A reference parameter is one that you declare by attaching an ampersand to the name of its data type. It is called a reference parameter because the called function can refer to the corresponding argument directly. Specifically, the function is allowed to inspect *and modify* the caller's argument.

When a function is invoked using a reference parameter, it is the *location* (memory address) of the argument, not its value, that is passed to the function. There is only one copy of the information, and it is used by both the caller and the called function. When a function is called, the argument and the parameter become synonyms for the same location in memory. Whatever value is left by the called function in this location is the value that the caller will find there. Therefore, you must be careful when using a reference parameter because any change made to it affects the argument in the calling code. Let's look at an example.

In Chapter 5, we wrote an Activity program that reads in a temperature from the user and prints the recommended activity. Here is its design.

Main	Level 0

Get temperature
Print activity

Get Temperature	Level 1

Prompt user for temperature
Read temperature
Echo print temperature

Print Activity

Print "The recommended activity is"
IF temperature > 85
    Print "swimming."
ELSE IF temperature > 70
    Print "tennis."
ELSE IF temperature > 32
    Print "golf."
ELSE IF temperature > 0
    Print "skiing."
ELSE
    Print "dancing."

Let's write the two level 1 modules as void functions, GetTemp and PrintActivity, so that the main function looks like the main module of our functional decomposition. Here is the resulting program.

```cpp
//****************************************************************
// Activity program
// This program outputs an appropriate activity
// for a given temperature
//****************************************************************
#include <iostream>

using namespace std;

void GetTemp( int& );                    // Function prototypes
void PrintActivity( int );

int main()
{
    int temperature;      // The outside temperature

    GetTemp(temperature);                // Function call
    PrintActivity(temperature);          // Function call
    return 0;
}


//****************************************************************

void GetTemp( int& temp )                // Reference parameter

// This function prompts for a temperature to be entered,
// reads the input value into temp, and echo prints it
```

```
{
    cout << "Enter the outside temperature:" << endl;
    cin >> temp;
    cout << "The current temperature is " << temp << endl;
}


//*****************************************************************


void PrintActivity( int temp )                  // Value parameter

// Given the value of temp, this function prints a message
// indicating an appropriate activity

{
    cout << "The recommended activity is ";
    if (temp > 85)
        cout << "swimming." << endl;
    else if (temp > 70)
        cout << "tennis." << endl;
    else if (temp > 32)
        cout << "golf." << endl;
    else if (temp > 0)
        cout << "skiing." << endl;
    else
        cout << "dancing." << endl;
}
```

In the Activity program, the arguments in the two function calls are both named temperature. The parameter in GetTemp is a reference parameter named temp. The parameter in PrintActivity is a value parameter, also named temp.

The main function tells GetTemp where to leave the temperature by giving it the location of the variable temperature when it makes the function call. We *must* use a reference parameter here so that GetTemp knows where to deposit the result. In a sense, the parameter temp is just a convenient placeholder in the function definition. When GetTemp is called with temperature as its argument, all the references to temp inside the function actually are made to temperature. If the function were to be called again with a different variable as an argument, all the references to temp would actually refer to that other variable until the function returned control to main.

In contrast, PrintActivity's parameter is a value parameter. When PrintActivity is called, main sends a copy of the value of temperature for the function to work with. It's appropriate to use a value parameter in this case because PrintActivity is not supposed to modify the argument temperature.

Because arguments and parameters can have different names, we can call a function at different times with different arguments. Suppose we wanted to change the

Activity program to print an activity for both the indoor and outdoor temperatures. We could declare integer variables in the `main` function named `indoorTemp` and `outdoorTemp`, then write the body of `main` as follows:

```
GetTemp(indoorTemp);
PrintActivity(indoorTemp);
GetTemp(outdoorTemp);
PrintActivity(outdoorTemp)
return 0;
```

In `GetTemp` and `PrintActivity`, the parameters would receive values from, or pass values to, either `indoorTemp` or `outdoorTemp`.

The following table summarizes the usage of arguments and parameters.

Item	Usage
Argument	Appears in a function *call*. The corresponding parameter may be either a reference or a value parameter.
Value parameter	Appears in a function *heading*. Receives a *copy* of the value of the corresponding argument.
Reference parameter	Appears in a function *heading*. Receives the *address* of the corresponding argument.

An Analogy

Before we talk more about parameter passing, let's look at an analogy from daily life. You're at the local discount catalog showroom to buy a Father's Day present. To place your order, you fill out an order form. The form has places to write in the quantity of each item and its catalog number, and places where the order clerk will fill in the prices. You write down what you want and hand the form to the clerk. You wait for the clerk to check whether the items are available and calculate the cost. He returns the form, and you see that the items are in stock and the price is $48.50. You pay the clerk and go on about your business.

This illustrates how function calls work. The clerk is like a void function. You, acting as the `main` function, ask him to do some work for you. You give him some information: the item numbers and quantities. These are his input parameters. You wait until he returns some information to you: the availability of the items and their prices. These are the clerk's output parameters. The clerk does this task all day long with different input values. Each order activates the same process. The shopper waits until the clerk returns information based on the specific input.

The order form is analogous to the arguments of a function call. The spaces on the form represent variables in the `main` function. When you hand the form to the clerk, some of the places contain information and some are empty. The clerk holds the form while doing his job so he can write information in the blank spaces. These blank spaces correspond to reference parameters; you expect the clerk to return results to you in the spaces.

When the `main` function calls another function, reference parameters allow the called function to access and change the variables in the argument list. When the called function finishes, `main` continues, making use of whatever new information the called function left in the variables.

The parameter list is like the set of shorthand or slang terms the clerk uses to describe the spaces on the order form. For example, he may think in terms of "units," "codes," and "receipts." These are his terms (parameters) for what the order form calls "quantity," "catalog number," and "price" (the arguments). But he doesn't waste time reading the names on the form every time; he knows that the first item is the units (quantity), the second is the code (catalog number), and so on. In other words, he looks only at the position of each space on the form. This is how arguments are matched to parameters—by their relative positions in the two lists.

Matching Arguments with Parameters

Earlier we said that with reference parameters, the argument and the parameter become synonyms for the same memory location. When a function returns control to its caller, the link between the argument and the parameter is broken. They are synonymous only during a particular call to the function. The only evidence that a matchup between the two ever occurred is that the contents of the argument may have changed (see Figure 7–2).

When flow of control is in the `main` function,
`temperature` can be accessed as shown by the arrow.

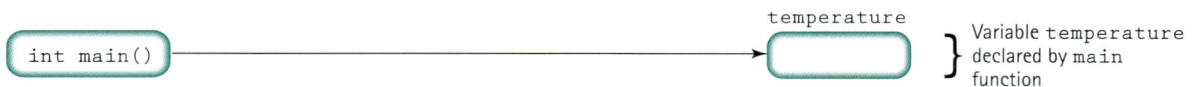

When flow of control is in function GetTemp, every
reference to `temp` accesses the variable `temperature`.

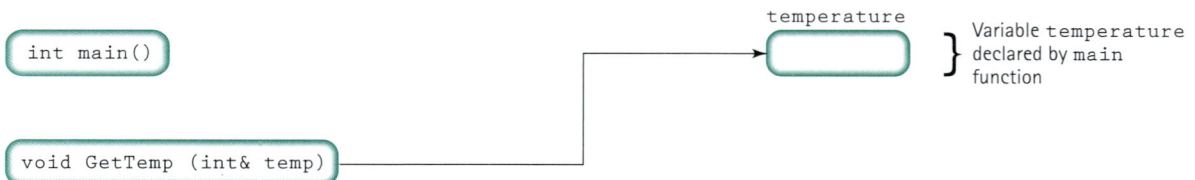

Figure 7–2   *Using a Reference Parameter to Access an Argument*

Only a variable can be passed as an argument to a reference parameter because a function can assign a new value to the argument. (In contrast, remember that an arbitrarily complicated expression can be passed to a value parameter.) Suppose that we have a function with the following heading:

```
void DoThis( float val,      // Value parameter
             int&  count )    // Reference parameter
```

Then the following function calls are all valid.

```
DoThis(someFloat, someInt);
DoThis(9.83, intCounter);
DoThis(4.9 * sqrt(y), myInt);
```

In the `DoThis` function, the first parameter is a value parameter, so any expression is allowed as the argument. The second parameter is a reference parameter, so the argument *must* be a variable name. The statement

```
DoThis(y, 3);
```

generates a compile-time error because the second argument isn't a variable name. Earlier we said the syntax template for an argument list is

ArgumentList

Expression , Expression . . .

But you must keep in mind that Expression is restricted to a variable name if the corresponding parameter is a reference parameter.

There is another important difference between value and reference parameters when it comes to matching arguments with parameters. With value parameters, we said that implicit type coercion occurs if the matched items have different data types (the value of the argument is coerced, if possible, to the data type of the parameter). In contrast, with reference parameters, the matched items *must* have exactly the same data type.

The following table summarizes the appropriate forms of arguments.

Parameter	Argument
Value parameter	A variable, constant, or arbitrary expression (type coercion may take place)
Reference parameter	A variable *only*, of exactly the same data type as the parameter

Finally, it is the programmer's responsibility to make sure that the argument list and parameter list match up semantically as well as syntactically. For example, suppose we had written the indoor/outdoor modification to the Activity program as follows.

```
int main()
{
    ⋮
    GetTemp(indoorTemp);
    PrintActivity(indoorTemp);
    GetTemp(outdoorTemp);
    PrintActivity(indoorTemp)    // Wrong argument
    return 0;
}
```

The argument list in the last function call matches the corresponding parameter list in its number and type of arguments, so no syntax error would be signaled. However, the output would be erroneous because the argument is the wrong temperature value. Similarly, if a function has two parameters of the same data type, you must be careful that the arguments are in the right order. If they are in the wrong order, no syntax error will result, but the answers will be wrong.

Theoretical Foundations

Argument-Passing Mechanisms

There are three major ways of passing arguments to and from subprograms. C++ supports only two of these mechanisms; however, it's useful to know about all three in case you have occasion to use them in another language.

C++ reference parameters employ a mechanism called *pass by address* or *pass by location*. A memory address is passed to the function. Another name for this is *pass by reference* because the function can refer directly to the caller's variable that is specified in the argument list.

C++ value parameters are an example of *pass by value*. The function receives a copy of the value of the caller's argument. Passing by value can be less efficient than passing by address because the value of an argument may occupy many memory locations (as we see in Chapter 11), whereas an address usually occupies only a single location. For the simple data types int, char, bool, and float, the efficiency of either mechanism is about the same.

A third method of passing arguments is called *pass by name*. The argument is passed to the function as a character string that must be interpreted by special runtime support software (called a *thunk*) supplied by the compiler. For example, if the name of a variable is passed to a function, the run-time interpreter looks up the name of the argument in a table of declarations to find the address of the variable. Passing by name can have unexpected results. If an argument has the same spelling as a local variable in the function, the function will refer to the local version of the variable instead of the variable in the calling code.

(continued) ▼

Argument-Passing Mechanisms

Some versions of passing by name allow an expression or even a code segment to be passed to a function. Each time the function refers to the parameter, an interpreter performs the action specified by the parameter. An interpreter is similar to a compiler and nearly as complex. Thus, passing by name is the least efficient of the three argument-passing mechanisms. Passing by name is supported by the ALGOL and LISP programming languages, but not by C++.

There are two different ways of matching arguments with parameters, although C++ supports only one of them. Most programming languages, C++ among them, match arguments and parameters by their relative positions in the argument and parameter lists. This is called *positional matching*, *relative matching*, or *implicit matching*. A few languages, such as Ada, also support *explicit* or *named matching*. In explicit matching, the argument list specifies the name of the parameter to be associated with each argument. Explicit matching allows arguments to be written in any order in the function call. The real advantage is that each call documents precisely which values are being passed to which parameters.

7.5 Designing Functions

We've looked at some examples of functions and defined the syntax of function prototypes and function definitions. But how do we design functions? First, we need to be more specific about what functions do. We've said that they allow us to organize our programs more like our functional decompositions, but what really is the advantage of doing that?

The body of a function is like any other segment of code, except that it is contained in a separate block within the program. Isolating a segment of code in a separate block means that its implementation details can be "hidden" from view. As long as you know how to call a function and what its purpose is, you can use it without looking at the code inside the function body. For example, you don't know how the code for a library function like `sqrt` is written (its implementation is hidden from view), yet you still can use it effectively.

The specification of what a function does and how it is invoked defines its **interface** (see Figure 7–3). By hiding a module implementation, or **encapsulating** the module, we can make changes to it without changing the `main`

Interface A connecting link at a shared boundary that permits independent systems to meet and act on or communicate with each other. Also, the formal description of the purpose of a subprogram and the mechanism for communicating with it.

Encapsulation Hiding a module implementation in a separate block with a formally specified interface.

Heading: `void PrintActivity ( int temp )`
Precondition: `temp` is a temperature value in a valid range
Postcondition: A message has been printed indicating an
appropriate activity given temperature `temp`

Implementation

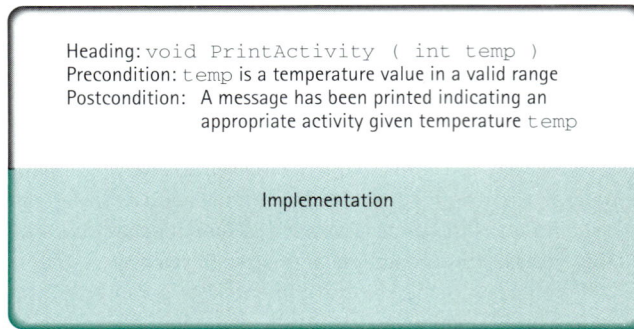

Figure 7–3   *Function Interface (Visible) and Implementation (Hidden)*

function, as long as the interface remains the same. For example, you might rewrite the body of a function using a more efficient algorithm.

Encapsulation is what we do in the functional decomposition process when we postpone the solution of a difficult subproblem. We write down its purpose, its precondition and postcondition, and what information it takes and returns, and then we write the rest of our design as if the subproblem had already been solved. We could hand this interface specification to someone else, and that person could develop a function for us that solves the subproblem. We needn't be concerned about how it works, as long as it conforms to the interface specification. Interfaces and encapsulation are the basis for *team programming*, in which a group of programmers work together to solve a large problem.

Thus, designing a function can (and should) be divided into two tasks: designing the interface and designing the implementation. We already know how to design an implementation—it is a segment of code that corresponds to an algorithm. To design the interface, we focus on the *what*, not the *how*. We must define the behavior of the function (what it does) and the mechanism for communicating with it.

You already know how to specify formally the behavior of a function. Because a function corresponds to a module, its behavior is defined by the precondition and postcondition of the module. All that remains is to define the mechanism for communicating with the function. To do so, make a list of the following items:

1. *Incoming values* that the function receives from the caller.
2. *Outgoing values* that the function produces and returns to the caller.
3. *Incoming/outgoing values*—values the caller has that the function changes (receives and returns).

Now decide which identifiers inside the module match the values in this list. These identifiers become the variables in the parameter list for the function. Then the parameters are declared in the function heading. All other variables that the function needs are local and must be declared within the body of the function. This process is repeated for all the modules at each level.

Let's look more closely at designing the interface. First we examine function preconditions and postconditions. After that, we consider in more detail the notion of incoming, outgoing, and incoming/outgoing parameters.

Writing Assertions as Program Comments

We have been writing module preconditions and postconditions as informal, English-language assertions. From now on, we include preconditions and postconditions as comments to document the interfaces of C++ functions. Here's an example:

```
void PrintAverage( float sum,
                   int   count )

// Precondition:
//     sum is assigned  &&  count > 0
// Postcondition:
//     The average sum/count has been output on one line

{
    cout << "Average is " << sum / float(count) << endl;
}
```

The precondition is an assertion describing everything that the function requires to be true at the moment the caller invokes the function. The postcondition describes the state of the program at the moment the function finishes executing.

You can think of the precondition and postcondition as a contract. The contract states that if the precondition is true at function entry, then the postcondition must be true at function exit. The *caller* is responsible for ensuring the precondition, and the *function code* must ensure the postcondition. If the caller fails to satisfy its part of the contract (the precondition), the contract is off; the function cannot guarantee that the postcondition will be true.

Above, the precondition warns the caller to make sure that sum has been assigned a meaningful value and to be sure that count is positive. If this precondition is true, the function guarantees it will satisfy the postcondition. If count isn't positive when PrintAverage is invoked, the effect of the function is undefined. (For example, if count equals 0, the postcondition surely isn't satisfied—the program crashes!)

Sometimes the caller doesn't need to satisfy any precondition before calling a function. In this case, the precondition can be written as the value true or simply omitted. In the following example, no precondition is necessary:

```
void Get2Ints( int& int1,
               int& int2 )

// Postcondition:
//     User has been prompted to enter two integers
//  && int1 == first input value
//  && int2 == second input value

{
    cout << "Please enter two integers: ";
    cin >> int1 >> int2;
}
```

In assertions written as C++ comments, we use either `&&` or AND to denote the logical AND operator, either `||` or OR to denote a logical OR, either `!` or NOT to denote a logical NOT, and `==` to denote "equals." (Notice that we do *not* use `=` to denote "equals." Even when we write program comments, we want to keep C++'s `==` operator distinct from the assignment operator.)

There is one final notation we use when we express assertions as program comments. Preconditions implicitly refer to values of variables at the moment the function is invoked. Postconditions implicitly refer to values at the moment the function returns. But sometimes you need to write a postcondition that refers to parameter values that existed at the moment the function was invoked. To signify "at the time of entry to the function," we attach the symbol `@entry` to the end of the variable name. Below is an example of the use of this notation. The `Swap` function exchanges, or swaps, the contents of its two parameters.

```cpp
void Swap( int& firstInt,
           int& secondInt )

// Precondition:
//      firstInt and secondInt are assigned
// Postcondition:
//      firstInt == secondInt@entry
//   && secondInt == firstInt@entry

{
    int temporaryInt;

    temporaryInt = firstInt;
    firstInt = secondInt;
    secondInt = temporaryInt;
}
```

Matters of Style

Function Preconditions and Postconditions

Preconditions and postconditions, when well written, are a concise but accurate description of the behavior of a function. A person reading your program should be able to see at a glance how to use the function by looking only at its interface (the function heading and the precondition and postcondition). The reader should never have to look into the code of the function body to understand the purpose of the function or how to use it.

A function interface describes what the function does, not the details of *how* it does it. For this reason, the postcondition should mention (by name) each outgoing parameter and its value but should not mention any local variables. Local variables are implementation details; they are irrelevant to the function's interface.

Documenting the Direction of Data Flow

Another helpful piece of documentation in a function interface is the direction of **data flow** for each parameter in the parameter list. Data flow is the flow of information between the function and its caller. We said earlier that each parameter can be classified as an *incoming* parameter, an *outgoing* parameter, or an

> **Data flow**   The flow of information from the calling code to a function and from the function back to the calling code.

incoming/outgoing parameter. (Some programmers refer to these as *input* parameters, *output* parameters, and *input/output* parameters.)

For an incoming parameter, the direction of data flow is one-way—into the function. The function inspects and uses the current value of the parameter but does not modify it. In the function heading, we attach the comment

```
/* in */
```

to the declaration of the parameter. (Remember that C++ comments come in two forms. The first, which we use most often, starts with two slashes and extends to the end of the line. The second form encloses a comment between /* and */ and allows us to embed a comment within a line of code.) Here is the `PrintAverage` function with comments added to the parameter declarations:

```
void PrintAverage( /* in */ float sum,
                   /* in */ int   count )

// Precondition:
//      sum is assigned  &&  count > 0
// Postcondition:
//      The average sum/count has been output on one line

{
    cout << "Average is " << sum / float(count) << endl;
}
```

Passing by value is appropriate for each parameter that is incoming only. As you can see in the function body, `PrintAverage` does not modify the values of the parameters `sum` and `count`. It merely uses their current values. The direction of data flow is one-way—into the function.

The data flow for an outgoing parameter is one-way—out of the function. The function produces a new value for the parameter without using the old value in any way. The comment /* out */ identifies an outgoing parameter. Here we've added comments to the `Get2Ints` function heading:

```
void Get2Ints( /* out */ int& int1,
               /* out */ int& int2 )
```

Passing by reference must be used for an outgoing parameter. If you look back at the body of `Get2Ints`, you'll see that the function stores new values into the two variables (by means of the input statement), replacing whatever values they originally contained.

Finally, the data flow for an incoming/outgoing parameter is two-way—into and out of the function. The function uses the old value and also produces a new value for the parameter. We use /* inout */ to document this two-way direction of data flow. Here is an example of a function that uses two parameters, one of them incoming only and the other one incoming/outgoing:

```
void Calc( /* in */     int   alpha,
           /* inout */ int& beta   )

// Precondition:
//     alpha and beta are assigned
// Postcondition:
//     beta == beta@entry * 7 - alpha

{
    beta = beta * 7 - alpha;
}
```

This function first inspects the incoming value of beta so that it can evaluate the expression to the right of the equal sign. Then it stores a new value into beta by using the assignment operation. The data flow for beta is therefore considered a two-way flow of information. A pass by value is appropriate for alpha (it's incoming only), but a pass by reference is required for beta (it's an incoming/outgoing parameter).

Matters of Style

Formatting Function Headings

From here on, we follow a specific style when coding our function headings. Comments appear next to the parameters to explain how each parameter is used. Also, embedded comments indicate which of the three data flow categories each parameter belongs to (In, Out, or Inout).

```
void Print( /* in */     float val,     // Value to be printed
            /* inout */ int&  count )   // Number of lines printed
                                        //    so far
```

Notice that the first parameter above is a value parameter. The second is a reference parameter, presumably because the function changes the value of the counter.

We use comments in the form of rows of asterisks (or dashes or some other character) before and after a function to make the function stand out from the surrounding code. Each function also has its own block of introductory comments, just like those at the start of a program, as well as its precondition and postcondition.

It's important to put as much care into documenting each function as you would into the documentation at the beginning of a program.

The following table summarizes the correspondence between a parameter's data flow and the appropriate argument-passing mechanism.

Data Flow for a Parameter	Argument-Passing Mechanism
Incoming	Pass by value
Outgoing	Pass by reference
Incoming/outgoing	Pass by reference

There are exceptions to the guidelines in this table. C++ requires that I/O stream objects be passed by reference because of the way streams and files are implemented. We encounter another exception in Chapter 12.

Software Engineering Tip

Conceptual Versus Physical Hiding of a Function Implementation

In many programming languages, the encapsulation of an implementation is purely conceptual. If you want to know how a function is implemented, you simply look at the function body. C++, however, permits function implementations to be written and stored separately from the `main` function.

Larger C++ programs are usually split up and stored into separate files on a disk. One file might contain just the source code for the `main` function; another file, the source code for one or two functions invoked by `main`; and so on. This organization is called a *multifile program*. To translate the source code into object code, the compiler is invoked for each file independently of the others, possibly at different times. A program called the *linker* then collects all the resulting object code into a single executable program.

When you write a program that invokes a function located in another file, it isn't necessary for that function's source code to be available. All that's required is for you to include a function prototype so that the compiler can check the syntax of the call to the function. After the compiler is done, the linker finds the object code for that function and links it with your `main` function's object code. We do this kind of thing all the time when we invoke library functions. C++ systems supply only the object code, not the source code, for library functions like `sqrt`. The source code for their implementations are physically hidden from view.

One advantage of physical hiding is that it helps the programmer avoid the temptation to take advantage of any unusual features of a function's implementation. For example, suppose we want to change the Activity program to read temperatures and output activities repeatedly. Knowing

(continued) ▼

Conceptual Versus Physical Hiding of a Function Implementation

that the `GetTemp` function doesn't perform range checking on the input value, we might be tempted to use –1000 as a sentinel for the loop:

```
int main()
{
    int temperature;

    GetTemp(temperature);
    while (temperature != -1000)
    {
        PrintActivity(temperature);
        GetTemp(temperature);
    }
    return 0;
}
```

This code works fine for now, but later another programmer decides to improve `GetTemp` so that it checks for a valid temperature range (as it should):

```
void GetTemp( /* out */ int& temp )

// This function prompts for a temperature to be entered, reads
// the input value, checks to be sure it is in a valid temperature
// range, and echo prints it

// Postcondition:
//      User has been prompted for a temperature value (temp)
//   && Error messages and additional prompts have been printed
//      in response to invalid data
//   && IF no valid data was encountered before EOF
//          Value of temp is undefined
//      ELSE
//          -50 <= temp <= 130  &&  temp has been printed

{
    cout << "Enter the outside temperature (-50 through 130): ";
    cin >> temp;
    while (cin &&                           // While not EOF and
           (temp < -50 || temp > 130))      //   temp is invalid ...
```

(continued) ▼

Conceptual Versus Physical Hiding of a Function Implementation

```
    {
        cout << "Temperature must be"
             << " -50 through 130." << endl;
        cout << "Enter the outside temperature: ";
        cin >> temp;
    }
    if (cin)                                    // If not EOF ...
        cout << "The current temperature is "
             << temp << endl;
}
```

Unfortunately, this improvement causes the `main` function to be stuck in an infinite loop because `GetTemp` won't let us enter the sentinel value –1000. If the original implementation of `GetTemp` had been physically hidden, we would not have relied on the knowledge that it does not perform error checking. Instead, we would have written the `main` function in a way that is unaffected by the improvement to `GetTemp`:

```
int main()
{
    int temperature;

    GetTemp(temperature);
    while (cin)                         // While not EOF ...
    {
        PrintActivity(temperature);
        GetTemp(temperature);
    }
    return 0;
}
```

Later in the book, you learn how to write multifile programs and hide implementations physically. In the meantime, conscientiously avoid writing code that depends on the internal workings of a function.

Problem–Solving Case Study

Total Cost of Mortgage

PROBLEM In Chapter 3, you wrote a mortgage calculator for your parents to help them decide whether to refinance their mortgage. This exercise got you to thinking. All ads from cars to appliances to furniture to houses state that you pay "only so much a month." How much are you really paying for a house or any product bought on the installment plan? You decide to embed your calculator in a program that tells you how much you actually are paying for whatever you are financing. Since you now know about loops, you decide to do the processing within a loop, so that the user can see how a change in the interest rate or length of the contract can affect what you are actually paying.

INPUT At the end of Chapter 4, Case Study Follow Up Exercise 5 had you change your calculator program to allow the user to input the various values. These values are input to this program.

> Total loan amount (float)
> Yearly interest rate (float)
> Number of years (integer)

OUTPUT The input values are echo printed in a table that also shows the amount actually paid over the term of the loan.

DISCUSSION This program is a simple event-controlled loop, within which the user is prompted to input the loan amount, the interest rate, and the number of years. You decide to use a sentinel-controlled loop here, with a negative value for the loan amount as the sentinel. This decision requires that you use a priming read, reading the first loan amount outside the loop and the following loan amounts at the end of the loop.

Main	**Level 0**

Open file for output
If file not opened ok
    Write error message
    Return 1
Print heading
Prompt for and read loan amount
WHILE loan amount is not negative
    Get rest of data
    Determine payment
    Print results
    Prompt for and read loan amount
Close output file

Open File for Output	**Level 1**

dataOut.open("mortgage.out")

Print Heading

Print "Loan Amount"
Print "No. Years"
Print "Payment"
Print "Total Paid"

Prompt for and Read loanAmount

Prompt user for loan amount
Get loanAmount

Get Rest of Data

Prompt for interest rate
Get yearlyInterest
Prompt for number of years
Get numberOfYears

Determine Payment

Set monthly interest rate to yearlyInterest / 1200
Set number of payments to numberOfYears * 12
Set payment to (loanAmount * pow(1 + monthlyRate ,
               numberOfPayments) * monthlyRate)/
               (pow(1 + monthlyRate , numberOfPayments) – 1)

Print Results

Print loan amount
Print number of years
Print interest rate
Print payment
Print (number of years*12*payment)

Close OutputFile

dataOut.close()

This looks like a very complicated design for such a simple problem. Do we really need to represent each module as a C++ function? The answer depends on your own style. Certain of the modules definitely should be functions, for example, DeterminePayment. Certain of the modules probably should not be functions; for example, OpenOutputFile and CloseOutputFile. The file operation modules are only one line of code each, so there is no need to encapsulate them into a C++ function. If the problem states that the names of the input and/or output files are to be read from the keyboard, then this process would become part of the opening module, making it plausible to represent the module in a function.

Whether to implement the other modules as functions is a matter of style. As we stated earlier, the question is whether or not using a function makes the program easier to understand. "Easier to understand" is open to individual interpretation. Here, we choose to make PrintHeading and PrintResults functions, but not the other modules. Case Study Follow Up Exercise 1 asks you to implement the other modules as functions and determine which is easier for you to understand.

MODULE STRUCTURE CHART

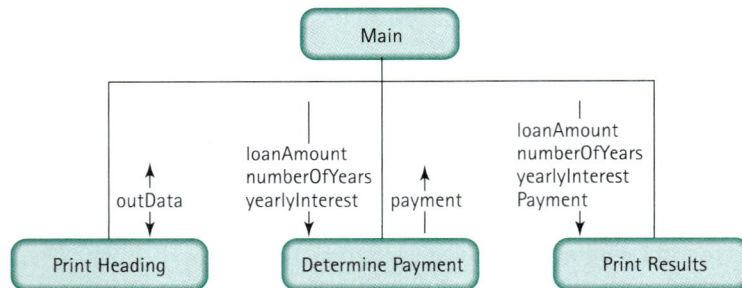

```
//*****************************************************************
// Mortgage Payment Tables program
// This program prints a table showing loan amount, interest rate,
// length of loan, monthly payments, and total cost of a mortgage.
//*****************************************************************

#include <iostream>
#include <cmath>
#include <iomanip>
#include <fstream>

using namespace std;

// Function prototypes
void PrintHeading(ofstream&);
void DeterminePayment(float, int, float, float&);
```

```cpp
void PrintResults(ofstream&, float, int, float, float);

int main()
{
    // Input variables
    float loanAmount;
    float yearlyInterest;
    int numberOfYears;
    float payment;

    // Declare and open output file
    ofstream dataOut;
    dataOut.open("mortgage.out");
    if ( !dataOut )
    { // no
        cout << "Can't open output file." << endl;
        return 1;
    }

    PrintHeading(dataOut);

    // Prompt for and read loan amount
    cout << "Input the total loan amount; "
         << "a negative value stops processing." << endl;
    cin >> loanAmount;

    // Loop calculating monthly payments
    while (loanAmount >= 0.0)
    {
        // Prompt for and read interest rate and number of years.
        cout << "Input the interest rate." << endl;
        cin >> yearlyInterest;
        cout << "Enter the number of years for the loan" << endl;
        cin >> numberOfYears;

        DeterminePayment(loanAmount, numberOfYears, yearlyInterest,
            payment);
        PrintResults(dataOut, loanAmount, numberOfYears,
            yearlyInterest, payment);
        // Prompt for and read loan amount
        cout << "Input the total loan amount; "
             << "a negative value stops processing."  << endl;
        cin >> loanAmount;
    }

    dataOut.close();
    return 0;
}
```

```
//**********************************************************************

void DeterminePayment
    ( /* in */ float loanAmount,      // Loan amount
      /* in */ int numberOfYears,     // Term of loan
      /* in */ float yearlyInterest,  // Interest rate
      /* inout */ float& payment )    // Monthly payment

// Calculates the monthly payment for a loan amount using the
// formula for compound interest.
// Precondition:
//     Arguments have been assigned values
// Postcondition:
//     payment contains the monthly payment as calculated by the
//     compound interest formula

{
    // local variables
    float monthlyRate;
    int numberOfPayments;

    monthlyRate = yearlyInterest / 1200;
    numberOfPayments = numberOfYears * 12;
    payment = (loanAmount * pow(1 + monthlyRate, numberOfPayments)
                * monthlyRate) /
                (pow(1 + monthlyRate, numberOfPayments) - 1);
}


//**********************************************************************

void PrintResults( /* inout */ ofstream& dataOut,    // Output file
                   /* in */    float loanAmount,      // Loan amount
                   /* in */    int numberOfYears,     // Term of loan
                   /* in */    float yearlyInterest,  // Interest rate
                   /* in */    float payment )        // Payment

// Prints the loan amount, number of years, yearly interest rate,
// and payment amount on file dataOut
// Precondition:
//     File dataOut has been opened successfully &&
//     All arguments have been assigned values
// Postcondition:
//     Loan amount, number of years, yearly interest rate, and
//     payment have been printed on dataOut with proper
//     documentation.
```

```
{
    dataOut << fixed << setprecision(2) << setw(12) << loanAmount
            << setw(12) << numberOfYears << setw(12)
            << yearlyInterest << setw(15) << payment
            << setw(12) << numberOfYears*12*payment << endl;
}


//******************************************************************


void PrintHeading( /* inout */ ofstream& dataOut )   // Output file

// Prints the heading on file dataOut for each column in the table.
// Precondition:
//    File dataOut has been opened successfully
// Postcondition:
//    "Loan Amount", "No. Years", "Interest Rate", "Payment",
//    "Total Paid" have been written on file dataOut

{
    dataOut << fixed << setprecision(2) << setw(12) << "Loan Amount"
            << setw(12) << "No. Years" << setw(15)
            << "Interest Rate" << setw(12) << "Payment"
            << setw(12) << "Total Paid" << endl;
}
```

Here is a sample run and the output.

```
C:\PPSC++\Mortgage\MortgageTables.exe                                    _ □ ×
Input the total loan amount; a negative value stops processing.
100000.00
Input the interest rate.
4.99
Enter the number of years for the loan
5
Input the total loan amount; a negative value stops processing.
3000.00
Input the interest rate.
18.0
Enter the number of years for the loan
2
Input the total loan amount; a negative value stops processing.
45000.00
Input the interest rate.
2.9
Enter the number of years for the loan
5
Input the total loan amount; a negative value stops processing.
-1_
```

```
mortgage.out - Notepad
File  Edit  Format  View  Help
Loan Amount    No. Years   Interest Rate    Payment   Total Paid
   100000.00           5            4.99    1886.67   113199.91
     3000.00           2           18.00     149.77     3594.54
    45000.00           5            2.90     806.59    48395.57
```

Testing There are three numeric inputs to this program. A negative loan amount ends the processing. The sample run used a variety of values for the loan amount, interest, and length of term. Case Study Follow Up Exercise 2 asks you to examine what happens if the interest and/or number of years is zero or negative.

Testing and Debugging

The parameters declared by a function and the arguments that are passed to the function by the caller must satisfy the interface to the function. Errors that occur with the use of functions often are due to an incorrect use of the interface between the calling code and the called function.

One source of errors is mismatched argument lists and parameter lists. The C++ compiler ensures that the lists have the same number of items and that they are compatible in type. It's the programmer's responsibility, however, to verify that each argument list contains the correct items. This is a matter of comparing the parameter declarations to the argument list in every call to the function. This job is much easier if the function heading gives each parameter a distinct name and describes its purpose in a comment. You can avoid mistakes in writing an argument list by using descriptive variable names in the calling code to suggest exactly what information is being passed to the function.

Another source of error is the failure to ensure that the precondition for a function is met before it is called. For example, if a function assumes that the input file is not at EOF when it is called, then the calling code must ensure that this is true before making the call to the function. If a function behaves incorrectly, review its precondition, then trace the program execution up to the point of the call to verify the precondition. You can waste a lot of time trying to locate an error in a correct function when the error is really in the part of the program prior to the call.

If the arguments match the parameters and the precondition is correctly established, then the source of the error is most likely in the function itself. Trace the function to verify that it transforms the precondition into the proper postcondition. Check that all local variables are initialized properly. Parameters that are supposed to return data to the caller must be declared as reference parameters (with an & symbol attached to the data type name).

An important technique for debugging a function is to use your system's debugger program, if one is available, to step through the execution of the function. If a debugger is not available, you can insert debug output statements to print the values of the arguments immediately before and after calls to the function. It also may help to print the values of all local variables at the end of the function. This information provides a snapshot of the function (a picture of its status at a particular moment in time) at its two most critical points, which is useful in verifying hand traces.

To test a function thoroughly, you must arrange the incoming values so that the precondition is pushed to its limits; then the postcondition must be verified. For example, if a function requires a parameter to be within a certain range, try calling the function with values in the middle of that range and at its extremes.

The `assert` Library Function

We have discussed how function preconditions and postconditions are useful for debugging (by checking that the precondition of each function is true prior to a function call, and by verifying that each function correctly transforms the precondition into the postcondition) and for testing (by pushing the precondition to its limits and even violating it). To state the preconditions and postconditions for our functions, we've been writing the assertions as program comments:

```
// Precondition:
//      studentCount > 0
```

All comments, of course, are ignored by the compiler. They are not executable statements; they are for humans to examine.

On the other hand, the C++ standard library gives us a way in which to write *executable assertions*. Through the header file `cassert`, the library provides a void function named `assert`. This function takes a logical (Boolean) expression as an argument and halts the program if the expression is false. Here's an example:

```
#include <cassert>
    ⋮
assert(studentCount > 0);
average = sumOfScores / studentCount;
```

The argument to the `assert` function must be a valid C++ logical expression. If its value is `true`, nothing happens; execution continues on to the next statement. If its value is `false`, execution of the program terminates immediately with a message stating (a) the assertion as it appears in the argument list, (b) the name of the file containing the program source code, and (c) the line number in the program. In the example above, if the value of `studentCount` is less than or equal to 0, the program halts after printing a message like this:

```
Assertion failed: studentCount > 0, file myprog.cpp, line 48
```

(This message is potentially confusing. It doesn't mean that studentCount *is* greater than 0. In fact, it's just the opposite. The message tells you that the assertion student-Count > 0 is *false*.)

Executable assertions have a profound advantage over assertions expressed as comments: the effect of a false assertion is highly visible (the program terminates with an error message). The assert function is therefore valuable in software testing. A program under development might be filled with calls to the assert function to help identify where errors are occurring. If an assertion is false, the error message gives the precise line number of the failed assertion.

Additionally, there is a way to "remove" the assertions without really removing them. If you use the preprocessor directive #define NDEBUG before including the header file cassert, like this:

```
#define NDEBUG
#include <cassert>
    ⋮
```

then all calls to the assert function are ignored when you run the program. (NDEBUG stands for "No debug," and a #define directive is a preprocessor feature that we don't discuss right now.) After program testing and debugging, programmers often like to "turn off" debugging statements yet leave them physically present in the source code in case they might need the statements later. Inserting the line #define NDEBUG turns off assertion checking without having to remove the assertions.

As useful as the assert function is, it has two limitations. First, the argument to the function must be expressed as a C++ logical expression. We can turn a comment such as

```
//   0.0 <= yearlyInterest && numberOfYears <= 30
```

into an executable assertion with the statement

```
assert(0.0 <= yearlyInterest && numberOfYears <= 30);
```

But there is no easy way to turn the comment

```
//   The file contains a loan amount,
//   interest rate, and number of years
```

into a C++ logical expression.

The second limitation is that the assert function is appropriate only for testing a program that is under development. A production program (one that has been completed and released to the public) must be robust and must furnish helpful error messages to the user of the program. You can imagine how baffled a user would be if the program suddenly quit and displayed an error message such as

```
Assertion failed: sysRes <= resCount, file newproj.cpp, line 298
```

Despite these limitations, you should consider using the assert function as a regular tool for testing and debugging your programs.

Testing and Debugging Hints

1. Follow documentation guidelines carefully when writing functions (see Appendix F). As your programs become more complex and therefore prone to errors, it becomes increasingly important to adhere to documentation and formatting standards. Even if the function name seems to reflect the process being done, describe that process in comments. Include comments stating the function precondition (if any) and postcondition to make the function interface complete. Use comments to explain the purposes of all parameters and local variables whose roles are not obvious.

2. Provide a function prototype near the top of your program for each function you've written. Make sure that the prototype and its corresponding function heading are an *exact* match (except for the absence of parameter names in the prototype).

3. Be sure to put a semicolon at the end of a function prototype. But do *not* put a semicolon at the end of the function heading in a function definition. Because function prototypes look so much like function headings, it's common to get one of them wrong.

4. Be sure the parameter list gives the data type of each parameter.

5. Use value parameters unless a result is to be returned through a parameter. Reference parameters can change the contents of the caller's argument; value parameters cannot.

6. In a parameter list, be sure the data type of each reference parameter ends with an ampersand (&). Without the ampersand, the parameter is a value parameter.

7. Make sure that the argument list of every function call matches the parameter list in number and order of items, and be very careful with their data types. The compiler will trap any mismatch in the number of arguments. But if there is a mismatch in data types, there may be no compile-time error. Specifically, with a pass by value, a type mismatch can lead to implicit type coercion rather than a compile-time error.

8. Remember that an argument matching a reference parameter *must* be a variable, whereas an argument matching a value parameter can be any expression that supplies a value of the same data type (except as noted above in Hint 7).

9. Become familiar with *all* the tools available to you when you're trying to locate the sources of errors—the algorithm walk-through, hand tracing, the system's debugger program, the `assert` function, and debug output statements.

Summary

C++ allows us to write programs in modules expressed as functions. The structure of a program, therefore, can parallel its functional decomposition even when the program is complicated. To make your `main` function look exactly like level 0 of your functional decomposition, simply write each lower-level module as a function. The `main` function then executes these other functions in logical sequence.

Functions communicate by means of two lists: the parameter list (which specifies the data type of each identifier) in the function heading, and the argument list in the calling code. The items in these lists must agree in number and position, and they should agree in data type.

Part of the functional decomposition process involves determining what data must be received by a lower-level module and what information must be returned from it. The names of these data items, together with the precondition and postcondition of a module, define its interface. The names of the data items become the parameter list, and the module name becomes the name of the function. With void functions, a call to the function is accomplished by writing the function's name as a statement, enclosing the appropriate arguments in parentheses.

C++ has two kinds of parameters: reference and value. Reference parameters have data types ending in & in the parameter list, whereas value parameters do not. Parameters that return values from a function must be reference parameters. All others should be value parameters. This minimizes the risk of errors, because only a copy of the value of an argument is passed to a value parameter, and thus the argument is protected from change.

In addition to the variables declared in its parameter list, a function may have local variables declared within it. These variables are accessible only within the block in which they are declared. Local variables must be initialized each time the function containing them is called because their values are destroyed when the function returns.

You may call functions from more than one place in a program. The positional matching mechanism allows the use of different variables as arguments to the same function. Multiple calls to a function, from different places and with different arguments, can simplify greatly the coding of many complex programs.

Quick Check

1. What elements of a functional decomposition correspond to functions in C++? (pp. 306–307)
2. What character do we use to indicate a reference parameter, and where does it appear in the parameter's declaration? (pp. 322–327)
3. Where do arguments appear and where do parameters appear? (pp. 327–330)
4. You are writing a function to return the first name from a string containing a full name. How many parameters does the function have, and which of them are reference and which are value parameters? (pp. 331–337)

5. What kind of parameter would you use for an incoming value from an argument? For an outgoing value? For a value that comes in, is changed, and returns to the argument? (pp. 331–337)

6. Where do declarations of functions that are called by `main` appear in the program, with respect to `main`? (pp. 315–318)

7. What parts of a program can access a local variable declared within a function's block? (pp. 318–320)

8. If the same function appears in multiple places in a functional decomposition, how do you convert it into code in a program? (pp. 315–319)

Answers

1. Modules   2. The & character appears at the end of the type name of the parameter.   3. Arguments appear in function calls and parameters appear in function headings.   4. It should have two parameters, one for each string. The full name parameter should be a value parameter, and the first name parameter should be a reference parameter.   5. Incoming values use value parameters. Values that return to the argument (`out` or `inout`) must be passed through reference parameters.   6. They must be declared before they are used, so they appear before `main`. However, the declaration may simply be a function prototype and the actual definition can then appear anywhere.   7. Only the statements within the block, following the declaration.   8. You code it once, placing it, or its prototype before any reference to it in the rest of the program, and call it from each place in the program that corresponds to its appearance in the functional decomposition.

Exam Preparation Exercises

1. What three things distinguish a `void` function from `main`?

2. A function prototype must specify the name of a function and the name and type of each of its parameters. True or false?

3. When and to where does control return from a `void` function?

4. Match the following terms with the definitions given below.
   a. Argument
   b. Parameter
   c. Function call
   d. Function prototype
   e. Function definition
   f. Local variable
   g. Value parameter
   h. Reference parameter
       i. A function declaration without a body.
       ii. A parameter that receives a copy of the argument's value.
       iii. A variable declared in a function heading.
       iv. A function declaration with a body.
       v. A variable or expression listed in a call to a function.
       vi. A statement that transfers control to a function.
       vii. A parameter that receives the location of the argument.
       viii. A variable declared within a block.

5. In the following function heading, which parameters are value parameters and which are reference parameters?

```
void ExamPrep (string& name, int age, float& salary,
char level)
```

6. If a function has six parameters, how many arguments must be in a call to the function?

7. What happens if a function assigns a new value to a value parameter? What happens if it assigns a new value to a reference parameter?

8. What's wrong with this function prototype?

```
void ExamPrep (phone& int, name string, age& int)
```

9. Arguments can appear in any order as long as they have the correct types and C++ will figure out the correspondence. True or false?

10. Define encapsulation.

11. For which direction(s) of data flow do you use reference parameters?

12. What is wrong with the following function?

```
void Square (int& x)
{
    x = x * x;
    return 0;
}
```

13. What is wrong with the following function?

```
void Power (int x, int y)
{
    int result;
    result = 1;
    while (y > 0)
    {
        result = result * x;
        y--;
    }
}
```

14. What is wrong with the following function?

```
void Power (int x, int y, int result)
{
    result = 1;
    while (y > 0)
    {
        result = result * x;
        y--;
    }
}
```

15. What is wrong with the following function?

```
void Power (int& x, int& y, int& result)
{
    result = 1;
    while (y > 0)
    {
        result = result * x;
        y--;
    }
}
```

16. A local variable can be referenced anywhere within the block in which it is declared. True or false?

17. Functions can be called from other functions in addition to `main`. True or false?

18. What would be the precondition for a function that reads a file of integers and returns their mean?

Programming Warm-Up Exercises

1. Write the heading for a void function called `Max` that has three `int` parameters, `num1`, `num2`, and `greatest`. The first two parameters receive data from the caller, and `greatest` returns a value. Document the data flow of the parameters with appropriate comments.

2. Write the function prototype for the function in Exercise 1.

3. Write the function definition of the function in Exercise 1 so that it returns the greatest of the two input parameters.

4. Write the heading for a void function called `GetLeast` that takes an `ifstream` parameter called `infile` as an input parameter that is changed, and that has a an `int` parameter called `lowest` that returns a value. Document the data flow of the parameters with appropriate comments.

5. Write the function prototype for the function in Exercise 4.

6. Write the function definition for the function in Exercise 4 so that it reads all of `infile` as a series of `int` values and returns the lowest integer input from `infile`.

7. Add comments to the preceding function definition that state its precondition and postcondition.

8. Write the heading for a function called `Reverse` that takes two string parameters. In the second parameter, the function returns a string that is the character-by-character reverse of the string in the first parameter. The parameters are called `original` and `lanigiro`. Document the data flow of the parameters with appropriate comments.

9. Write the function prototype for the function in Exercise 8.

10. Write the function definition for the function in Exercise 8.

11. Add comments to the preceding function definition that state its precondition and postcondition.

12. Write a void function, `LowerCount`, that reads a line from `cin`, and returns an `int` (`count`) containing the number of lowercase letters in the line. In Appendix C you will find the description of function `islower`, which returns `true` if its `char` parameter is a lowercase character. Document the data flow of the parameters with appropriate comments.

13. Add comments to the function definition that you wrote for Exercise 12 that state its precondition and postcondition.

14. Write a `void` function, `GetNonemptyLine`, that takes an `ifstream` (`infile`) as an in/out parameter, and reads lines from the file until it finds a line that contains characters. It should then return the line via a `string` parameter called `line`. Document the data flow of the parameters with appropriate comments.

15. Write a `void` function, `SkipToEmptyLine`, that takes an `ifstream` (`infile`) as an in/out parameter, and which reads lines from the file until it finds a line that contains no characters. It should then return the number of lines skipped via a `int` parameter called `skipped`. Document the data flow of the parameters with appropriate comments.

16. Write a `void` function, `TimeAdd`, that takes parameters representing two times in days, hours, and minutes, and adds them to get a new time. Each part of the time is an `int`, and hours range from 0 to 23, while minutes range from 0 to 59. There is no limit on the range of days. We assume that the time to be added is positive. The values in the parameters representing the first time are replaced by the result of adding the two times. Here is an example call in which 3 days, 17 hours, 49 minutes is added to 12 days, 22 hours, and 14 minutes.

```
days = 12;
hours = 22;
minutes = 14;
TimeAdd(days, hours, minutes, 3, 17, 49)
```

After the call, the values in the variables are:

```
days = 16
hours = 16
minutes = 3
```

Document the data flow of the parameters with appropriate comments.

17. Extend function `TimeAdd` in Exercise 16 to include seconds.

18. Write a void function, `SeasonPrint`, that takes `int` parameters representing a month and a day and outputs to `cout` the name of the season. For the purposes of this exercise, Spring begins on March 21, Summer begins June 21, Fall begins September 21, and Winter begins December 21. Note that the year begins and ends during Winter. The function can assume that the values in the `month` and `day` parameters have been validated before it is called. Document the data flow of the parameters with appropriate comments.

Programming Problems

1. Rewrite the program from Programming Problem 1 of Chapter 6 using functions. The program is to print a bar chart of the hourly temperatures for one day, given the data on a file. You should have a function to print the chart's heading, and another function that prints the bar of stars for a given temperature value. Note that the second function does not print the value to the left of the bar graph. The main program coordinates the process of inputting values, and calling these functions as necessary.

   Now that your programs are becoming more complex, it is even more important for you to use proper indentation and style, meaningful identifiers, and appropriate comments.

2. You're working for a company that lays ceramic floor tile, and they need a program that estimates the number of boxes of tile for a job. A job is estimated by taking the dimensions of each room in feet and inches, and converting these dimensions into a multiple of the tile size (rounding up any partial multiple) before multiplying to get the number of tiles for the room. A box contains 20 tiles, so the total number needed should be divided by 20 and rounded up to get the number of boxes. The tiles are assumed to be square.

   The program should initially prompt the user for the size of the tile in inches, and the number of rooms to be input. It should then input the dimensions for each room, and output the tiles needed for that room. After the last room is input, the program also should output the total number of tiles needed, the number of boxes needed, and how many extra tiles will be left over.

   Here is an example of how a run might appear:

```
Enter number of rooms: 2
Enter size of tile in inches: 12
Enter room width (feet and inches, separated by a space): 17 4
Enter room length (feet and inches, separated by a space): 9 3
Room requires 180 tiles.
Enter room width (feet and inches, separated by a space): 11 6
Enter room length (feet and inches, separated by a space): 11 9
Room requires 144 tiles.
Total tiles required is 324.
Number of boxes needed is 17.
There will be 16 extra tiles.
```

   Use functional decomposition to solve this problem, and code the solution using functions wherever it makes sense to do so. Your program should check for invalid data such as non-positive dimensions, number of rooms less than one, number of inches greater than 11, and so on. It should prompt for corrected input whenever invalid input is detected. Now that your programs are becoming more complex, it is even more important for you to use proper indentation and style, meaningful identifiers, and appropriate comments.

3. Programming Problem 6 in Chapter 4 asked you to write a program to compute the score for one frame in an a game of tenpin bowling. Here you will extend this algorithm to compute the score for an entire game for one player. A game consists of 10 frames, but the tenth frame has some special cases that were not described in Chapter 4.

A frame is played by first setting up the 10 pins. The player then rolls the ball to knock them down. If all 10 are knocked down on the first throw, it is called a strike, and the frame is over. If fewer than 10 are knocked down on the first throw, the number knocked down is recorded and the player gets a second throw. If the remaining pins are all knocked down on the second throw, it is called a spare. The frame ends after the second throw, even if there are pins left standing. If the second throw fails to knock all of the pins down, then the number that it knocked down is recorded, and the score for the frame is just the number of pins knocked down by the two throws. However, in the case of a strike or a spare, the score for the frame depends on throws in the next frame and possibly the frame after that.

If the frame is a strike then the score is equal to 10 points plus the number of pins knocked down in the next two throws. Thus, the maximum score for a frame is thirty, which occurs when the frame is a strike and the two following frames are also strikes. If the frame is a spare, then the score is those 10 points plus the number of pins knocked down on the next throw.

The last frame is played somewhat differently. If the player gets a strike, then he or she gets two more throws so that the score for the strike can be computed. Similarly, if it is a spare, then one extra throw is given. If the first two throws fail to knock down all of the pins then the score for the last frame is just the number knocked down, and there is no extra throw. Here is an example of how the I/O might appear for the start of a run:

```
Enter throw for frame 1: 10
Strike!
Enter throw for frame 2: 7
Enter throw for frame 2: 3
Spare!
Score for frame 1 is 20. Total is 20.
Enter throw for frame 3: 5
Score for frame 2 is 15. Total is 35.
Enter throw for frame 3: 2
Score for frame 3 is 7. Total is 42.
Enter score for frame 4: 12
Input error. Please enter number of pins in range of 0 to 10.
Enter score for frame 4:
```

Your program should input the number of pins knocked down by each throw, and output the score for each frame as it is computed. The program must recognize when a frame has ended (either due to a strike or a second throw). The program also should check for erroneous input. For example, a throw may be in the range of 0 through 10 pins, and the total of the two throws in any of the first nine frames must be less than or equal to 10. Use functional decomposition to solve this problem and code the solution using functions as appropriate. Be sure to use proper formatting and appropriate comments in your code. The output should be clearly labeled and neatly formatted, and the error messages should be informative.

4. Write a simple telephone directory program in C++ that looks up phone numbers in a file containing a list of names and phone numbers. The user should be prompted to enter a first and last name, and the program then outputs the corresponding number, or indicates that the name isn't in the directory. After each lookup, the program should ask the user whether they want to look up another number, and then either repeat the process or exit the program. The data on the file should be organized so that each line contains a first name, a last name, and a phone number, separated by blanks. You can return to the beginning of the file by closing it and opening it again.

Use functional decomposition to solve the problem and code the solution using functions as appropriate. Be sure to use proper formatting and appropriate comments in your code. The output should be clearly labeled and neatly formatted, and the error messages should be informative.

5. Extend the program in Problem 4 to look up addresses also. Change the file format so that the name and phone number appear on one line, and the address appears on the following line for each entry. The program should ask the user whether they want to look up a phone number, an address, or both, then perform the lookup and output the requested information. The program should recognize an invalid request and prompt the user to enter the request again. As in Problem 4, the program should allow the user to keep entering queries until they indicate that they are done.

6. Programming Problem 1 in Chapter 4 asked you to write a program that inputs a letter and outputs the corresponding word in the International Civil Aviation Organization phonetic alphabet. This problem asks you to turn that program into a function, and use it to convert a string input by the user into the series of words that would be used to spell it out phonetically. For example:

```
Enter string: program
Phonetic version is: Papa Romeo Oscar Golf Romeo Alpha Mike
```

For ease of reference, the ICAO alphabet is repeated here from Chapter 4:

A   Alpha
B   Bravo
C   Charlie
D   Delta
E   Echo
F   Foxtrot
G   Golf

H	Hotel
I	India
J	Juliet
K	Kilo
L	Lima
M	Mike
N	November
O	Oscar
P	Papa
Q	Quebec
R	Romeo
S	Sierra
T	Tango
U	Uniform
V	Victor
W	Whiskey
X	X-ray
Y	Yankee
Z	Zulu

Be sure to use proper formatting and appropriate comments in your code. Provide appropriate prompts to the user. The output should be clearly labeled and neatly formatted.

7. You've been asked to write a program to grade a multiple-choice exam. The exam has 20 questions, each answered with a letter in the range of 'a' through 'f'. The data are stored on a file (exams.dat) where the first line is the key, consisting of a string of 20 characters. The remaining lines on the file are exam answers, and consist of a student ID number, a space, and a string of 20 characters. The program should read the key, then read each exam and output the ID number and score to file scores.dat. Erroneous input should result in an error message. For example, given the data:

```
abcdefabcdefabcdefab
1234567 abcdefabcdefabcdefab
9876543 abddefbbbdefcbcdefac
5554446 abcdefabcdefabcdef
4445556 abcdefabcdefabcdefabcd
3332221 abcdefghijklmnopqrst
```

The program would output on scores.dat:

```
1234567    20
9876543    15
5554446    Too few answers
4445556    Too many answers
3332221    Invalid answers
```

Use functional decomposition to solve the problem and code the solution using functions as appropriate. Be sure to use proper formatting and appropriate comments in your code. The output should be neatly formatted, and the error messages should be informative.

Case Study Follow-Up Answers

1. Revise the code for the case study program implementing the input modules as functions. Compare the two programs. Which do you find easier to read?

2. Experiment with the mortgage program by using the following input values:

Loan Amount	100000.00
Number of years	0
Interest rate	0
Loan Amount	50000.00
Number of months	−1
Interest rate	−1

Describe what happens.

3. Add error checking to the Mortgage program to take care of the problems that surfaced in Exercise 2.

4. Add a column to the output of the Mortgage program that shows how much interest has been paid.

Scope, Lifetime, and More on Functions

Knowledge Goals

- *To know what a global reference is.*
- *To understand and be able to avoid unwanted side effects.*
- *To know when to use a value-returning function.*

Skill Goals

To be able to:

- *Determine which variables in a program are local.*
- *Determine which variables are accessible in a given block.*
- *Determine the lifetime of each variable in a program.*
- *Design and code a value-returning function for a specified task.*
- *Invoke a value-returning function properly.*

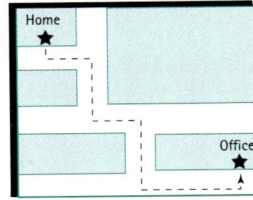

As programs get larger and more complicated, the number of identifiers in a program increases. We invent function names, variable names, constant identifiers, and so on. Some of these identifiers we declare inside blocks. Other identifiers—function names, for example—we declare outside of any block. This chapter examines the C++ rules by which a function may access identifiers that are declared outside its own block. Using these rules, we return to the discussion of interface design that we began in Chapter 7.

Finally, we look at the second kind of subprogram provided by C++: the *value-returning function*. Unlike void functions, which return results (if any) through the parameter list, a value-returning function returns a single result—the function value—to the expression from which it was called. In this chapter, you learn how to write user-defined value-returning functions.

8.1 Scope of Identifiers

As we saw in Chapter 7, local variables are those declared inside a block, such as the body of a function. Recall that local variables cannot be accessed outside the block that contains them. The same access rule applies to declarations of named constants: Local constants may be accessed only in the block in which they are declared.

Any block, not only a function body, can contain variable and constant declarations. For example, this If statement contains a block that declares a local variable n:

```
if (alpha > 3)
{
    int n;

    cin >> n;
    beta = beta + n;
}
```

As with any local variable, n cannot be accessed by any statement outside the block containing its declaration.

If we listed all the places from which an identifier could be accessed legally, we would describe that identifier's **scope of visibility** or **scope of access**, often just called its scope.

> **Scope**   The region of program code where it is legal to reference (use) an identifier.

C++ defines several categories of scope for any identifier. We begin by describing three of these categories.

1. *Class scope.* This term refers to the data type called a *class*, which we introduced briefly in Chapter 4. We postpone a detailed discussion of class scope until Chapter 11.

2. *Local scope.* The scope of an identifier declared inside a block extends from the point of declaration to the end of that block. Also, the scope of a function parameter (formal parameter) extends from the point of declaration to the end of the block that is the body of the function.

3. *Global scope.* The scope of an identifier declared outside all functions and classes extends from the point of declaration to the end of the entire file containing the program code.

C++ function names have global scope. (There is an exception to this rule, which we discuss in Chapter 11 when we examine C++ classes.) Once a function name has been declared, the function can be invoked by any other function in the rest of the program. In C++, there is no such thing as a local function—that is, you cannot nest a function definition inside another function definition.

Global variables and constants are those declared outside all functions. In the following code fragment, gamma is a global variable and can be accessed directly by statements in main and SomeFunc.

```cpp
int gamma;     // Global variable

int main()
{
    gamma = 3;
      ⋮
}


void SomeFunc()
{
    gamma = 5;
      ⋮
}
```

When a function declares a local identifier with the same name as a global identifier, the local identifier takes precedence within the function. This principle is called **name precedence** or **name hiding**.

Name precedence   The precedence that a local identifier in a function has over a global identifier with the same name in any references that the function makes to that identifier; also called *name hiding*.

Here's an example that uses both local and global declarations:

```cpp
#include <iostream>

using namespace std;

void SomeFunc( float );

const int a = 17;              // A global constant
int b;                         // A global variable
int c;                         // Another global variable

int main()
{
    b = 4;                     // Assignment to global b
    c = 6;                     // Assignment to global c
    SomeFunc(42.8);
    return 0;
}

void SomeFunc( float c )       // Prevents access to global c
{
    float b;                   // Prevents access to global b

    b = 2.3;                   // Assignment to local b
    cout << "a = " << a;       // Output global a (17)
    cout << " b = " << b;      // Output local b (2.3)
    cout << " c = " << c;      // Output local c (42.8)
}
```

In this example, function SomeFunc accesses global constant a but declares its own local variable b and parameter c. Thus, the output would be

```
a = 17 b = 2.3 c = 42.8
```

Local variable b takes precedence over global variable b, effectively hiding global b from the statements in function SomeFunc. Parameter c also blocks access to global variable c from within the function. Function parameters act just like local variables in this respect; that is, parameters have local scope.

Scope Rules

When you write C++ programs, you rarely declare global variables. There are negative aspects to using global variables, which we discuss later. But when a situation crops up in which you have a compelling need for global variables, it pays to know how C++

handles these declarations. The rules for accessing identifiers that aren't declared locally are called scope rules.

In addition to local and global access, the C++ scope rules define what happens when blocks are nested within other blocks. Anything declared in a block that contains a nested block is nonlocal to the inner block. (Global identifiers are nonlocal with respect to all blocks in the program.) If a block accesses any identifier declared outside its own block, it is a *nonlocal access.*

> **Scope rules** The rules that determine where in the program an identifier may be accessed, given the point where that identifier is declared.
>
> **Nonlocal identifier** With respect to a given block, any identifier declared outside that block.

Here are the detailed scope rules, excluding class scope and certain language features we have not yet discussed:

1. A function name has global scope. Function definitions cannot be nested within function definitions.

2. The scope of a function parameter is identical to the scope of a local variable declared in the outermost block of the function body.

3. The scope of a global variable or constant extends from its declaration to the end of the file, except as noted in Rule 5.

4. The scope of a local variable or constant extends from its declaration to the end of the block in which it is declared. This scope includes any nested blocks, except as noted in Rule 5.

5. The scope of an identifier does not include any nested block that contains a locally declared identifier with the same name (local identifiers have name precedence).

Here is a sample program that demonstrates C++ scope rules. To simplify the example, only the declarations and headings are spelled out. Note how the While-loop body labeled Block3, located within function `Block2`, contains its own local variable declarations.

```cpp
// ScopeRules program

#include <iostream>

using namespace std;

void Block1( int, char& );
void Block2();

int   a1;          // One global variable
char  a2;          // Another global variable

int main()
```

```
{
    ⋮
}

//*********************************************************************

void Block1( int    a1,              // Prevents access to global a1
             char& b2 )              // Has same scope as c1 and d2
{
    int c1;              // A variable local to Block1
    int d2;              // Another variable local to Block1
    ⋮
}

//*********************************************************************

void Block2()
{
    int a1;              // Prevents access to global a1
    int b2;              // Local to Block2; no conflict with b2 in Block1

    while ( ... )
    {                    // Block3
        int c1;          // Local to Block3; no conflict with c1 in Block1
        int b2;          // Prevents nonlocal access to b2 in Block2; no
                         //    conflict with b2 in Block1

        ⋮
    }
}
```

Let's look at the ScopeRules program in terms of the blocks it defines and see just what these rules mean. Figure 8–1 shows the headings and declarations in the Scope-Rules program with the scopes of visibility indicated by boxes.

Anything inside a box can refer to anything in a larger surrounding box, but outside-in references aren't allowed. Thus, a statement in Block3 could access any identifier declared in Block2 or any global variable. A statement in Block3 could not access identifiers declared in Block1 because it would have to enter the Block1 box from outside.

Notice that the parameters for a function are inside the function's box, but the function name itself is outside. If the name of the function were inside the box, no function could call another function. This demonstrates merely that function names are globally accessible.

Imagine the boxes in Figure 8–1 as rooms with walls made of two-way mirrors, with the reflective side facing out and the see-through side facing in. If you stood in the room for Block3, you would be able to see out through all the surrounding rooms to the declarations of the global variables (and anything between). You would not be able to

```
int a1;
char a2;

int main()
{

}

void Block1(          int    a1,
                      char& b2 )
{

        int c1;
        int d2;

}

void Block2()
{

        int a1;
        int b2;

        while (...)
        {                 // Block3

                int c1;
                int b2;

        }

}
```

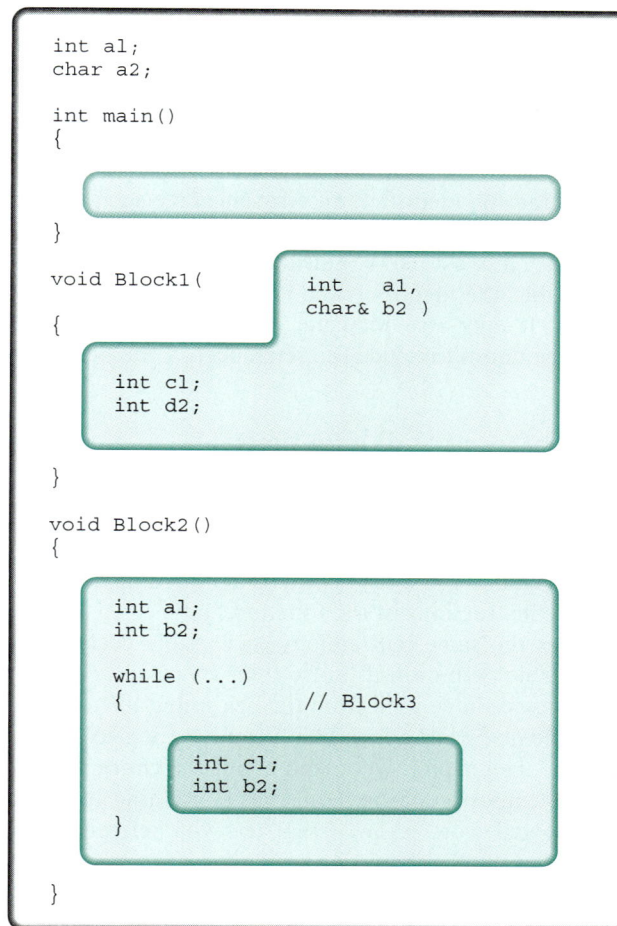

Figure 8–1   *Scope Diagram for ScopeRules Program*

see into any other rooms (such as Block 1), however, because their mirrored outer surfaces would block your view. Because of this analogy, the term *visible* is often used in describing a scope of access. For example, variable a2 is visible throughout the program, meaning that it can be accessed from anywhere in the program.

Figure 8–1 does not tell the whole story; it represents only scope rules 1 through 4. We also must keep rule 5 in mind. Variable a1 is declared in three different places in the ScopeRules program. Because of name precedence, Block2 and Block3 access the a1 declared in Block2 rather than the global a1. Similarly, the scope of the variable b2 declared in Block2 does *not* include the "hole" created by Block3, because Block3 declares its own variable b2.

Name precedence is implemented by the compiler as follows. When an expression refers to an identifier, the compiler first checks the local declarations. If the identifier isn't local, the compiler works its way outward through each level of nesting until it finds an identifier with the same name. There it stops. If there is an identifier with the same name declared at a level even further out, it is never reached. If the compiler reaches the global declarations (including identifiers inserted by #include directives) and still can't find the identifier, an error message such as "UNDECLARED IDENTIFIER" is issued.

Such a message most likely indicates a misspelling or an incorrect capitalization, or it could mean that the identifier was not declared before the reference to it or was not declared at all. It may also indicate, however, that the blocks are nested so that the identifier's scope doesn't include the reference.

Variable Declarations and Definitions

In Chapter 7, you learned that C++ terminology distinguishes between a function declaration and a function definition. A function prototype is a declaration only—that is, it doesn't cause memory space to be reserved for the function. In contrast, a function declaration that includes the body is called a function definition. The compiler reserves memory for the instructions in the function body.

C++ applies the same terminology to variable declarations. A variable declaration becomes a variable definition if it also reserves memory for the variable. All of the variable declarations we have used from the beginning have been variable definitions. What would a variable declaration look like if it were *not* also a definition?

In the previous chapter, we talked about the concept of a multifile program, a program that physically occupies several files containing individual pieces of the program. C++ has a reserved word extern that lets you reference a global variable located in another file. A "normal" declaration such as

```
int someInt;
```

causes the compiler to reserve a memory location for someInt. On the other hand, the declaration

```
extern int someInt;
```

is known as an *external declaration*. It states that someInt is a global variable located in another file and that no storage should be reserved for it here. System header files such as iostream contain external declarations so that user programs can access important variables defined in system files. For example, iostream includes declarations like these:

```
extern istream cin;
extern ostream cout;
```

These declarations allow you to reference `cin` and `cout` as global variables in your program, but the variable definitions are located in another file supplied by the C++ system.

In C++ terminology, the statement

```
extern int someInt;
```

is a declaration but not a definition of `someInt`. It associates a variable name with a data type so that the compiler can perform type checking. But the statement

```
int someInt;
```

is both a declaration and a definition of `someInt`. It is a definition because it reserves memory for `someInt`. In C++, you can declare a variable or a function many times, but there can be only one definition.

Except in situations in which it's important to distinguish between declarations and definitions of variables, we'll continue to use the more general phrase *variable declaration* instead of the more specific *variable definition*.

Namespaces

For some time, we have been including the following `using` directive in our programs:

```
using namespace std;
```

What exactly is a namespace? As a general concept, *namespace* is another word for *scope*. However, as a specific C++ language feature, a namespace is a mechanism by which the programmer can create a named scope. For example, the standard header file `cstdlib` contains function prototypes for several library functions, one of which is the absolute value function, `abs`. The declarations are contained within a *namespace definition* as follows:

```
// In header file cstdlib:

namespace std
{
    ⋮
    int abs( int );
    ⋮
}
```

A namespace definition consists of the word `namespace`, then an identifier of the programmer's choice, and then the *namespace body* between braces. Identifiers declared within the namespace body are said to have *namespace scope*. Such identifiers cannot be accessed outside the body except by using one of three methods.

The first method, introduced in Chapter 2, is to use a qualified name: the name of the namespace, followed by the scope resolution operator (::), followed by the desired identifier. Here is an example:

```
#include <cstdlib>

int main()
{
    int alpha;
    int beta;
       ⋮
    alpha = std::abs(beta);     // A qualified name
       ⋮
}
```

The general idea is to inform the compiler that we are referring to the abs declared in the std namespace, not some other abs (such as a global function named abs that we might have written ourselves).

The second method is to use a statement called a *using declaration* as follows:

```
#include <cstdlib>

int main()
{
    int alpha;
    int beta;
    using std::abs;      // A using declaration
       ⋮
    alpha = abs(beta);
       ⋮
}
```

This using declaration allows the identifier abs to be used throughout the body of main as a synonym for the longer std::abs.

The third method—one with which we are familiar—is to use a using directive (not to be confused with a using declaration).

```
#include <cstdlib>

int main()
{
    int alpha;
    int beta;
    using namespace std;      // A using directive
       ⋮
```

```
   alpha = abs(beta);
     ⋮
}
```

With a `using` directive, *all* identifiers from the specified namespace are accessible, but only in the scope in which the `using` directive appears. Above, the `using` directive is in local scope (it's within a block), so identifiers from the `std` namespace are accessible only within `main`. On the other hand, if we put the `using` directive outside all functions (as we have been doing), like this:

```
#include <cstdlib>

using namespace std;

int main()
{
     ⋮
}
```

then the `using` directive is in global scope; consequently, identifiers from the `std` namespace are accessible globally.

Placing a `using` directive in global scope can be a convenience. For example, all of the functions we write can refer to identifiers such as `abs`, `cin`, and `cout` without our having to insert a `using` directive locally in each function. However, global `using` directives are considered a bad idea when creating large, multifile programs. Programmers often make use of several libraries, not just the C++ standard library, when developing complex software. Two or more libraries may, just by coincidence, use the same identifier for completely different purposes. If global `using` directives are employed, *name clashes* (multiple definitions of the same identifier) can occur because all the identifiers have been brought into global scope. (C++ programmers refer to this as "polluting the global namespace.") Over the next several chapters, we continue to use global `using` directives for the `std` namespace because our programs are relatively small and therefore name clashes aren't likely.

Given the concept of namespace scope, we refine our description of C++ scope categories as follows.

1. *Class scope.* This term refers to the data type called a *class.* We postpone a detailed discussion of class scope until Chapter 11.

2. *Local scope.* The scope of an identifier declared inside a block extends from the point of declaration to the end of that block. Also, the scope of a function parameter (formal parameter) extends from the point of declaration to the end of the block that is the body of the function.

3. *Namespace scope.* The scope of an identifier declared in a namespace definition extends from the point of declaration to the end of the namespace body, *and* its scope includes the scope of a `using` directive specifying that namespace.

4. *Global* (or *global namespace*) *scope.* The scope of an identifier declared outside all namespaces, functions, and classes extends from the point of declaration to the end of the entire file containing the program code.

Note that these are general descriptions of scope categories and not scope rules. The descriptions do not account for name hiding (the redefinition of an identifier within a nested block).

8.2 Lifetime of a Variable

A concept related to but separate from the scope of a variable is its lifetime—the period of time during program execution when an identifier actually has memory allocated to it. We have said that storage for local variables is created (allocated) at the moment control enters a function. Then the variables are "alive" while the function is executing, and finally the storage is destroyed (deallocated) when the function exits. In contrast, the lifetime of a global variable is the same as the lifetime of the entire program. Memory is allocated only once, when the program begins executing, and is deallocated only when the entire program terminates. Observe that scope is a *compile-time* issue, but lifetime is a *run-time* issue.

> **Lifetime** The period of time during program execution when an identifier has memory allocated to it.
>
> **Automatic variable** A variable for which memory is allocated and deallocated when control enters and exits the block in which it is declared.
>
> **Static variable** A variable for which memory remains allocated throughout the execution of the entire program.

In C++, an **automatic variable** is one whose storage is allocated at block entry and deallocated at block exit. A **static variable** is one whose storage remains allocated for the duration of the entire program. All global variables are static variables. By default, variables declared within a block are automatic variables. However, you can use the reserved word `static` when you declare a local variable. If you do so, the variable is a static variable and its lifetime persists from function call to function call:

```
void SomeFunc()
{
    float   someFloat;      // Destroyed when function exits
    static int someInt;     // Retains its value from call to call
       ⋮
}
```

It is usually better to declare a local variable as `static` than to use a global variable. Like a global variable, its memory remains allocated throughout the lifetime of the entire program. But unlike a global variable, its local scope prevents other functions in the program from tinkering with it.

Initializations in Declarations

One of the most common things we do in programs is first declare a variable and then, in a separate statement, assign an initial value to the variable. Here's a typical example:

```
int sum;

sum = 0;
```

C++ allows you to combine these two statements into one. The result is known as an *initialization in a declaration.* Here we initialize `sum` in its declaration:

```
int sum = 0;
```

In a declaration, the expression that specifies the initial value is called an *initializer.* Above, the initializer is the constant 0. Implicit type coercion takes place if the data type of the initializer is different from the data type of the variable.

An automatic variable is initialized to the specified value each time control enters the block:

```
void SomeFunc( int someParam )
{
    int i = 0;                      // Initialized each time
    int n = 2 * someParam + 3;      // Initialized each time
        :
}
```

In contrast, initialization of a static variable (either a global variable or a local variable explicitly declared `static`) occurs once only, the first time control reaches its declaration. Here's an example in which two local static variables are initialized only once (the first time the function is called):

```
void AnotherFunc( int param )
{
    static char ch = 'A';           // Initialized once only
    static int  m  = param + 1;     // Initialized once only
        :
}
```

Although an initialization gives a variable an initial value, it is perfectly acceptable to reassign it another value during program execution.

There are differing opinions about initializing a variable in its declaration. Some programmers never do it, preferring to keep an initialization close to the executable statements that depend on that variable. For example,

```
int loopCount;
    :
loopCount = 1;
while (loopCount <= 20)
{
    :
}
```

Other programmers maintain that one of the most frequent causes of program errors is forgetting to initialize variables before using their contents; initializing each variable in its declaration eliminates these errors. As with any controversial topic, most programmers seem to take a position somewhere between these two extremes.

8.3 Interface Design

We return now to the issue of interface design, which we first discussed in Chapter 7. Recall that the data flow through a function interface can take three forms: incoming only, outgoing only, and incoming/outgoing. Any item that can be classified as purely incoming should be coded as a value parameter. Items in the remaining two categories (outgoing and incoming/outgoing) must be reference parameters; the only way the function can deposit results into the caller's arguments is to have the addresses of those arguments. For emphasis, we repeat the following table from Chapter 7.

Data Flow for a Parameter	Argument-Passing Mechanism
Incoming	Pass by value
Outgoing	Pass by reference
Incoming/outgoing	Pass by reference

As we said in the last chapter, there are exceptions to the guidelines in this table. C++ requires that I/O stream objects be passed by reference because of the way streams and files are implemented. We encounter another exception in Chapter 12.

Sometimes it is tempting to skip the interface design step when writing a function, letting it communicate with other functions by referencing global variables. Don't! Without the interface design step, you would actually be creating a poorly structured and undocumented interface. Except in well-justified circumstances, the use of global variables is a poor programming practice that can lead to program errors. These errors are extremely hard to locate and usually take the form of unwanted side effects.

Side Effects

Suppose you made a call to the `sqrt` library function in your program:

```
y = sqrt(x);
```

Side effect   Any effect of one function on another that is not a part of the explicitly defined interface between them.

You expect the call to `sqrt` to do one thing only: compute the square root of the variable `x`. You'd be surprised if `sqrt` also changed the value of your variable `x` because `sqrt`, by definition, does not make such changes. This would be an example of an unexpected and unwanted side effect.

Side effects are sometimes caused by a combination of reference parameters and careless coding in a function. Perhaps an assignment statement in the function stores a temporary result into one of the reference parameters, accidentally changing the value of an argument back in the calling code. As we mentioned before, using value parameters avoids this type of side effect by preventing the change from reaching the argument.

Side effects also can occur when a function accesses a global variable. An error in the function might cause the value of a global variable to be changed in an unexpected way, causing an error in other functions that access that variable.

The symptoms of a side-effect error are misleading because the trouble shows up in one part of the program when it really is caused by something in another part. To avoid such errors, the only external effect that a function should have is to transfer information through the well-structured interface of the parameter list (see Figure 8–2). If functions access nonlocal variables *only* through their parameter lists, and if all incoming-only parameters are value parameters, then each function is essentially isolated from other parts of the program and side effects cannot occur.

When a function is free of side effects, we can treat it as an independent module and reuse it in other programs. It is hazardous or impossible to reuse functions with side effects.

Here is a short example of a program that runs but produces incorrect results because of global variables and side effects.

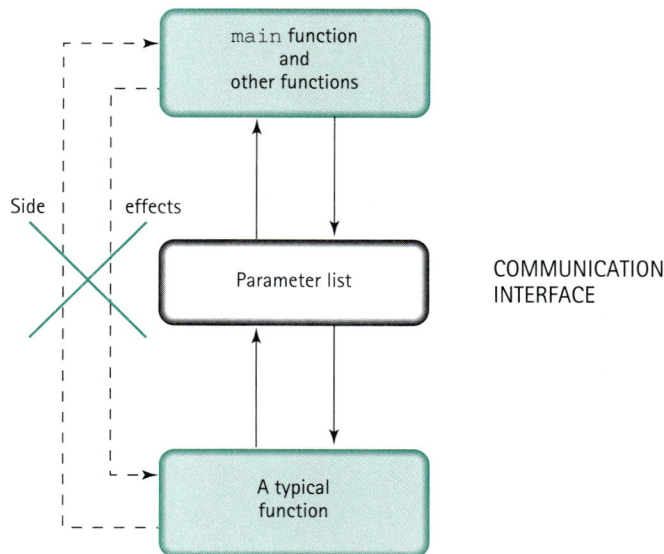

Figure 8–2   *Side Effects*

```cpp
//*******************************************************************
// Trouble program
// This is an example of poor program design, which
// causes an error when the program is executed
//*******************************************************************
#include <iostream>

using namespace std;

void CountInts();

int count;          // Supposed to count input lines, but does it?
int intVal;         // Holds one input integer

int main()
{
    count = 0;
    cin >> intVal;
    while (cin)
    {
        count++;
        CountInts();
        cin >> intVal;
    }
    cout << count << " lines of input processed." << endl;
    return 0;
}

//*******************************************************************

void CountInts()

// Counts the number of integers on one input line (where 99999
// is a sentinel on each line) and prints the count
// Note: main() has already read the first integer on a line

{
    count = 0;                                  // Side effect
    while (intVal != 99999)
    {
        count++;                                // Side effect
        cin >> intVal;
    }
    cout << count << " integers on this line." << endl;
}
```

The Trouble program is supposed to count and print the number of integers on each line of input. After the last line has been processed, it should print the number of lines. Strangely enough, each time the program is run, it reports that the number of lines of input is the same as the number of integers in the last line of input. This is because the `CountInts` function accesses the global variable `count` and uses it to store the number of integers on each input line.

There is no reason for `count` to be a global variable. If a local variable `count` is declared in `main` and another local variable `count` is declared in `CountInts`, the program works correctly. There is no conflict between the two variables because each is visible only inside its own block.

The Trouble program also demonstrates one common exception to the rule of not accessing global variables. Technically, `cin` and `cout` are global objects declared in the header file `iostream`. The `CountInts` function reads and writes directly to these streams. To be absolutely correct, `cin` and `cout` should be passed as arguments to the function. However, `cin` and `cout` are fundamental I/O facilities supplied by the standard library, and it is conventional for C++ functions to access them directly.

Global Constants

Contrary to what you might think, it is acceptable to reference named constants globally. Because the values of global constants cannot be changed while the program is running, no side effects can occur.

There are two advantages to referencing constants globally: ease of change, and consistency. If you need to change the value of a constant, it's easier to change only one global declaration than to change a local declaration in every function. By declaring a constant in only one place, we also ensure that all parts of the program use exactly the same value.

This is not to say that you should declare *all* constants globally. If a constant is needed in only one function, then it makes sense to declare it locally within that function.

At this point, you may want to turn to the Problem-Solving Case Study at the end of this chapter. This case study further illustrates the interface design process and the use of value and reference parameters.

May We Introduce

Ada Lovelace

On December 10, 1815 (the same year in which George Boole was born), a daughter—Augusta Ada Byron—was born to Anna Isabella (Annabella) Byron and George Gordon, Lord Byron. In England at that time, Byron's fame derived not only from his poetry but also from his wild, scandalous behavior. The marriage was strained from the beginning, and Annabella left Byron shortly after Ada's birth. By April of 1816, the two had signed separation papers. Byron left

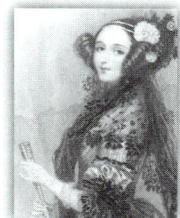

(continued) ▼

Ada Lovelace

England, never to return. Throughout the rest of his life, he regretted being unable to see his daughter. At one point, he wrote of her:

I see thee not. I hear thee not.
But none can be so wrapt in thee.

Before he died in Greece at age 36, he exclaimed, "Oh my poor dear child! My dear Ada! My God, could I but have seen her!"

Meanwhile, Annabella, who would eventually become a baroness in her own right, and who was educated as both a mathematician and a poet, carried on with Ada's upbringing and education. Annabella gave Ada her first instruction in mathematics, but it soon became clear that Ada was gifted in the subject and should receive more extensive tutoring. Ada received further training from Augustus DeMorgan, famous today for one of the basic theorems of Boolean algebra, the logical foundation for modern computers. By age 8, Ada had also demonstrated an interest in mechanical devices and was building detailed model boats.

When she was 18, Ada visited the Mechanics Institute to hear Dr. Dionysius Lardner's lectures on the Difference Engine, a mechanical calculating machine being built by Charles Babbage. She became so interested in the device that she arranged to be introduced to Babbage. It was said that, upon seeing Babbage's machine, Ada was the only person in the room to understand immediately how it worked and to recognize its significance. Ada and Charles Babbage became lifelong friends. She worked with him, helping to document his designs, translating writings about his work, and developing programs for his machines. In fact, today Ada is recognized as the first computer programmer in history, and the modern Ada programming language is named in her honor.

When Babbage designed his Analytical Engine, Ada foresaw that it could go beyond arithmetic computations and become a general manipulator of symbols, and that it would thus have far-reaching capabilities. She even suggested that such a device could eventually be programmed with rules of harmony and composition so that it could produce "scientific" music. In effect, Ada foresaw the field of artificial intelligence more than 150 years ago.

In 1842, Babbage gave a series of lectures in Turin, Italy, on his Analytical Engine. One of the attendees was Luigi Menabrea, who was so impressed that he wrote an account of Babbage's lectures. At age 27, Ada decided to translate the account into English with the intent of adding a few of her own notes about the machine. In the end, her notes were twice as long as the original material, and the document, "The Sketch of the Analytical Engine," became the definitive work on the subject.

It is obvious from Ada's letters that her "notes" were entirely her own and that Babbage was sometimes making unsolicited editorial changes. At one point, Ada wrote to him,

I am much annoyed at your having altered my Note. You know I am always willing to make any required alterations myself, but that I cannot endure another person to meddle with my sentences.

(continued) ▼

Ada Lovelace

Ada gained the title Countess of Lovelace when she married Lord William Lovelace. The couple had three children, whose upbringing was left to Ada's mother while Ada pursued her work in mathematics. Her husband was supportive of her work, but for a woman of that day, such behavior was considered almost as scandalous as some of her father's exploits.

Ada Lovelace died of cancer in 1852, just one year before a working Difference Engine was built in Sweden from one of Babbage's designs. Like her father, Ada lived only to age 36, and even though they led very different lives, she had undoubtedly admired him and taken inspiration from his unconventional, rebellious nature. In the end, Ada asked to be buried beside him at the family's estate.

8.4 Value-Returning Functions

In Chapter 7 and the first part of this chapter, we have been writing our own void functions. We now look at the second kind of subprogram in C++, the value-returning function. You already know several value-returning functions supplied by the C++ standard library: `sqrt`, `abs`, `fabs`, and others. From the caller's perspective, the main difference between void functions and value-returning functions is the way in which they are called. A call to a void function is a complete statement; a call to a value-returning function is part of an expression.

From a design perspective, value-returning functions are used when there is only one result returned by a function and that result is to be used directly in an expression. For example, suppose we are writing a program that calculates a prorated refund of tuition for students who withdraw in the middle of a semester. The amount to be refunded is the total tuition times the remaining fraction of the semester (the number of days remaining divided by the total number of days in the semester). The people who use the program want to be able to enter the dates on which the semester begins and ends and the date of withdrawal, and they want the program to calculate the fraction of the semester that remains.

Because each semester at this particular school begins and ends within one calendar year, we can calculate the number of days in a period by determining the day number of each date and subtracting the starting day number from the ending day number. The day number is the number associated with each day of the year if you count sequentially from January 1. December 31 has the day number 365, except in leap years, when it is 366. For example, if a semester begins on 1/3/01 and ends on 5/17/01, the calculation is as follows.

The day number of 1/3/01 is 3
The day number of 5/17/01 is 137
The length of the semester is $137 - 3 + 1 = 135$

We add 1 to the difference of the days because we count the first day as part of the period.

The algorithm for calculating the day number for a date is complicated by leap years and by months of different lengths. We could code this algorithm as a void function named ComputeDay. The refund could then be computed by the following code segment.

```
ComputeDay(startMonth, startDay, startYear, start);
ComputeDay(lastMonth, lastDay, lastYear, last);
ComputeDay(withdrawMonth, withdrawDay, withdrawYear, withdraw);
fraction = float(last - withdraw + 1) / float(last - start + 1);
refund = tuition * fraction;
```

The first three arguments to ComputeDay are received by the function, and the last one is returned to the caller. Because ComputeDay returns only one value, we can write it as a value-returning function instead of a void function. Let's look at how the calling code would be written if we had a value-returning function named Day that returned the day number of a date in a given year.

```
start = Day(startMonth, startDay, startYear);
last = Day(lastMonth, lastDay, lastYear);
withdraw = Day(withdrawMonth, withdrawDay, withdrawYear);
fraction = float(last - withdraw + 1) / float(last - start + 1);
refund = tuition * fraction;
```

The second version of the code segment is much more intuitive. Because Day is a value-returning function, you know immediately that all its parameters receive values and that it returns just one value (the day number for a date).

Let's look at the function definition for Day. Don't worry about how Day works; for now, you should concentrate on its syntax and structure.

```
int Day( /* in */ int month,         // Month number, 1 - 12
         /* in */ int dayOfMonth,    // Day of month, 1 - 31
         /* in */ int year       )   // Year. For example, 2001

// This function computes the day number within a year, given
// the date. It accounts correctly for leap years. The
// calculation is based on the fact that months average 30 days
// in length. Thus, (month - 1) * 30 is roughly the number of
// days in the year at the start of any month. A correction
// factor is used to account for cases where the average is
// incorrect and for leap years. The day of the month is then
// added to produce the day number

// Precondition:
//     1 <= month <= 12
```

```
//   && dayOfMonth is in valid range for the month
//   && year is assigned
// Postcondition:
//    Return value is day number in the range 1 - 365
//                    (or 1 - 366 for a leap year)

{
    int correction = 0;    // Correction factor to account for leap
                           //   year and months of different lengths

    // Test for leap year

    if (year % 4 == 0 && (year % 100 != 0 || year % 400 == 0))
        if (month >= 3)            // If date is after February 29
            correction = 1;        //   then add one for leap year

    // Correct for different-length months

    if (month == 3)
        correction = correction - 1;
    else if (month == 2 || month == 6 || month == 7)
        correction = correction + 1;
    else if (month == 8)
        correction = correction + 2;
    else if (month == 9 || month == 10)
        correction = correction + 3;
    else if (month == 11 || month == 12)
        correction = correction + 4;
    return (month - 1) * 30 + correction + dayOfMonth;
}
```

The first thing to note is that the function definition looks like a void function, except for the fact that the heading begins with the data type int instead of the word void. The second thing to observe is the Return statement at the end, which includes an integer expression between the word return and the semicolon.

A value-returning function returns one value, not through a parameter but by means of a Return statement. The data type at the beginning of the heading declares the type of value that the function returns. This data type is called the *function type,* although a more precise term is **function value type** (or *function return type* or *function result type*).

> **Function value type**   The data type of the result value returned by a function.

The last statement in the Day function evaluates the expression

```
(month - 1) * 30 + correction + dayOfMonth
```

and returns the result as the function value (see Figure 8–3).

```
int main()
{

     _____
     _____
     _____
     ____
     _____

     cout << Day(3,18,2002);
     _____
     _____
     ____
     ____
     ____
     _____
     _____
     _____

}
```

```
int Day( int month,
         int dayOfMonth,
         int year        )
{
     _____
     _____

     return (month-1) * 30 +
            correction +
            dayOfMonth;
}
```

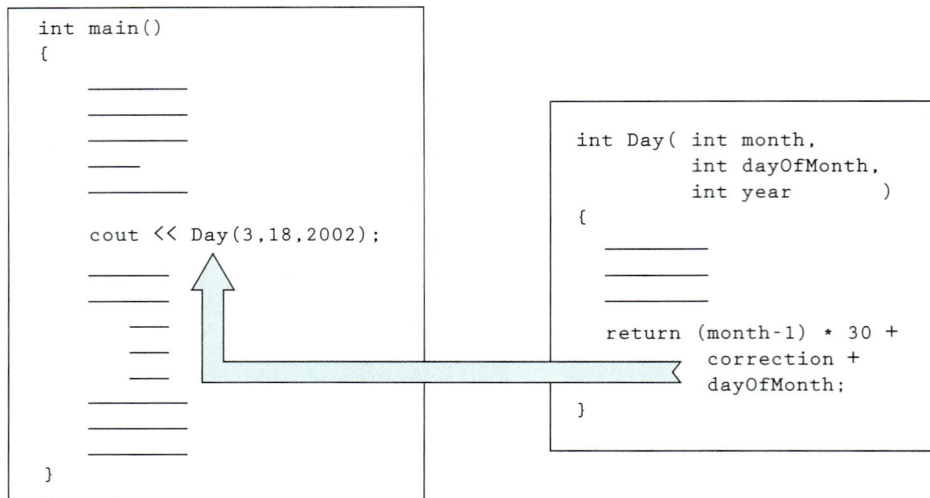

Figure 8-3   *Returning a Function Value to the Expression That Called the Function*

You now have seen two forms of the Return statement. The form

```
return;
```

is valid *only* in void functions. It causes control to exit the function immediately and return to the caller. The second form is

```
return Expression;
```

This form is valid *only* in a value-returning function. It returns control to the caller, sending back the value of Expression as the function value. (If the data type of Expression is different from the declared function type, its value is coerced to the correct type.)

In Chapter 7, we presented a syntax template for the function definition of a void function. We now update the syntax template to cover both void functions and value-returning functions:

FunctionDefinition

```
DataType FunctionName ( ParameterList )
{
     Statement
        ⋮
}
```

If DataType is the word `void`, the function is a void function; otherwise, it is a value-returning function. Notice from the shading in the syntax template that DataType is optional. If you omit the data type of a function, `int` is assumed. We mention this point only because you sometimes encounter programs where DataType is missing from the function heading. Many programmers do not consider this practice to be good programming style.

The parameter list for a value-returning function has exactly the same form as for a void function: a list of parameter declarations, separated by commas. Also, a function prototype for a value-returning function looks just like the prototype for a void function except that it begins with a data type instead of `void`.

Let's look at two more examples of value-returning functions. The C++ standard library provides a power function, `pow`, that raises a floating-point number to a floating-point power. The library does not supply a power function for `int` values, so let's build one of our own. The function receives two integers, x and n (where $n \geq 0$), and computes x^n. We use a simple approach, multiplying repeatedly by x. Because the number of iterations is known in advance, a count-controlled loop is appropriate. The loop counts down to 0 from the initial value of n. For each iteration of the loop, x is multiplied by the previous product.

```
int Power( /* in */ int x,      // Base number
           /* in */ int n )     // Power to raise base to

// This function computes x to the n power

// Precondition:
//     x is assigned  &&  n >= 0  &&  (x to the n) <= INT_MAX
// Postcondition:
//     Return value is x to the n power

{
    int result;      // Holds intermediate powers of x

    result = 1;
    while (n > 0)
    {
        result = result * x;
        n--;
    }
    return result;
}
```

Notice the notation we use in the postcondition of a value-returning function. Because a value-returning function returns a single value, it is most concise if you simply state what that value equals. Except in complicated examples, the postcondition looks like this:

```
// Postcondition
//     Return value is ...
```

Another function that is used frequently in calculating probabilities is the factorial. For example, 5 factorial (written 5! in mathematical notation) is $5 \times 4 \times 3 \times 2 \times 1$. Zero factorial, by definition, equals 1. This function has one integer parameter. As with the `Power` function, we use repeated multiplication, but we decrement the multiplier on each iteration.

```
int Factorial( /* in */ int n )     // Number whose factorial is
                                     //    to be computed
// This function computes n!

// Precondition:
//      n >= 0   &&   n! <= INT_MAX
// Postcondition:
//      Return value is n!

{
    int result;     // Holds partial products

    result = 1;
    while (n > 0)
    {
        result = result * n;
        n--;
    }
    return result;
}
```

A call to the `Factorial` function might look like this:

```
combinations = Factorial(n) / (Factorial(m) * Factorial(n - m));
```

Boolean Functions

Value-returning functions are not restricted to returning numerical results. We can also use them, for example, to evaluate a condition and return a Boolean result. Boolean functions can be useful when a branch or loop depends on some complex condition. Rather than code the condition directly into the If or While statement, we can call a Boolean function to form the controlling expression.

Suppose we are writing a program that works with triangles. The program reads three angles as floating-point numbers. Before performing any calculations on those angles, however, we want to check that they really form a triangle by adding the angles to confirm that their sum equals 180 degrees. We can write a value-returning function that takes the three angles as parameters and returns a Boolean result. Such a function would look like this (recall from Chapter 5 that you should test floating-point numbers only for near equality):

```
#include <cmath>     // For fabs()
    ⋮
bool IsTriangle( /* in */ float angle1,     // First angle
                 /* in */ float angle2,     // Second angle
                 /* in */ float angle3 )    // Third angle

// This function checks to see if its three incoming values
// add up to 180 degrees, forming a valid triangle

// Precondition:
//     angle1, angle2, and angle3 are assigned
// Postcondition:
//     Return value is true, if (angle1 + angle2 + angle3) is
//                             within 0.00000001 of 180.0 degrees
//                  is false, otherwise

{
    return (fabs(angle1 + angle2 + angle3 - 180.0) < 0.00000001);
}
```

The following program shows how the IsTriangle function is called. (The function definition is shown without its documentation to save space.)

```
//************************************************************
// Triangle program
// This program exercises the IsTriangle function
//************************************************************
#include <iostream>
#include <cmath>       // For fabs()

using namespace std;

bool IsTriangle( float, float, float );

int main()
{
    float angleA;     // Three potential angles of a triangle
    float angleB;
    float angleC;

    cout << "Enter 3 angles: ";
    cin >> angleA;
    while (cin)
    {
        cin >> angleB >> angleC;
        if (IsTriangle(angleA, angleB, angleC))
```

```
                    cout << "The 3 angles form a valid triangle." << endl;
                else
                    cout << "Those angles do not form a triangle." << endl;
                cout << "Enter 3 angles: ";
                cin >> angleA;
            }
            return 0;
    }


    //****************************************************************************

    bool IsTriangle( /* in */ float angle1,
                     /* in */ float angle2,
                     /* in */ float angle3 )
    {
        return (fabs(angle1 + angle2 + angle3 - 180.0) < 0.00000001);
    }
```

In the `main` function of the Triangle program, the If statement is much easier to understand with the function call than it would be if the entire condition were coded directly. When a conditional test is at all complicated, a Boolean function is in order.

The C++ standard library provides a number of helpful functions that let you test the contents of `char` variables. To use them, you #include the header file `cctype`. Here are some of the available functions; Appendix C contains a more complete list.

Header File	Function	Function Type	Function Value
`<cctype>`	`isalpha(ch)`	int	Nonzero, if ch is a letter ('A'–'Z', 'a'–'z'); 0, otherwise
`<cctype>`	`isalnum(ch)`	int	Nonzero, if ch is a letter or a digit ('A'–'Z', 'a'–'z', '0'–'9'); 0, otherwise
`<cctype>`	`isdigit(ch)`	int	Nonzero, if ch is a digit ('0'–'9'); 0, otherwise
`<cctype>`	`islower(ch)`	int	Nonzero, if ch is a lowercase letter ('a'–'z'); 0, otherwise
`<cctype>`	`isspace(ch)`	int	Nonzero, if ch is a whitespace character (blank, newline, tab, carriage return, form feed); 0, otherwise
`<cctype>`	`isupper(ch)`	int	Nonzero, if ch is an uppercase letter ('A'–'Z'); 0, otherwise

Although they return `int` values, the "`is...`" functions behave like Boolean functions. They return an `int` value that is nonzero (coerced to `true` in an If or While condition) or 0 (coerced to `false` in an If or While condition). These functions are convenient to use and make programs more readable. For example, the test

```
if (isalnum(inputChar))
```

is easier to read and less prone to error than if you coded the test the long way:

```
if (inputChar >= 'A' && inputChar <= 'Z' ||
    inputChar >= 'a' && inputChar <= 'z' ||
    inputChar >= '0' && inputChar <= '9'    )
```

In fact, this complicated logical expression doesn't work correctly on some machines. We'll see why when we examine character data in Chapter 10.

Matters of Style

Naming Value-Returning Functions

In Chapter 7, we said that it's good style to use imperative verbs when naming void functions. The reason is that a call to a void function is a complete statement and should look like a command to the computer:

```
PrintResults(a, b, c);
DoThis(x);
DoThat();
```

This naming scheme, however, doesn't work well with value-returning functions. A statement such as

```
z = 6.7 * ComputeMaximum(d, e, f);
```

sounds awkward when you read it aloud: "Set z equal to 6.7 times the *compute maximum* of d, e, and f."

With a value-returning function, the function call represents a value within an expression. Things that represent values, such as variables and value-returning functions, are best given names that are nouns or, occasionally, adjectives. See how much better this statement sounds when you pronounce it out loud:

```
z = 6.7 * Maximum(d, e, f);
```

(continued) ▼

Naming Value-Returning Functions

You would read this as "Set z equal to 6.7 times the *maximum* of d, e, and f." Other names that suggest values rather than actions are `SquareRoot`, `Cube`, `Factorial`, `StudentCount`, `SumOfSquares`, and `SocialSecurityNum`. As you see, they are all nouns or noun phrases.

Boolean value-returning functions (and variables) are often named using adjectives or phrases beginning with *Is*. Here are a few examples:

```
while (Valid(m, n))
if (Odd(n))
if (IsTriangle(s1, s2, s3))
```

When you are choosing a name for a value-returning function, try to stick with nouns or adjectives so that the name suggests a value, not a command to the computer.

Interface Design and Side Effects

The interface to a value-returning function is designed in much the same way as the interface to a void function. We simply write down a list of what the function needs and what it must return. Because value-returning functions return only one value, there is only one item labeled "outgoing" in the list: the function return value. Everything else in the list is labeled "incoming," and there aren't any "incoming/outgoing" parameters.

Returning more than one value from a value-returning function (by modifying the caller's arguments) is a side effect and should be avoided. If your interface design calls for multiple values to be returned, then you should use a void function instead of a value-returning function.

A rule of thumb is never to use reference parameters in the parameter list of a value-returning function, but to use value parameters exclusively. Let's look at an example that demonstrates the importance of this rule. Suppose we define the following function:

```
int SideEffect( int& n )
{
    int result = n * n;

    n++;                        // Side effect
    return result;
}
```

This function returns the square of its incoming value, but it also increments the caller's argument before returning. Now suppose we call this function with the following statement:

```
y = x + SideEffect(x);
```

If x is originally 2, what value is stored into y? The answer depends on the order in which your compiler generates code to evaluate the expression. If the compiled code first calls the function, then the answer is 7. If it accesses x first in preparation for adding it to the function result, the answer is 6. This uncertainty is precisely why reference parameters shouldn't be used with value-returning functions. A function that causes an unpredictable result has no place in a well-written program.

An exception is the case in which an I/O stream object is passed to a value-returning function. Remember that C++ allows a stream object to be passed only to a reference parameter. Within a value-returning function, the only operation that should be performed is testing the state of the stream (for EOF or I/O errors). A value-returning function should not perform input or output operations. Such operations are considered to be side effects of the function. (We should point out that not everyone agrees with this point of view. Some programmers feel that performing I/O within a value-returning function is perfectly acceptable. You will find strong opinions on both sides of this issue.)

There is another advantage to using only value parameters in a value-returning function definition: You can use constants and expressions as arguments. For example, we can call the IsTriangle function using literals and other expressions:

```
if (IsTriangle(30.0, 60.0, 30.0 + 60.0))
    cout << "A 30-60-90 angle combination forms a triangle.";
else
    cout << "Something is wrong.";
```

When to Use Value-Returning Functions

There aren't any formal rules for determining when to use a void function and when to use a value-returning function, but here are some guidelines:

1. If the module must return more than one value or modify any of the caller's arguments, do not use a value-returning function.

2. If the module must perform I/O, do not use a value-returning function. (This guideline is not universally agreed upon.)

3. If there is only one value returned from the module and it is a Boolean value, a value-returning function is appropriate.

4. If there is only one value returned and that value is to be used immediately in an expression, a value-returning function is appropriate.

5. When in doubt, use a void function. You can recode any value-returning function as a void function by adding an extra outgoing parameter to carry back the computed result.

6. If both a void function and a value-returning function are acceptable, use the one you feel more comfortable implementing.

Value-returning functions were included in C++ to provide a way of simulating the mathematical concept of a function. The C++ standard library supplies a set of commonly used mathematical functions through the header file cmath. A list of these appears in Appendix C.

Background Information

Ignoring a Function Value

A peculiarity of the C++ language is that it lets you ignore the value returned by a value-returning function. For example, you could write the following statement in your program without any complaint from the compiler:

```
sqrt(x);
```

When this statement is executed, the value returned by `sqrt` is promptly discarded. This function call has absolutely no effect except to waste the computer's time by calculating a value that is never used.

Clearly, the above call to `sqrt` is a mistake. No programmer would write that statement intentionally. But C++ programmers occasionally write value-returning functions in a way that allows the caller to ignore the function value. Here is a specific example from the C++ standard library.

The library provides a function named `remove`, the purpose of which is to delete a disk file from the system. It takes a single argument—a C string specifying the name of the file—and it returns a function value. This function value is an integer notifying you of the status: 0 if the operation succeeded, and nonzero if it failed. Here is how you might call the `remove` function:

```
status = remove("junkfile.dat");
if (status != 0)
    PrintErrorMsg();
```

On the other hand, if you assume that the system always succeeds at deleting a file, you can ignore the returned status by calling `remove` as though it were a void function:

```
remove("junkfile.dat");
```

The `remove` function is sort of a hybrid between a void function and a value-returning function. Conceptually, it is a void function; its principal purpose is to delete a file, not to compute a value to be returned. Literally, however, it's a value-returning function. It does return a function value—the status of the operation (which you can choose to ignore).

In this book, we don't write hybrid functions. We prefer to keep the concept of a void function distinct from a value-returning function. But there are two reasons why every C++ programmer should know about the topic of ignoring a function value. First, if you accidentally call a value-returning function as if it were a void function, the compiler won't prevent you from making the mistake. Second, you sometimes encounter this style of coding in other people's programs and in the C++ standard library. Several of the library functions are technically value-returning functions, but the function value is used merely to return something of secondary importance such as a status value.

Problem–Solving Case Study

Health Profile

PROBLEM   Your grandmother has just come back from the doctor's office and is confused about all the numbers that were used to evaluate her health. The nurse weighed her, took her blood pressure, noted her cholesterol from her lab work, told her to sit down, and said that the doctor would be in shortly. After half an hour the doctor came in, looked at her chart, smiled, and said that she was fine. In looking over the report they gave your grandmother, you realize that there could be a market for a program to explain this information to medical patients. You have a project due in your software engineering class, so you decide to write a program to do exactly that.

Before you can state the input and output from this program, you need to do some research on the Web. You find that there are two important parts to a cholesterol reading: HDL (good) and LDL (bad). The ratio of the two is also important. You find several references that provide interpretations for a range of input values. The interpretation of your weight is dependent on the ratio of your weight to your size as represented by the body mass index (BMI). Great, you already have a program to calculate the BMI! Blood pressure is made up of two values: systolic and diastolic. When talking about blood pressure, the readings are usually given as "something" over "something," such as 120/80. The first value is the systolic pressure, and the second value is the diastolic pressure. Now, you have enough information to determine the input for your program.

INPUT   Patient's name, HDL, LDL, weight in pounds, height in inches, systolic pressure, and diastolic pressure.

OUTPUT   Patient's name and an interpretation of the cholesterol, weight, and blood pressure readings are written on file "Profile."

DISCUSSION   The decomposition of this problem into tasks is very straightforward. The data values are prompted for, entered, and evaluated. The only question is whether to enter the data all at once and evaluate it or have each evaluation module enter its own data. The principle of information hiding suggests that we embed the data gathering within the functions that evaluate the data.

Here are the interpretations you found on the Internet concerning cholesterol.

HDL	Interpretation
< 40	Too low
>= 40 and < 60	Is okay
>= 60	Excellent

LDL	Interpretation
< 100	Optimal
>=100 and < 130	Near optimal
>=130 and < 160	Borderline high
>=160 and < 190	High
>= 190	Very high

Fortunately, you already have a BMI calculator that can simply be turned into a function (with the food suggestions removed). What about blood pressure readings? Again, here is what you found on the Internet concerning blood pressure readings.

Systolic	Interpretation
< 120	Optimal
< 130	Normal
< 140	Normal high
< 160	Stage 1 hypertension
< 180	Stage 2 hypertension
>= 180	Stage 3 hypertension

Diastolic	Interpretation
< 80	Optimal
< 85	Normal
< 90	High normal
< 100	Stage 1 hypertension
< 110	Stage 2 hypertension
>= 110	Stage 3 hypertension

Main   **Level 0**

```
Open output file
If output file not opened ok
    Write error message
    Return 1
Get name
Evaluate cholesterol
Evaluate BMI
Evaluate blood pressure
Close output file
```

Get Name
out: Function value   **Level 1**

```
Prompt for first name
Get first name
Prompt for last name
Get last name
Prompt for middle initial
Get middle initial
return first + ' ' + middle + ". " + last
```

Evaluate Cholesterol(Inout: healthProfile; In: name)

> Prompt for name's input
> Get data
> Evaluate input according to charts
> Print message

Name has been added to the parameter list so that the user can prompt for the specific patient's data. The first two lines and the last line can be directly translated into C++.

Evaluate Input(In: HDL, LDL)

> if (HDL < 40)
>   Print on healthProfile "HDL is too low"
> else if (HDL < 60)
>   Print on healthProfile "HDL is okay"
> else
>   Print on healthProfile "HDL is excellent"
>
> if (LDL < 100)
>   Print on healthProfile "LDL is optimal"
> else if (LDL < 130)
>   Print on healthProfile "LDL is near optimal"
> else if (LDL < 160)
>   Print on healthProfile "LDL is borderline high"
> else if (LDL < 190)
>   Print on healthProfile "LDL is high"
> else
>   Print on healthProfile "LDL is very high"
>
> if (ratio < 3.22)
>   Print on healthProfile "Ratio of LDL to HDL is good"
> else
>   Print on healthProfile "Ratio of LDL to HDL is not good"

The algorithm for Evaluate BMI is in Chapter 5, and Evaluate Blood Pressure is identical in form, so we leave the writing of its design as Case Study Follow-Up Exercise 1.

Which modules should be functions and which should be coded inline? GetName should obviously be a value-returning function; EvaluateCholesterol, EvaluateBMI, and EvaluateBloodPressure clearly should be void functions. The question is whether the EvaluateInput modules should be coded as separate functions. If we were coding this problem in a language that allowed us to embed a function within a function, good style would suggest that we make the EvaluateInput modules separate functions. However, C++ does not allow nested functioning. The EvaluateInput modules would have to be coded at the same level as the functions that call them. Thus, these modules should be coded in line. Another reason for doing so is that EvaluateCholesterol, Evaluate-BMI, and EvaluateBloodPressure are tightly knit functions with a clearly stated purpose and interface.

MODULE STRUCTURE CHART

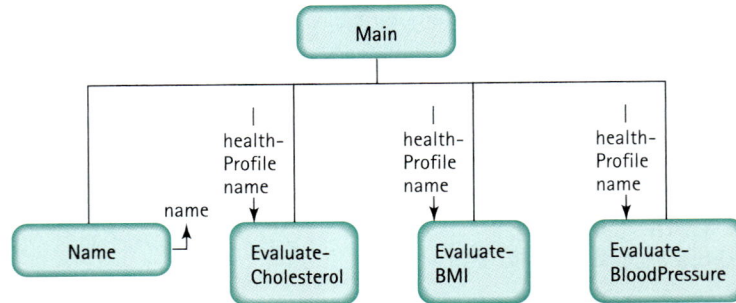

```
//***********************************************************************
// Profile Program
// This program inputs a name, weight, height, blood pressure
// readings, and cholesterol values.  Appropriate health messages
// are written for each of the input values on file healthProfile.
// To save space, we omit from each function the precondition
// comments that document the assumptions made about valid input
// parameter data. These would be included in a program intended
// for actual use.
//***********************************************************************

#include <fstream>
#include <iostream>
#include <string>

using namespace std;

// Function prototypes
string Name();
void EvaluateCholesterol( ofstream& healthProfile, string name);
void EvaluateBMI( ofstream& healthProfile, string name);
void EvaluateBloodPressure( ofstream& healthProfile, string name);
```

```
int main()
{
    // Declare and open the output file
    ofstream healthProfile;
    healthProfile.open("Profile");
    if ( !healthProfile )
    { // No
        cout << "Can't open output file." << endl;
        return 1;
    }
    string name;
    name = Name();

    // Write patient's name on output file
    healthProfile << "Patient's name " << name << endl;

    // Evaluate the patient's statistics
    EvaluateCholesterol(healthProfile, name);
    EvaluateBMI(healthProfile, name);
    EvaluateBloodPressure(healthProfile, name);
    healthProfile << endl;

    healthProfile.close();
    return 0;
}

//*********************************************************************

string Name()

// Name function
// This function inputs a name and returns it in first,
// middle initial, and last order
// Postcondition:
//     Return value is the string composed of the first name,
//     blank, middle initial, period, blank, last name

{
    // Declare the patient's name
    string firstName;
    string lastName;
    char middleInitial;

    // Prompt for and enter the patient's name
    cout << "Enter the patient's first name: ";
    cin >> firstName;
    cout << "Enter the patient's last name: ";
    cin >> lastName;
```

```cpp
        cout << "Enter the patient's middle initial: ";
        cin >> middleInitial;
        return firstName + ' '  + middleInitial + ". " + lastName;
}


//******************************************************************


void EvaluateCholesterol
    ( /* inout */ ofstream& healthProfile,    // Output file
      /* in */    string name )               // Patient's name

// This function inputs HDL (good cholesterol) and LDL (bad
// cholesterol) and prints out a health message based on their
// values on file healthProfile.
// Precondition:
//     Output file has been successfully opened
// Postcondition:
//     Appropriate health messages for the input values of
//     HDL, LDL, and their ratio have been printed on file
//     healthProfile.

{
    int HDL;
    int LDL;

    // Prompt for and enter HDL and LDL
    cout << "Enter HDL for " << name << ": ";
    cin >> HDL;
    cout << "Enter LDL for " << name << ": ";
    cin >> LDL;
    float ratio = LDL/HDL;      // Calculate ratio of LDL to HDL

    healthProfile << "Cholesterol Profile " << endl;
    // Print message based on HDL value
    if (HDL < 40)
        healthProfile << "    HDL is too low" << endl;
    else if (HDL < 60)
        healthProfile << "    HDL is okay" << endl;
    else
        healthProfile << "    HDL is excellent" << endl;
    // Print message based on LDL value
    if (LDL < 100)
        healthProfile << "    LDL is optimal" << endl;
    else if (LDL < 130)
        healthProfile << "    LDL is near optimal" << endl;
```

```
        else if (LDL < 160)
            healthProfile << "   LDL is borderline high" << endl;
        else if (LDL < 190)
            healthProfile << "   LDL is high" << endl;
        else
            healthProfile << "   LDL is very high" << endl;

        if (ratio < 3.22)
            healthProfile << "   Ratio of LDL to HDL is good"
                          << endl;
        else
            healthProfile << "   Ratio of LDL to HDL is not good"
                          << endl;
}


//*******************************************************************


void EvaluateBMI
    ( /* inout */ ofstream& healthProfile,    // Output file
      /* in */     string name )              // Patient's name

// This function inputs weight in pounds and height in inches and
// calculates the body mass index (BMI prints a health message
// based on the BMI. Input in English weights
// Precondition:
//     Output file has been successfully opened
// Postcondition:
//     Appropriate health messages for the BMI based on input values
//     of weight and height have been printed on file healthProfile

{
    const int BMI_CONSTANT = 703; // Constant in English formula
    float pounds;
    float inches;

    // Enter the patient's weight and height
    cout << "Enter the weight in pounds for " << name << ": ";
    cin >> pounds;
    cout << "Enter the height in inches for " << name << ": ";
    cin >> inches;
    float bodyMassIndex = pounds * BMI_CONSTANT / (inches * inches);
    healthProfile << "Body Mass Index Profile" << endl;

    // Print bodyMassIndex
    healthProfile << "   Body mass index is " << bodyMassIndex
```

```
                             << ". " << endl;
            healthProfile << "    Interpretation of BMI " << endl;

            // Print interpretation of BMI
            if (bodyMassIndex <20)
                healthProfile << "    Underweight: BMI is too low"
                            << endl;
            else if (bodyMassIndex <=25)
                healthProfile << "    Normal: BMI is average"  << endl;
            else if (bodyMassIndex <= 30)
                healthProfile << "    Overweight: BMI is too high"
                            << endl;
            else
                healthProfile << "    Obese: BMI is dangerously high"
                            << endl;
        }


//***************************************************************************


void EvaluateBloodPressure
        ( /* inout */ ofstream& healthProfile,    // Output file
          /* in */    string name )               // Patient's name

// This function gets blood pressure readings (systolic/diastolic)
// and prints out a  health message based on their values
// on file healthProfile
// Precondition:
//      Output file has been successfully opened
// Postcondition:
//      Appropriate health messages for the blood pressure readings,
//      based on input values of systolic and diastolic pressure have
//      been printed on file healthProfile

{
        // Declare the blood pressure readings
        int systolic;
        int diastolic;

        // Enter the patient's blood pressure readings
        cout << "Enter the systolic blood pressure reading for"
            << name << ": ";
        cin  >> systolic;
```

```cpp
cout << "Enter the diastolic blood pressure reading for "
     << name << ": ";
cin >> diastolic;

// Print interpretation of systolic reading
healthProfile << "Blood Pressure Profile " << endl;
if (systolic < 120)
    healthProfile << "    Systolic reading is optimal" << endl;
else if (systolic < 130)
    healthProfile << "    Systolic reading is normal" << endl;
else if (systolic < 140)
    healthProfile << "    Systolic reading is high normal"
                  << endl;
else if (systolic < 160)
    healthProfile <<
        "    Systolic indicates hypertension Stage 1" << endl;
else if (systolic < 180)
    healthProfile <<
        "    Systolic indicates hypertension Stage 2" << endl;
else
    healthProfile <<
        "    Systolic indicates hypertension Stage 3" << endl;

// Print interpretation of diastolic reading
if (diastolic < 80)
    healthProfile << "    Diastolic reading is optimal" << endl;
else if (diastolic < 85)
    healthProfile << "    Diastolic reading is normal" << endl;
else if (diastolic < 90)
    healthProfile << "    Diastolic reading is high normal"
                  << endl;
else if (diastolic < 100)
    healthProfile <<
        "    Diastolic indicates hypertension Stage 1" << endl;
else if (diastolic < 110)
    healthProfile <<
        "    Diastolic indicates hypertension Stage 2" << endl;
else
    healthProfile <<
        "    Diastolic indicates hypertension Stage 3" << endl;
}
```

Here is sample input and output.

```
C:\PPSC++\HealthProfile\HealthProfile.exe                                    -□×
Enter the patient's first name: Stephen
Enter the patient's last name: Stark
Enter the patient's middle initial: S
Enter HDL for Stephen S. Stark: 60
Enter LDL for Stephen S. Stark: 120
Enter the weight in pounds for Stephen S. Stark: 180
Enter the height in inches for Stephen S. Stark: 72
Enter the systolic blood pressure reading for Stephen S. Stark: 130
Enter the diastolic blood pressure reading for Stephen S. Stark: 80
```

```
Profile - Notepad                                                            -□×
File  Edit  Format  View  Help
Patient's name Stephen S. Stark
Cholesterol Profile
    HDL is excellent
    LDL is near optimal
    Ratio of LDL to HDL is good
Body Mass Index Profile
    Body mass index is 24.4097.
    Interpretation of BMI
    Normal: BMI is average
Blood Pressure Profile
    Systolic reading is high normal
    Diastolic reading is normal
```

TESTING There are nine inputs to this program: two strings and a character in Name, two integer values in EvaluateChelesterol, two floating point values in EvaluateBMI, and two integer values in EvaluateBloodPressure. The code in Name duplicates the code in program Name in Chapter 4, so we can assume that it is correct. Each of the other functions needs to be checked separately, choosing values that occur at the break points in the If statements of each function.

We have not included any data validation in this case study because the values are input from a patient's chart. Although the values can be assumed to be correct on the chart, we cannot assume that they are input correctly. Case Study Follow-Up Exercise 3 asks you to add data validation to this program.

Software Engineering Tip

Control Abstraction, Functional Cohesion,
and Communication Complexity

The Profile program contains four functions, which makes the main function look complex. Yet if you look at the individual modules, the most complicated control structure is an If statement with If statements nested within it.

The complexity of a program is hidden by reducing each of the major control structures to an abstract action performed by a function call. In the Profile program, for example, evaluating a patient's BMI is an abstract action that appears as a call to evaluate BMI. The logical properties of the action are separated from its implementation. This aspect of a design is called control abstraction.

Control abstraction   The separation of the logical properties of an action from its implementation.

Functional cohesion   The principle that a module should perform exactly one abstract action.

Communication complexity   A measure of the quantity of data passing through a module's interface.

Control abstraction can serve as a guideline for deciding which modules to code as functions and which to code directly. If a module contains a control structure, it is a good candidate for being implemented as a function. But even if a module does not contain a control structure, you still want to consider other factors. Is it lengthy, or is it called from more than one place? If so, you should use a function.

Somewhat related to control abstraction is the concept of functional cohesion, which states that a module should perform exactly one abstract action.

If you can state the action that a module performs in one sentence with no conjunctions (*and*s), then it is highly cohesive. A module that has more than one primary purpose lacks cohesion. Apart from `main`, all the functions in the Profile program have good cohesion.

A module that only partially fulfills a purpose also lacks cohesion. Such a module should be combined with whatever other modules are directly related to it. For example, it would make no sense to have a separate function that prints the first digit of a date because printing a date is one abstract action.

A third and related aspect of a module's design is its communication complexity, the amount of data that passes through a module's interface—for example, the number of arguments. A module's communication complexity is often an indicator of its cohesiveness. Usually, if a module requires a large number of arguments, it either is trying to accomplish too much or is only partially fulfilling a purpose. You should step back and see if there is an alternative way of dividing up the problem so that a minimal amount of data is communicated between modules. The modules in Profile have low communication complexity.

Testing and Debugging

One of the advantages of a modular design is that you can test it long before the code has been written for all of the modules. If we test each module individually, then we can assemble the modules into a complete program with much greater confidence that the program is correct. In this section, we introduce a technique for testing a module separately.

Stubs and Drivers

Suppose you were given the code for a module and your job was to test it. How would you test a single module by itself? First of all, it must be called by something (unless it is the main function). Second, it may have calls to other modules that aren't available to you. To test the module, you must fill in these missing links.

When a module contains calls to other modules, we can write dummy functions called stubs to satisfy those calls.

Stub A dummy function that assists in testing part of a program. A stub has the same name and interface as a function that actually would be called by the part of the program being tested, but it is usually much simpler.

A stub usually consists of an output statement that prints a message such as "Function such-and-such just got called." Even though the stub is a dummy, it allows us to determine whether the function is called at the right time by the main function or another function.

A stub also can be used to print the set of values that are passed to it; this tells us whether or not the module being tested is supplying the correct information. Sometimes a stub assigns new values to its reference parameters to simulate data being read or results being computed in order to give the calling module something on which to keep working. Because we can choose the values that are returned by the stub, we have better control over the conditions of the test run.

Here is a stub that simulates the Name function in the Profile program by returning an arbitrarily chosen string.

```cpp
string Name()
// Stub for Name function in the Profile program

{
    cout << "Name was called here. Returning \"John J. Smith\"."
        << endl;
    return "John J. Smith";
}
```

This stub is simpler than the function it simulates, which is typical because the object of using a stub is to provide a simple, predictable environment for testing a module.

In addition to supplying a stub for each call within the module, you must provide a dummy program—a **driver**—to call the module itself. A driver program contains the bare minimum of code required to call the module being tested.

> **Driver** A simple main function that is used to call a function being tested. The use of a driver permits direct control of the testing process.

By surrounding a module with a driver and stubs, you gain complete control of the conditions under which it executes. This allows you to test different situations and combinations that may reveal errors. For example, the following program is a driver for the EvaluateCholesterol function in the Profile program.

```cpp
//*************************************************************
// EvaluateCholesterol Driver program
// This program provides an environment for testing the
// EvaluateCholesterol function in isolation from the Profile
// program
//*************************************************************

#include <iostream>
#include <fstream>

using namespace std;

// Function prototype
void EvaluateCholesterol(ofstream&, string);

int main()
{
    ofstream healthProfile;
    healthProfile.open("Profile");
    string name = "John J. Smith";
    for (int test = 1; test <= 8; test++)
        EvaluateCholesterol(healthProfile, name);
    healthProfile.close();
    return 0;
}

//*************************************************************

void EvaluateCholesterol
        ( /* inout */ ofstream& healthProfile,    // Output file
          /* in */    string name )               // Patient's name
```

```cpp
// This function inputs HDL (good cholesterol) and LDL (bad
// cholesterol) and prints out a health message based on their
// values on file healthProfile.
// Precondition:
//     Output file has been successfully opened
// Postcondition:
//     Appropriate health messages for the input values of
//        HDL, LDL, and their ratio have been printed on file
//        healthProfile.

{
    int HDL;
    int LDL;

    // Prompt for and enter HDL and LDL
    cout << "Enter HDL for " << name << ": ";
    cin >> HDL;
    cout << "Enter LDL for " << name << ": ";
    cin >> LDL;
    float ratio = LDL/HDL; // Calculate ratio of LDL to HDL

    healthProfile << "Cholesterol Profile " << endl;
    // Print message based on HDL value
    if (HDL < 40)
        healthProfile << "   HDL is too low" << endl;
    else if (HDL < 60)
        healthProfile << "   HDL is okay" << endl;
    else
        healthProfile << "   HDL is excellent" << endl;
    // Print message based on LDL value
    if (LDL < 100)
        healthProfile << "   LDL is optimal" << endl;
    else if (LDL < 130)
        healthProfile << "   LDL is near optimal" << endl;
    else if (LDL < 160)
        healthProfile << "   LDL is borderline high" << endl;
    else if (LDL < 190)
        healthProfile << "   LDL is high" << endl;
    else
        healthProfile << "   LDL is very high" << endl;
```

```
    if (ratio < 3.22)
        healthProfile << "   Ratio of LDL to HDL is good"
                      << endl;
    else
        healthProfile << "   Ratio of LDL to HDL is not good"
                      << endl;
}
```

The driver calls the function eight times, which allows the points in the If statements to be executed. Here is a screen shot of the input and the output.

```
C:\PPSC++\Driver\Driver.exe
Enter HDL for John J. Smith: 39
Enter LDL for John J. Smith: 99
Enter HDL for John J. Smith: 59
Enter LDL for John J. Smith: 99
Enter HDL for John J. Smith: 69
Enter LDL for John J. Smith: 99
Enter HDL for John J. Smith: 39
Enter LDL for John J. Smith: 129
Enter HDL for John J. Smith: 39
Enter LDL for John J. Smith: 159
Enter HDL for John J. Smith: 39
Enter LDL for John J. Smith: 189
Enter HDL for John J. Smith: 39
Enter LDL for John J. Smith: 190
Enter HDL for John J. Smith: 39
Enter LDL for John J. Smith: 99
```

```
Profile - Notepad
File  Edit  Format  View  Help
Cholesterol Profile
   HDL is too low
   LDL is optimal
   Ratio of LDL to HDL is good
Cholesterol Profile
   HDL is okay
   LDL is optimal
   Ratio of LDL to HDL is good
Cholesterol Profile
   HDL is excellent
   LDL is optimal
   Ratio of LDL to HDL is good
Cholesterol Profile
   HDL is too low
   LDL is near optimal
   Ratio of LDL to HDL is good
Cholesterol Profile
   HDL is too low
   LDL is borderline high
   Ratio of LDL to HDL is not good
Cholesterol Profile
   HDL is too low
   LDL is high
   Ratio of LDL to HDL is not good
Cholesterol Profile
   HDL is too low
   LDL is very high
   Ratio of LDL to HDL is not good
Cholesterol Profile
   HDL is too low
   LDL is optimal
   Ratio of LDL to HDL is good
```

Stubs and drivers are important tools in team programming. The programmers develop the overall design and the interfaces between the modules. Each programmer then designs and codes one or more of the modules and uses drivers and stubs to test the code. When all of the modules have been coded and tested, they are assembled into what should be a working program.

For team programming to succeed, it is essential that all of the module interfaces be defined explicitly and that the coded modules adhere strictly to the specifications for those interfaces. Obviously, global variable references must be carefully avoided in a team-programming situation because it is impossible for each person to know how the rest of the team is using every variable.

Testing and Debugging Hints

1. Make sure that variables used as arguments to a function are declared in the block where the function call is made.

2. Carefully define the precondition, postcondition, and parameter list to eliminate side effects. Variables used only in a function should be declared as local variables. *Do not* use global variables in your programs. (Exception: It is acceptable to reference `cin` and `cout` globally.)

3. If the compiler displays a message such as "UNDECLARED IDENTIFIER," check that the identifier isn't misspelled (and that it is, in fact, declared), that the identifier is declared before it is referenced, and that the scope of the identifier includes the reference to it.

4. If you intend to use a local name that is the same as a nonlocal name, a misspelling in the local declaration will wreak havoc. The C++ compiler won't complain, but will cause every reference to the local name to go to the nonlocal name instead.

5. Remember that the same identifier cannot be used in both the parameter list and the outermost local declarations of a function.

6. With a value-returning function, be sure the function heading and prototype begin with the correct data type for the function return value.

7. With a value-returning function, don't forget to use a statement

   `return` Expression;

   to return the function value. Make sure the expression is of the correct type, or implicit type coercion will occur.

8. Remember that a call to a value-returning function is part of an expression, whereas a call to a void function is a separate statement. (C++ softens this distinction, however, by letting you call a value-returning function as if it were a void function, ignoring the return value. Be careful here.)

9. In general, don't use reference parameters in the parameter list of a value-returning function. A reference parameter must be used, however, when an I/O stream object is passed as a parameter.

10. If necessary, use your system's debugger (or use debug output statements) to indicate when a function is called and if it is executing correctly. The values of the arguments can be displayed immediately before the call to the function (to show the incoming values) and immediately after (to show the outgoing values). You also may want to display the values of local variables in the function itself to indicate what happens each time it is called.

Summary

The scope of an identifier refers to the parts of the program in which it is visible. C++ function names have global scope, as do the names of variables and constants that are declared outside all functions and namespaces. Variables and constants declared within a block have local scope; they are not visible outside the block. The parameters of a function have the same scope as local variables declared in the outermost block of the function.

With rare exceptions, it is not considered good practice to declare global variables and reference them directly from within a function. All communication between the modules of a program should be through the argument and parameter lists (and via the function value sent back by a value-returning function). The use of global constants, on the other hand, is considered to be an acceptable programming practice because it adds consistency and makes a program easier to change while avoiding the pitfalls of side effects. Well-designed and well-documented functions that are free of side effects can often be reused in other programs. Many programmers keep a library of functions that they use repeatedly.

The lifetime of a variable is the period of time during program execution when memory is allocated to it. Global variables have static lifetime (memory remains allocated for the duration of the program's execution). By default, local variables have automatic lifetime (memory is allocated and deallocated at block entry and block exit). A local variable may be given static lifetime by using the word `static` in its declaration. This variable has the lifetime of a global variable but the scope of a local variable.

C++ allows a variable to be initialized in its declaration. For a static variable, the initialization occurs once only—when control first reaches its declaration. An automatic variable is initialized each time control reaches the declaration.

C++ provides two kinds of subprograms, void functions and value-returning functions, for us to use. A value-returning function is called from within an expression and returns a single result that is used in the evaluation of the expression. For the function value to be returned, the last statement executed by the function must be a Return statement containing an expression of the appropriate data type.

All the scope rules, as well as the rules about reference and value parameters, apply to both void functions and value-returning functions. It is considered poor programming practice, however, to use reference parameters in a value-returning function definition. Doing so increases the potential for unintended side effects. (An exception is when I/O stream objects are passed as parameters. Other exceptions are noted in later chapters.)

We can use stubs and drivers to test functions in isolation from the rest of a program. They are particularly useful in the context of team-programming projects.

Quick Check

1. If a function references a variable that is not declared in its block or its parameter list, is the reference global or local? (pp. 362–368)

2. How do references to global variables contribute to the potential for unwanted side effects? (pp. 374–377)
3. If a module has three /* in */ parameters and one /* out */ parameter, should it be implemented by a void or a value-returning function? (p. 389)
4. A program has two functions, Quick1 and Quick2. The program itself declares variables check and qc. Function Quick1 declares variables called quest and qc. Function Quick2 declares one variable called quest and a static variable called forever. Which of these variables are local? (pp. 362–368)
5. In Quick Check question 4, which variables are accessible within function Quick1? (pp. 362–368)
6. In Quick Check question 4, what is the lifetime of each of the six variables? (pp. 372–374)
7. What distinguishes a value-returning function from a void function? (pp. 379–384)
8. Given the following function heading, how would you write a call to it that will pass it the value 98.6 and assign the result to the variable fever? (pp. 384–387)

```
bool TempCheck (/* in */ float temp)
```

Answers

1. Global.   2. They enable a function to affect the state of the program through a means other than the well-defined interface of the parameter list.   3. A value-returning function.   4. Variables declared within the functions are local. In Quick1, quest and qc. In Quick2, quest and for-ever.   5. check, quest, and the locally-declared qc.   6. check and qc in the program, together with forever, are static. The variables in Quick1, and the variable quest in Quick2 are auto-matic.   7. Using a type-name in place of void, and using a return statement to pass a value back to the caller.   8. fever = TempCheck(98.6);

Exam Preparation Exercises

1. A function parameter is local to the entire block that is the body of the function. True or false?
2. A reference parameter has the same scope as a global variable. True or false?
3. A global variable can be referenced anywhere within the program. True or false?
4. Function names have global scope. True or false?
5. Match the following terms with the definitions given below.
   a. Scope
   b. Name precedence
   c. Scope rules
   d. Nonlocal identifier
   e. Lifetime
   f. Automatic variable
   g. Static variable

    h. Side effect
        i. The semantics that specify where we can reference nonlocal identifiers.
        ii. A variable for which memory is allocated for the duration of the program.
        iii. When one function affects another in a manner that isn't defined by their interface.
        iv. The precedence that a local identifier has over a global identifier with the same name.
        v. The region of program code where it is legal to reference an identifier.
        vi. A variable that has memory allocated at block entry and deallocated at block exit.
        vii. An identifier declared outside of the current block.
        viii. The period in which an identifier has memory allocated to it.

6. Identify the side effect in the following function.

```cpp
int ExamPrep (int param1, int& param2)
{
    if (param2 = param1)
        return param2;
    else if (param2 > param1)
        return param1;
    else
        return param1 * param2;
}
```

7. Identify the side effect in the following program (which uses poor style for naming variables).

```cpp
#include <iostream>

using namespace std;

string a;
int w;

bool GetYesOrNo();

int main ()
{
    cout << "Enter name:";
    cin >> a;
    w = 0;
    cout << "Are there weight data?";
    if (GetYesOrNo());
    {
        cout << "Enter weight:";
```

```
        cin >> w;
    }
    cout << "Name is " << a << "  weight is " << w << endl;
}


bool GetYesOrNo()
{
    cout << "Enter yes or no: ";
    cin >> a;
    return a == "yes";
}
```

8. What is the scope of a namespace that is specified in a using directive outside of all functions?

9. What is the scope of the `std` namespace in the following code?

```
// Include directives and function prototypes here

int main()
{
    using namespace std;
    // Rest of main body is here
}
// Function definitions are here
```

10. What is the lifetime of each of the following?
    a. A global variable.
    b. A local variable in a function.
    c. A local, static variable in a function.

11. Rewrite the following declaration and initialization as a single statement.

```
float pi;
pi = 3.14159265;
```

12. If a local, static variable is initialized in its declaration within a function, when does the variable get initialized and how often?

13. If a local, non-static variable is initialized in its declaration within a function, when does the variable get initialized and how often?

14. A value-returning function can have just one `return` statement. True or false?

15. What's wrong with the following function?

```
bool Greater (int a, int b)
{
    if (a > b)
        return true;
}
```

16. What's wrong with the following function?

```
int Average (int a, int b, int c)
{
    return (a + b + c)/3.0;
}
```

17. What's wrong with the following function?

```
void Maximum (int a, int b, int& max)
{
    if (a > b)
        max = a;
    else
        max = b;
    return max;
}
```

18. Using a reference parameter in a value-returning function makes what kind of programming error more likely?

Programming Warm-Up Exercises

1. The following program is written in a very poor style that uses global variables instead of parameters and arguments, resulting in unwanted side effects. Rewrite it using good style.

```
#include <iostream>
using namespace std;
int Power ();
int pow;
int x;
int result;
int main ()
{
cout << "Enter power: ";
cin >> pow;
cout << "Enter value to be raised to power: ";
cin >> x;
cout << Power(x, pow);
}
int Power()
{
result = 1;
while (pow > 0)
{
result = result * x;
pow--;
```

```
    }
    return result;
}
```

2. Write the heading for a `bool` function `Equals` that has two `/* in */` `float` parameters, x and y.

3. Write the function prototype for the function in Exercise 2.

4. Write a body for the function in Exercise 2 that compares x and y, returning `true` if their difference is less than 0.00000001, and `false` otherwise.

5. Write the heading and function prototype for a float function called ConeVolume that takes two `/* in */` float parameters, radius and height.

6. Write the body for the function heading in Exercise 5. The body computes the volume of a cone using the following formula.

$$\frac{1}{3}\pi \times radius^2 \times height$$

7. Rewrite `void` function described in Programming Warm-Up Exercises 4 and 6 in Chapter 7 as a value-returning function. The function is called `GetLeast` and it takes an `ifstream` parameter called `infile` as an input parameter that is changed. It returns an `int` value that is the lowest value read from the file.

8. Rewrite the `void` function called `Reverse` described in Programming Warm-Up Exercises 8 and 10 in Chapter 7 as a value-returning function. It should take a `string` parameter as input. The function returns a string that is the character-by-character reverse of the string in the parameter. The parameter is called `original`.

9. Rewrite the void function, `LowerCount` described in Programming Warm-Up Exercise 12 of Chapter 7 as a value-returning function. The function reads a line from `cin`, and returns an `int` containing the number of lowercase letters in the line. In Appendix C you will find the description of function `islower`, which returns `true` if its `char` parameter is a lowercase character.

10. Write a value-returning `float` function called `SquareKm` that takes two `float` parameters, length and width, and the return value is in square kilometers. The parameters are the length and width of an area in miles. The conversion factor for kilometers from miles is 1.6.

11. Write a value-returning `bool` function called `Exhausted` that takes an `int` parameter called `filmRolls`. The function keeps track of how many rolls of film have been processed by the chemistry in a photo-processing machine. When the total number of rolls exceeds 1000, it returns `true`. Each time it is called, the value in the parameter is added to the total. When the total exceeds 1000, the variable containing the total is reset to zero before the function returns, under the assumption that the exhausted chemistry will be replaced before more rolls are processed.

12. Write a value returning `string` function called `MonthAbbrev` that takes an `int` value as a parameter. The parameter, `month`, represents the number of the month. The function returns a string containing the three-letter abbreviation for

the corresponding month number. Assume that the month number is in the range of 1 to 12.

13. Modify the function in Exercise 12 to handle month numbers that are not in the valid range by returning the string `"Inv"`.

14. Write a value-returning `float` function called `RunningAvg` that takes a `float` variable, `value`, as its input and returns the running average of all the values that have been passed to the function since the program first called it.

Programming Problems

1. You are working on a project that requires climate data for a location. The maximum daily change in barometric pressure is one aspect of climate that your company needs. You have a file (`barometric.dat`) with hourly barometer readings taken over the course of a year. Each line of the file contains the readings for a single day, separated by blanks. Each reading is expressed in inches of mercury, so it is a decimal number ranging from about 28.00 to 32.00. For each line of data, you need to determine the maximum and minimum reading, and output the difference between those readings to file `differences.dat`. Each output value should be on a separate line of the file. Once the file has been read, the program also should output the greatest and least difference for the year on `cout`. Develop the program using functional decomposition, and use proper style and documentation in your code. Your program should make appropriate use of value-returning functions in solving this problem.

2. Extend the program in Problem 1 so that it also outputs the maximum and minimum barometric reading for each day on file `differences.dat`, and then outputs the maximum and minimum reading for the year on `cout` at the end of the run.

3. You're working for a lumber company, and they would like a program that calculates the cost of lumber for an order. The company sells pine, fir, cedar, maple, and oak lumber. Lumber is priced by board feet. One board foot equals one square foot, one inch thick. The price per board foot is given in the following table:

Pine	0.89
Fir	1.09
Cedar	2.26
Maple	4.50
Oak	3.10

The lumber is sold in different dimensions (specified in inches of width and height, and feet of length) that need to be converted to board feet. For example, a 2 × 4 × 8 piece is 2 inches wide, 4 inches high, and 8 feet long, and is equivalent to 5.333 board feet. An entry from the user will be in the form of a letter and four integer numbers. The integers are: number of pieces, width, height, and length. The letter will be one of P, F, C, M, O (corresponding to the five kinds of wood) or T, meaning Total. When the letter is T, there are no integers following it on the line. The program should print out the price for each entry, and print the total after T is entered. Here is an example run:

Enter item: P 10 2 4 8
10 2×4×8 Pine, cost: $47.47
Enter item: M 1 1 12 8
1 1×12×8 Maple, cost: $36.00
Enter item: T
Total cost: $83.47

Develop the program using functional decomposition, and use proper style and documentation in your code. Your program should make appropriate use of value-returning functions in solving this problem. Be sure that the user prompts are clear, and that the output is labeled appropriately.

4. Write a program that determines the day of the week for a given date. You can invent your own complex algorithm that takes into account the special leap year rules, and changes in calendars, but this is a case where it makes sense to look for things that are familiar. Who else might need to compute values from dates over a wide span of time? Historians work with dates, but generally don't compute from them. Astronomers, however, need to know the difference in time between orbital events in the solar system that span hundreds of years. Consulting an astronomy text, you will find that there is a standard way of representing a date, called the Julian Day Number (JDN). This is the number of days that have elapsed since January 1, 4713 BC. Given the JDN for a date, there is a simple formula that tells the day of the week:

```
DayOfWeek = (JDN + 1) % 7
```

The result is in the range of 0 to 6, with 0 representing Sunday.

The only remaining problem is how to compute the JDN, which is not so simple. The algorithm computes several intermediate results that are added together to give the JDN. We look at the computation of each of these three intermediate values in turn.

If the date comes from the Gregorian calendar (later than October 15, 1582), then compute `intRes1` with the following formula, otherwise let `intRes1` be zero.

```
intRes1 = 2 - year / 100 + year / 400        (integer division)
```

The second intermediate result is computed as follows:

```
intRes2 = int(365.25 * Year)
```

We compute the third intermediate value with this formula:

```
intRes3 = int(30.6001 * (month + 1))
```

Finally, the JDN is computed this way:

```
JDN = intRes1 + intRes2 + intRes3 + day + 1720994.5
```

Your program should make appropriate use of value-returning functions in solving this problem. These formulas require nine significant digits; you may have to use the integer type `long` and the floating-point type `double`. Your program should prompt appropriately for input of the date, and properly label the output. Use proper coding style with comments to document the algorithm as needed.

5. Reusing functions from Problem 4 as appropriate, write a C++ program that computes the number of days between two dates. If your design for Problem 4 used good functional decomposition, this should be a trivial program to write. You merely need to input two dates, convert them to their JDNs, and take the difference of the JDNs.

Your program should make appropriate use of value-returning functions in solving this problem. These formulas require nine significant digits; you may have to use the integer type `long` and the floating-point type `double`. Your program should prompt appropriately for input of the date, and properly label the output. Use proper coding style with comments to document the algorithm as needed.

Case Study Follow-Up

1. Write the algorithm for the EvaluateBloodPressure module.
2. Write a driver and test function `EvaluateBloodPressure`, making sure that every branch is taken.
3. Add a Boolean function to the three Evaluate modules, which is true if the data are ok and false otherwise. Test the input within each module for negative or zero input values, which should be considered errors. If an error occurs, state in which module it occurs and set the error flag.
4. Rewrite the main program to test this flag after each call and exit the program if an error occurs.

Additional Control Structures

Knowledge Goals

- *To know how to choose the most appropriate looping statement for a given problem.*
- *To understand the purpose of the Break and Continue statements.*

Skill Goals

To be able to:

- *Write a Switch statement for a multiway branching problem.*
- *Write a Do-While statement and contrast it with a While statement.*
- *Write a For statement to implement a count-controlled loop.*

In the preceding chapters, we introduced C++ statements for sequence, selection, loop, and subprogram structures. In some cases, we introduced more than one way of implementing these structures. For example, selection may be implemented by an If-Then structure or an If-Then-Else structure. The If-Then is sufficient to implement any selection structure, but C++ provides the If-Then-Else for convenience because the two-way branch is frequently used in programming.

This chapter introduces five new statements that are also nonessential to, but nonetheless convenient for, programming. One, the Switch statement, makes it easier to write selection structures that have many branches. Two new looping statements, For and Do-While, make it easier to program certain types of loops. The other two statements, Break and Continue, are control statements that are used as part of larger looping and selection structures.

9.1 The Switch Statement

The Switch statement is a selection control structure that allows us to list any number of branches. In other words, it is a control structure for multiway branches. A Switch is similar to nested If statements. The value of the **switch expression**—an expression whose value is matched with a label attached to a branch—determines which one of the branches is executed. For example, look at the following statement:

> **Switch expression** The expression whose value determines which switch label is selected. It cannot be a floating-point or string expression.

```
switch (letter)
{
    case 'X' : Statement1;
               break;
    case 'L' :
    case 'M' : Statement2;
               break;
    case 'S' : Statement3;
               break;
    default  : Statement4;
}
Statement5;
```

In this example, `letter` is the switch expression. The statement means "If `letter` is 'X', execute Statement1 and break out of the Switch statement, continuing with Statement5. If `letter` is 'L' or 'M', execute Statement2 and continue with Statement5. If `letter` is 'S', execute Statement3 and continue with Statement5. If `letter` is none of the characters mentioned, execute Statement4 and continue with Statement5." The Break statement causes an immediate exit from the Switch statement. We'll see shortly what happens if we omit the Break statements.

The syntax template for the Switch statement is

SwitchStatement

```
switch ( IntegralOrEnumExpression )
{
    SwitchLabel ... Statement
            ⋮
}
```

IntegralOrEnumExpression is an expression of integral type—char, short, int, long, bool—or of enum type (we discuss enum in the next chapter). The optional SwitchLabel in front of a statement is either a *case label* or a *default label:*

SwitchLabel

```
{ case ConstantExpression :
  default :
```

In a case label, ConstantExpression is an integral or enum expression whose operands must be literal or named constants. The following are examples of constant integral expressions (where CLASS_SIZE is a named constant of type int):

```
3
CLASS_SIZE
'A'
2 * CLASS_SIZE + 1
```

The data type of ConstantExpression is coerced, if necessary, to match the type of the switch expression.

In our opening example that tests the value of letter, the following are the case labels:

```
case 'X' :
case 'L' :
case 'M' :
case 'S' :
```

As that example shows, a single statement may be preceded by more than one case label. Each case value may appear only once in a given Switch statement. If a value appears more than once, a syntax error results. Also, there can be only one default label in a Switch statement.

The flow of control through a Switch statement goes like this. First, the switch expression is evaluated. If this value matches one of the values in a case label, control branches to the statement following that case label. From there, control proceeds sequentially until either a Break statement or the end of the Switch statement is encountered. If the value of the switch expression doesn't match any case value, then one of two things happens. If there is a default label, control branches to the statement following that label. If there is no default label, all statements within the Switch are skipped and control simply proceeds to the statement following the entire Switch statement.

The following Switch statement prints an appropriate comment based on a student's grade (grade is of type char):

```cpp
switch (grade)
{
    case 'A' :
    case 'B' : cout << "Good Work";
               break;
    case 'C' : cout << "Average Work";
               break;
    case 'D' :
    case 'F' : cout << "Poor Work";
               numberInTrouble++;
               break;           // Unnecessary, but a good habit
}
```

Notice that the final Break statement is unnecessary. But programmers often include it anyway. One reason is that it's easier to insert another case label at the end if a Break statement is already present.

If grade does not contain one of the specified characters, none of the statements within the Switch is executed. Unless a precondition of the Switch statement is that grade is definitely one of 'A', 'B', 'C', 'D', or 'F', it would be wise to include a default label to account for an invalid grade:

```cpp
switch (grade)
{
    case 'A' :
    case 'B' : cout << "Good Work";
               break;
    case 'C' : cout << "Average Work";
               break;
    case 'D' :
    case 'F' : cout << "Poor Work";
               numberInTrouble++;
               break;
    default  : cout << grade << " is not a valid letter grade.";
               break;
}
```

A Switch statement with a Break statement after each case alternative behaves exactly like an If-Then-Else-If control structure. For example, our Switch statement is equivalent to the following code:

```
if (grade == 'A' || grade == 'B')
    cout << "Good Work";
else if (grade == 'C')
    cout << "Average Work";
else if (grade == 'D' || grade == 'F')
{
    cout << "Poor Work";
    numberInTrouble++;
}
else
    cout << grade << " is not a valid letter grade.";
```

Is either of these two versions better than the other? There is no absolute answer to this question. For this particular example, our opinion is that the Switch statement is easier to understand because of its two-dimensional, table-like form. But some may find the If-Then-Else-If version easier to read. When implementing a multiway branching structure, our advice is to write down both a Switch and an If-Then-Else-If and then compare them for readability. Keep in mind that C++ provides the Switch statement as a matter of convenience. Don't feel obligated to use a Switch statement for every multiway branch.

Finally, we said we would look at what happens if you omit the Break statements inside a Switch statement. Let's rewrite our letter grade example without the Break statements:

```
switch (grade)     // Wrong version
{
    case 'A' :
    case 'B' : cout << "Good Work";
    case 'C' : cout << "Average Work";
    case 'D' :
    case 'F' : cout << "Poor Work";
              numberInTrouble++;
    default  : cout << grade << " is not a valid letter grade.";
}
```

If `grade` happens to be 'H', control branches to the statement at the default label and the output is

```
H is not a valid letter grade.
```

Unfortunately, this case alternative is the only one that works correctly. If `grade` is 'A', the resulting output is this:

```
Good WorkAverage WorkPoor WorkA is not a valid letter grade.
```

Remember that after a branch is taken to a specific case label, control proceeds sequentially until either a Break statement or the end of the Switch statement is encountered. Forgetting a Break statement in a case alternative is a very common source of errors in C++ programs.

May We Introduce

Admiral Grace Murray Hopper

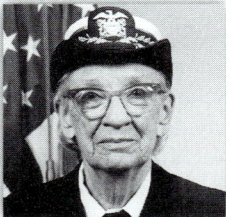

From 1943 until her death on New Year's Day in 1992, Admiral Grace Murray Hopper was intimately involved with computing. In 1991, she was awarded the National Medal of Technology "for her pioneering accomplishments in the development of computer programming languages that simplified computer technology and opened the door to a significantly larger universe of users."

Admiral Hopper was born Grace Brewster Murray in New York City on December 9, 1906. She attended Vassar and received a Ph.D. in mathematics from Yale. For the next ten years, she taught mathematics at Vassar.

In 1943, Admiral Hopper joined the U.S. Navy and was assigned to the Bureau of Ordnance Computation Project at Harvard University as a programmer on the Mark I. After the war, she remained at Harvard as a faculty member and continued work on the Navy's Mark II and Mark III computers. In 1949, she joined Eckert-Mauchly Computer Corporation and worked on the UNIVAC I. It was there that she made a legendary contribution to computing: She discovered the first computer "bug"—a moth caught in the hardware.

Admiral Hopper had a working compiler in 1952, at a time when the conventional wisdom was that computers could do only arithmetic. Although not on the committee that designed the computer language COBOL, she was active in its design, implementation, and use. COBOL (which stands for Common Business-Oriented Language) was developed in the early 1960s and still is widely used in business data processing.

Admiral Hopper retired from the Navy in 1966, only to be recalled within a year to full-time active duty. Her mission was to oversee the Navy's efforts to maintain uniformity in programming languages. It has been said that just as Admiral Hyman Rickover was the father of the nuclear navy, Rear Admiral Hopper was the mother of computerized data automation in the Navy. She served with the Naval Data Automation Command until she retired again in 1986 with the rank of rear admiral. At the time of her death, she was a senior consultant at Digital Equipment Corporation.

During her lifetime, Admiral Hopper received honorary degrees from more than 40 colleges and universities. She was honored by her peers on several occasions, including the first Computer Sciences Man of the Year award given by the Data Processing Management Association, and the Contributions to Computer Science Education Award given by the Special Interest Group for Computer Science Education of the ACM (Association for Computing Machinery).

(continued) ▼

Admiral Grace Murray Hopper

Admiral Hopper loved young people and enjoyed giving talks on college and university campuses. She often handed out colored wires, which she called nanoseconds because they were cut to a length of about one foot—the distance that light travels in a nanosecond (billionth of a second). Her advice to the young was, "You manage things, you lead people. We went overboard on management and forgot about leadership."

When asked which of her many accomplishments she was most proud of, she answered, "All the young people I have trained over the years."

9.2 The Do-While Statement

The Do-While statement is a looping control structure in which the loop condition is tested at the end (bottom) of the loop. This format guarantees that the loop body executes at least once. The syntax template for the Do-While is this:

DoWhileStatement

```
do
      Statement
while ( Expression );
```

As usual in C++, Statement is either a single statement or a block. Also, note that the Do-While ends with a semicolon.

The statement

```
do
{
      Statement1;
      Statement2;
      ⋮
      StatementN;
} while (Expression);
```

means "Execute the statements between `do` and `while` as long as Expression still has the value `true` at the end of the loop."

Let's compare a While loop and a Do-While loop that do the same task: They find the first period in a file of data. Assume that there is at least one period in the file.

While Solution

```
dataFile >> inputChar;
while (inputChar != '.')
    dataFile >> inputChar;
```

Do-While Solution

```
do
    dataFile >> inputChar;
while (inputChar != '.');
```

The While solution requires a priming read so that `inputChar` has a value before the loop is entered. This isn't required for the Do-While solution because the input statement within the loop is executed before the loop condition is evaluated.

Let's look at another example. Suppose a program needs to read a person's age interactively. The program requires that the age be positive. The following loops ensure that the input value is positive before the program proceeds any further.

While Solution

```
cout << "Enter your age: ";
cin >> age;
while (age <= 0)
{
    cout << "Your age must be positive." << endl;
    cout << "Enter your age: ";
    cin >> age;
}
```

Do-While Solution

```
do
{
    cout << "Enter your age: ";
    cin >> age;
    if (age <= 0)
        cout << "Your age must be positive." << endl;
} while (age <= 0);
```

Notice that the Do-While solution does not require the prompt and input steps to appear twice—once before the loop and once within it—but it does test the input value twice.

We can also use the Do-While to implement a count-controlled loop *if* we know in advance that the loop body should always execute at least once. Below are two versions of a loop to sum the integers from 1 through n.

While Solution

```
sum = 0;
counter = 1;
```

```
while (counter <= n)
{
    sum = sum + counter;
    counter++;
}
```

Do-While Solution

```
sum = 0;
counter = 1;
do
{
    sum = sum + counter;
    counter++;
} while (counter <= n);
```

If n is a positive number, both of these versions are equivalent. But if n is 0 or negative, the two loops give different results. In the While version, the final value of sum is 0 because the loop body is never entered. In the Do-While version, the final value of sum is 1 because the body executes once and *then* the loop test is made.

Because the While statement tests the condition before executing the body of the loop, it is called a *pretest loop*. The Do-While statement does the opposite and thus is known as a *posttest loop*. Figure 9–1 compares the flow of control in the While and Do-While loops.

After we look at two other new looping constructs, we offer some guidelines for determining when to use each type of loop.

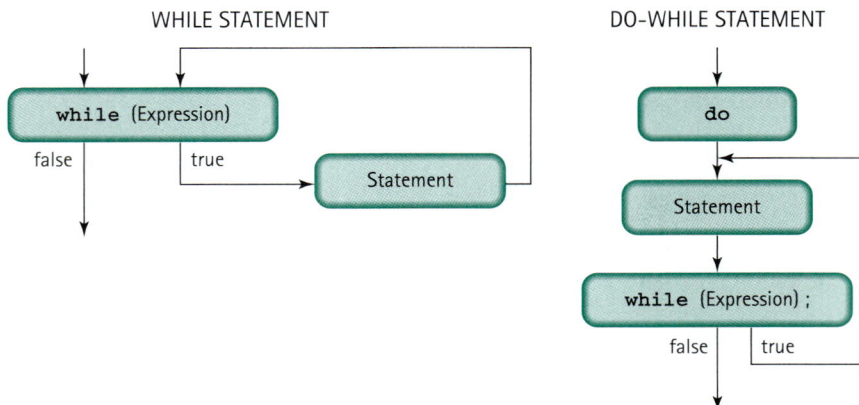

Figure 9–1   *Flow of Control: While and Do-While*

9.3 The For Statement

The For statement is designed to simplify the writing of count-controlled loops. The following statement prints out the integers from 1 through n:

```
for (count = 1; count <= n; count++)
    cout << count << endl;
```

This For statement means "Initialize the loop control variable `count` to 1. While `count` is less than or equal to n, execute the output statement and increment `count` by 1. Stop the loop after `count` has been incremented to n + 1."

In C++, a For statement is merely a compact notation for a While loop. In fact, the compiler essentially translates a For statement into an equivalent While loop as follows:

The syntax template for a For statement is

ForStatement

```
for (InitStatement Expression1 ; Expression2 )
    Statement
```

Expression1 is the While condition. InitStatement can be one of the following: the null statement (just a semicolon), a declaration statement (which always ends in a semicolon), or an expression statement (an expression ending in a semicolon). Therefore, there is always a semicolon before Expression1. (This semicolon isn't shown in the syntax template because InitStatement always ends with its own semicolon.)

Most often, a For statement is written such that InitStatement initializes a loop control variable and Expression2 increments or decrements the loop control variable. Here are two loops that execute the same number of times (50):

```
for (loopCount = 1; loopCount <= 50; loopCount++)
    :
```

```
for (loopCount = 50; loopCount >= 1; loopCount--)
    :
```

Just like While loops, Do-While and For loops may be nested. For example, the nested For structure

```
for (lastNum = 1; lastNum <= 7; lastNum++)
{
    for (numToPrint = 1; numToPrint <= lastNum; numToPrint++)
        cout << numToPrint;
    cout << endl;
}
```

prints the following triangle of numbers.

```
1
12
123
1234
12345
123456
1234567
```

Although For statements are used primarily for count-controlled loops, C++ allows you to write *any* While loop by using a For statement. To use For loops intelligently, you should know the following facts.

1. In the syntax template, InitStatement can be the null statement, and Expression2 is optional. If Expression2 is omitted, there is no statement for the compiler to insert at the bottom of the loop. As a result, you could write the While loop

```
while (inputVal != 999)
    cin >> inputVal;
```

as the equivalent For loop

```
for ( ; inputVal != 999; )
    cin >> inputVal;
```

2. According to the syntax template, Expression1—the While condition—is optional. If you omit it, the expression true is assumed. The loop

```
for ( ; ; )
    cout "Hi" << endl;
```

is equivalent to the While loop

```
while (true)
    cout << "Hi" << endl;
```

Both of these are infinite loops that print "Hi" endlessly.

3. The initializing statement, InitStatement, can be a declaration with initialization:

```
for (int i = 1; i <= 20; i++)
    cout << "Hi" << endl;
```

Here, the variable i has local scope, even though there are no braces creating a block. The scope of i extends only to the end of the For statement. Like any local variable, i is inaccessible outside its scope (that is, outside the For statement). Because i is local to the For statement, it's possible to write code like this:

```
for (int i = 1; i <= 20; i++)
    cout << "Hi" << endl;
for (int i = 1; i <= 100; i++)
    cout << "Ed" << endl;
```

This code does *not* generate a compile-time error (such as "MULTIPLY DEFINED IDENTIFIER"). We have declared two distinct variables named i, each of which is local to its own For statement.*

As you have seen by now, the For statement in C++ is a very flexible structure. Its use can range from a simple count-controlled loop to a general-purpose, "anything goes" While loop. Some programmers squeeze a lot of work into the heading (the first line) of a For statement. For example, the program fragment

```
cin >> ch;
while (ch != '.')
    cin >> ch;
```

can be compressed into the following For loop:

```
for (cin >> ch; ch != '.'; cin >> ch)
    ;
```

Because all the work is done in the For heading, there is nothing for the loop body to do. The body is simply the null statement.

With For statements, our advice is to keep things simple. The trickier the code is, the harder it will be for another person (or you!) to understand your code and track down errors. In this book, we use For loops for count-controlled loops only.

---

*In versions of C++ prior to the ISO/ANSI language standard, i would not be local to the body of the loop. Its scope would extend to the end of the block surrounding the For statement. In other words, it would be as if i had been declared outside the loop. If you are using an older version of C++ and your compiler tells you something like "MULTIPLY DEFINED IDENTIFIER" in code similar to the pair of For statements above, simply choose a different variable name in the second For loop.

Here is a program that contains both a For statement and a Switch statement. It analyzes the first 100 characters read from the standard input device and reports how many of the characters were letters, periods, question marks, and exclamation marks. For the first category (letters), we use the library function isalpha, one of the "is..." functions we described in Chapter 8. To conserve space, we have omitted the interface documentation for the functions.

```cpp
//*****************************************************************
// CharCounts program
// This program counts the number of letters, periods, question
// marks, and exclamation marks found in the first 100 input
// characters
// Assumption: Input consists of at least 100 characters
//*****************************************************************
#include <iostream>
#include <cctype>          // For isalpha()

using namespace std;

void IncrementCounter( char, int&, int&, int&, int& );
void PrintCounters( int, int, int, int );

int main()
{
    char inChar;              // Current input character
    int  loopCount;           // Loop control variable
    int  letterCount = 0;     // Number of letters
    int  periodCount = 0;     // Number of periods
    int  questCount = 0;      // Number of question marks
    int  exclamCount = 0;     // Number of exclamation marks

    cout << "Enter your text:" << endl;
    for (loopCount = 1; loopCount <= 100; loopCount++)
    {
        cin.get(inChar);
        IncrementCounter(inChar, letterCount, periodCount,
                         questCount, exclamCount);
    }
    PrintCounters(letterCount, periodCount, questCount,
                  exclamCount);
    return 0;
}
```

```
//***************************************************************

void IncrementCounter( /* in */     char ch,
                       /* inout */ int& letterCount,
                       /* inout */ int& periodCount,
                       /* inout */ int& questCount,
                       /* inout */ int& exclamCount )
{
    if (isalpha(ch))
        letterCount++;
    else
        switch (ch)
        {
            case '.' : periodCount++;
                       break;
            case '?' : questCount++;
                       break;
            case '!' : exclamCount++;
                       break;
            default  : ;                // Unnecessary, but OK
        }
}


//***************************************************************

void PrintCounters( /* in */ int letterCount,
                    /* in */ int periodCount,
                    /* in */ int questCount,
                    /* in */ int exclamCount )
{
    cout << endl;
    cout << "Input contained" << endl
         << letterCount << " letters" << endl
         << periodCount << " periods" << endl
         << questCount << " question marks" << endl
         << exclamCount << " exclamation marks" << endl;
}
```

9.4 The Break and Continue Statements

The Break statement, which we introduced with the Switch statement, is also used with loops. A Break statement causes an immediate exit from the innermost Switch, While, Do-While, or For statement in which it appears. Notice the word *innermost*. If break is in a loop that is nested inside another loop, control exits the inner loop but not the outer.

One of the more common ways of using `break` with loops is to set up an infinite loop and use If tests to exit the loop. Suppose we want to input ten pairs of integers, performing data validation and computing the square root of the sum of each pair. For data validation, assume that the first number of each pair must be less than 100 and the second must be greater than 50. Also, after each input, we want to test the state of the stream for EOF. Here's a loop using Break statements to accomplish the task:

```
loopCount = 1;
while (true)
{
    cin >> num1;
    if ( !cin || num1 >= 100)
        break;
    cin >> num2;
    if ( !cin || num2 <= 50)
        break;
    cout << sqrt(float(num1 + num2)) << endl;
    loopCount++;
    if (loopCount > 10)
        break;
}
```

Note that we could have used a For loop to count from 1 to 10, breaking out of it as necessary. However, this loop is both count-controlled and event-controlled, so we prefer to use a While loop.

The above loop contains three distinct exit points. Some people vigorously oppose this style of programming, as it violates the single-entry, single-exit philosophy we discussed with regard to multiple returns from a function. Is there any advantage to using an infinite loop in conjunction with `break`? To answer this question, let's rewrite the loop without using Break statements. The loop must terminate when `num1` is invalid or `num2` is invalid or `loopCount` exceeds 10. We'll use Boolean flags to signal invalid data in the While condition:

```
num1Valid = true;
num2Valid = true;
loopCount = 1;
while (num1Valid && num2Valid && loopCount <= 10)
{
    cin >> num1;
    if ( !cin || num1 >= 100)
        num1Valid = false;
    else
```

```
    {
        cin >> num2;
        if ( !cin || num2 <= 50)
            num2Valid = false;
        else
        {
            cout << sqrt(float(num1 + num2)) << endl;
            loopCount++;
        }
    }
}
```

One could argue that the first version is easier to follow and understand than this second version. The primary task of the loop body—computing the square root of the sum of the numbers—is more prominent in the first version. In the second version, the computation is obscured by being buried within nested Ifs. The second version also has a more complicated control flow.

The disadvantage of using break with loops is that it can become a crutch for those who are too impatient to think carefully about loop design. It's easy to overuse (and abuse) the technique. Here's an example, printing the integers 1 through 5:

```
i = 1;
while (true)
{
    cout << i;
    if (i == 5)
        break;
    i++;
}
```

There is no real justification for setting up the loop this way. Conceptually, it is a pure count-controlled loop, and a simple For loop does the job:

```
for (i = 1; i <= 5; i++)
    cout << i;
```

The For loop is easier to understand and is less prone to error.

A good rule of thumb is: Use break within loops only as a last resort. Specifically, use it only to avoid baffling combinations of multiple Boolean flags and nested Ifs.

Another statement that alters the flow of control in a C++ program is the Continue statement. This statement, valid only in loops, terminates the current loop iteration (but not the entire loop). It causes an immediate branch to the bottom of the loop—skipping the rest of the statements in the loop body—in preparation for the next iteration. Here is an example of a reading loop in which we want to process only the positive numbers in an input file:

```
for (dataCount = 1; dataCount <= 500; dataCount++)
{
    dataFile >> inputVal;
    if (inputVal <= 0)
        continue;
    cout << inputVal;
      ⋮
}
```

If `inputVal` is less than or equal to 0, control branches to the bottom of the loop. Then, as with any For loop, the computer increments `dataCount` and performs the loop test before going on to the next iteration.

The Continue statement is not used often, but we present it for completeness (and because you may run across it in other people's programs). Its primary purpose is to avoid obscuring the main process of the loop by indenting the process within an If statement. For example, the above code would be written without a Continue statement as follows:

```
for (dataCount = 1; dataCount <= 500; dataCount++)
{
    dataFile >> inputVal;
    if (inputVal > 0)
    {
        cout << inputVal;
          ⋮
    }
}
```

Be sure to note the difference between `continue` and `break`. The Continue statement means "Abandon the current iteration of the loop, and go on to the next iteration." The Break statement means "Exit the entire loop immediately."

9.5 Guidelines for Choosing a Looping Statement

Here are some guidelines to help you decide when to use each of the three looping statements (While, Do-While, and For).

1. If the loop is a simple count-controlled loop, the For statement is a natural. Concentrating the three loop control actions—initialize, test, and increment/decrement—into one location (the heading of the For statement) reduces the chances of forgetting to include one of them.

2. If the loop is an event-controlled loop whose body should execute at least once, a Do-While statement is appropriate.

3. If the loop is an event-controlled loop and nothing is known about the first execution, use a While (or perhaps a For) statement.

4. When in doubt, use a While statement.

5. An infinite loop with Break statements sometimes clarifies the code but more often reflects an undisciplined loop design. Use it only after careful consideration of While, Do-While, and For.

Problem–Solving Case Study

The Rich Uncle

PROBLEM   Your rich uncle has just died, and in his desk you find two wills. One of them, dated several months ago, leaves you and your relatives a substantial part of his fortune; the other, dated last week, gives it all to his next-door neighbor. Being suspicious that the second will is a forgery, you decide to write a program to analyze writing style and thus compare the wills. The program reads and categorizes each character. When the entire file has been read, it prints a summary table showing the percentage of uppercase letters, lowercase letters, decimal digits, blanks, and end-of-sentence punctuation marks in the data file. The names of the input and output files are read from the keyboard. The name of the input file should be printed on the output.

INPUT   Text on a file whose name is read from the keyboard.

OUTPUT   A table giving the name of each category and what percentage of the total the category represents on the file whose name is read from the keyboard.

DISCUSSION   Doing this task by hand would be tedious but quite straightforward. You would set up five places to make hash marks, one for each of the categories of symbols to be counted. You would then read the text character by character, determine in which category to put each character, and make a hash mark in the appropriate place.

You can look at a character and tell immediately which category to mark. You can simulate "looking" with an If statement with branches for the uppercase letters, the lowercase letters, the digits, a blank, and end-of-sentence punctuation marks. An uppercase letter is defined as one between 'A' and 'Z' inclusive; a lowercase letter is defined as one between 'a' and 'z' inclusive. *But wait:* Before you start writing algorithms to recognize these categories, shouldn't you look in the library to see if they already exist? Sure enough, header file `<cctype>` contains functions to recognize uppercase letters, lowercase letters, and digits.

There is a function that recognizes white space. Will that do for counting blanks? Function `isspace` returns true if the character is a blank, newline, tab, carriage return, or form feed. The problem specifies a count of the number of blanks. A newline might function as the end of a word like a blank, but the problem doesn't ask for the number of words; it asks for the number of blanks.

There is a function to recognize punctuation, but not end-of-sentence punctuation. The problem doesn't state what end-of-sentence marks are. What kinds of sentences are there? Regular sentences, ending in a period; questions, ending in a question mark; and exclamations, ending in an exclamation mark.

ASSUMPTIONS   File is not empty.

Main	Level 0

```
Open files for processing
If files not opened ok
     Write error message
     return 1
Get a character
DO
     Increment character counter(character)
     Get a character
WHILE (more data)
Print table
Close files
```

Open Files(Inout: text, table)	Level 1

```
Prompt for input file name
Read file name
Open input file
Prompt for output file name
Read file name
Open output file
Print input file name on output file
```

Increment Counters(Inout: upperCaseCounter, lowerCaseCounter, blankCounter, digitCounter, punctuationCounter; In: character)

```
IF (isupper(character))
     Increment uppercaseCounter
ELSE IF (islower(character))
     Increment lowercaseCounter
ELSE IF (character == ' ')
     Increment blankCounter
ELSE IF (isdigit(character))
     Increment digitCounter
ELSE IF ((character == '.') || (character == '?') || (character == '!'))
     Increment punctuationCounter
```

At this point you realize that the instructions do not indicate whether the percentages are to be taken of the total number of characters read, including those that do not fit any of the categories, or of the total number of characters that fall into the five categories. You decide to assume that all characters should be counted. Thus, you add an ELSE branch to this module that increments a counter (called allElseCounter) for all characters that do not fall into one of the five categories. This assumption needs to be added to the program.

Calculate and Print Percentages (Inout: tables, upperCaseCounter, lowerCaseCounter, blankCounter, digitCounter, punctuationCounter, allElseCounter)

Set Total to sum of 6 counters
Print 'Percentage of uppercase letters:',
uppercaseCounter / Total * 100
Print 'Percentage of lowercase letters:',
lowercaseCounter / Total * 100
Print 'Percentage of decimal digits:',
digitCounter / Total * 100
Print 'Percentage of blanks:',
blankCounter / Total * 100
Print 'Percentage of end-of-sentence punctuation:',
punctuationCounter / Total * 100

MODULE STRUCTURE CHART

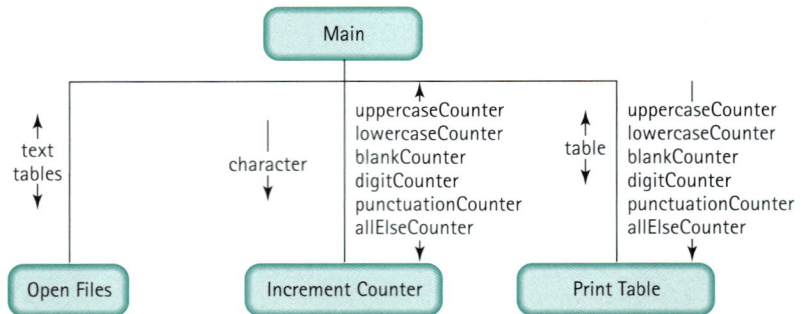

```
// *******************************************************************
// Rich Uncle Program
// A table is printed to show the percentage of characters in the
// file that belong to five categories: uppercase characters,
// lowercase characters, decimal digits, blanks, and
// end-of-sentence punctuation marks
// Assumptions: Input file is not empty and percentages are based
// on total number of characters in the file
```

```
// To save space, we omit from each function the precondition
// comments that document the assumptions made about valid input
// parameter data. These would be included in a program intended
// for actual use
//*******************************************************************

#include <fstream>
#include <iostream>
#include <iomanip>
#include <cctype>

using namespace std;

// Function prototypes
void OpenFiles(ifstream&, ofstream&);
void IncrementCounter(char, int&, int&, int&, int&, int&, int&);
void PrintTable(ofstream& table, int, int, int, int, int, int);

int main()
{
    // Prepare files for reading and writing
    ifstream text;
    ofstream table;
    char character;

    // Declare and initialize counters
    int uppercaseCounter = 0;       // Number of uppercase letters
    int lowercaseCounter = 0;       // Number of lowercase letters
    int blankCounter = 0;           // Number of blanks
    int digitCounter = 0;           // Number of digits
    int punctuationCounter = 0;     // Number of end '.', '?', '!'
    int allElseCounter = 0;         // Remaining characters

    OpenFiles(text, table);
    if ( !text || !table)
    {
        cout << "Files did not open successfully." << endl;
        return 1;
    }
    text.get(character);            // Input one character
    do
    { // Process each character
            IncrementCounter(character, uppercaseCounter,
            lowercaseCounter, blankCounter, digitCounter,
            punctuationCounter, allElseCounter);
        text.get(character);
    } while (text);
```

```
            PrintTable(table, uppercaseCounter, lowercaseCounter,
                blankCounter, digitCounter, punctuationCounter,
                allElseCounter);

            text.close();
            table.close();
            return 0;
    }


//**********************************************************************


void IncrementCounter(
        /* in */      char character),          // Character being examined
        /* inout */   int& uppercaseCounter,    // Uppercase letters
        /* inout */   int& lowercaseCounter,    // Lowercase letters
        /* inout */   int& blankCounter,        // Blanks
        /* inout */   int& digitCounter,        // Digits
        /* inout */   int& punctuationCounter,  // '.', '?', '!'
        /* inout */   int& allElseCounter )     // Everything else

// Function IncrementCounter examines character and increments the
// appropriate counter
// Postondition:
//      The category to which the character belongs has been
//      incremented

{
        if (isupper(character))
            uppercaseCounter++;
        else if (islower(character))
            lowercaseCounter++;
        else if (character == ' ')
            blankCounter++;
        else if (isdigit(character))
            digitCounter++;
        else if ((character == '.') || (character == '?') ||
                (character == '!'))
            punctuationCounter++;
        else
            allElseCounter++;
}
```

```
//*********************************************************************

void PrintTable(
    /* inout */ ofstream& table,         // Output file
    /* in */ int uppercaseCounter,       // Uppercase letters
    /* in */ int lowercaseCounter,       // Lowercase letters
    /* in */ int blankCounter,           // Blanks
    /* in */ int digitCounter,           // Digits
    /* in */ int punctuationCounter,     // '.', '?', '!'
    /* in */ int allElseCounter )        // Everything else

// Function PrintTable prints the percentages represented by each
// of the five categories
// Postcondition:
//     The output has been written on file table, appropriately
//     labeled

{
    // Calculate total number of characters
    float total = uppercaseCounter + lowercaseCounter
        + blankCounter + digitCounter + punctuationCounter
        + allElseCounter;

    // Write output on stream table
    table << fixed << setprecision(3)
        << "Percentage of uppercase characters: "
        << uppercaseCounter / total * 100 << endl;
    table << fixed << setprecision(3)
        << "Percentage of lowercase characters: "
        << lowercaseCounter / total * 100 << endl;
    table << fixed << setprecision(3) << "Percentage of blanks: "
        << blankCounter / total * 100 << endl;
    table << fixed << setprecision(3) << "Percentage of digits: "
        << digitCounter / total * 100 << endl;
    table << fixed << setprecision(3)
        << "Percentage of end-of-sentence "
        << "punctuation " << punctuationCounter / total * 100
        << endl;
}


//*********************************************************************

void OpenFiles( /* inout */ ifstream& text,   // Input file
                /* inout */ ofstream& table ) // Output file
```

```
// Function OpenFiles reads in the names of the input file and the
// output file and opens them for processing.
// Postcondition:
//     Files have been opened AND the input file name has been
//     written on the output file
{
    string inFileName;      // User specified input file name
    string outFileName;     // User specified output file name
    cout << "Enter the name of the file to be processed" << endl;

    cin >> inFileName;
    text.open(inFileName.c_str());

    cout << "Enter the name of the output file" << endl;
    cin >> outFileName;
    table.open(outFileName.c_str());

    // Write label on output file
    table << "Analysis of characters on input file " << inFileName
          << endl;
}
```

TESTING To be tested thoroughly, the Rich Uncle program must be run with all possible combinations of the categories of characters being counted. Listed below is the minimum set of cases that must be tested.

1. All the categories of characters are present.

2. Four of the categories are present; one is not. (This alone will require five test runs.)

3. Only characters that fall into one of the five categories are present.

4. Other characters are present.

The output listed below was run on a file of over 4,000 characters. (No, it isn't a will, but it is sufficient for testing.)

```
CharacterCount.out - Notepad
File  Edit  Format  View  Help
Analysis of characters on input file history.in
Percentage of uppercase characters: 2.978
Percentage of lowercase characters: 75.609
Percentage of blanks: 16.805
Percentage of digits: 0.331
Percentage of end-of-sentence punctuation 1.040
```

Testing and Debugging

The same testing techniques we used with While loops apply to Do-While and For loops. There are, however, a few additional considerations with these loops.

The body of a Do-While loop always executes at least once. Thus, you should try data sets that show the result of executing a Do-While loop the minimal number of times.

With a data-dependent For loop, it is important to test for proper results when the loop executes zero times. This occurs when the starting value is greater than the ending value (or less than the ending value if the loop control variable is being decremented).

When a program contains a Switch statement, you should test it with enough different data sets to ensure that each branch is selected and executed correctly. You should also test the program with a switch expression whose value is not in any of the case labels.

Testing and Debugging Hints

1. In a Switch statement, make sure there is a Break statement at the end of each case alternative. Otherwise, control "falls through" to the code in the next case alternative.

2. Case labels in a Switch statement are made up of values, not variables. They may, however, include named constants and expressions involving only constants.

3. A switch expression cannot be a floating-point or string expression, and case constants cannot be floating-point or string constants.

4. If there is a possibility that the value of the switch expression might not match one of the case constants, you should provide a `default` alternative. In fact, it is a good practice to always include a `default` alternative.

5. Double-check long Switch statements to make sure that you haven't omitted any branches.

6. The Do-While loop is a posttest loop. If there is a possibility that the loop body should be skipped entirely, use a While statement or a For statement.

7. The For statement heading (the first line) always has three pieces within the parentheses. Most often, the first piece initializes a loop control variable, the second piece tests the variable, and the third piece increments or decrements the variable. The three pieces must be separated by semicolons. Any of the pieces can be omitted, but the semicolons still must be present.

8. With nested control structures, the Break statement can exit only one level of nesting—the innermost Switch or loop in which the `break` is located.

Summary

The Switch statement is a multiway selection statement. It allows the program to choose among a set of branches. A Switch containing Break statements can always be simulated by an If-Then-Else-If structure. If a Switch can be used, however, it often makes the code easier to read and understand. A Switch statement cannot be used with floating-point or string values in the case labels.

The Do-While is a general-purpose looping statement. It is like the While loop except that its test occurs at the end of the loop, guaranteeing at least one execution of the loop body. As with a While loop, a Do-While continues as long as the loop condition is `true`. A Do-While is convenient for loops that test input values and repeat if the input is not correct.

The For statement is also a general-purpose looping statement, but its most common use is to implement count-controlled loops. The initialization, testing, and incrementation (or decrementation) of the loop control variable are centralized in one location, the first line of the For statement.

The For, Do-While, and Switch statements are the ice cream and cake of C++. We can live without them if we absolutely must, but they are very nice to have.

Quick Check

1. If a problem calls for a pure count-controlled loop, would you use a While, a Do-While, or a For statement to implement the loop? (pp. 433–434)
2. When it is executed within a loop, to where does a Break statement transfer control? Where does control proceed from a Continue statement? (pp. 430–433)
3. In converting an If-Else-If multiway branching structure to a Switch statement, what part of the Switch is used to implement the final Else branch of the If-Else-If? (pp. 418–422)
4. Which looping statement always executes its body at least once? (pp. 423–425)
5. Write a For statement that counts from –10 to 10. (pp. 426–430)

Answers

1. A For statement. 2. The Break statement immediately exits the loop. The Continue statement sends control to the end of the loop. 3. The `default` branch. 4. Do-While. 5. `for (int count = -10; count <= 10; count++)`

Exam Preparation Exercises

1. A switch expression may be of type `bool`, `char`, `int`, or `long`, but not of type `float`. True or false?
2. A variable declared in the initialization statement of a For loop has global scope. True of false?
3. Any While loop can be directly rewritten as a Do-While merely by changing the statement syntax and moving the exit condition to the end of the loop. True or false?

4. A Break statement is not allowed in a For loop, but a Continue statement is. True or false?

5. Which of the looping statements in C++ are pretest loops and which are posttest loops?

6. What happens when you forget to include the Break statements in a Switch statement?

7. If you omit all of the clauses within a For loop (`for ( ; ; )`), what would be the condition in an equivalent While loop?

8. How many times is the inner loop body executed in the following nested loop?

```
for (int x = 1; x <= 10; x++)
   for (int y = 1; y <= 10; y++)
      for (int z = 1; z <= 10; z++)
         cout << x + y + z;
```

9. Which looping statement would you choose for a problem in which the decision to repeat a process depends on an event, and the event cannot occur until the process is executed at least once?

10. Which looping statement would you choose for a problem in which the decision to repeat the process depends on an iteration counter and on the state of an input file, and the process may be skipped if the file is empty?

11. What is output by the following code segment if `wood` contains `'O'`?

```
switch (wood)
{
   case 'P' : cout << "Pine";
   case 'F' : cout << "Fir";
   case 'C' : cout << "Cedar";
   case 'O' : cout << "Oak";
   case 'M' : cout << "Maple";
   default  : cout << "Error";
}
```

12. What is output by the following code segment if `month` contains 8?

```
switch (month)
{
   case 1 : cout << "January"; break;
   case 2 : cout << "February"; break;
   case 3 : cout << "March"; break;
   case 4 : cout << "April"; break;
   case 5 : cout << "May"; break;
   case 6 : cout << "June"; break;
   case 7 : cout << "July"; break;
   case 8 : cout << "August"; break;
   case 9 : cout << "September"; break;
```

```
case 10 : cout << "October"; break;
case 11 : cout << "November"; break;
case 12 : cout << "December"; break;
default : cout << "Error";
}
```

13. What is output by the following code segment?

```
outCount = -1;
do
{
  inCount = 3;
  do
  {
    cout << outCount + inCount << endl;
    inCount --
  } while (inCount > 0);
  outCount++;
} while (outCount < 2);
```

14. What is output by the following code segment?

```
for (int outCount = -1; outCount < 2; outCount++)
  for (int inCount = 3; inCount > 0; inCount--)
    cout << outCount + inCount << endl;
```

15. Rewrite the code segment in Exercise 14 using While loops.

16. What is printed by the following code segment?

```
for (int count = 1; count <= 4; count++)
  switch (count)
  {
    case 4 : cout << " cow?"; break;
    case 2 : cout << " now"; break;
    case 1 : cout << "How"; break;
    case 3 : cout << " brown"; break;
  }
```

17. Write a single simple statement that has the same effect on cout as the code segment in Exercise 16.

18. What does the following code segment (which is written in poor style) output?

```
count = 1;
for ( ; ; count++)
  if (count < 3)
    cout << count;
  else
    break;
```

Programming Warm-Up Exercises

1. Write a Switch statement that outputs the day of the week to cout according to the int value in day that ranges from 0 to 6, with 0 being Sunday.

2. Extend the Switch statement in Exercise 1 so that it outputs "Error" if the value in day is not in the range of 0 through 6.

3. Rewrite the Switch statement in Exercise 2 so that it is within a value-returning function that returns the string with the day of the week, given day as its parameter.

4. Write a For loop that uses the function written in Exercise 3 to output the days of the week, each on a separate line, starting from Saturday and working backward to Sunday.

5. Change the For loop in Exercise 4 so that it outputs the days of the week in forward order, starting on Wednesday and going through Tuesday.

6. Write a Do-While loop that prompts for and inputs a user entry of "Y" or "N". If the user fails to enter a correct value, the loop outputs an error message and then repeats the request for them to enter the value.

7. Write a value-returning function that takes an integer parameter and returns an integer result. The function adds up the positive integers, starting at one, until the sum equals or exceeds the value in the parameter, and it then returns the last integer added to the sum. Use a Do-While loop to do the summing.

8. Write a nested For loop that prints out a multiplication table for the integers 1 through 10.

9. Write a nested For loop that prints a filled right triangle of stars, one star on the first line, two on the next, and so on, up to the tenth line having ten stars.

10. Rewrite the nested loop in Exercise 9 with Do-While loops.

11. Rewrite the nested loop in Exercise 9 with While loops.

12. Write a void function, using For loops, that prints a hollow rectangle of stars whose width and height are specified by two int parameters. The top and bottom of the rectangle is a solid row of stars, each row between the top and bottom consists of a star, then *width–2* spaces, and another star.

13. Write a nested For loop that outputs the hours and minutes in the period from 3:15 to 7:30.

14. Extend the loop in Exercise 13 to also output seconds.

15. How many lines do the loops in Exercises 13 and 14 output?

Programming Problems

1. Programming Problem 6 in Chapter 7 asked you to write a program that inputs a string and outputs the corresponding words in the International Civil Aviation Organization that would be used to spell it out phonetically. For example:

```
Enter string: program
Phonetic version is: Papa Romeo Oscar Golf Romeo Alpha Mike
```

Rewrite the function in this program that returns the word corresponding to a specified letter, using a Switch statement instead of an If structure. For ease of reference, the ICAO alphabet from Chapter 7 is repeated here:

A   Alpha
B   Bravo
C   Charlie
D   Delta
E   Echo
F   Foxtrot
G   Golf
H   Hotel
I   India
J   Juliet
K   Kilo
L   Lima
M   Mike
N   November
O   Oscar
P   Papa
Q   Quebec
R   Romeo
S   Sierra
T   Tango
U   Uniform
V   Victor
W   Whiskey
X   X-ray
Y   Yankee
Z   Zulu

Be sure to use proper formatting and appropriate comments in your code. Provide appropriate prompts to the user. The output should be clearly labeled and neatly formatted.

2. Programming Problem 2 in Chapter 4 asked you write a C++ program that asks the user to enter their weight and the name of a planet. The program was then to output how much the user would weigh on that planet. Rewrite that program so that the selection of the factor to use in computing the weight is made with a Switch statement instead of an If structure. The computation should be done in a value-returning function and called from `main`.

For ease of reference, the information for the original problem is repeated here. The following table gives the factor by which the weight must be multiplied for each planet. The program should output an error message if the user doesn't type a correct planet name. The prompt and the error message should make it clear to the user how a planet name must be entered. Be sure to use proper formatting and appropriate comments in your code. The output should be clearly labeled and neatly formatted.

Mercury	0.4155
Venus	0.8975
Earth	1.0
Moon	0.166
Mars	0.3507
Jupiter	2.5374
Saturn	1.0677
Uranus	0.8947
Neptune	1.1794
Pluto	0.0899

3. You are working for a company that has traveling salespeople. The salespeople call in their sales to a fulfillment desk, where the sales are all entered into a file. Each sale is recorded as one line on the file `sales.dat` as a salesperson ID number, an item number, and a quantity, all separated by blanks. There are 10 salespeople, with ID's of 1 through 10. The company sells eight different products, with ID's of 7 through 14 (some older products have been discontinued). The unit prices of the products are:

Product Number	Unit Price
7	345.00
8	853.00
9	471.00
10	933.00
11	721.00
12	663.00
13	507.00
14	259.00

You have been asked to write a program that reads in the sales file, and generates a separate file for each salesperson containing just their sales. Each line from the sales file is copied to the appropriate salesperson file (`salespers1.dat` through `salespers10.dat`), with the salesperson ID omitted. The total for the sale (quantity times unit price) is appended to the record. At the end of processing, the total sales for each salesperson should be output with informative labels to `cout`. Use functional decomposition to design the program. Be sure that the program handles invalid ID numbers. If a salesperson ID is invalid, write out an error message to `cout`. If a product number is invalid, write the error message to the salesperson's file and don't compute a total for that sale. There should be ample opportunity to use Switch statements and value-returning functions in this application.

4. Write a number-guessing game in which the computer selects a random number in the range of 0 to 100, and the user gets up to 20 attempts to guess it. At the end of each game, the user should be told whether they won or lost, and then be asked whether they want to play again. When the user quits, the program should

output the total number of wins and losses. To make the game more interesting, the program should vary the wording of the messages that it outputs for winning, for losing, and for asking for another game. Make up 10 different messages for each of these cases, and use random numbers to choose among them. See Appendix C.7 for information on the C++ random number generator functions. This application should provide a good opportunity for you to use a Do-While statement and Switch statements. Use functional decomposition to solve the problem, write your C++ code using good style and documenting comments, and have fun thinking up some messages that will surprise the user.

5. Write a functional decomposition and a C++ program that reads a time in numeric form and prints it in English. The time is input as hours and minutes, separated by a space. Hours are specified in 24-hour time (15 is 3 PM), but the output should be in 12-hour AM/PM form. Note that noon and midnight are special cases. Here are some examples:

Enter time: 12 00
Noon

Enter time: 0 00
Midnight

Enter time: 6 44
Six forty four AM

Enter time: 18 11
Six eleven PM

Write your C++ code using good style and documenting comments. This application should provide you with ample opportunity to use Switch statements.

6. Extend the program in Problem 5 so that it asks the user if he or she wants to enter another time, and then repeats the process until the response to the question is "no". You should be able to code this easily using a Do-While statement.

Case Study Follow-Up

1. What changes would be necessary in the Rich Uncle program if uppercase letters and lowercase letters were to be counted as members of the same category?
2. You decide that you are interested in counting the number of words in the text. How might you estimate this number?
3. Given that you can calculate the number of words in the text, how can you calculate the average word length?
4. Can you think of any other characteristics of a person's writing style that you might be able to measure?

Simple Data Types: Built-In and User-Defined

Goals

Knowledge Goals

- To know all of the simple data types provided by the C++ language.
- To be familiar with specialized C++ operators and expressions.
- To understand the difference between external and internal representations of character data.
- To understand how floating-point numbers are represented in the computer.
- To understand how the limited numeric precision of the computer can affect calculations.
- To understand the concepts of type promotion and type demotion.

Skill Goals

To be able to:

- Select the most appropriate simple data type for a given variable.
- Declare and use an enumeration type.
- Use the For and Switch statements with user-defined enumeration types.
- Distinguish a named user-defined type from an anonymous user-defined type.
- Create a user-written header file.

This chapter represents a transition point in your study of computer science and C++ programming. So far, we have emphasized simple variables, control structures, and named processes (functions). After this chapter, the focus shifts to ways to structure (organize) data and to the algorithms necessary to process data in these structured forms. In order to make this transition, we must examine the concept of data types in greater detail.

Until now, we have worked primarily with the data types `int`, `char`, `bool`, and `float`. These four data types are adequate for solving a wide variety of problems. But certain programs need other kinds of data. In this chapter, we take a closer look at all of the simple data types that are part of the C++ language. As part of this look, we discuss the limitations of the computer in doing calculations. We examine how these limitations can cause numerical errors and how to avoid such errors.

There are times when even the built-in data types cannot adequately represent all the data in a program. C++ has several mechanisms for creating *user-defined* data types; that is, we can define new data types ourselves. This chapter introduces one of these mechanisms, the enumeration type. In subsequent chapters, we introduce additional user-defined data types.

10.1 Built-In Simple Types

In Chapter 2, we defined a data type as a specific set of data values (which we call the *domain*) along with a set of operations on those values. For the `int` type, the domain is the set of whole numbers from `INT_MIN` through `INT_MAX`, and the allowable operations we have seen so far are +, −, *, /, %, ++, −−, and the relational and logical operations. The domain of the `float` type is the set of all real numbers that a particular computer is capable of representing, and the operations are the same as those for the `int` type except that modulus (%) is excluded. For the `bool` type, the domain is the set consisting of the two values `true` and `false`, and the allowable operations are the logical (!, &&, ||) and relational operations. The `char` type, though used primarily to manipulate character data, is classified as an integral type because it uses integers in memory to stand for characters. Later in the chapter we see how this works.

The `int`, `char`, `bool`, and `float` types have a property in common. The domain of each type is made up of indivisible, or atomic, data values. Data types with this property are called **simple** (or **atomic**) **data types**. When we say that a value is atomic, we mean that it has no component parts that can be accessed individually. For example, a single character of type `char` is atomic, but the string "Good Morning" is not (it is composed of 12 individual characters).

Simple (atomic) data type   A data type in which each value is atomic (indivisible).

Another way of describing a simple type is to say that only one value can be associated with a variable of that type. In contrast, a *structured type* is one in which an entire collection of values is associated with a single variable of that type. For example, a `string` object represents a collection of characters that are given a single name. Beginning in Chapter 11, we look at structured types.

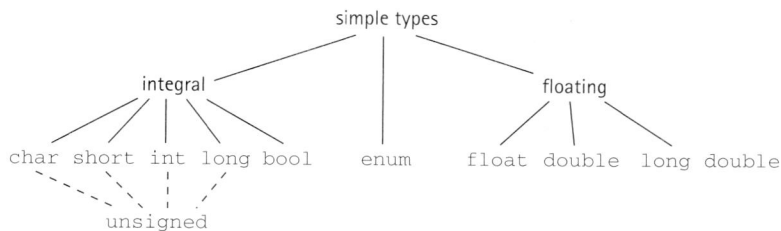

Figure 10–1 *C++ Simple Types*

Figure 10–1 displays the simple types that are built into the C++ language. This figure is a portion of the complete diagram of C++ data types that you saw in Figure 3–1.

In this figure, one of the types—enum—is not actually a single data type in the sense that int and float are data types. Instead, it is a mechanism with which we can define our own simple data types. We look at enum later in the chapter.

The integral types char, short, int, and long represent nothing more than integers of different sizes. Similarly, the floating-point types float, double, and long double simply refer to floating-point numbers of different sizes. What do we mean by *sizes*?

In C++, sizes are measured in multiples of the size of a char. By definition, the size of a char is 1. On most—but not all—computers, the 1 means one byte. (Recall from Chapter 1 that a byte is a group of eight consecutive bits [1s or 0s].)

Let's use the notation *sizeof*(SomeType) to denote the size of a value of type Some-Type. Then, by definition, *sizeof*(char) = 1. Other than char, the sizes of data objects in C++ are machine dependent. On one machine, it might be the case that

sizeof(char) = 1
sizeof(short) = 2
sizeof(int) = 4
sizeof(long) = 8

On another machine, the sizes might be as follows:

sizeof(char) = 1
sizeof(short) = 2
sizeof(int) = 2
sizeof(long) = 4

Despite these variations, the C++ language guarantees that the following statements are true:

- $1 = sizeof(\text{char}) \leq sizeof(\text{short}) \leq sizeof(\text{int}) \leq sizeof(\text{long})$.
- $1 \leq sizeof(\text{bool}) \leq sizeof(\text{long})$.
- $sizeof(\text{float}) \leq sizeof(\text{double}) \leq sizeof(\text{long double})$.
- A char is at least 8 bits.
- A short is at least 16 bits.
- A long is at least 32 bits.

> **Range of values** The interval within which values of a numeric type must fall, specified in terms of the largest and smallest allowable values.

For numeric data, the size of a data object determines its **range of values**. Let's look in more detail at the sizes, ranges of values, and literal constants for each of the built-in types.

Integral Types

Before looking at how the sizes of integral types affect their possible values, we remind you that the reserved word `unsigned` may precede the name of certain integral types—`unsigned char`, `unsigned short`, `unsigned int`, `unsigned long`. Values of these types are nonnegative integers with values from 0 through some machine-dependent maximum value. Although we rarely use unsigned types in this book, we include them in this discussion for thoroughness.

Ranges of Values   The following table displays sample ranges of values for the `char`, `short`, `int`, and `long` data types and their `unsigned` variations.

Type	Size in Bytes*	Minimum Value*	Maximum Value*
char	1	−128	127
unsigned char	1	0	255
short	2	−32,768	32,767
unsigned short	2	0	65,535
int	2	−32,768	32,767
unsigned int	2	0	65,535
long	4	−2,147,483,648	2,147,483,647
unsigned long	4	0	4,294,967,295

* These values are for one particular machine. Your machine's values may be different.

C++ systems provide the header file `climits`, from which you can determine the maximum and minimum values for your machine. This header file defines the constants `CHAR_MAX` and `CHAR_MIN`, `SHRT_MAX` and `SHRT_MIN`, `INT_MAX` and `INT_MIN`, and `LONG_MAX` and `LONG_MIN`. The unsigned types have a minimum value of 0 and maximum values defined by `UCHAR_MAX`, `USHRT_MAX`, `UINT_MAX`, and `ULONG_MAX`. To find out the values specific to your computer, you could print them out like this:

```
#include <climits>
using namespace std;
    ⋮
cout << "Max. long = " << LONG_MAX << endl;
cout << "Min. long = " << LONG_MIN << endl;
    ⋮
```

Literal Constants   In C++, the valid `bool` constants are `true` and `false`. Integer constants can be specified in three different number bases: decimal (base 10), octal (base 8), and hexadecimal (base 16). Just as the decimal number system has 10 digits—0 through 9—the octal system has eight digits—0 through 7. The hexadecimal system has digits 0, 1, 2, 3, 4, 5, 6, 7, 8, 9, A, B, C, D, E, and F, which correspond to the decimal values 0 through 15. Octal and hexadecimal values are used in system software (compilers, linkers, and operating systems, for example) to refer directly to individual bits in a memory cell and to control hardware devices. These manipulations of low-level objects in a computer are the subject of more advanced study and are outside the scope of this book.

The following table shows examples of integer constants in C++. Notice that an L or a U (either uppercase or lowercase) can be added to the end of a constant to signify `long` or `unsigned`, respectively.

Constant	Type	Remarks
1658	int	Decimal (base–10) integer.
03172	int	Octal (base–8) integer. Begins with 0 (zero). Decimal equivalent is 1658.
0x67A	int	Hexadecimal (base–16) integer. Begins with 0 (zero), then either x or X. Decimal equivalent is 1658.
65535U	unsigned int	Unsigned constants end in U or u.
421L	long	Explicit `long` constant. Ends in L or l.
53100	long	Implicit `long` constant, assuming the machine's maximum `int` is, say, 32767.
389123487UL	unsigned long	Unsigned `long` constants end in UL or LU in any combination of uppercase and lowercase letters.

Notice that this table presents only numeric constants for the integral types. We discuss `char` constants later in a separate section.

Here is the syntax template for an integer constant:

IntegerConstant

$$
\left\{
\begin{array}{l}
\text{DecimalConstant} \\
\text{OctalConstant} \\
\text{HexConstant}
\end{array}
\right\}
\left(
\left\{ \begin{array}{l} L \\ l \end{array} \right\} \left\{ \begin{array}{l} U \\ u \end{array} \right\}
\left\{ \begin{array}{l} U \\ u \end{array} \right\} \left\{ \begin{array}{l} L \\ l \end{array} \right\}
\right)
$$

DecimalConstant is a nonzero digit followed, optionally, by a sequence of decimal digits:

DecimalConstant

NonzeroDigit DigitSeq

NonzeroDigit, DigitSeq, and Digit are defined as follows:

NonzeroDigit

$$
\begin{cases}
1 \\
2 \\
3 \\
4 \\
5 \\
6 \\
7 \\
8 \\
9
\end{cases}
$$

DigitSeq

Digit Digit ...

Digit

$$
\begin{cases}
0 \\
\text{NonzeroDigit}
\end{cases}
$$

The second form of integer constant, OctalConstant, has the following syntax:

OctalConstant

0 OctalDigit ...

OctalDigit

$$
\begin{cases}
0 \\
1 \\
2 \\
3 \\
4 \\
5 \\
6 \\
7
\end{cases}
$$

Finally, HexConstant is defined as

HexConstant

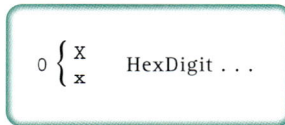

HexDigit

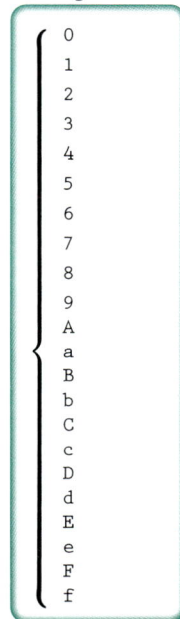

Floating-Point Types

Ranges of Values Below is a table that gives sample ranges of values for the three floating-point types, `float`, `double`, and `long double`. In this table we show, for each type, the maximum positive value and the minimum positive value (a tiny fraction that is very close to 0). Negative numbers have the same range but the opposite sign. Ranges of values are expressed in exponential (scientific) notation, where 3.4E+38 means 3.4×10^{38}.

Type	Size in Bytes*	Minimum Positive Value*	Maximum Positive Value*
`float`	4	3.4E–38	3.4E+38
`double`	8	1.7E–308	1.7E+308
`long double`	10	3.4E–4932	1.1E+4932

*These values are for one particular machine. Your machine's values may be different.

The standard header file `cfloat` defines the constants `FLT_MAX` and `FLT_MIN`, `DBL_MAX` and `DBL_MIN`, and `LDBL_MAX` and `LDBL_MIN`. To determine the ranges of values for your machine, you could write a short program that prints out these constants.

Literal Constants When you use a floating-point constant such as 5.8 in a C++ program, its type is assumed to be `double` (double precision). If you store the value into a `float` variable, the computer coerces its type from `double` to `float` (single precision). If you insist on a constant being of type `float` rather than `double`, you can append an F or an f at the end of the constant. Similarly, a suffix of L or 1 signifies a `long double` constant. Here are some examples of floating-point constants in C++:

Constant	Type	Remarks
6.83	double	By default, floating-point constants are of type `double`.
6.83F	float	Explicit `float` constants end in F or f.
6.83L	long double	Explicit `long double` constants end in L or 1.
4.35E-9	double	Exponential notation, meaning 4.35×10^{-9}.

Here's the syntax template for a floating-point constant in C++:

FloatingPtConstant

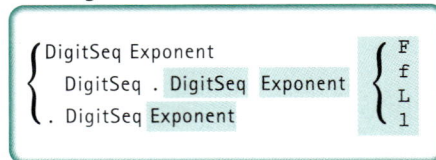

DigitSeq is the same as defined in the section on integer constants—a sequence of decimal (base–10) digits. The form of Exponent is the following:

Exponent

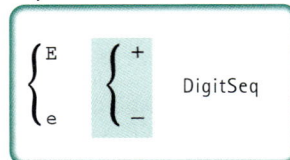

10.2 Additional C++ Operators

C++ has a rich, sometimes bewildering, variety of operators that allow you to manipulate values of the simple data types. Operators you have learned about so far include the assignment operator (=), the arithmetic operators (+, -, *, /, %), the increment and decrement operators (++, --), the relational operators (==, !=, <, <=, >, >=), and the logical operators (!, &&, ||). In certain cases, a pair of parentheses is also considered to be an operator—namely, the function call operator,

```
ComputeSum(x, y);
```

and the type cast operator,

```
y = float(someInt);
```

C++ also has many specialized operators that are seldom found in other programming languages. Here is a table of these additional operators. As you inspect the table, don't panic—a quick scan will do.

Operator	Remarks
Combined assignment operators	
+= Add and assign	
-= Subtract and assign	
*= Multiply and assign	
/= Divide and assign	
Increment and decrement operators	
++ Pre-increment	Example: ++someVar
++ Post-increment	Example: someVar++
-- Pre-decrement	Example: --someVar
-- Post-decrement	Example: someVar--
Bitwise operators	Integer operands only
<< Left shift	
>> Right shift	
& Bitwise AND	
| Bitwise OR	
^ Bitwise EXCLUSIVE OR	
~ Complement (invert all bits)	
More combined assignment operators	Integer operands only
%= Modulus and assign	
<<= Shift left and assign	
>>= Shift right and assign	
&= Bitwise AND and assign	
|= Bitwise OR and assign	
^= Bitwise EXCLUSIVE OR and assign	
Other operators	
() Cast	
sizeof Size of operand in bytes	Form: sizeof Expr or sizeof(Type)
?: Conditional operator	Form: Expr1 ? Expr2 : Expr3

The operators in this table, along with those you already know, comprise most—but not all—of the C++ operators. We introduce a few more operators in later chapters as the need arises.

Assignment Operators and Assignment Expressions

C++ has several assignment operators. The equal sign (=) is the basic assignment operator. When combined with its two operands, it forms an **assignment expression** (*not* an assignment statement). Every assignment expression has a *value* and a *side effect*, namely, that the value is stored into the object denoted by the left-hand side. For example, the expression

> **Assignment expression**   A C++ expression with (1) a value and (2) the side effect of storing the expression value into a memory location.
>
> **Expression statement**   A statement formed by appending a semicolon to an expression.

```
delta = 2 * 12
```

has the value 24 and the side effect of storing this value into `delta`.

In C++, any expression becomes an **expression statement** when it is terminated by a semicolon. All three of the following are valid C++ statements, although the first two have no effect whatsoever at run time:

```
23;
2 * (alpha + beta);
delta = 2 * 12;
```

The third expression statement *is* useful because of its side effect of storing 24 into `delta`.

Because an assignment is an expression, not a statement, you can use it anywhere an expression is allowed. Here is a statement that stores the value 20 into `firstInt`, the value 30 into `secondInt`, and the value 35 into `thirdInt`:

```
thirdInt = (secondInt = (firstInt = 20) + 10) + 5;
```

Some C++ programmers use this style of coding, but others find it hard to read and error-prone.

In Chapter 5, we cautioned against the mistake of using the = operator in place of the == operator:

```
if (alpha = 12)   // Wrong
    ⋮
else
    ⋮
```

The condition in the If statement is an assignment expression, not a relational expression. The value of the expression is 12 (interpreted in the If condition as `true`), so the else-clause is never executed. Worse yet, the side effect of the assignment expression is to store 12 into `alpha`, destroying its previous contents.

In addition to the = operator, C++ has several combined assignment operators (+=, *=, and the others listed in our table of operators). These operators have the following semantics:

Statement	Equivalent Statement
`i += 5;`	`i = i + 5;`
`pivotPoint *= n + 3;`	`pivotPoint = pivotPoint * (n + 3);`

The combined assignment operators are another example of "ice cream and cake." They are sometimes convenient for writing a line of code more compactly, but you can do just fine without them.

Increment and Decrement Operators

The increment and decrement operators (++ and - -) operate only on variables, not on constants or arbitrary expressions. Suppose a variable `someInt` contains the value 3. The expression ++`someInt` denotes preincrementation. The side effect of incrementing `someInt` occurs first, so the resulting value of the expression is 4. In contrast, the expression `someInt`++ denotes post-incrementation. The value of the expression is 3, and *then* the side effect of incrementing `someInt` takes place. The following code illustrates the difference between pre- and post-incrementation:

```
int1 = 14;
int2 = ++int1;
// Assert: int1 == 15  &&  int2 == 15

int1 = 14;
int2 = int1++;
// Assert: int1 == 15  &&  int2 == 14
```

Using side effects in the middle of larger expressions is always a bit dangerous. It's easy to make semantic errors, and the code may be confusing to read. Look at this example:

```
a = (b = c++)  *  --d / (e += f++);
```

Some people make a game of seeing how much they can do in the fewest keystrokes possible. But they should remember that serious software development requires writing code that other programmers can read and understand. Overuse of side effects hinders this goal. By far the most common use of ++ and - - is to do the incrementation or decrementation as a separate expression statement:

```
count++;
```

Here, the value of the expression is unused, but we get the desired side effect of incrementing `count`. In this example, it doesn't matter whether you use pre-incrementation or post-incrementation. The choice is up to you.

Bitwise Operators

The bitwise operators listed in the operator table (`<<`, `>>`, `&`, `|`, and so forth) are used for manipulating individual bits within a memory cell. This book does not explore the use of these operators; the topic of bit-level operations is most often covered in a course on computer organization and assembly language programming. However, we point out two things about the bitwise operators.

First, the built-in operators `<<` and `>>` are the left shift and right shift operators, respectively. Their purpose is to take the bits within a memory cell and shift them to the left or right. Of course, we have been using these operators all along, but in an entirely different context—program input and output. The header file `iostream` uses an advanced C++ technique called *operator overloading* to give additional meanings to these two operators. An overloaded operator is one that has multiple meanings, depending on the data types of its operands. When looking at the `<<` operator, the compiler determines by context whether a left shift operation or an output operation is desired. Specifically, if the first (left-hand) operand denotes an output stream, then it is an output operation. If the first operand is an integer variable, it is a left shift operation.

Second, we repeat our caution from Chapter 5: Do not confuse the `&&` and `||` operators with the `&` and `|` operators. The statement

```
if (i == 3 & j == 4)    // Wrong
    k = 20;
```

is syntactically correct because `&` is a valid operator (the bitwise AND operator). The program containing this statement compiles correctly but executes incorrectly. Although we do not examine what the bitwise AND and OR operators do, just be careful to use the relational operators `&&` and `||` in your logical expressions.

The Cast Operation

You have seen that C++ is very liberal about letting the programmer mix data types in expressions, in assignment operations, in argument passing, and in returning a function value. However, implicit type coercion takes place when values of different data types are mixed together. Instead of relying on implicit type coercion in a statement such as

```
intVar = floatVar;
```

we have recommended using an explicit type cast to show that the type conversion is intentional:

```
intVar = int(floatVar);
```

In C++, the cast operation comes in two forms:

```
intVar = int(floatVar);       // Functional notation
intVar = (int) floatVar;      // Prefix notation. Parentheses required
```

The first form is called functional notation because it looks like a function call. It isn't really a function call (there is no user-defined or predefined subprogram named `int`), but it has the syntax and visual appearance of a function call. The second form, prefix notation, doesn't look like any familiar language feature in C++. In this notation, the parentheses surround the name of the data type, not the expression being converted. Prefix notation is the only form available in the C language; C++ added the functional notation.

Although most C++ programmers use the functional notation for the cast operation, there is one restriction on its use. The data type name must be a single identifier. If the type name consists of more than one identifier, you *must* use prefix notation. For example,

```
myVar = unsigned int(someFloat);     // No
myVar = (unsigned int) someFloat;    // Yes
```

The `sizeof` Operator

The `sizeof` operator is a unary operator that yields the size, in bytes, of its operand. The operand can be a variable name, as in

```
sizeof someInt
```

or the operand can be the name of a data type, enclosed in parentheses:

```
sizeof(float)
```

You could find out the sizes of various data types on your machine by using code like this:

```
cout << "Size of a short is " << sizeof(short) << endl;
cout << "Size of an int is " << sizeof(int) << endl;
cout << "Size of a long is " << sizeof(long) << endl;
```

The `?:` Operator

The last operator in our operator table is the `?:` operator, sometimes called the conditional operator. It is a ternary (three-operand) operator with the following syntax:

ConditionalExpression

Expression1 ? Expression2 : Expression3

Here's how it works. First, the computer evaluates Expression1. If the value is `true`, then the value of the entire expression is Expression2; otherwise, the value of the entire expression is Expression3. (Only one of Expression2 and Expression3 is evaluated.) A classic example of its use is to set a variable `max` equal to the larger of two variables `a` and `b`. Using an If statement, we would do it this way:

```
if (a > b)
    max = a;
else
    max = b;
```

With the `? :` operator, we can use the following assignment statement:

```
max = (a > b) ? a : b;
```

Here is another example. The absolute value of a number x is defined as

$$|x| = \begin{cases} x, & \text{if } x \geq 0 \\ -x, & \text{if } x < 0 \end{cases}$$

To compute the absolute value of a variable `x` and store it into `y`, you could use the `? :` operator as follows:

```
y = (x >= 0) ? x : -x;
```

In both the `max` and the absolute value examples, we used parentheses around the expression being tested. These parentheses are unnecessary because, as we'll see shortly, the conditional operator has very low precedence. But it is customary to include the parentheses for clarity.

Operator Precedence

Below is a summary of operator precedence for the C++ operators we have encountered so far, excluding the bitwise operators. (Appendix B contains the complete list.) In the table, the operators are grouped by precedence level, and a horizontal line separates each precedence level from the next-lower level.

Precedence (highest to lowest)		
Operator	**Associativity**	**Remarks**
( )	Left to right	Function call and function-style cast
++ --	Right to left	++ and - - as postfix operators
++ -- ! Unary + Unary -	Right to left	++ and - - as prefix operators
(cast) sizeof	Right to left	
* / %	Left to right	
+ -	Left to right	
< <= > >=	Left to right	
== !=	Left to right	
&&	Left to right	
||	Left to right	
? :	Right to left	
= += -= *= /=	Right to left	

The column labeled *Associativity* describes grouping order. Within a precedence level, most operators group from left to right. For example,

a - b + c

means

(a - b) + c

and not

a - (b + c)

Certain operators, though, group from right to left—specifically, the unary operators, the assignment operators, and the ? : operator. Look at the assignment operators, for example. The expression

sum = count = 0

means

```
sum = (count = 0)
```

This associativity makes sense because the assignment operation is naturally a right-to-left operation.

A word of caution: Although operator precedence and associativity dictate the *grouping* of operators with their operands, C++ does not define the *order* in which subexpressions are evaluated. Therefore, using side effects in expressions requires extra care. For example, if i currently contains 5, the statement

```
j = ++i + i;
```

stores either 11 or 12 into j, depending on the particular compiler being used. Let's see why. There are three operators in the expression statement above: =, ++, and +. The ++ operator has the highest precedence, so it operates just on i, not the expression i + i. The addition operator has higher precedence than the assignment operator, giving implicit parentheses as follows:

```
j = (++i + i);
```

So far, so good. But now we ask this question: In the addition operation, is the left operand or the right operand evaluated first? The C++ language doesn't dictate the order. If a compiler generates code to evaluate the left operand first, the result is 6 + 6, or 12. Another compiler might generate code to evaluate the right operand first, yielding 6 + 5, or 11. To be assured of left-to-right evaluation in this example, you should force the ordering with two separate statements:

```
++i;
j = i + i;
```

The moral here is that if you use multiple side effects in expressions, you increase the risk of unexpected or inconsistent results. For the newcomer to C++, it's better to avoid unnecessary side effects altogether.

10.3 Working with Character Data

We have been using char variables to store character data, such as the character 'A' or 'e' or '+':

```
char someChar;
    ⋮
someChar = 'A';
```

However, because `char` is defined to be an integral type and `sizeof(char)` equals 1, we also can use a `char` variable to store a small (usually one-byte) integer constant. For example,

```
char counter;
    ⋮
counter = 3;
```

On computers with a very limited amount of memory space, programmers sometimes use the `char` type to save memory when they are working with small integers.

A natural question to ask is, How does the computer know the difference between integer data and character data when the data is sitting in a memory cell? The answer is, The computer *can't* tell the difference! To explain this surprising fact, we must look more closely at how character data is stored in a computer.

Character Sets

Each computer uses a particular character set, the set of all possible characters with which it is capable of working. Two character sets widely in use today are the ASCII character set and the EBCDIC character set. ASCII is used by the vast majority of all computers, whereas EBCDIC is found primarily on IBM mainframe computers. ASCII consists of 128 different characters, and EBCDIC has 256 characters. Appendix E shows the characters that are available in these two character sets.

A more recently developed character set called *Unicode* allows many more distinct characters than either ASCII or EBCDIC. Unicode was invented primarily to accommodate the larger alphabets and symbols of various international human languages. In C++, the data type `wchar_t` rather than `char` is used for Unicode characters. In fact, `wchar_t` can be used for other, possibly infrequently used, "wide character" sets in addition to Unicode. In this book, we do not examine Unicode or the `wchar_t` type. We continue to focus our attention on the `char` type and the ASCII and EBCDIC character sets.

Whichever character set is being used, each character has an **external representation**—the way it looks on an I/O device like a printer—and an **internal representation**—the way it is stored inside the computer's memory unit. If you use the `char` constant 'A' in a C++ program, its external representation is the letter *A*. That is, if you print it out you see an *A*, as you would expect. Its internal representation, though, is an integer value. The 128 ASCII characters have internal representations 0 through 127; the EBCDIC characters, 0 through 255. For example, the ASCII table in Appendix E shows that the character 'A' has internal representation 65, and the character 'b' has internal representation 98.

> **External representation**   The printable (character) form of a data value.
>
> **Internal representation**   The form in which a data value is stored inside the memory unit.

Let's look again at the statement

```
someChar = 'A';
```

Assuming our machine uses the ASCII character set, the compiler translates the constant 'A' into the integer 65. We could also have written the statement as

```
someChar = 65;
```

Both statements have exactly the same effect—that of storing 65 into `someChar`. However, the second version is *not* recommended. It is not as understandable as the first version, and it is nonportable (the program won't work correctly on a machine that uses EBCDIC, which uses a different internal representation—193—for 'A').

Earlier we mentioned that the computer cannot tell the difference between character and integer data in memory. Both are stored internally as integers. However, when we perform I/O operations, the computer does the right thing—it uses the external representation that corresponds to the data type of the expression being printed. Look at this code segment, for example:

```
// This example assumes use of the ASCII character set
int   someInt = 97;
char  someChar = 97;

cout << someInt << endl;
cout << someChar << endl;
```

When these statements are executed, the output is

```
97
a
```

When the `<<` operator outputs `someInt`, it prints the sequence of characters 9 and 7. To output `someChar`, it prints the single character a. Even though both variables contain the value 97 internally, the data type of each variable determines how it is printed.

What do you think is output by the following sequence of statements?

```
char ch = 'D';

ch++;
cout << ch;
```

If you answered E, you are right. The first statement declares `ch` and initializes it to the integer value 68 (assuming ASCII). The next statement increments `ch` to 69, and then its external representation (the letter *E*) is printed. Extending this idea of incrementing a `char` variable, we could print the letters *A* through *G* as follows:

```
char ch;

for (ch = 'A'; ch <= 'G'; ch++)
    cout << ch;
```

This code initializes `ch` to 'A' (65 in ASCII). Each time through the loop, the external representation of `ch` is printed. On the final loop iteration, the *G* is printed and `ch` is incremented to 'H' (72 in ASCII). The loop test is then false, so the loop terminates.

C++ `char` Constants

In C++, `char` constants come in two different forms. The first form, which we have been using regularly, is a single printable character enclosed by apostrophes (single quotes):

```
'A'    '8'    ')'    '+'
```

Notice that we said *printable* character. Character sets include both printable characters and *control characters* (or *nonprintable characters*). Control characters are not meant to be printed but are used to control the screen, printer, and other hardware devices. If you look at the ASCII character table, you see that the printable characters are those with integer values 32–126. The remaining characters (with values 0–31 and 127) are non-printable control characters. In the EBCDIC character set, the control characters are those with values 0–63 and 250–255 (and some that are intermingled with the printable characters). One control character you already know about is the newline character, which causes the screen cursor to advance to the next line.

To accommodate control characters, C++ provides a second form of `char` constant: the *escape sequence*. An escape sequence is one or more characters preceded by a back-slash (\). You are familiar with the escape sequence \n, which represents the newline character. Here is the complete description of the two forms of `char` constant in C++:

1. A single printable character—except an apostrophe (') or backslash (\)—enclosed by apostrophes.
2. One of the following escape sequences, enclosed by apostrophes:

\n	Newline (Line feed in ASCII)
\t	Horizontal tab
\v	Vertical tab
\b	Backspace
\r	Carriage return
\f	Form feed
\a	Alert (a bell or beep)
\\	Backslash
\'	Single quote (apostrophe)
\"	Double quote (quotation mark)
\0	Null character (all 0 bits)
\ddd	Octal equivalent (one, two, or three octal digits specifying the integer value of the desired character)
\xddd	Hexadecimal equivalent (one or more hexadecimal digits specifying the integer value of the desired character)

Even though an escape sequence is written as two or more characters, each escape sequence represents a single character in the character set. The alert character (\a) is the same as what is called the BEL character in ASCII and EBCDIC. To ring the bell (well, these days, beep the beeper) on your computer, you can output the alert character like this:

```
cout << '\a';
```

In the list of escape sequences above, the entries labeled *Octal equivalent* and *Hexadecimal equivalent* let you refer to any character in your machine's character set by specifying its integer value in either octal or hexadecimal form.

Note that you can use an escape sequence within a string just as you can use any printable character within a string. The statement

```
cout << "\aWhoops!\n";
```

beeps the beeper, displays Whoops!, and terminates the output line. The statement

```
cout << "She said \"Hi\"";
```

outputs She said "Hi" and does not terminate the output line.

Programming Techniques

What kinds of things can we do with character data in a program? In the last chapter, we counted different categories of characters. The possibilities are endless and depend, of course, on the particular problem we are solving. But several techniques are so widely used that it's worth taking a look at them.

Comparing Characters   In previous chapters, you have seen examples of comparing characters for equality. We have used tests such as

```
if (ch == 'a')
```

and

```
while (inputChar != '\n')
```

Characters also can be compared by using <, <=, >, and >=. For example, if the variable firstLetter contains the first letter of a person's last name, we can test to see if the last name starts with *A* through *H* by using this test:

```
if (firstLetter >= 'A' && firstLetter <= 'H')
```

On one level of thought, a test like this is reasonable if you think of < as meaning "comes before" in the character set and > as meaning "comes after." On another level, the test makes even more sense when you consider that the underlying representation of a character is an integer number. The machine literally compares the two integer values using the mathematical meaning of less than or greater than.

When you write a logical expression to check whether a character lies within a certain range of values, you sometimes have to keep in mind the character set your machine uses. In Chapter 8, we hinted that a test like

```
if (ch >= 'a' && ch <= 'z')
```

works correctly on some machines but not on others. In ASCII, this If test behaves correctly because the lowercase letters occupy 26 consecutive positions in the character set. In EBCDIC, however, there is a gap between the lowercase letters i and j that includes nonprintable characters, and there is another gap between r and s. (There are similar gaps between the uppercase letters I and J and between R and S.) If your machine uses EBCDIC, you must rephrase the If test to be sure you include *only* the desired characters. A better approach, though, is to take advantage of the "is. . ." functions supplied by the standard library through the header file `cctype`. If you replace the above If test with this one:

```
if (islower(ch))
```

then your program is more portable; the test works correctly on any machine, regardless of its character set. It's a good idea to become well acquainted with these character-testing library functions (Appendix C). They can save you time and help you to write more portable programs.

Converting Digit Characters to Integers Suppose you want to convert a digit that is read in character form to its numeric equivalent. Because the digit characters '0' through '9' are consecutive in both the ASCII and EBCDIC character sets, subtracting '0' from any digit in character form gives the digit in numeric form:

```
'0' - '0' = 0
'1' - '0' = 1
'2' - '0' = 2
    ⋮
```

For example, in ASCII, '0' has internal representation 48 and '2' has internal representation 50. Therefore, the expression

```
'2' - '0'
```

equals 50 – 48 and evaluates to 2.

Why would you want to do this? Recall that when the extraction operator (>>) reads data into an `int` variable, the input stream fails if an invalid character is encountered. (And once the stream has failed, no further input will succeed). Suppose you're writing a program that prompts an inexperienced user to enter a number from 1 through 5. If the input variable is of type `int` and the user accidentally types a letter of the alphabet, the program is in trouble. To defend against this possibility, you might read the user's response as a character and convert it to a number, performing error checking along the way. Here's a code segment that demonstrates the technique:

```cpp
#include <cctype>     // For isdigit()
using namespace std;
   ⋮
void GetResponse( /* out */ int& response )

// Postcondition:
//      User has been prompted to enter a digit from 1
//      through 5 (repeatedly, and with error messages,
//      if data is invalid)
//   && 1 <= response <= 5

{
    char inChar;
    bool badData = false;

    do
    {
        cout << "Enter a number from 1 through 5: ";
        cin >> inChar;
        if ( !isdigit(inChar) )
            badData = true;                    // It's not a digit
        else
        {
            response = int(inChar - '0');
            if (response < 1 || response > 5)
                badData = true;                // It's a digit, but
        }                                      // it's out of range
        if (badData)
            cout << "Please try again." << endl;
    } while (badData);
}
```

Converting to Lowercase and Uppercase   When working with character data, you sometimes find that you need to convert a lowercase letter to uppercase, or vice versa. Fortunately, the programming technique required to do these conversions is easy—a simple call to a library function is all it takes. Through the header file cctype, the standard library provides not only the "is..." functions we have discussed, but also two value-returning functions named toupper and tolower. Here are their descriptions:

Header File	Function	Function Type	Function Value
`<cctype>`	`toupper(ch)`	`char`*	Uppercase equivalent of `ch`, if `ch` is a lowercase letter; `ch`, otherwise
`<cctype>`	`tolower(ch)`	`char`	Lowercase equivalent of `ch`, if `ch` is an uppercase letter; `ch`, otherwise

*Technically, both the argument and the return value are of type `int`. But conceptually, the functions operate on character data.

Notice that the value returned by each function is just the original character if the condition is not met. For example, `tolower('M')` returns the character 'm', whereas `tolower('+')` returns '+'.

A common use of these two functions is to let the user respond to certain input prompts by using either uppercase or lowercase letters. For example, if you want to allow either *Y* or *y* for a "Yes" response from the user, and either *N* or *n* for "No," you might do this:

```
#include <cctype>     // For toupper()
using namespace std;
     ⋮
cout << "Enter Y or N: ";
cin >> inputChar;
if (toupper(inputChar) == 'Y')
{
     ⋮
}
else if (toupper(inputChar) == 'N')
{
     ⋮
}
else
     PrintErrorMsg();
```

Below is a function named `Lower`, which is our implementation of the `tolower` function. (You wouldn't actually want to waste time by writing this function because `tolower` is already available to you.) This function returns the lowercase equivalent of an uppercase letter. In ASCII, each lowercase letter is exactly 32 positions beyond the corresponding uppercase letter. And in EBCDIC, the lowercase letters are 64 positions *before* their corresponding uppercase letters. To make our `Lower` function work on both ASCII-based and EBCDIC-based machines, we define a constant DISTANCE to have the value

```
'a' - 'A'
```

In ASCII, the value of this expression is 32. In EBCDIC, the value is –64.

```cpp
#include <cctype>      // For isupper()
using namespace std;
   ⋮
char Lower( /* in */ char ch )

// Postcondition:
//      Function value == lowercase equivalent of ch, if ch is
//                          an uppercase letter
//                       == ch, otherwise

{
    const int DISTANCE = 'a' - 'A';    // Fixed distance between
                                       // uppercase and lowercase
                                       // letters
    if (isupper(ch))
        return ch + DISTANCE;
    else
        return ch;
}
```

Accessing Characters Within a String In the last section, we gave the outline of a code segment that prompts the user for a "Yes" or "No" response. The code accepted a response of 'Y' or 'N' in uppercase or lowercase letters. If a problem requires the user to type the entire word *Yes* or *No* in any combination of uppercase and lowercase letters, the code becomes more complicated. Reading the user's response as a string into a string object named inputStr, we would need a lengthy If-Then-Else-If structure to compare inputStr to "yes", "Yes", "yEs", "yeS", and so on.

As an alternative, let's inspect only the first character of the input string, comparing it with 'Y', 'y', 'N', or 'n', and then ignore the rest of the string. The string class allows you to access an individual character in a string by giving its position number in square brackets:

StringObject [Position]

Within a string, the first character is at position 0, the second is at position 1, and so forth. Therefore, the value of Position must be greater than or equal to 0 and less than or equal to the string length minus 1. For example, if inputStr is a string object and ch is a char variable, the statement

```cpp
ch = inputStr[2];
```

accesses the character at position 2 of the string (the third character) and copies it into
ch.

Now we can sketch out the code for reading a "Yes" or "No" response, checking
only the first letter of that response.

```
string inputStr;
    ⋮
cout << "Enter Yes or No: ";
cin >> inputStr;
if (toupper(inputStr[0]) == 'Y')
{
    ⋮
}
else if (toupper(inputStr[0]) == 'N')
{
    ⋮
}
else
    PrintErrorMsg();
```

Here is another example of accessing characters within a string. The following program asks the user to type the name of a month and then outputs how many days there
are in that month. The input can be in either uppercase or lowercase characters, and the
program allows approximate input. For example, the inputs February, FEBRUARY,
fEbRu, feb, fe, f, and fyz34x are all interpreted as February because that is the only
month that begins with *f*. However, the input Ma is rejected because it could represent
either March or May. To conserve space, we have omitted the interface documentation
for the DaysInMonth function in this program.

```
//***************************************************************
// NumDays program
// This program repeatedly prompts for a month and outputs the
// number of days in that month. Approximate input is allowed: only
// the characters needed to determine the month are examined
//***************************************************************
#include <iostream>
#include <cctype>        // For toupper()
#include <string>        // For string type

using namespace std;

string DaysInMonth( string );

int main()
{
    string month;      // User's input value
```

```cpp
    do
    {
        cout << "Name of the month (or q to quit) : ";
        cin >> month;
        if (month != "q")
            cout << "No. of days in " << month << " is "
                << DaysInMonth(month) << endl;
    } while (month != "q");
    return 0;
}

//**********************************************************************

string DaysInMonth( /* in */ string month )
{
    string::size_type i;                    // Loop control variable
    string badData = "** Invalid month **"; // Bad data message

    // Convert to all uppercase

    for (i = 0; i < month.length(); i++)
        month[i] = toupper(month[i]);

    // Make sure length is at least 3 for upcoming tests

    month = month + "   ";

    // Examine first character, then others if needed

    switch (month[0])
    {
        case 'J' : if (month[1] == 'A' ||       // January
                        month[2] == 'L'   )     // July
                        return "31";
                    else if (month[2] == 'N')   // June
                        return "30";
                    else
                        return badData;
        case 'F' : return "28 or 29";           // February
        case 'M' : if (month[2] == 'R' ||       // March
                        month[2] == 'Y'   )     // May
                        return "31";
                    else
                        return badData;
        case 'A' : if (month[1] == 'P')         // April
                        return "30";
```

```
            else if (month[1] == 'U')   // August
                return "31";
            else
                return badData;
    case 'S' :                          // September
    case 'N' : return "30";             // November
    case 'O' :                          // October
    case 'D' : return "31";             // December
    default  : return badData;
    }
}
```

10.4 More on Floating-Point Numbers

We have used floating-point numbers off and on since we introduced them in Chapter 2, but we have not examined them in depth. Floating-point numbers have special properties when used on the computer. Thus far, we've almost ignored these properties, but now it's time to consider them in detail.

Representation of Floating-Point Numbers

Let's assume we have a computer in which each memory location is the same size and is divided into a sign plus five decimal digits. When a variable or constant is defined, the location assigned to it consists of five digits and a sign. When an `int` variable or constant is defined, the interpretation of the number stored in that place is straightforward. When a `float` variable or constant is defined, the number stored there has both a whole number part and a fractional part, so it must be coded to represent both parts.

Let's see what such coded numbers might look like. The range of whole numbers we can represent with five digits is −99,999 through +99,999:

−99999 through +99999

Our **precision** (the number of digits we can represent) is five digits, and each number within that range can be represented exactly.

> Precision   The maximum number of significant digits.

What happens if we allow one of those digits (the leftmost one, for example) to represent an exponent?

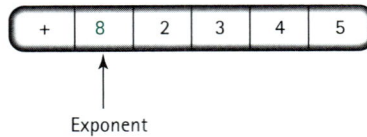

Exponent

Then +82345 represents the number $+2345 \times 10^8$. The range of numbers we now can represent is much larger:

-9999×10^9 through 9999×10^9

or

$-9,999,000,000,000$ through $+9,999,000,000,000$

However, our precision is now only four digits; that is, only four-digit numbers can be represented exactly in our system. What happens to numbers with more digits? The four leftmost digits are represented correctly, and the rightmost digits, or least significant digits, are lost (assumed to be 0). Figure 10–2 shows what happens. Note that 1,000,000 can be represented exactly but $-4,932,416$ cannot, because our coding scheme limits us to four **significant digits**.

> **Significant digits**   Those digits from the first nonzero digit on the left to the last nonzero digit on the right (plus any 0 digits that are exact).

To extend our coding scheme to represent floating-point numbers, we must be able to represent negative exponents. Examples are

$$7394 \times 10^{-2} = 73.94$$

and

$$22 \times 10^{-4} = .0022$$

NUMBER	POWER OF TEN NOTATION	CODED REPRESENTATION	VALUE
+99,999	$+9999 \times 10^1$	Sign: + Exp: 1, 9 9 9 9	+99,990
−999,999	-9999×10^2	Sign: − Exp: 2, 9 9 9 9	−999,900
+1,000,000	-1000×10^3	Sign: + Exp: 3, 1 0 0 0	+1,000,000
−4,932,416	-4932×10^3	Sign: − Exp: 3, 4 9 3 2	−4,932,000

Figure 10–2   *Coding Using Positive Exponents*

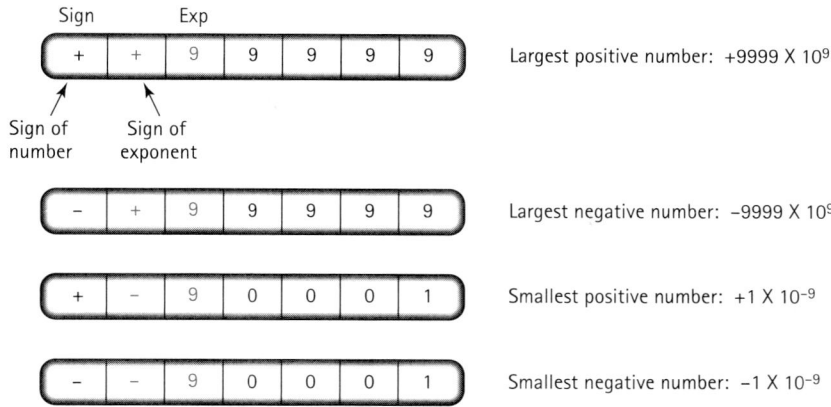

Figure 10–3   *Coding Using Positive and Negative Exponents*

Because our scheme does not include a sign for the exponent, let's change it slightly. The existing sign becomes the sign of the exponent, and we add a sign to the far left to represent the sign of the number itself (see Figure 10–3).

All the numbers between -9999×10^9 and 9999×10^9 can now be represented accurately to four digits. Adding negative exponents to our scheme allows us to represent fractional numbers as small as 1×10^{-9}.

Figure 10-4 shows how we would encode some floating-point numbers. Note that our precision is still only four digits. The numbers 0.1032, −5.406, and 1,000,000 can be represented exactly. The number 476.0321, however, with seven significant digits, is represented as 476.0; the *321* cannot be represented. (We should point out that some

Figure 10–4   *Coding of Some Floating-Point Numbers*

computers perform *rounding* rather than simple truncation when discarding excess digits. Using our assumption of four significant digits, such a machine would store 476.0321 as 476.0 but would store 476.0823 as 476.1. We continue our discussion assuming simple truncation rather than rounding.)

Arithmetic with Floating-Point Numbers

When we use integer arithmetic, our results are exact. Floating-point arithmetic, however, is seldom exact. To understand why, let's add the three floating-point numbers x, y, and z using our coding scheme.

First, we add x to y and then we add z to the result. Next, we perform the operations in a different order, adding y to z, and then adding x to that result. The associative law of arithmetic says that the two answers should be the same—but are they? Let's use the following values for x, y, and z:

$$x = -1324 \times 10^3 \quad y = 1325 \times 10^3 \quad z = 5424 \times 10^0$$

Here is the result of adding z to the sum of x and y:

(x)	-1324×10^3
(y)	$\underline{1325 \times 10^3}$
	$1 \times 10^3 \quad = 1000 \times 10^0$

(x+y)	1000×10^0
(z)	$\underline{5424 \times 10^0}$
	$6424 \times 10^0 \quad \leftarrow (x+y)+z$

Now here is the result of adding x to the sum of y and z:

(y)	1325000×10^0
(z)	$\underline{5424 \times 10^0}$
	$1330424 \times 10^0 \quad = 1330 \times 10^3 \text{ (truncated to four digits)}$

(y+z)	1330×10^3
(x)	$\underline{-1324 \times 10^3}$
	$6 \times 10^3 \quad = 6000 \times 10^0 \leftarrow x + (y + z)$

Representational error Arithmetic error that occurs when the precision of the true result of an arithmetic operation is greater than the precision of the machine.

These two answers are the same in the thousands place but are different thereafter. The error behind this discrepancy is called **representational error**.

Because of representational errors, it is unwise to use a floating-point variable as a loop control variable. Because precision may be lost in calculations involving floating-point numbers, it is difficult to predict when (or even *if*) a loop control variable of type `float` (or `double` or `long double`) will equal the termination value. A count-controlled loop with a floating-point control variable can behave unpredictably.

Also because of representational errors, you should never compare floating-point numbers for exact equality. Rarely are two floating-point numbers exactly equal, and thus you should compare them only for near equality. If the difference between the two numbers is less than some acceptable small value, you can consider them equal for the purposes of the given problem.

Implementation of Floating-Point Numbers in the Computer

All computers limit the precision of floating-point numbers, although modern machines use binary rather than decimal arithmetic. In our representation, we used only 5 digits to simplify the examples, and some computers really are limited to only 4 or 5 digits of precision. A more typical system might provide 6 significant digits for `float` values, 15 digits for `double` values, and 19 for the `long double` type. We have shown only a single-digit exponent, but most systems allow 2 digits for the `float` type and up to 4-digit exponents for type `long double`.

When you declare a floating-point variable, part of the memory location is assumed to contain the exponent, and the number itself (called the *mantissa*) is assumed to be in the balance of the location. The system is called floating-point representation because the number of significant digits is fixed, and the decimal point conceptually is allowed to float (move to different positions as necessary). In our coding scheme, every number is stored as four digits, with the leftmost digit being nonzero and the exponent adjusted accordingly. Numbers in this form are said to be *normalized*. The number 1,000,000 is stored as

+	+	3	1	0	0	0

and 0.1032 is stored as

+	−	4	1	0	3	2

Normalization provides the maximum precision possible.

Model Numbers   Any real number that can be represented exactly as a floating-point number in the computer is called a *model number*. A real number whose value cannot be represented exactly is approximated by the model number closest to it. In our system with four digits of precision, 0.3021 is a model number. The values 0.3021409, 0.3021222, and 0.30209999999 are examples of real numbers that are represented in the computer by the same model number. The following table shows all of the model numbers for an even simpler floating-point system that has one digit in the mantissa and an exponent that can be −1, 0, or 1. Zero is a special case, because it has the same value regardless of the exponent.

0.1×10^{-1}	0.1×10^{0}	$0.1 \times 10^{+1}$
0.2×10^{-1}	0.2×10^{0}	$0.2 \times 10^{+1}$
0.3×10^{-1}	0.3×10^{0}	$0.3 \times 10^{+1}$
0.4×10^{-1}	0.4×10^{0}	$0.4 \times 10^{+1}$
0.5×10^{-1}	0.5×10^{0}	$0.5 \times 10^{+1}$
0.6×10^{-1}	0.6×10^{0}	$0.6 \times 10^{+1}$
0.7×10^{-1}	0.7×10^{0}	$0.7 \times 10^{+1}$
0.8×10^{-1}	0.8×10^{0}	$0.8 \times 10^{+1}$
0.9×10^{-1}	0.9×10^{0}	$0.9 \times 10^{+1}$

The difference between a real number and the model number that represents it is a form of representational error called *rounding error*. We can measure rounding error in two ways. The *absolute error* is the difference between the real number and the model number. For example, the absolute error in representing 0.3021409 by the model number 0.3021 is 0.0000409. The *relative error* is the absolute error divided by the real number and sometimes is stated as a percentage. For example, 0.0000409 divided by 0.3021409 is 0.000135, or 0.0135%.

The maximum absolute error depends on the *model interval*—the difference between two adjacent model numbers. In our example, the interval between 0.3021 and 0.3022 is 0.0001. The maximum absolute error in this system, for this interval, is less than 0.0001. Adding digits of precision makes the model interval (and thus the maximum absolute error) smaller.

The model interval is not a fixed number; it varies with the exponent. To see why the interval varies, consider that the interval between 3021.0 and 3022.0 is 1.0, which is 10^4 times larger than the interval between 0.3021 and 0.3022. This makes sense, because 3021.0 is simply 0.3021 times 10^4. Thus, a change in the exponent of the model numbers adjacent to the interval has an equivalent effect on the size of the interval. In practical terms, this means that we give up significant digits in the fractional part in order to represent numbers with large integer parts. Figure 10–5 illustrates this by graphing all of the model numbers listed in the preceding table.

We also can use relative and absolute error to measure the rounding error resulting from calculations. For example, suppose we multiply 1.0005 by 1000. The correct result is 1000.5, but because of rounding error, our four-digit computer produces 1000.0 as its

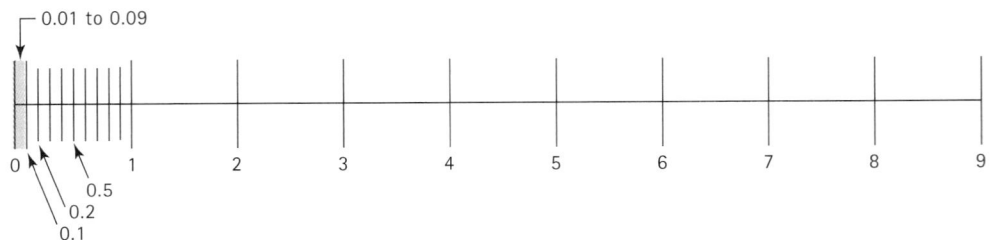

Figure 10–5 *A Graphical Representation of Model Numbers*

result. The absolute error of the computed result is 0.5, and the relative error is 0.05%. Now suppose we multiply 100,050.0 by 1000. The correct result is 100,050,000, but the computer produces 100,000,000 as its result. If we look at the relative error, it is still a modest 0.05%, but the absolute error has grown to 50,000. Notice that this example is another case of changing the size of the model interval.

Whether it is more important to consider the absolute error or the relative error depends on the situation. It is unacceptable for an audit of a company to discover a $50,000 accounting error; the fact that the relative error is only 0.05% is not important. On the other hand, a 0.05% relative error is acceptable in representing prehistoric dates because the error in measurement techniques increases with age. That is, if we are talking about a date roughly 10,000 years ago, an absolute error of 5 years is acceptable; if the date is 100,000,000 years ago, then an absolute error of 50,000 years is equally acceptable.

Comparing Floating-Point Numbers   We have cautioned against comparing floating-point numbers for exact equality. Our exploration of representational errors in this chapter reveals why calculations may not produce the expected results even though it appears that they should. In Chapter 5, we wrote an expression that compares two floating-point variables r and s for near equality using the floating-point absolute value function fabs:

```
fabs(r - s) < 0.00001
```

From our discussion of model numbers, you now can recognize that the constant 0.00001 in this expression represents a maximum absolute error. We can generalize this expression as

```
fabs(r - s) < ERROR_TERM
```

where ERROR_TERM is a value that must be determined for each programming problem.

What if we want to compare floating-point numbers with a relative error measure? We must multiply the error term by the value in the problem to which the error is relative. For example, if we want to test whether r and s are "equal" within 0.05% of s, we write the following expression:

```
fabs(r - s) < 0.0005 * s
```

Keep in mind that the choice of the acceptable error and whether it should be absolute or relative depends on the problem being solved. The error terms we have shown in our example expressions are completely arbitrary and may not be appropriate for most problems. In solving a problem that involves the comparison of floating-point numbers, you typically want an error term that is as small as possible. Sometimes the choice is specified in the problem description or is reasonably obvious. Some cases require careful analysis of both the mathematics of the problem and the representational limits of the particular computer. Such analyses are the domain of a branch of mathematics called *numerical analysis* and are beyond the scope of this text.

Underflow and Overflow In addition to representational errors, there are two other problems to watch out for in floating-point arithmetic: *underflow* and *overflow*.

Underflow is the condition that arises when the value of a calculation is too small to be represented. Going back to our decimal representation, let's look at a calculation involving small numbers:

$$
\begin{array}{r}
4210 \times 10^{-8} \\
\times\ 2000 \times 10^{-8} \\
\hline
8420000 \times 10^{-16} = 8420 \times 10^{-13}
\end{array}
$$

This value cannot be represented in our scheme because the exponent -13 is too small. Our minimum is -9. One way to resolve the problem is to set the result of the calculation to 0.0. Obviously, any answer depending on this calculation will not be exact.

Overflow is a more serious problem because there is no logical recourse when it occurs. For example, the result of the calculation

$$
\begin{array}{r}
9999 \times 10^{9} \\
\times\ 1000 \times 10^{9} \\
\hline
9999000 \times 10^{18} = 9999 \times 10^{21}
\end{array}
$$

cannot be stored, so what should we do? To be consistent with our response to underflow, we could set the result to 9999×10^{9} (the maximum representable value in this case). Yet this seems intuitively wrong. The alternative is to stop with an error message.

C++ does not define what should happen in the case of overflow or underflow. Different implementations of C++ solve the problem in different ways. You might try to cause an overflow with your system and see what happens. Some systems may print a run-time error message such as "FLOATING POINT OVERFLOW." On other systems, you may get the largest number that can be represented.

Although we are discussing problems with floating-point numbers, integer numbers also can overflow both negatively and positively. Most implementations of C++ ignore integer overflow. To see how your system handles the situation, you should try adding 1 to INT_MAX and -1 to INT_MIN. On most systems, adding 1 to INT_MAX sets the result to INT_MIN, a negative number.

Sometimes you can avoid overflow by arranging computations carefully. Suppose you want to know how many different five-card poker hands can be dealt from a deck of cards. What we are looking for is the number of *combinations* of 52 cards taken 5 at a time. The standard mathematical formula for the number of combinations of n things taken r at a time is

$$
\frac{n!}{r!(n-r)!}
$$

We could use the `Factorial` function we wrote in Chapter 8 and write this formula in an assignment statement:

```
hands = Factorial(52) / (Factorial(5) * Factorial(47));
```

The only problem is that 52! is a very large number (approximately 8.0658×10^{67}). And 47! is also large (approximately 2.5862×10^{59}). Both of these numbers are well beyond the capacity of most systems to represent exactly as integers (52! requires 68 digits of precision). Even though they can be represented on many machines as floating-point numbers, most of the precision is still lost. By rearranging the calculations, however, we can achieve an exact result on any system with 9 or more digits of precision. How? Consider that most of the multiplications in computing 52! are canceled when the product is divided by 47!

$$\frac{52!}{5! \times 47!} = \frac{52 \times 51 \times 50 \times 49 \times 48 \times 47 \times 46 \times 45 \times 44 \times \dots}{(5 \times 4 \times 3 \times 2 \times 1) \times (47 \times 46 \times 45 \times 44 \times \dots)}$$

So, we really only have to compute

```
hands = 52 * 51 * 50 * 49 * 48 / Factorial(5);
```

which means the numerator is 311,875,200 and the denominator is 120. On a system with 9 or more digits of precision, we get an exact answer: 2,598,960 poker hands.

Cancellation Error   Another type of error that can happen with floating-point numbers is called *cancellation error*, a form of representational error that occurs when numbers of widely differing magnitudes are added or subtracted. Let's look at an example:

$$(1 + 0.00001234 - 1) = 0.00001234$$

The laws of arithmetic say this equation should be true. But is it true if the computer does the arithmetic?

$$
\begin{array}{r}
100000000 \times 10^{-8} \\
+ \quad\quad 1234 \times 10^{-8} \\
\hline
100001234 \times 10^{-8}
\end{array}
$$

To four digits, the sum is 1000×10^{-3}. Now the computer subtracts 1:

$$
\begin{array}{r}
1000 \times 10^{-3} \\
-1000 \times 10^{-3} \\
\hline
0
\end{array}
$$

The result is 0, not .00001234.

Sometimes you can avoid adding two floating-point numbers that are drastically different in size by carefully arranging the calculations. Suppose a problem requires many small floating-point numbers to be added to a large floating-point number. The result is more accurate if the program first sums the smaller numbers to obtain a larger number and then adds the sum to the large number.

Background Information

Practical Implications of Limited Precision

A discussion of representational, overflow, underflow, and cancellation errors may seem purely academic. In fact, these errors have serious practical implications in many problems. We close this section with three examples illustrating how limited precision can have costly or even disastrous effects.

During the Mercury space program, several of the spacecraft splashed down a considerable distance from their computed landing points. This delayed the recovery of the spacecraft and the astronaut, putting both in some danger. Eventually, the problem was traced to an imprecise representation of the Earth's rotation period in the program that calculated the landing point.

As part of the construction of a hydroelectric dam, a long set of high-tension cables had to be constructed to link the dam to the nearest power distribution point. The cables were to be several miles long, and each one was to be a continuous unit. (Because of the high power output from the dam, shorter cables couldn't be spliced together.) The cables were constructed at great expense and strung between the two points. It turned out that they were too short, however, so another set had to be manufactured. The problem was traced to errors of precision in calculating the length of the catenary curve (the curve that a cable forms when hanging between two points).

An audit of a bank turned up a mysterious account with a large amount of money in it. The account was traced to an unscrupulous programmer who had used limited precision to his advantage. The bank computed interest on its accounts to a precision of a tenth of a cent. The tenths of cents were not added to the customers' accounts, so the programmer had the extra tenths for all the accounts summed and deposited into an account in his name. Because the bank had thousands of accounts, these tiny amounts added up to a large amount of money. And because the rest of the bank's programs did not use as much precision in their calculations, the scheme went undetected for many months.

The moral of this discussion is twofold: (1) The results of floating-point calculations are often imprecise, and these errors can have serious consequences; and (2) if you are working with extremely large numbers or extremely small numbers, you need more information than this book provides and should consult a numerical analysis text.

Software Engineering Tip

Choosing a Numeric Data Type

A first encounter with all the numeric data types of C++ may leave you feeling overwhelmed. To help in choosing an alternative, you may even feel tempted to toss a coin. You should resist this temptation, because each data type exists for a reason. Here are some guidelines:

1. In general, int is preferable.

    As a rule, you should use floating-point types *only* when absolutely necessary—that is, when you definitely need fractional values. Not only is floating-point arithmetic subject to representational errors, it also is significantly slower than integer arithmetic on most computers.

    For ordinary integer data, use int instead of char or short. It's easy to make overflow errors with these smaller data types. (For character data, though, the char type is appropriate.)

2. Use long only if the range of int values on your machine is too restrictive.

    Compared to int, the long type requires more memory space and execution time.

3. Use double and long double only if you need enormously large or small numbers, or if your machine's float values do not carry enough digits of precision.

    The cost of using double and long double is increased memory space and execution time.

4. Avoid the unsigned forms of integral types.

    These types are primarily for manipulating bits within a memory cell, a topic this book does not cover. You might think that declaring a variable as unsigned prevents you from accidentally storing a negative number into the variable. However, the C++ compiler does *not* prevent you from doing so. Later in this chapter, we explain why.

By following these guidelines, you'll find that the simple types you use most often are int and float, along with char for character data and bool for Boolean data. Only rarely do you need the longer and shorter variations of these fundamental types.

10.5 User-Defined Simple Types

The concept of a data type is fundamental to all of the widely used programming languages. One of the strengths of the C++ language is that it allows programmers to create new data types, tailored to meet the needs of a particular program. Much of the remainder of this book is about user-defined data types. In this section, we examine how to create our own simple types.

The Typedef Statement

The *Typedef statement* allows you to introduce a new name for an existing type. Its syntax template is

TypedefStatement

```
typedef ExistingTypeName NewTypeName ;
```

Before the `bool` data type was part of the C++ language, many programmers used code like the following to simulate a Boolean type:

```
typedef int Boolean;
const int TRUE = 1;
const int FALSE = 0;
    ⋮
Boolean dataOK;
    ⋮
dataOK = TRUE;
```

In this code, the Typedef statement causes the compiler to substitute the word `int` for every occurrence of the word `Boolean` in the rest of the program.

The Typedef statement provides a very limited way of defining our own data types. In fact, Typedef does not create a new data type at all: It merely creates an additional name for an existing data type. As far as the compiler is concerned, the domain and operations of the above `Boolean` type are identical to the domain and operations of the `int` type.

Despite the fact that Typedef cannot truly create a new data type, it is a valuable tool for writing self-documenting programs. Before `bool` was a built-in type, program code that used the identifiers `Boolean`, `TRUE`, and `FALSE` was more descriptive than code that used `int`, 1, and 0 for Boolean operations.

Names of user-defined types obey the same scope rules that apply to identifiers in general. Most types, like `Boolean` above, are defined globally, although it is reasonable to define a new type within a subprogram if that is the only place it is used. The guidelines that determine where a named constant should be defined apply also to data types.

Enumeration Types

C++ allows the user to define a new simple type by listing (enumerating) the literal values that make up the domain of the type. These literal values must be *identifiers*, not numbers. The identifiers are separated by commas, and the list is enclosed in braces. Data types defined in this way are called **enumeration types**. Here's an example:

> **Enumeration type** A user-defined data type whose domain is an ordered set of literal values expressed as identifiers.

```
enum Days {SUN, MON, TUE, WED, THU, FRI, SAT};
```

This declaration creates a new data type named Days. Whereas Typedef merely creates a synonym for an existing type, an enumeration type like Days is truly a new type and is distinct from any existing type.

The values in the Days type—SUN, MON, TUE, and so forth—are called **enumerators**. The enumerators are *ordered*, in the sense that SUN < MON < TUE ... < FRI < SAT. Applying relational operators to enumerators is like applying them to characters: The relation that is tested is whether an enumerator "comes before" or "comes after" in the ordering of the data type.

> **Enumerator** One of the values in the domain of an enumeration type.

Earlier we saw that the internal representation of a char constant is a nonnegative integer. The 128 ASCII characters are represented in memory as the integers 0 through 127. Values in an enumeration type are also represented internally as integers. By default, the first enumerator has the integer value 0, the second has the value 1, and so forth. Our declaration of the Days enumeration type is similar to the following set of declarations:

```
typedef int Days;
const int SUN = 0;
const int MON = 1;
const int TUE = 2;
   ⋮
const int SAT = 6;
```

If there is some reason that you want different internal representations for the enumerators, you can specify them explicitly like this:

```
enum Days {SUN = 4, MON = 18, TUE = 9, ...  };
```

There is rarely any reason to assign specific values to enumerators. With the Days type, we are interested in the days of the week, not in the way the machine stores them internally. We do not discuss this feature any further, although you may occasionally see it in C++ programs.

Notice the style we use to capitalize enumerators. Because enumerators are, in essence, named constants, we capitalize the entire identifier. This is purely a style choice. Many C++ programmers use both uppercase and lowercase letters when they invent names for the enumerators.

Here is the syntax template for the declaration of an enumeration type. It is a simplified version; later in the chapter we expand it.

EnumDeclaration

```
enum Name { Enumerator , Enumerator ... } ;
```

Each enumerator has the following form:

Enumerator

Identifier = ConstIntExpression

where the optional ConstIntExpression is an integer expression composed only of literal or named constants.

The identifiers used as enumerators must follow the rules for any C++ identifier. For example,

```
enum Vowel {'A', 'E', 'I', 'O', 'U'};      // Error
```

is not legal because the items are not identifiers. The declaration

```
enum Places {1st, 2nd, 3rd};      // Error
```

is not legal because identifiers cannot begin with digits. In the declarations

```
enum Starch {CORN, RICE, POTATO, BEAN};
enum Grain {WHEAT, CORN, RYE, BARLEY, SORGHUM};      // Error
```

type `Starch` and type `Grain` are legal individually, but together they are not. Identifiers in the same scope must be unique. `CORN` cannot be defined twice.

Suppose you are writing a program for a veterinary clinic. The program must keep track of different kinds of animals. The following enumeration type might be used for this purpose.

Type identifier   Literal values in the domain
        ↓

```
enum Animals {RODENT, CAT, DOG, BIRD, REPTILE, HORSE, BOVINE, SHEEP};
```

```
Animals inPatient;
Animals outPatient;
```
} Creation of two variables of type `Animals`

`RODENT` is a literal, one of the values in the data type `Animals`. Be sure you understand that `RODENT` is not a variable name. Instead, `RODENT` is one of the values that can be stored into the variables `inPatient` and `outPatient`. Let's look at the kinds of operations we might want to perform on variables of enumeration types.

Assignment   The assignment statement

```
inPatient = DOG;
```

does not assign to inPatient the character string "DOG", nor the contents of a variable named DOG. It assigns the *value* DOG, which is one of the values in the domain of the data type Animals.

Assignment is a valid operation, as long as the value being stored is of type Animals. Both of the statements

```
inPatient = DOG;
outPatient = inPatient;
```

are acceptable. Each expression on the right-hand side is of type Animals—DOG is a literal of type Animals, and inPatient is a variable of type Animals. Although we know that the underlying representation of DOG is the integer 2, the compiler prevents us from using this assignment:

```
inPatient = 2;    // Not allowed
```

Here is the precise rule:

> *Implicit type coercion is defined from an enumeration type to an integral type but not from an integral type to an enumeration type.*

Applying this rule to the statements

```
someInt = DOG;    // Valid
inPatient = 2;    // Error
```

we see that the first statement stores 2 into someInt (because of implicit type coercion), but the second produces a compile-time error. The restriction against storing an integer value into a variable of type Animals is to keep you from accidentally storing an out-of-range value:

```
inPatient = 65;    // Error
```

Incrementation   Suppose that you want to "increment" the value in inPatient so that it becomes the next value in the domain:

```
inPatient = inPatient + 1;    // Error
```

This statement is illegal for the following reason. The right-hand side is OK because implicit type coercion lets you add inPatient to 1; the result is an int value. But the assignment operation is not valid because you can't store an int value into inPatient. The statement

```
inPatient++;    // Error
```

is also invalid because the compiler considers it to have the same semantics as the assignment statement above. However, you can escape the type coercion rule by using an *explicit* type conversion—a type cast—as follows:

```
inPatient = Animals(inPatient + 1);    // Correct
```

When you use the type cast, the compiler assumes that you know what you are doing and allows it.

Incrementing a variable of an enumeration type is very useful in loops. Sometimes we need a loop that processes all the values in the domain of the type. We might try the following For loop:

```
Animals patient;

for (patient=RODENT; patient <= SHEEP; patient++)   // Error
    ⋮
```

However, as we explained above, the compiler will complain about the expression patient++. To increment patient, we must use an assignment expression and a type cast:

```
for (patient=RODENT; patient <= SHEEP; patient=Animals(patient + 1))
    ⋮
```

The only caution here is that when control exits the loop, the value of patient is 1 *greater than* the largest value in the domain (SHEEP). If you want to use patient outside the loop, you must reassign it a value that is within the appropriate range for the Animals type.

Comparison   The most common operation performed on values of enumeration types is comparison. When you compare two values, their ordering is determined by the order in which you listed the enumerators in the type declaration. For instance, the expression

```
inPatient <= BIRD
```

has the value true if inPatient contains the value RODENT, CAT, DOG, or BIRD.

You can also use values of an enumeration type in a Switch statement. Because RODENT, CAT, and so on are literals, they can appear in case labels:

```
switch (inPatient)
{
    case RODENT  :
    case CAT     :
    case DOG     :
    case BIRD    : cout << "Cage ward";
                   break;
```

```
     case REPTILE : cout << "Terrarium ward";
                       break;
     case HORSE   :
     case BOVINE  :
     case SHEEP   : cout << "Barn";
}
```

Input and Output   Stream I/O is defined only for the basic built-in types (int, float, and so on), not for user-defined enumeration types. Values of enumeration types must be input or output indirectly.

To input values, one strategy is to read a string that spells one of the constants in the enumeration type. The idea is to input the string and translate it to one of the literals in the enumeration type by looking at only as many letters as are necessary to determine what it is.

For example, the veterinary clinic program could read the kind of animal as a string, then assign one of the values of type Animals to that patient. *Cat, dog, horse,* and *sheep* can be determined by their first letter. *Bovine, bird, rodent,* and *reptile* cannot be determined until the second letter is examined. The following program fragment reads in a string representing an animal name and converts it to one of the values in type Animals.

```
#include <cctype>    // For toupper()
#include <string>    // For string type
    ⋮
string animalName;
    ⋮
cin >> animalName;
switch (toupper(animalName[0]))
{
    case 'R' : if (toupper(animalName[1]) == 'O')
                   inPatient = RODENT;
               else
                   inPatient = REPTILE;
               break;
    case 'C' : inPatient = CAT;
               break;
    case 'D' : inPatient = DOG;
               break;
    case 'B' : if (toupper(animalName[1]) == 'I')
                   inPatient = BIRD;
               else
                   inPatient = BOVINE;
               break;
    case 'H' : inPatient = HORSE;
```

```
                              break;
         default :   inPatient = SHEEP;
    }
```

Enumeration type values cannot be printed directly either. Printing is done by using a Switch statement that prints a character string corresponding to the value.

```
switch (inPatient)
{
    case RODENT   : cout << "Rodent";
                      break;
    case CAT      : cout << "Cat";
                      break;
    case DOG      : cout << "Dog";
                      break;
    case BIRD     : cout << "Bird";
                      break;
    case REPTILE  : cout << "Reptile";
                      break;
    case HORSE    : cout << "Horse";
                      break;
    case BOVINE   : cout << "Bovine";
                      break;
    case SHEEP    : cout << "Sheep";
}
```

You might ask, Why not use just a pair of letters or an integer number as a code to represent each animal in a program? The answer is that we use enumeration types to make our programs more readable; they are another way to make the code more self-documenting.

Returning a Function Value   We have been using value-returning functions to compute and return values of built-in types such as int, float, and char:

```
int Factorial( int );
float CargoMoment( int );
```

C++ allows a function return value to be of *any* data type—built-in or user-defined—except an array (a data type we examine in later chapters).

In the last section, we wrote a Switch statement to convert an input string into a value of type Animals. Let's write a value-returning function that performs this task. Notice how the function heading declares the data type of the return value to be Animals.

```
Animals StrToAnimal( /* in */ string str )
{
    switch (toupper(str[0]))
```

```
        {
            case 'R' : if (toupper(str[1]) == 'O')
                            return RODENT;
                       else
                            return REPTILE;
            case 'C' : return CAT;
            case 'D' : return DOG;
            case 'B' : if (toupper(str[1]) == 'I')
                            return BIRD;
                       else
                            return BOVINE;
            case 'H' : return HORSE;
            default  :  return SHEEP;
        }
    }
```

In this function, why didn't we include a Break statement after each case alternative? Because when one of the alternatives executes a Return statement, control immediately exits the function. It's not possible for control to "fall through" to the next alternative.

Here is a sample of code that calls the StrToAnimal function:

```
enum Animals {RODENT, CAT, DOG, BIRD, REPTILE, HORSE, BOVINE, SHEEP};

Animals StrToAnimal( string );
   ⋮
int main()
{
    Animals inPatient;
    Animals outPatient;
    string  inputStr;
     ⋮
    cin >> inputStr;
    inPatient = StrToAnimal(inputStr);
     ⋮
    cin >> inputStr;
    outPatient = StrToAnimal(inputStr);
     ⋮
}
```

Named and Anonymous Data Types

The enumeration types we have looked at, Animals and Days, are called **named types** because their declarations included names for the types. Variables of these new data types are declared separately using the type identifiers Animals and Days.

Named type A user-defined type whose declaration includes a type identifier that gives a name to the type.

C++ also lets us introduce a new type directly in a variable declaration. Instead of the declarations

```
enum CoinType {NICKEL, DIME, QUARTER, HALF_DOLLAR};
enum StatusType {OK, OUT_OF_STOCK, BACK_ORDERED};

CoinType    change;
StatusType status;
```

we could write

```
enum {NICKEL, DIME, QUARTER, HALF_DOLLAR} change;
enum {OK, OUT_OF_STOCK, BACK_ORDERED} status;
```

A new type declared in a variable declaration is called an **anonymous type** because it does not have a name—that is, it does not have a type identifier associated with it.

Anonymous type   A type that does not have an associated type identifier.

If we can create a data type in a variable declaration, why bother with a separate type declaration that creates a named type? Named types, like named constants, make a program more readable, more understandable, and easier to modify. Also, declaring a type and declaring a variable of that type are two distinct concepts; it is best to keep them separate.

We now give a more complete syntax template for an enumeration type declaration. This template shows that the type name is optional (yielding an anonymous type) and that a list of variables may optionally be included in the declaration.

EnumDeclaration

```
enum Name { Enumerator , Enumerator ... } VariableName , VariableName ... ;
```

User-Written Header Files

As you create your own user-defined data types, you often find that a data type can be useful in more than one program. For example, you may be working on several programs that need an enumeration type consisting of the names of the 12 months of the year. Instead of typing the statement

```
enum Months
{
    JANUARY, FEBRUARY, MARCH, APRIL, MAY, JUNE,
    JULY, AUGUST, SEPTEMBER, OCTOBER, NOVEMBER, DECEMBER
};
```

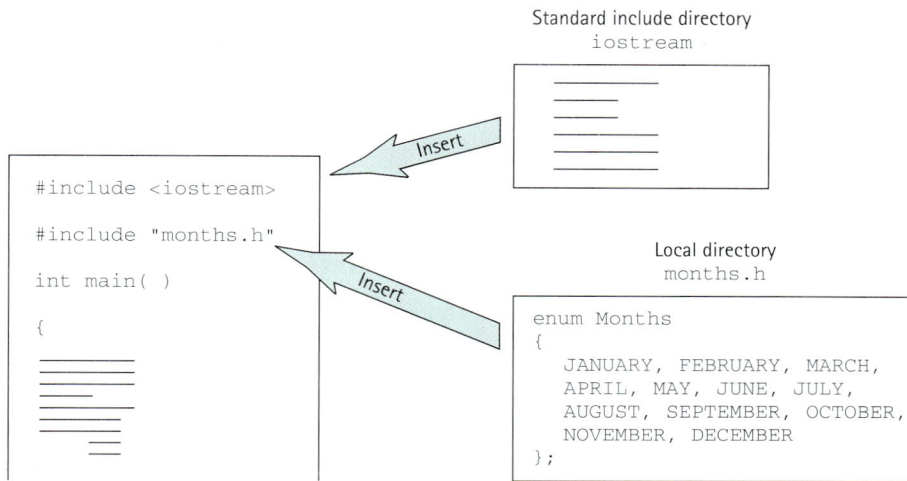

Figure 10–6   *Including Header Files*

at the beginning of every program that uses the Months type, you can put this statement into a separate file named, say, months.h. Then you use months.h just as you use system-supplied header files such as iostream and cmath. By using an #include directive, you ask the C++ preprocessor to insert the contents of the file physically into your program. (Although many C++ systems use the filename extension .h [or no extension at all] to denote header files, other systems use extensions such as .hpp or .hxx.)

When you enclose the name of a header file in angle brackets, as in

```
#include <iostream>
```

the preprocessor looks for the file in the standard *include directory,* a directory that contains all the header files supplied by the C++ system. On the other hand, you can enclose the name of a header file in double quotes, like this:

```
#include "months.h"
```

In this case, the preprocessor looks for the file in the programmer's current directory. This mechanism allows us to write our own header files that contain type declarations and constant declarations. We can use a simple #include directive instead of retyping the declarations in every program that needs them (see Figure 10–6.)

10.6 More on Type Coercion

As you have learned over the course of several chapters, C++ performs implicit type coercion whenever values of different data types are used in the following:

1. Arithmetic and relational expressions

2. Assignment operations

3. Argument passing

4. Return of the function value from a value-returning function

For item 1—mixed type expressions—the C++ compiler follows one set of rules for type coercion. For items 2, 3, and 4, the compiler follows a second set of rules. Let's examine each of these two rules.

Type Coercion in Arithmetic and Relational Expressions

> **Promotion (widening)** The conversion of a value from a "lower" type to a "higher" type according to a programming language's precedence of data types.

Suppose that an arithmetic expression consists of one operator and two operands—for example, `3.4*sum` or `var1/var2`. If the two operands are of different data types, then one of them is temporarily **promoted** (or **widened**) to match the data type of the other. To understand exactly what promotion means, let's look at the rule for type coercion in an arithmetic expression.*

Step 1: Each `char`, `short`, `bool`, or enumeration value is promoted (widened) to `int`. If both operands are now `int`, the result is an `int` expression.

Step 2: If step 1 still leaves a mixed type expression, the following precedence of types is used:

lowest ————————————————————————————→ highest

`int, unsigned int, long, unsigned long, float, double, long double`

The value of the operand of "lower" type is promoted to that of the "higher" type, and the result is an expression of that type.

A simple example is the expression `someFloat+2`. This expression has no `char`, `short`, `bool`, or enumeration values in it, so step 1 still leaves a mixed type expression. In step 2, `int` is a "lower" type than `float`, so the value 2 is coerced temporarily to the `float` value, say, 2.0. Then the addition takes place, and the type of the entire expression is `float`.

This description of type coercion also holds for relational expressions such as

`someInt <= someFloat`

The value of `someInt` is temporarily coerced to floating-point representation before the comparison takes place. The only difference between arithmetic expressions and relational expressions is that the resulting type of a relational expression is always `bool`—the value `true` or `false`.

---

*The rule we give for type coercion is a simplified version of the rule found in the C++ language definition. The complete rule has more to say about unsigned types, which we rarely use in this book.

Here is a table that describes the result of promoting a value from one simple type to another in C++:

From	To	Result of Promotion
double	long double	Same value, occupying more memory space
float	double	Same value, occupying more memory space
Integral type	Floating-point type	Floating-point equivalent of the integer value; fractional part is zero
Integral type	Its unsigned counterpart	Same value, if original number is nonnegative; a radically different positive number, if original number is negative
Signed integral type	Longer signed integral type	Same value, occupying more memory space
unsigned integral type	Longer integral type (either signed or unsigned)	Same nonnegative value, occupying more memory space

NOTE: The result of promoting a char to an int is compiler dependent. Some compilers treat char as unsigned char, so promotion always yields a nonnegative integer. With other compilers, char means signed char, so promotion of a negative value yields a negative integer.

The note at the bottom of the table suggests a potential problem if you are trying to write a portable C++ program. If you use the char type only to store character data, there is no problem. C++ guarantees that each character in a machine's character set (such as ASCII) is represented as a nonnegative value. Using character data, promotion from char to int gives the same result on any machine with any compiler.

But if you try to save memory by using the char type for manipulating small signed integers, then promotion of these values to the int type can produce different results on different machines! That is, one machine may promote negative char values to negative int values, whereas the same program on another machine might promote negative char values to *positive* int values. The moral is this: Unless you are squeezed to the limit for memory space, do not use char to manipulate small signed numbers. Use char only to store character data.

Type Coercion in Assignments, Argument Passing, and Return of a Function Value

In general, promotion of a value from one type to another does not cause loss of information. Think of promotion as moving your baseball cards from a small shoe box to a larger shoe box. All of the cards still fit into the new box and there is room to spare. On the other hand, **demotion** (or **narrowing**) of data values can potentially cause loss of information. Demotion is like moving a shoe box full of baseball cards into a smaller box—something has to be thrown out.

> **Demotion (narrowing)**   The conversion of a value from a "higher" type to a "lower" type according to a programming language's precedence of data types. Demotion may cause loss of information.

Consider an assignment operation

$$v = e$$

where v is a variable and e is an expression. Regarding the data types of v and e, there are three possibilities:

1. If the types of v and e are the same, no type coercion is necessary.
2. If the type of v is "higher" than that of e (using the type precedence we explained with promotion), then the value of e is promoted to v's type before being stored into v.
3. If the type of v is "lower" than that of e, the value of e is demoted to v's type before being stored into v.

Demotion, which you can think of as shrinking a value, may cause loss of information:

- Demotion from a longer integral type to a shorter integral type (such as `long` to `int`) results in discarding the leftmost (most significant) bits in the binary number representation. The result may be a drastically different number.
- Demotion from a floating-point type to an integral type causes truncation of the fractional part (and an undefined result if the whole-number part will not fit into the destination variable). The result of truncating a negative number is machine dependent.
- Demotion from a longer floating-point type to a shorter floating-point type (such as `double` to `float`) may result in a loss of digits of precision.

Our description of type coercion in an assignment operation also holds for argument passing (the mapping of arguments onto parameters) and for returning a function value with a Return statement. For example, assume that `INT_MAX` on your machine is 32767 and that you have the following function:

```
void DoSomething( int n )
{
    ⋮
}
```

If the function is called with the statement

```
DoSomething(50000);
```

then the value 50000 (which is implicitly of type `long` because it is larger than `INT_MAX`) is demoted to a completely different, smaller value that fits into an `int` location. In a similar fashion, execution of the function

```
int SomeFunc( float x )
{
    ⋮
    return 70000;
}
```

causes demotion of the value 70000 to a smaller `int` value because `int` is the declared type of the function return value.

One interesting consequence of implicit type coercion is the futility of declaring a variable to be `unsigned`, hoping that the compiler will prevent you from making a mistake like this:

```
unsignedVar = -5;
```

The compiler does not complain at all. It generates code to coerce the `int` value to an `unsigned int` value. If you now print out the value of `unsignedVar`, you'll see a strange-looking positive integer. As we have pointed out before, `unsigned` types are most appropriate for advanced techniques that manipulate individual bits within memory cells. It's best to avoid using `unsigned` for ordinary numeric computations.

Problem–Solving Case Study
Stylistical Analysis of Text

PROBLEM The Rich Uncle problem in Chapter 9 and the Case Study Follow-Up Exercises intrigued you, so you decide to change and enhance the program. Rather than calculating percentages of groups of characters, you will just show counts. You also will determine the average word length and the average sentence length. Because you have just learned about enumerated types and Switch statements, you decide to redo the design using these constructs.

DISCUSSION The Case Study Follow-Up exercise answers in Chapter 9 suggest that the number of new lines, punctuation marks, and blanks give a good approximation to the number of words. However, if any of these characters appear consecutively, only the first should be counted as an end-of-word symbol. You can use a Boolean variable endOfWord that is set to true when an end-of-word symbol is found. The word counter should only be incremented when endOfWord is false, after which endOfWord is set to true. When an alphanumeric character is read, endOfWord is set to false.

INPUT Text on the file whose name is read from the keyboard.

OUTPUT A table giving the file whose name is read from the keyboard, showing the following values.

Total number of alphanumeric characters
Number of uppercase letters
Number of lowercase letters

Number of digits
Number of characters ignored
Number of words
Number of sentences
Average word length
Average sentence length

Main	Level 0

Open files for processing
    If files not opened ok
    Write error message
    return 1
Get a character
DO
    ProcessCharacter(character)
    Get a character
WHILE (more data)
Print table

The Open Files module in the Rich Uncle program can be used directly. In fact, only the Process Character module needs to be decomposed, although the Print Table module will be changed somewhat.

PROCESS CHARACTER   In the Rich Uncle program you used an If statement to determine to which category a character belongs. In this program you will use a Switch statement with case labels of an enumerated type. The categories are uppercase, lowercase, digits, end-of-word, end-of-sentence, and ignore.

enum Features {UPPER, LOWER, DIGIT, EOW, EOS, IGNORE};

This module is where the endOfWord switch must be set. It should be set to false when it is declared and set to true when an end-of-word symbol is found and reset to false when an alphanumeric character is found. In order for this process to work properly, endOfWord must be marked as a static variable. A static variable is a local variable that maintains its value from invocation to invocation.

(In: character; InOut: uppercaseCounter, lowercaseCounter, digitCounter, wordCounter, sentenceCounter, ignoreCounter)	Level 1

Set (static) endOfWord to false

SWITCH (Decode(character))
    UPPER :   Increment uppercaseCounter
            Set endOfWord to false
    LOWER :   Increment lowercaseCounter
            Set endOfWord to false

DIGIT :   Increment digitCounter
           Set endOfWord to false
EOW :   IF NOT endOfWord
               Increment wordCounter
               Set endOfWord to true;
EOS: Increment sentenceCounter
IGNORE: Increment ignoreCounter

Decode(In: character)   **Level 2**

Out: Function value—Feature

```
IF isupper(character))
    return UPPER
ELSE IF islower(character)
    return LOWER
ELSE IF isdigit(character)
    return DIGIT
ELSE
    SWITCH (character)
        '.' :
        '?' :
        '!' : return EOS;

        ' ' :
        ',' :
        ';' :
        ':' :
        '\n' : return EOW;
return IGNORE;
```

Notice that a Switch statement can be used in the last else branch because characters can be used as case labels. If either of the first two are matched, control flows into the third case, which has a `return` beside it that causes execution to jump to the end of the Switch statement. The same is true of the fourth through seventh case labels, which flow through into the last case label, which has a `return` beside it.

As you look at this algorithm, you realize that the end-of-sentence markers are also end-of-word markers! Yet, you also want to keep the counts separate. You decide to take care of this problem in module Print Results by adding the number of sentences to the number of words.

Print Table (Inout: table, uppercaseCounter, lowercaseCounter, digitCounter, sentenceCounter, wordCounter, ignoreCounter)   **Level 1**

Set totalAlphaNum to uppercaseCounter + lowercaseCounter + digitCounter

Print on table "Total number of alphanumeric characters: " totalAlphaNum
Print on table "Number of uppercase letters: " uppercaseCounter
Print on table "Number of lowercase letters: " lowercaseCounter
Print on table "Number of digits: " digitCounter
Print on table "Number of characters ignored: " ignoreCounter

Set wordCounter to wordCounter + sentenceCounter

Print on table "Number of Words: " wordCounter
Print on table "Number of Sentences: " sentenceCounter
Print on table "Average word length: " float(totalAlphaNum)/ wordCounter
Print on table "Average sentence length: "
     float(wordCounter) / sentenceCounter

MODULE STRUCTURE CHART

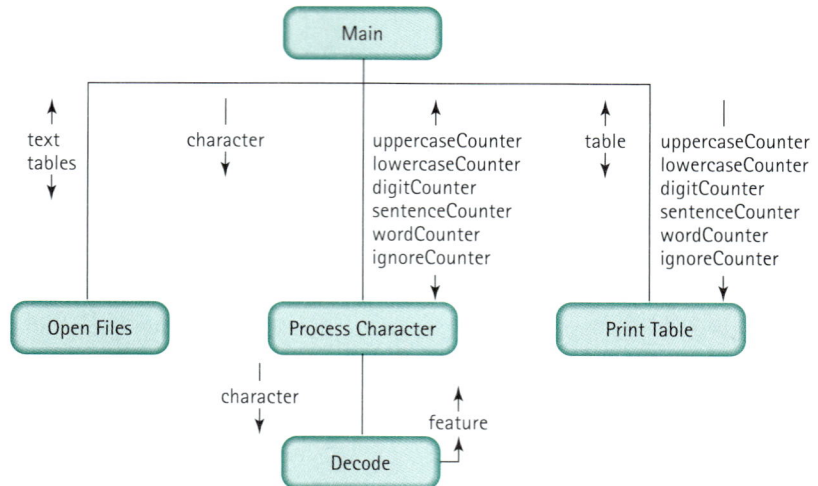

```cpp
//****************************************************************
// Style Program
// A stylistic analysis of the following features of text is
// computed:
//    number of words
//    average word length
//    number of sentences
//    average sentence length
//    number of uppercase letters
//    number of lowercase letters
//    number of digits
// To save space, we omit from each function the precondition
// comments that document the assumptions made about valid input
// parameter data. These would be included in a program intended
// for actual use
//****************************************************************

#include <fstream>
#include <iostream>
#include <iomanip>
#include <cctype>

using namespace std;

enum Features {UPPER, LOWER, DIGIT, IGNORE, EOW, EOS};

// Function prototypes
void OpenFiles(ifstream&, ofstream&);
Features Decode(char character);
void ProcessCharacter(char, int&, int&, int&, int&, int&, int&);
void PrintTable(ofstream& table, int, int, int, int, int, int);

int main()
{
    // Prepare files for reading and writing
    ifstream text;
    ofstream table;
    OpenFiles(text, table);
    if (!text || !table )
    {
        cout << "Files did not open successfully." << endl;
        return 1;
    }

    char character;                    // Input character

    // Declare and initialize counters
    int uppercaseCounter = 0;
```

```cpp
        int lowercaseCounter = 0;
        int digitCounter = 0;
        int wordCounter = 0;
        int sentenceCounter = 0;
        int ignoreCounter = 0;


        text.get(character);              // Input one character
        do
        { // Process each character
            ProcessCharacter(character, uppercaseCounter,
                lowercaseCounter, digitCounter, sentenceCounter,
                wordCounter, ignoreCounter);
            text.get(character);          // Input one character
        } while (text);

        PrintTable(table, uppercaseCounter, lowercaseCounter,
            digitCounter, sentenceCounter, wordCounter, ignoreCounter);
        text.close();
        table.close();
        return 0;
}


//******************************************************************

Features Decode( /* in */ char character ) // Character decoded

// Function Decode examines the character and returns its type
// Postcondition:
//      Return value is the enumerated type to which character
//      belongs

{
    if (isupper(character))
        return UPPER;
    else if (islower(character))
        return LOWER;
    else if (isdigit(character))
        return DIGIT;
    else
        switch  (character)
        {
            case '.'  :
            case '?'  :
            case '!'  :  return EOS;
```

```
            case ' '  :
            case ','  :
            case ';'  :
            case ':'  :
            case '\n' :  return EOW;

        }
    return IGNORE;
}


//********************************************************************

void OpenFiles( /* inout */ ifstream& text,    // Input file
                /* inout */ ofstream& table )  // Output file

// Function OpenFiles reads in the names of the input file and the
// output file and opens them for processing; input file name is
// written on the output file
// Postcondition:
//     Files have been opened AND the input file name has been
//     written on the output file

{
    string inFileName;
    string outFileName;
    cout << "Enter the name of the file to be processed" << endl;
    cin >> inFileName;
    text.open(inFileName.c_str());
    cout << "Enter the name of the output file" << endl;
    cin >> outFileName;
    table.open(outFileName.c_str());
    table << "Analysis of characters on input file " << inFileName
          << endl << endl;
}


//********************************************************************

void PrintTable
    ( /* inout */ ofstream& table,        // Output file
      /* in */ int uppercaseCounter,      // Uppercase letters
      /* in */ int lowercaseCounter,      // Lowercase letters
      /* in */ int digitCounter,          // Digits
      /* in */ int sentenceCounter,       // '.', '?', '!'
      /* in */ int wordCounter,           // Words
```

```cpp
        /* in */ int ignoreCounter )        // Everything else

// Function PrintTable prints the percentages represented by each
// of the five categories
// Postcondition:
//      The output has been written on file table, appropriately
//      labeled

{

    int totalAlphaNum;
    totalAlphaNum = uppercaseCounter + lowercaseCounter
        + digitCounter;

    // Print results on file table
    table << "Total number of alphanumeric characters: "
        << totalAlphaNum << endl;
    table << "Number of uppercase letters: " << uppercaseCounter
        << endl;
    table << "Number of lowercase letters: " << lowercaseCounter
        << endl;
    table << "Number of digits: " << digitCounter << endl;
    table << "Number of characters ignored: " << ignoreCounter
        << endl;

    // Add number of end-of-sentence markers to the word count
    wordCounter = wordCounter + sentenceCounter;

    // Write rest of results on file table
    table << "Number of Words: " <<  wordCounter << endl;
    table << "Number of Sentences: " << sentenceCounter << endl;
    table << "Average word length: " << fixed << setprecision(2)
        << float(totalAlphaNum)/ wordCounter  << endl;
    table << "Average sentence length: " << fixed << setprecision(2)
        << float(wordCounter) / sentenceCounter << endl;

}


//*****************************************************************


void ProcessCharacter
    ( /* in  */    char character,        // Character to be
                                          // processed
      /* inout */ int& uppercaseCounter,  // Uppercase letters
      /* inout */ int& lowercaseCounter,  // Lowercase letters
```

```
    /* inout */ int& digitCounter,       // Digits
    /* inout */ int& sentenceCounter,    // '.', '?', '!'
    /* inout */ int& wordCounter,        // Words
    /* inout */ int& ignoreCounter )     // Everything else

// Function ProcessCharacter examines character and increments the
// appropriate counter.
// Postcondition:
//     The category to which the character belongs has been
//     incremented

{
    static bool endOfWord = false;

    switch (Decode(character))
    {
        case UPPER :  uppercaseCounter++;
                      endOfWord = false;
                      break;
        case LOWER :  lowercaseCounter++;
                      endOfWord = false;
                      break;
        case DIGIT :  digitCounter++;
                      endOfWord = false;
                      break;
        case EOW   :  if (!endOfWord)
                      {
                          wordCounter++;
                          endOfWord = true;
                      }
                      break;
        case EOS   :  sentenceCounter++;
                      break;
        case IGNORE:  ignoreCounter++;
                      break;
    }
}
```

TESTING   Let's take a sample of text, calculate the statistics by hand, and compare the results with the output from the program.

Input

The Abacus (which appeared in the sixteenth century) was the first calculator. In the middle of the seventeenth century Blaise Pascal, a French mathematician, built and sold gear-driven mechanical machines which performed whole number addition and subtraction. (Yes, the language Pascal is named for him.)

Later in the seventeenth century a German mathematician Gottfried Wilhelm von Leibniz built the first mechanical device designed to do all four whole number operations: addition, subtraction, multiplication and division. The state of mechanical gears and levers at that time was such that the Leibniz machine was not very reliable.

Output from the program:

```
TempHistory.out - Notepad                                    _ □ X
File  Edit  Format  View  Help
Analysis of characters on input file TempHistory.in

Total number of alphanumeric characters: 527
Number of uppercase letters: 15
Number of lowercase letters: 512
Number of digits: 0
Number of characters ignored: 5
Number of words: 100
Number of Sentences: 5
Average word length: 5.27
Average sentence length: 20.00
```

The number of words, average word length, and average sentence length is wrong. You recount the number of words and again come up with 96. You took care of the case where end-of-sentence markers end words by adding the number of sentences to the number of words. But endOfWord wasn't set when end-of-sentence markers were found. You correct the problem in function ProcessCharacter like this:

```
case EOS    :   sentenceCounter++;
                endOfWord = true;
                break;
```

You rerun the program and get this output.

```
temp5.out - Notepad
File  Edit  Format  View  Help
Analysis of characters on input file tempHis.in

Total number of alphanumeric characters: 527
Number of uppercase letters: 15
Number of lowercase letters: 512
Number of digits: 0
Number of characters ignored: 5
Number of words: 95
Number of Sentences: 5
Average word length: 5.55
Average sentence length: 19.00
```

The number of words is still off by one. Now you see it. You counted "gear-driven" as two words; the program counts it as one. You are asked to examine a solution to this problem in the Case Study Follow-Up Exercises.

Testing and Debugging

Floating-Point Data

When a problem requires the use of floating-point numbers that are extremely large, small, or precise, it is important to keep in mind the limitations of the particular system you are using. When testing a program that performs floating-point calculations, determine the acceptable margin of error beforehand, and then design your test data to try to push the program beyond those limits. Carefully check the accuracy of the computed results. (Remember that when you hand-calculate the correct results, a pocket calculator may have *less* precision than your computer system.) If the program produces acceptable results when given worst-case data, it probably performs correctly on typical data.

Coping with Input Errors

Several times in this book, we've had our programs test for invalid data and write an error message. Writing an error message is certainly necessary, but it is only the first step. We must also decide what the program should do next. The problem itself and the severity of the error should determine what action is taken in any error condition. The approach taken also depends on whether or not the program is being run interactively.

In a program that reads its data only from an input file, there is no interaction with the person who entered the data. The program, therefore, should try to adjust for the bad data items, if at all possible.

If the invalid data item is not essential, the program can skip it and continue; for example, if a program averaging test grades encounters a negative test score, it could simply skip the negative score. If an educated guess can be made about the probable value of the bad data, it can be set to that value before being processed. In either event, a message should be written stating that an invalid data item was encountered and outlining the steps that were taken. Such messages form an *exception report*.

If the data item is essential and no guess is possible, processing should be terminated. A message should be written to the user with as much information as possible about the invalid data item.

In an interactive environment, the program can prompt the user to supply another value. The program should indicate to the user what is wrong with the original data. Another possibility is to write out a list of actions and ask the user to choose among them.

These suggestions on how to handle bad data assume that the program recognizes bad data values. There are two approaches to error detection: passive and active. Passive error detection leaves it to the system to detect errors. This may seem easier, but the programmer relinquishes control of processing when an error occurs. An example of passive error detection is the system's division-by-zero error.

Active error detection means having the program check for possible errors and determine an appropriate action if an error occurs. An example of active error detection would be to read a value and use an If statement to see if the value is 0 before dividing it into another number.

Testing and Debugging Hints

1. Avoid using unnecessary side effects in expressions. The test

   ```
   if ((x = y) < z)
       ⋮
   ```

   is less clear and more prone to error than the equivalent sequence of statements

   ```
   x = y;
   if (y < z)
       ⋮
   ```

   Also, if you accidentally omit the parentheses around the assignment operation, like this:

   ```
   if (x = y < z)
   ```

   then, according to C++ operator precedence, x is *not* assigned the value of y. It is assigned the value 1 or 0 (the coerced value of the Boolean result of the relational expression y < z).

2. Programs that rely on a particular machine's character set may not run correctly on another machine. Check to see what character-handling functions are supplied by

the standard library. Functions such as `tolower`, `toupper`, `isalpha`, and `iscntrl` automatically account for the character set being used.

3. Don't directly compare floating-point values for equality. Instead, check them for near equality. The tolerance for near equality depends on the particular problem you are solving.

4. Use integers if you are dealing with whole numbers only. Any integer can be represented exactly by the computer, as long as it is within the machine's allowable range of values. Also, integer arithmetic is faster than floating-point arithmetic on most machines.

5. Be aware of representational, cancellation, overflow, and underflow errors. If possible, try to arrange calculations in your program to keep floating-point numbers from becoming too large or too small.

6. If your program increases the value of a positive integer and the result suddenly becomes a negative number, you should suspect integer overflow. On most computers, adding 1 to `INT_MAX` yields `INT_MIN`, a negative number.

7. Except when you really need to, avoid mixing data types in expressions, assignment operations, argument passing, and the return of a function value. If you must mix types, explicit type casts can prevent unwelcome surprises caused by implicit type coercion.

8. Consider using enumeration types to make your programs more readable, understandable, and modifiable.

9. Avoid anonymous data typing. Give each user-defined type a name.

10. Enumeration type values cannot be input or output directly.

11. Type demotion can lead to decreased precision or corruption of data.

Summary

A data type is a set of values (the domain) along with the operations that can be applied to those values. Simple data types are data types whose values are atomic (indivisible).

The integral types in C++ are `char`, `short`, `int`, `long`, and `bool`. The most commonly used integral types are `int` and `char`. The `char` type can be used for storing small (usually one-byte) numeric integers or, more often, for storing character data. Character data includes both printable and nonprintable characters. Nonprintable characters—those that control the behavior of hardware devices—are expressed in C++ as escape sequences such as `\n`. Each character is represented internally as a nonnegative integer according to the particular character set (such as ASCII or EBCDIC) that a computer uses.

The floating-point types built into the C++ language are `float`, `double`, and `long double`. Floating-point numbers are represented in the computer with a mantissa and an exponent. This representation permits numbers that are much larger or much smaller than those that can be represented with the integral types. Floating-point representation also allows us to perform calculations on numbers with fractional parts.

However, there are drawbacks to using floating-point numbers in arithmetic calculations. Representational errors, for example, can affect the accuracy of a program's computations. When using floating-point numbers, keep in mind that if two numbers are vastly different from each other in size, adding or subtracting them can produce the wrong answer. Remember, also, that the computer has a limited range of numbers that it can represent. If a program tries to compute a value that is too large or too small, an error message may result when the program executes.

C++ allows the programmer to define additional data types. The Typedef statement is a simple mechanism for renaming an existing type, although the result is not truly a new data type. An enumeration type, created by listing the identifiers that make up the domain, is a new data type that is distinct from any existing type. Values of an enumeration type may be assigned, compared in relational expressions, used as case labels in a Switch statement, passed as arguments, and returned as function values. Enumeration types are extremely useful in the writing of clear, self-documenting programs. In succeeding chapters, we look at language features that let us create even more powerful user-defined types.

Quick Check

1. Is `bool` considered an integral type or an enum type? (pp. 452–455)
2. What is the difference between the `&&` operator and the `&` operator? (pp. 456–460)
3. How do we represent nonprintable characters as literals in a C++ program? (pp. 464–468)
4. If we were to enlarge the exponent portion of a floating-point representation, what part of the representation would shrink, and what would be the effect of this change? (pp. 475–481)
5. What do we call the error that results when the precision of a calculation is greater than what the precision of the computer can support? (pp. 478–479)
6. If we assign an `int` to a `long`, is the type conversion a promotion or a demotion? (pp. 495–499)
7. Would you use an `int` or a `long` to represent a social security number? (pp. 450–452)
8. Write an enumeration type definition for the four seasons. (pp. 486–493)
9. Write a For loop heading that iterates through the Seasons type defined in Quick Check question 8. (pp. 489–490)
10. Can an anonymous user-defined type be a parameter in a function? (pp. 493–494)
11. In an include directive, how is the file name of a header file in the current directory written differently from the name of a header file in the standard include directory? (pp. 494–495)

Answers

1. It is an integral type.   2. `&&` is a logical AND of a pair of `bool` values, while `&` is a bitwise AND of a pair of integral values.   3. Using escape sequences, or by using their integer values.   4. The mantissa would shrink. The change would increase the range of the representation but decrease its precision.   5. Representational error.   6. A promotion.   7. A `long`, unless the system supports 64-bit `int` values.   8. `enum Seasons {SPRING, SUMMER, WINTER, AUTUMN};`
9. `for (quarter = SPRING;`
      `quarter <= AUTUMN;`
      `quarter = Seasons(quarter + 1))`
10. No.   11. It is enclosed in quotes rather than angle braces.

Exam Preparation Exercises

1. All of the integral types in C++ can be signed or unsigned. True or false?
2. The difference between an assignment expression and an assignment statement is a semicolon. True or false?
3. The sizeof operator can be used to determine whether a machine's `int` type is 32 or 64 bits long. True or false?
4. Floating point numbers are seldom exactly equal. True or false?
5. The values of enumerator types must be written in uppercase letters. True or false?
6. What are the five integral types in C++?
7. What happens if the leading digit of an integer literal is a zero? What if the zero is followed by an X?
8. Which group of C++ operators has the lowest precedence of all?
9. What is the difference in effect of writing `count++` versus `++count`?
10. In what situation is it necessary to use prefix notation for the cast operation instead of functional notation?
11. What functions could you use to simplify the following expression?

    `(reply == 'N' || reply == 'n' || reply == 'Y' || reply == 'y')`

12. If `string` variable `name` contains `"Abigail"`, what does the expression `name[3]` equal?
13. If a computer has a floating point type with five digits of decimal precision, and a one-digit exponent, what would be the result of adding 3.8281×10^4 and 2.4531×10^0?
14. Explain the difference between relative and absolute error in comparing two floating point numbers for equality.
15. What is wrong with the following pair of enumeration type declarations?

    `enum Colors {RED, ORANGE, YELLOW, GREEN, BLUE, INDIGO, VIOLET};`
    `enum Flowers{ROSE, DAFFODIL, LILY, VIOLET, COSMOS, ORCHID};`

16. Given the declaration of Colors in Exercise 15, what is the value of the expression `(YELLOW + 1)`?

17. Given the code segment:

```
enum Flowers{ROSE, DAFFODIL, LILY, VIOLET, COSMOS, ORCHID};
Flowers choice;
choice = LILY;
choice++;
```

Why does the compiler give an invalid type error message for the last line?

18. Why is it impossible to use an anonymous type with a function parameter?

Programming Warm-Up Exercises

1. Write the integer value 5
   a. as a literal of type int
   b. as a literal of type long
   c. as a literal of type unsigned long
   d. in base 8 (octal)
   e. in base 16 (hexadecimal)
2. Write the floating point value 3.14159265
   a. as a literal of type float
   b. as a literal of type double
   c. as a literal of type long double
   d. as a literal of type double using an exponent of 0.
3. Write assignment expression statements that do the following:
   a. add 7 to the variable days
   b. multiply the value in variable radius by 6.2831853
   c. subtract 40 from variable workHours
   d. divide variable average by variable count
4. Write an expression whose result is the number of bits in a value of type long.
5. Use the C++ precedence rules to remove any unnecessary parentheses from the following expressions:
   a. `((a * b) + (c * d))`
   b. `((a * b) / (c * d))`
   c. `((a + b) + ((c / (d + e)) * f))`
   d. `(((a + b) / (c + d)) * (e + f))`
   e. `((-a + b) <= (c * d)) && ((a + b) >= (c - d))`
6. Write a code segment that inputs a character, and if it is a numeric character, converts it to an int value.
7. Write a For loop that scans through a string called inLine, counting the occurrences of the character 'e'.
8. Write a value-returning function with a nested Switch statement that returns the number corresponding to a month name that is supplied via a string parameter. The month name may be in uppercase or lowercase, or a mixture.
9. Write an If statement that adds 12 to hour if the first letter in string ampm is a 'P' or a 'p'.

10. Write an expression that returns `true` if the float variable `balance` is equal to `audit` with an absolute error of 0.001 or less.
11. Write an expression that returns `true` if the float variable `year` is equal to `epoch` within 0.00001% of the value in `epoch`. (Think carefully here.)
12. Declare an enumeration type consisting of the nine planets in their order by distance from the Sun (Mercury first, Pluto last).
13. Write a value-returning function that converts the name of a planet given as a `string` parameter to a value of the enumeration type declared in Exercise 12. If the string isn't a proper planet name, return EARTH.
14. Write a value-returning function that converts a planet of the enumeration type declared in Exercise 12 into the corresponding string. The planet is an input parameter and the string is returned by the function. If the input is not a valid planet, return `"Error"`.
15. Write a For statement that prints out the names of the planets in order, using the enumeration type declared in Exercise 12, and the function declared in Exercise 14.

Programming Problems

1. Programming Problem 2 in Chapter 4 asked you write a C++ program that asks the user to enter their weight and the name of a planet. In Chapter 9, Programming Problem 2 asked you to rewrite the program using a Switch statement. Now, rewrite the program so it uses an enumerated type to represent the planet. If you did Programming Warm-Up Exercises 12 through 15, this rewrite should be quite easy.

For ease of reference, the information for the original problem is repeated here. The following table gives the factor by which the weight must be multiplied for each planet. The program should output an error message if the user doesn't type a correct planet name. The prompt and the error message should make it clear to the user how a planet name must be entered. Be sure to use proper formatting and appropriate comments in your code. The output should be clearly labeled and neatly formatted.

Mercury	0.4155
Venus	0.8975
Earth	1.0
Moon	0.166
Mars	0.3507
Jupiter	2.5374
Saturn	1.0677
Uranus	0.8947
Neptune	1.1794
Pluto	0.0899

2. Programming Problem 3 in Chapter 9 asked you to write a program that generates sales-report files for a set of traveling salespeople. There, we used an integer in the range of 1 through 10 to represent ID numbers for the salespeople. Rewrite the program so that it uses an enumeration type whose values are the names of the salespeople (you can make up the names). The sales file format should replace the salesperson ID number with a string that is the person's last name, so that a line of the file contains a name, an item number, and a quantity. For convenience, the other information concerning the problem is repeated here.

The company sells eight different products, with ID's of 7 through 14 (some older products have been discontinued). The unit prices of the products are:

Product Number	Unit Price
7	345.00
8	853.00
9	471.00
10	933.00
11	721.00
12	663.00
13	507.00
14	259.00

The program reads in the sales file, and generates a separate file for each salesperson containing just his or her sales. Each line from the sales file is copied to the appropriate salesperson file, with the salesperson name omitted. The file names should be the name of the salesperson with .dat appended (you may have to adjust names that don't work as filenames on your computer, such as hyphenated names or names with apostrophes). The total for the sale (quantity times unit price) is appended to the record. At the end of processing, the total sales for each salesperson should be output with informative labels to cout. Use functional decomposition to design the program. Be sure that the program handles invalid salesperson names. If a salesperson name is invalid, write out an error message to cout. If a product number is invalid, write the error message to the salesperson's file and don't compute a total for the sale.

3. You are taking a geology class and the professor wants you to write a program to help students learn the periods of geologic time. The program should let the user enter a range of prehistoric dates (in millions of years), and then output the periods that are included in that range. Each time this is done, the user is asked if they want to continue. The goal of the exercise is for the student to try to figure out when each period began, so that he or she can make a chart of geologic time. Within the program, represent the periods with an enumeration type made up of their names. You will probably want to create a function that determines the period corresponding to a date, and another that returns the string corre-

sponding to each identifier in the enumeration. Then you can use a For loop to output the series of periods in the range. The periods of geologic time are:

Period Name	Starting Date (millions of years)
Quaternary	2.5
Tertiary	65
Cretaceous	136
Jurassic	192
Triassic	225
Permian	280
Carboniferous	345
Devonian	395
Silurian	435
Ordovician	500
Cambrian	570
Precambrian	4500 or earlier

Use functional decomposition to solve the problem. Be sure to use good coding style and documenting comments. The prompts and error messages that are output should be clear and informative.

4. The educational program that you wrote for Problem 4 was a big success. The geology professor wants you to write another program to help teach geologic time. In this program, the computer picks a date in geologic time and presents it to the student. The student guesses which period corresponds to the date. The student is allowed to continue guessing until he or she gets the right answer. Then the program asks the student whether he or she wants to try again, and repeats the process if the answer is "yes." You should again use an enumeration type consisting of the names of the periods. In this case, you'll probably want to make a function that returns the period corresponding to a string containing the name of a period (the program should work with any style of capitalization of the names). You also may want a function that returns the period for a given date.

Use functional design to solve the problem. Be sure to use good coding style and documenting comments. The prompts, and error messages that are output should be clear and informative. You may want to add some interest to the program by keeping track of the number of guesses taken by the user, and offering differing levels of praise and encouragement depending on how well the user is doing.

5. Write a C++ program that determines the largest number for which your computer can represent its factorial exactly using the `long double` type. The factorial is the product of all numbers from one to the given number. For example, ten factorial (written 10!) is:

$$1 * 2 * 3 * 4 * 5 * 6 * 7 * 8 * 9 * 10 = 3628800$$

As you can see, the factorial grows to be a large number very quickly. Your program should keep multiplying the prior factorial by the next integer, then subtract one and check whether the difference between the factorial and the factorial minus one is less than one—an error tolerance. When the maximum precision of the type is reached, and least significant digits are truncated to allow the most significant digits of the product to be stored, then subtracting one should have no effect on the value. Because floating point representations may not be exact, however, the expression

```
abs((number - 1) - number)
```

may not exactly equal 1. That's why you need to include a small error tolerance in the comparison.

Use functional decomposition to solve the problem. Code the program using good style and documenting comments. To keep the user informed of progress, you may wish to output all of the intermediate factorial values. The greatest number and its factorial should be clearly labeled as such.

Case Study Follow-Up

1. In the Style program, modules ProcessCharacter and PrintTable take six counters as parameters, making a very long parameter list. Could this have been handled any other way?
2. How could you determine whether a hyphen should be counted as an end-of-word symbol or a break in the word due to spacing?
3. Implement the change outlined in your answer to Exercise 2.
4. endOfWord is reset to false every time an alphanumeric character is read. Thus, it is being set to itself over and over again. Can you think of a scheme that would allow you to set it only once?
5. Should error detection be added to program Style? Explain.

Structured Types, Data Abstraction, and Classes

Knowledge Goals

- *To understand the general concept of a C++ union type.*
- *To understand the difference between specification and implementation of an abstract data type.*
- *To understand how encapsulation and information hiding are enforced by the C++ compiler.*

Skill Goals

To be able to:

- *Declare a* `struct` *(record) data type, a data structure whose components may be heterogeneous.*
- *Access a member of a* `struct` *variable.*
- *Define a hierarchical record structure.*
- *Access values stored in a hierarchical record.*
- *Declare a C++* `class` *type.*
- *Declare class objects, given the declaration of a* `class` *type.*
- *Write client code that invokes class member functions.*
- *Implement class member functions.*
- *Organize the code for a C++ class into two files: the specification (* `.h` *) file and the implementation file.*
- *Write a C++ class constructor.*

In the last chapter, we examined the concept of a data type and looked at how to define simple data types. In this chapter, we expand the definition of a data type to include structured types, which represent collections of components that are referred to by a single name. We begin with a discussion of structured types in general and then examine two structured types provided by the C++ language: the struct and the union.

Next, we introduce the concept of *data abstraction,* the separation of a data type's logical properties from its implementation. Data abstraction is important because it allows us to create data types not otherwise available in a programming language. Another benefit of data abstraction is the ability to produce *off-the-shelf software*—pieces of software that can be used over and over again in different programs either by the creator of the software or by any programmer wishing to use them.

The primary concept for practicing data abstraction is the *abstract data type.* In this chapter, we examine abstract data types in depth and introduce the C++ language feature designed expressly for creating abstract data types: the *class*. We conclude with two case studies that demonstrate data abstraction, abstract data types, and C++ classes.

11.1 Simple Versus Structured Data Types

In Chapter 10, we examined simple, or atomic, data types. A value in a simple type is a single data item; it cannot be broken down into component parts. For example, each int value is a single integer number and cannot be further decomposed. In contrast, a **structured data type** is one in which each value is a *collection* of component items. The entire collection is given a single name, yet each component can still be accessed individually. An example of a structured data type in C++ is the string class, used for creating and manipulating strings. When you declare a variable myString to be of type string, myString does not represent just one atomic data value; it represents an entire collection of characters. But each of the components in the string can be accessed individually (by using an expression such as my-String[3], which accesses the char value at position 3).

> **Structured data type** A data type in which each value is a collection of components and whose organization is characterized by the method used to access individual components. The allowable operations on a structured data type include the storage and retrieval of individual components.

Simple data types, both built-in and user-defined, are the building blocks for structured types. A structured type gathers together a set of component values and usually imposes a specific arrangement on them (see Figure 11–1). The method used to access the individual components of a structured type depends on how the components are arranged. As we discuss various ways of structuring data, we look at the corresponding access mechanisms.

Figure 11–2 shows the structured types available in C++. This figure is a portion of the complete diagram presented in Figure 3–1.

In this chapter, we examine the struct, union, and class types. Array data types are the topic of Chapter 12.

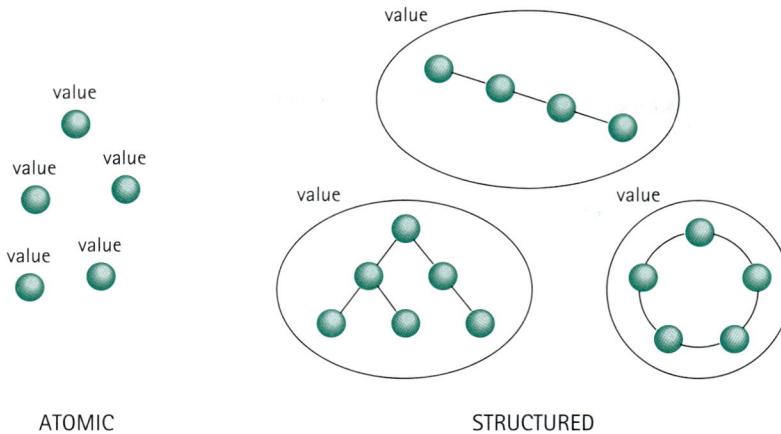

Figure 11–1   *Atomic (Simple) and Structured Data Types*

11.2 Records (Structs)

In computer science, a **record** is a heterogeneous structured data type. By *heterogeneous*, we mean that the individual components of a record can be of different data types. Each component of a record is called a **field** of the record, and each field is given a name called the *field name.* C++ uses its own terminology with records. A record is called a **structure**, the fields of a record are called **members** of the structure, and each member has a *member name.**

> **Record (structure, in C++)**   A structured data type with a fixed number of components that are accessed by name. The components may be heterogeneous (of different types).
>
> **Field (member, in C++)**   A component of a record.

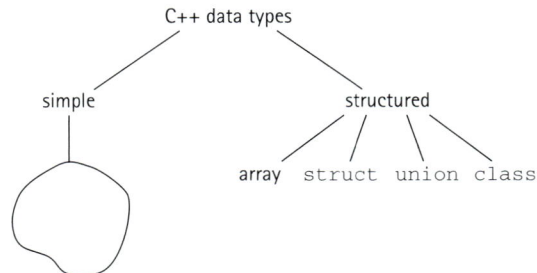

Figure 11–2   *C++ Structured Types*

---

*Technically, a C++ struct is almost identical to the class type that we introduce later in this chapter. However, in C a struct has the properties of a record, and most C++ programmers continue to use the struct in its traditional role of directly representing a record. In this book we retain this standard practice.

In C++, record data types are most commonly declared according to the following syntax:

StructDeclaration

```
struct TypeName
{
    MemberList
};
```

where TypeName is an identifier giving a name to the data type, and MemberList is defined as

MemberList

```
DataType MemberName ;
DataType MemberName ;
    ⋮
```

The reserved word struct is an abbreviation for *structure*. Because the word *structure* has many other meanings in computer science, we'll use *struct* or *record* to avoid any possible confusion about what we are referring to.

You probably recognize the syntax of a member list as being nearly identical to a series of variable declarations. Be careful: A struct declaration is a type declaration, and we still must declare variables of this type for any memory locations to be associated with the member names. As an example, let's use a struct to describe a student in a class. We want to store the first and last names, the overall grade point average prior to this class, the grade on programming assignments, the grade on quizzes, the final exam grade, and the final course grade.

```
// Type declarations

enum GradeType {A, B, C, D, F};

struct StudentRec
{
    string     firstName;
    string     lastName;
    float      gpa;              // Grade point average
    int        programGrade;     // Assume 0..400
    int        quizGrade;        // Assume 0..300
    int        finalExam;        // Assume 0..300
    GradeType  courseGrade;
};

// Variable declarations
```

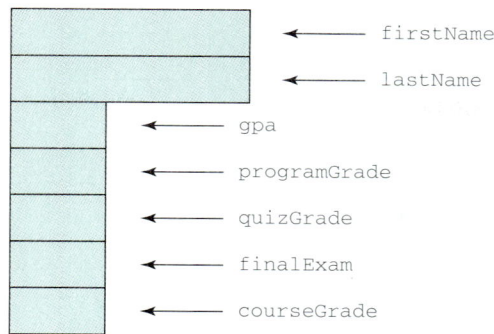

Figure 11–3   *Pattern for a Struct*

```
StudentRec  firstStudent;
StudentRec  student;
int         grade;
```

Notice, both in this example and in the syntax template, that a `struct` declaration ends with a semicolon. By now, you have learned not to put a semicolon after the right brace of a compound statement (block). However, the member list in a `struct` declaration is not considered to be a compound statement; the braces are simply required syntax in the declaration. A `struct` declaration, like all C++ declaration statements, must end with a semicolon.

`firstName`, `lastName`, `gpa`, `programGrade`, `quizGrade`, `finalExam`, and `courseGrade` are member names within the `struct` type `StudentRec`. These member names make up the member list. Note that each member name is given a type. Also, member names must be unique within a `struct` type, just as variable names must be unique within a block.

`firstName` and `lastName` are of type `string`. `gpa` is a `float` member. `programGrade`, `quizGrade`, and `finalExam` are `int` members. `courseGrade` is of an enumeration data type made up of the grades A through D and F.

None of these struct members are associated with memory locations until we declare a variable of the `StudentRec` type. `StudentRec` is merely a pattern for a struct (see Figure 11–3). The variables `firstStudent` and `student` are variables of type `StudentRec`.

Accessing Individual Components

To access an individual member of a struct variable, you give the name of the variable, followed by a dot (period), and then the member name. This expression is called a **member selector**. The syntax template is

> **Member selector**   The expression used to access components of a struct variable. It is formed by using the struct variable name and the member name, separated by a dot (period).

MemberSelector

> StructVariable . MemberName

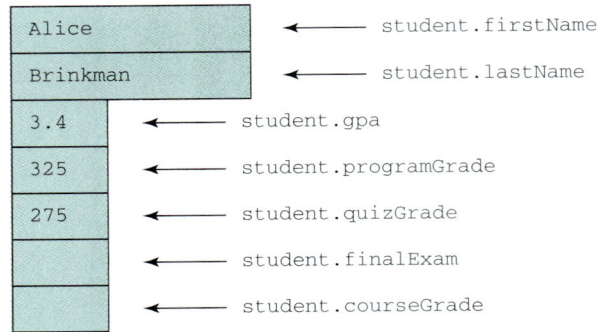

Figure 11–4   *Struct Variable* student *with Member Selectors*

This syntax for selecting individual components of a struct is often called *dot notation*. To access the grade point average of firstStudent, we would write

firstStudent.gpa

To access the final exam score of student, we would write

student.finalExam

The component of a struct accessed by the member selector is treated just like any other variable of the same type. It may be used in an assignment statement, passed as an argument, and so on. Figure 11–4 shows the struct variable student with the member selector for each member. In this example, we assume that some processing has already taken place, so values are stored in some of the components.

Let's demonstrate the use of these member selectors. Using our student variable, the following code segment reads in a final exam grade; adds up the program grade, the quiz grade, and the final exam grade; and then assigns a letter grade to the result.

```
cin >> student.finalExam;
grade = student.finalExam + student.programGrade +
        student.quizGrade;
if (grade >= 900)
    student.courseGrade = A;
else if (grade >= 800)
    student.courseGrade = B;
else   .
       .
       .
```

Aggregate Operations on Structs

In addition to accessing individual components of a struct variable, we can in some
cases use **aggregate operations**. An aggregate
operation is one that manipulates the struct
as an entire unit.

> **Aggregate operation**   An operation on a data structure as a whole, as opposed to an operation on an individual component of the data structure.

The following table summarizes the
aggregate operations that are allowed on struct variables.

Aggregate Operation	Allowed on Structs?
I/O	No
Assignment	Yes
Arithmetic	No
Comparison	No
Argument passage	Yes, by value or by reference
Return as a function's return value	Yes

According to the table, one struct variable can be assigned to another. However, both
variables must be declared to be of the same type. For example, given the declarations

```
StudentRec student;
StudentRec anotherStudent;
```

the statement

```
anotherStudent = student;
```

copies the entire contents of the struct variable `student` to the variable `anotherStu-
dent`, member by member.

On the other hand, aggregate arithmetic operations and comparisons are not
allowed (primarily because they wouldn't make sense):

```
student = student * anotherStudent;     // Not allowed
if (student < anotherStudent)           // Not allowed
```

Furthermore, aggregate I/O is not permitted:

```
cin >> student;                         // Not allowed
```

We must input or output a struct variable one member at a time:

```
cin >> student.firstName;
cin >> student.lastName;
⋮
```

According to the table, an entire struct can be passed as an argument, either by value or by reference, and a struct can be returned as the value of a value-returning function. Let's define a function that takes a `StudentRec` variable as a parameter.

The task of this function is to determine if a student's grade in a course is consistent with his or her overall grade point average (GPA). We define *consistent* to mean that the course grade corresponds correctly to the rounded GPA. The GPA is calculated on a four-point scale, where A is 4, B is 3, C is 2, D is 1, and F is 0. If the rounded GPA is 4 and the course grade is A, then the function returns `true`. If the rounded GPA is 4 and the course grade is not A, then the function returns `false`. Each of the other grades is tested in the same way.

The `Consistent` function is coded below. The parameter `aStudent`, a struct variable of type `StudentRec`, is passed by value.

```cpp
bool Consistent( /* in */ StudentRec aStudent )

// Precondition:
//      0.0 <= aStudent.gpa <= 4.0
// Postcondition:
//      Function value == true, if the course grade is consistent
//                                  with the overall GPA
//                        == false, otherwise

{
    int roundedGPA = int(aStudent.gpa + 0.5);

    switch (roundedGPA)
    {
        case 0: return (aStudent.courseGrade == F);
        case 1: return (aStudent.courseGrade == D);
        case 2: return (aStudent.courseGrade == C);
        case 3: return (aStudent.courseGrade == B);
        case 4: return (aStudent.courseGrade == A);
    }
}
```

More About Struct Declarations

To complete our initial look at C++ structs, we give a more complete syntax template for a `struct` type declaration:

StructDeclaration

```
struct TypeName
{
    MemberList
} VariableList ;
```

As you can see in the syntax template, two items are optional: TypeName (the name of the `struct` type being declared), and VariableList (a list of variable names between the right brace and the semicolon). Our examples thus far have declared a type name but have not included a variable list. The variable list allows you not only to declare a `struct` type but also to declare variables of that type, all in one statement. For example, you could write the declarations

```
struct StudentRec
{
    string firstName;
    string lastName;
      ⋮
};

StudentRec firstStudent;
StudentRec student;
```

more compactly in the form

```
struct StudentRec
{
    string firstName;
    string lastName;
      ⋮
} firstStudent, student;
```

In this book, we avoid combining variable declarations with type declarations, preferring to keep the two notions separate.

If you omit the type name but include the variable list, you create an anonymous type:

```
struct
{
    int    firstMember;
    float secondMember;
} someVar;
```

Here, `someVar` is a variable of an anonymous type. No other variables of that type can be declared because the type has no name. Therefore, `someVar` cannot participate in aggregate operations such as assignment or argument passage. The cautions given in Chapter 10 against anonymous typing of enumeration types apply to `struct` types as well.

Binding Like Items

In Chapters 9 and 10, we had a number of counters that had to be passed to two separate functions. For example, here is the call to the `ProcessCharacter` function in Chapter 10:

```
ProcessCharacter(character, uppercaseCounter,
    lowercaseCounter, digitCounter, sentenceCounter,
    wordCounter, ignoreCounter);
```

We can make the interface much simpler if we bind these counters together into a record as follows:

```
struct Counters
{
    int uppercaseCounter;
    int lowercaseCounter;
    int digitCounter;
    int sentenceCounter;
    int wordCounter;
    int ignoreCounter;
};
```

The prototypes for `ProcessCharacter` and `PrintTable` become

```
Counters counters;
void ProcessCharacter
        ( /* in */     char character,        // Character to be processed
          /* inout */ Counters& counters );// Category counters
void PrintTable
        ( /* inout */ ofstream& table,       // Output file
          /* inout */ Counters counters);   // Category counters
```

In fact, we can make the code simpler yet by adding a function to initialize the counters.

```
void InitializeCounters
        ( /* inout */ Counters& counters);  // Category counters
```

Of course the bodies of `ProcessCharacter` and `PrintTable` will have to be rewritten, and the body of `InitializeCounters` will have to be written. We won't take the space to show all of this code, but from the implementation of `Initialize-Counters` shown here, you can see the kinds of changes that are necessary in the other functions.

```
void InitializeCounters
        ( /* inout */ Counters& counters) // Category counters
// Counters for different categories are set to zero
// Postcondition:
//      Each field in struct variable counters has been set to zero
```

```
{
    counters.uppercaseCounter = 0;
    counters.lowercaseCounter = 0;
    counters.digitCounter = 0;
    counters.wordCounter = 0;
    counters.sentenceCounter = 0;
    counters.ignoreCounter = 0;
}
```

See how much simpler the code for the main function becomes?

```
int main()
{
    // Prepare files for reading and writing
    ifstream text;
    ofstream table;
    OpenFiles(text, table);
    if ( !text || !table)
    {
        cout << "Files did not open successfully." << endl;
        return 1;
    }
    char character;                 // Input character
    Counters counters;              // Contains category counters
    InitializeCounters(counters);   // Sets counters to zero
    text.get(character);            // Input one character
    do
    { // Process each character
        ProcessCharacter(character, counters);
        text.get(character);        // Input one character
    } while (text);
    PrintTable(table, counters);
    text.close();
    table.close();
    return 0;
}
```

Hierarchical Records

We have seen examples in which the components of a record are simple variables and
strings. A component of a record can also be
another record. Records whose components
are themselves records are called hierarchical
records.

> **Hierarchical record**   A record in which at least one of the components is itself a record.

Let's look at an example in which a hierarchical structure is appropriate. A small
machine shop keeps information about each of its machines. There is descriptive

information, such as the identification number, a description of the machine, the purchase date, and the cost. Statistical information is also kept, such as the number of down days, the failure rate, and the date of last service. What is a reasonable way of representing all this information? First, let's look at a flat (nonhierarchical) record structure that holds this information.

```
struct MachineRec
{
    int     idNumber;
    string  description;
    float   failRate;
    int     lastServicedMonth;  // Assume 1..12
    int     lastServicedDay;    // Assume 1..31
    int     lastServicedYear;   // Assume 1900..2050
    int     downDays;
    int     purchaseDateMonth;  // Assume 1..12
    int     purchaseDateDay;    // Assume 1..31
    int     purchaseDateYear;   // Assume 1900..2050
    float   cost;
};
```

The `MachineRec` type has 11 members. There is so much detailed information here that it is difficult to quickly get a feeling for what the record represents. Let's see if we can reorganize it into a hierarchical structure that makes more sense. We can divide the information into two groups: information that changes and information that does not. There are also two dates to be kept: date of purchase and date of last service. These observations suggest use of a record describing a date, a record describing the statistical data, and an overall record containing the other two as components. The following type declarations reflect this structure.

```
struct Date
{
    int month;  // Assume 1..12
    int day;    // Assume 1..31
    int year;   // Assume 1900..2050
};
struct Statistics
{
    float   failRate;
    Date    lastServiced;
    int     downDays;
};
```

```
struct MachineRec
{
    int             idNumber;
    string          description;
    Statistics      history;
    Date            purchaseDate;
    float           cost;
};


MachineRec machine;
```

The contents of a machine record are now much more obvious. Two of the components of the `struct` type `MachineRec` are themselves structs: `purchaseDate` is of `struct` type `Date`, and `history` is of `struct` type `Statistics`. One of the components of `struct` type `Statistics` is a struct of type `Date`.

How do we access the components of a hierarchical structure such as this one? We build the accessing expressions (member selectors) for the members of the embedded structs from left to right, beginning with the struct variable name. Here are some expressions and the components they access:

Expression	Component Accessed
`machine.purchaseDate`	`Date` struct variable
`machine.purchaseDate.month`	`month` member of a `Date` struct variable
`machine.purchaseDate.year`	`year` member of a `Date` struct variable
`machine.history.lastServiced.year`	`year` member of a `Date` struct variable contained in a struct of type `Statistics`

Figure 11–5 is a pictorial representation of `machine` with values. Look carefully at how each component is accessed.

11.3 Unions

In Figure 11–2, we presented a diagram showing the four structured types available in C++. We have discussed `struct` types and now look briefly at *union* types.

In C++, a union is defined to be a struct that holds only one of its members at a time during program execution. Here is a declaration of a `union` type and a union variable:

```
union WeightType
{
    long  wtInOunces;
```

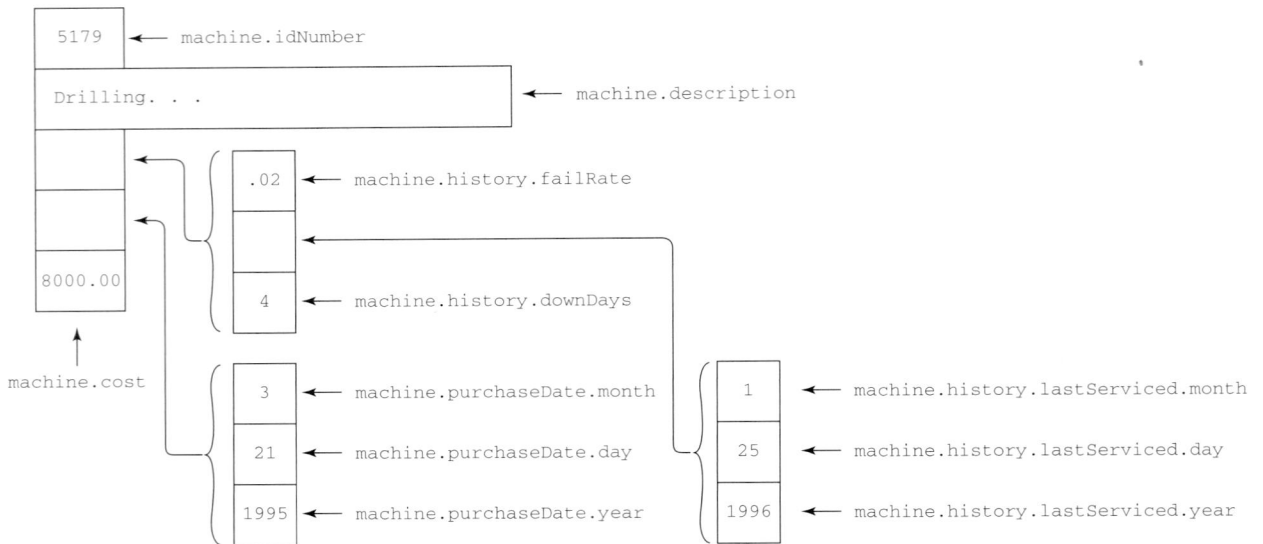

Figure 11–5   *Hierarchical Records in* machine *Variable*

```
    int    wtInPounds;
    float  wtInTons;
};
```

```
WeightType weight;
```

The syntax for declaring a union type is identical to the syntax that we showed earlier for the struct type, except that the word union is substituted for struct.

At run time, the memory space allocated to the variable weight does *not* include room for three distinct components. Instead, weight can contain only one of the following: *either* a long value *or* an int value *or* a float value. The assumption is that the program will never need a weight in ounces, a weight in pounds, and a weight in tons simultaneously while executing. The purpose of a union is to conserve memory by forcing several values to use the same memory space, one at a time. The following code shows how the weight variable might be used.

```
weight.wtInTons = 4.83;
    ⋮
// Weight in tons is no longer needed. Reuse the memory space.

weight.wtInPounds = 35;
    ⋮
```

After the last assignment statement, the previous `float` value 4.83 is gone, replaced by the `int` value 35.

It's quite reasonable to argue that a union is not a data structure at all. It does not represent a collection of values; it represents only a single value from among several *potential* values. On the other hand, unions are grouped together with the structured types because of their similarity to structs.

There is much more to be said about unions, including subtle issues related to their declaration and usage. However, these issues are more appropriate in an advanced study of data structures and systems programming. We have introduced unions only to present a complete picture of the structured types provided by C++ and to acquaint you with the general idea in case you encounter unions in other C++ programs.

11.4 Data Abstraction

As the software we develop becomes more complex, we design algorithms and data structures in parallel. We progress from the logical or abstract data structure envisioned at the top level through the refinement process until we reach the concrete coding in C++. We have illustrated two ways of representing the logical structure of a machine record in a shop inventory. The first used a record in which all the components were defined (made concrete) at the same time. The second used a hierarchical record in which the dates and statistics describing a machine's history were defined in lower-level records.

Let's look again at the two different ways in which we represented our logical data structure.

```
// *************** Version 1 ***************

struct MachineRec
{
    int    idNumber;
    string description;
    float  failRate;
    int    lastServicedMonth;  // Assume 1..12
    int    lastServicedDay;    // Assume 1..31
    int    lastServicedYear;   // Assume 1900..2050
    int    downDays;
    int    purchaseDateMonth;  // Assume 1..12
    int    purchaseDateDay;    // Assume 1..31
    int    purchaseDateYear;   // Assume 1900..2050
    float  cost;
};
```

```
// *************** Version 2 ***************

struct Date
{
    int month;    // Assume 1..12
    int day;      // Assume 1..31
    int year;     // Assume 1900..2050
};
struct Statistics
{
    float      failRate;
    Date       lastServiced;
    int        downDays;
};
struct MachineRec
{
    int             idNumber;
    string          description;
    Statistics      history;
    DateType        purchaseDate;
    float           cost;
};
```

Which of these two representations is better? The second one is better for two reasons.

First, it groups elements together logically. The statistics and the dates are entities within themselves. We may want a date or a machine history in another record structure. If we define the dates and statistics only within MachineRec (as in the first structure), we would have to define them again for every other data structure that needs them, giving us multiple definitions of the same logical entity.

Second, the details of the entities (statistics and dates) are pushed down to a lower level in the second structure. The principle of deferring details to as low a level as possible should be applied to designing data structures as well as to designing algorithms. How a machine history or a date is represented is not relevant to our concept of a machine record, so the details need not be specified until it is time to write the algorithms to manipulate those members.

Pushing the implementation details of a data type to a lower level separates the logical description from the implementation. This concept is analogous to control abstraction, which we discussed in Chapter 8. The separation of the logical properties of a data type from its implementation details is called **data abstraction**, which is a goal of effective programming and the foundation upon which abstract data types are built. (We explore the concept of abstract data types in the next section.)

> **Data abstraction** The separation of a data type's logical properties from its implementation.

Eventually, all the logical properties must be defined in terms of concrete data types and routines written to manipulate them. If the implementation is properly designed, we can use the same routines to manipulate the structure in a wide variety of applications. For example, if we have a routine to compare dates, we can use that routine to compare dates representing days on which equipment was bought or maintained, or dates representing people's birthdays. The concept of designing a low-level structure and writing routines to manipulate it is the basis for C++ `class` types, which we examine later in the chapter.

11.5 Abstract Data Types

We live in a complex world. Throughout the course of each day, we are constantly bombarded with information, facts, and details. To cope with complexity, the human mind engages in *abstraction*—the act of separating the essential qualities of an idea or object from the details of how it works or is composed.

With abstraction, we focus on the *what*, not the *how*. For example, our understanding of automobiles is largely based on abstraction. Most of us know *what* the engine does (it propels the car), but fewer of us know—or want to know—precisely *how* the engine works internally. Abstraction allows us to discuss, think about, and use automobiles without having to know everything about how they work.

In the world of software design, it is now recognized that abstraction is an absolute necessity for managing immense, complex software projects. In introductory computer science courses, programs are usually small (perhaps 50 to 200 lines of code) and understandable in their entirety by one person. However, large commercial software products composed of hundreds of thousands—even millions—of lines of code cannot be designed, understood, or tested thoroughly without using abstraction in various forms. To manage complexity, software developers regularly use two important abstraction techniques: control abstraction and data abstraction.

In Chapter 8, we defined control abstraction as the separation of the logical properties of an action from its implementation. We engage in control abstraction whenever we write a function that reduces a complicated algorithm to an abstract action performed by a function call. By invoking a library function, as in the expression

```
4.6 + sqrt(x)
```

we depend only on the function's *specification,* a written description of what it does. We can use the function without having to know its *implementation* (the algorithms that accomplish the result). By invoking the `sqrt` function, our program is less complex because all the details involved in computing square roots are absent.

Abstraction techniques also apply to data. Every data type consists of a set of values (the domain) along with a collection of allowable operations on those values. In the preceding section, we described data abstraction as the separation of a data type's logical properties from its implementation details. Data abstraction comes into play when we need a data type that is not built into the programming language. We can define the new data type as an **abstract data type (ADT)**, concentrating only on its logical properties and deferring the details of its implementation.

> **Abstract data type** A data type whose properties (domain and operations) are specified independently of any particular implementation.

As with control abstraction, an abstract data type has both a specification (the *what*) and an implementation (the *how*). The specification of an ADT describes the characteristics of the data values as well as the behavior of each of the operations on those values. The user of the ADT needs to understand only the specification, not the implementation, in order to use it. Here's a very informal specification of a list ADT:

TYPE
    IntList
DOMAIN
    Each IntList value is a collection of up to 100 separate integer numbers.
OPERATIONS
    Insert an item into the list.
    Delete an item from the list.
    Search the list for an item.
    Return the current length of the list.
    Sort the list into ascending order.
    Print the list.

Notice the complete absence of implementation details. We have not mentioned how the data might actually be stored in a program or how the operations might be implemented. Concealing the implementation details reduces complexity for the user and also shields the user from changes in the implementation.

Below is the specification of another ADT, one that might be useful for representing time in a program.

TYPE
    Time
DOMAIN
    Each Time value is a time of day in the form of hours, minutes, and seconds.
OPERATIONS
    Set the time.
    Print the time.
    Increment the time by one second.
    Compare two times for equality.
    Determine if one time is "less than" (comes before) another.

The specification of an ADT defines abstract data values and abstract operations for the user. Ultimately, of course, the ADT must be implemented in program code. To implement an ADT, the programmer must do two things:

> **Data representation** The concrete form of data used to represent the abstract values of an abstract data type.

1. Choose a concrete **data representation** of the abstract data, using data types that already exist.

2. Implement each of the allowable operations in terms of program instructions.

To implement the IntList ADT, we could choose a concrete data representation consisting of two items: a 100-element data structure (such as an *array*, the topic of the next chapter) and an `int` variable that keeps track of the current length of the list. To implement the IntList operations, we must create algorithms based on the chosen data representation. In the next two chapters, we discuss in detail the array data structure and its use in implementing list ADTs.

To implement the Time ADT, we might use three `int` variables for the data representation—one for the hours, one for the minutes, and one for the seconds. Or we might use three strings as the data representation. The specification of the ADT does not confine us to any particular data representation. As long as we satisfy the specification, we are free to choose among alternative data representations and their associated algorithms. Our choice may be based on time efficiency (the speed at which the algorithms execute), space efficiency (the economical use of memory space), or simplicity and readability of the algorithms. Over time, you will acquire knowledge and experience that help you decide which implementation is best for a particular context.

Theoretical Foundations

Categories of Abstract Data Type Operations

In general, the basic operations associated with an abstract data type fall into three categories: constructors, transformers, and observers.

An operation that creates a new instance of an ADT (such as a list) is a constructor. Operations that insert an item into a list and delete an item from a list are transformers. An operation that takes one list and appends it to the end of a second list is also a transformer.

A Boolean function that returns `true` if a list is empty and `false` if it contains any components is an example of an observer. A Boolean function that tests to see if a certain value is in the list is another observer.

Some operations are combinations of observers and constructors. An operation that takes two lists and merges them into a (new) third list is both an observer (of the two existing lists) and a constructor (of the third list).

In addition to the three basic categories of ADT operations, a fourth category is sometimes defined: iterators.

An example of an iterator is an operation that returns the first item in a list when it is called initially and returns the next one with each successive call.

Constructor   An operation that creates a new instance (variable) of an ADT.

Transformer   An operation that builds a new value of the ADT, given one or more previous values of the type.

Observer   An operation that allows us to observe the state of an instance of an ADT without changing it.

Iterator   An operation that allows us to process—one at a time—all the components in an instance of an ADT.

11.6 C++ Classes

In previous chapters, we have treated data values as passive quantities to be acted upon by functions. In Chapter 10, we viewed category counters as passive data, and we implemented operations as functions that took their values as parameters. Similarly, earlier in this chapter we treated a student record as a passive quantity, using a struct as the data representation and implementing the operation Consistent as a function receiving a struct as a parameter (see Figure 11-6).

This separation of operations and data does not correspond very well with the notion of an abstract data type. After all, an ADT consists of *both* data values and operations on those values. It is preferable to view an ADT as defining an *active* data structure—one that combines both data and operations into a single, cohesive unit (see Figure 11-7). C++ supports this view by providing a built-in structured type known as a **class**.

In Figure 11-2, we listed the four structured types available in the C++ language: the array, the struct, the union, and the class. A class is a structured type provided specifically for representing abstract data types. A class is similar to a struct but is nearly always designed so that its components (**class members**) include not only data but also functions that manipulate that data.* Here is a C++ class declaration corresponding to the Time ADT that we defined in the previous section:

> **Class**   A structured type in a programming language that is used to represent an abstract data type.
>
> **Class member**   A component of a class. Class members may be either data or functions.

```
class Time
{
public:
    void Set( int, int, int );
    void Increment();
```

OPERATIONS   DATA

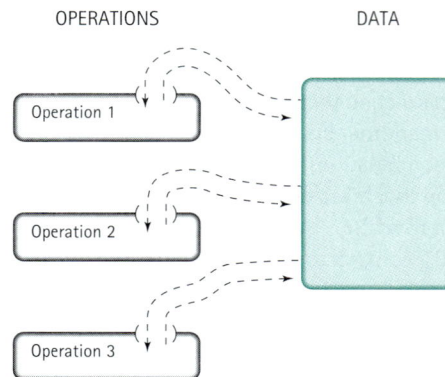

┌──────────────┐
│ Operation 1 │
└──────────────┘

┌──────────────┐
│ Operation 2 │
└──────────────┘

┌──────────────┐
│ Operation 3 │
└──────────────┘

Figure 11–6   *Data and Operations as Separate Entities*

As we noted earlier, in C++ a struct is almost identical to a class. But because of its heritage from the C struct construct, most programmers use class to implement an ADT, and limit their use of struct to applications where a record is needed that has no associated operations.

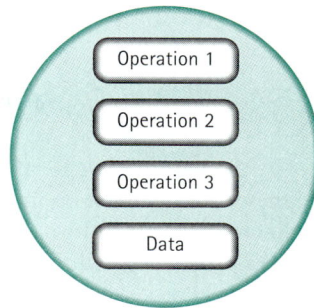

Figure 11–7   *Data and Operations Bound into a Single Unit*

```
    void Write() const;
    bool Equal( Time ) const;
    bool LessThan( Time ) const;
private:
    int hrs;
    int mins;
    int secs;
};
```

(For now, you should ignore the word `const` appearing in some of the function proto-types. We explain this use of `const` later in the chapter.)

The `Time` class has eight members—five member functions (`Set`, `Increment`, `Write`, `Equal`, `LessThan`) and three member variables (`hrs`, `mins`, `secs`). As you might guess, the three member variables form the concrete data representation for the Time ADT. The five member functions correspond to the operations we listed for the Time ADT: set the time (to the hours, minutes, and seconds passed as arguments to the `Set` function), increment the time by one second, print the time, compare two times for equality, and determine if one time is less than another. Although the `Equal` function compares two `Time` variables for equality, its parameter list has only one parameter—a `Time` variable. Similarly, the `LessThan` function has only one parameter, even though it compares two times. We'll see the reason later.

Like a `struct` declaration, the declaration of `Time` defines a data type but does not create variables of the type. Class variables (more often referred to as **class objects** or **class instances**) are created by using ordinary variable declarations:

> **Class object (class instance)**   A variable of a `class` type.

```
Time startTime;
Time endTime;
```

> **Client** Software that declares and manipulates objects of a particular class.

Any software that declares and manipulates `Time` objects is called a **client** of the class.

As you look at the preceding declaration of the `Time` class, you can see the reserved words `public` and `private`, each followed by a colon. Data and/or functions declared between the words `public` and `private` constitute the public interface; clients can access these class members directly. Class members declared after the word `private` are considered private information and are inaccessible to clients. If client code attempts to access a private item, the compiler signals an error.

Private class members can be accessed only by the class's member functions. In the `Time` class, the private variables `hrs`, `mins`, and `secs` can be accessed only by the member functions `Set`, `Increment`, `Write`, `Equal`, and `LessThan`, not by client code. This separation of class members into private and public parts is a hallmark of ADT design. To preserve the properties of an ADT correctly, an instance of the ADT should be manipulated *only* through the operations that form the public interface. We have more to say about this issue later in the chapter.

Matters of Style
Declaring Public and Private Class Members

C++ does not require you to declare public and private class members in a fixed order. Several variations are possible.

By default, class members are private; the word `public` must be used to "open up" any members for public access. Therefore, we could write the `Time` class declaration as follows:

```
class Time
{
    int hrs;
    int mins;
    int secs;
public:
    void Set( int, int, int );
    void Increment();
    void Write() const;
    bool Equal( Time ) const;
    bool LessThan( Time ) const;
};
```

By default, the variables `hrs`, `mins`, and `secs` are private. The public part extends from the word `public` to the end of the class declaration.

(continued) ▼

Declaring Public and Private Class Members

Even with the private part located first, some programmers use the reserved word `private` to be as explicit as possible:

```cpp
class Time
{
private:
    int hrs;
    int mins;
    int secs;
public:
    void Set( int, int, int );
    void Increment();
    void Write() const;
    bool Equal( Time ) const;
    bool LessThan( Time ) const;
};
```

Our preference is to locate the public part first so as to focus attention on the public interface and deemphasize the private data representation:

```cpp
class Time
{
public:
    void Set( int, int, int );
    void Increment();
    void Write() const;
    bool Equal( Time ) const;
    bool LessThan( Time ) const;
private:
    int hrs;
    int mins;
    int secs;
};
```

We use this style throughout the remainder of the book.

Regarding public versus private accessibility, we can now describe more fully the difference between C++ structs and classes. C++ defines a struct to be a class whose members are all, by default, public. In contrast, members of a class are, by default, private. Furthermore, it is most common to use only data, not functions, as members of a struct. Note that you *can* declare struct members to be private and you *can* include member functions in a struct, but then you might as well use a class! Hence, most programmers use the struct in the manner that is traditional from C, as a way to represent a record structure, and implement ADTs only with classes.

Classes, Class Objects, and Class Members

It is important to restate that a class is a type, not a data object. Like any type, a class is a pattern from which you create (or *instantiate*) many objects of that type. Think of a type as a cookie cutter and objects of that type as the cookies.

The declarations

```
Time time1;
Time time2;
```

create two objects of the Time class: time1 and time2. Each object has its own copies of hrs, mins, and secs, the private data members of the class. At a given moment during program execution, time1's copies of hrs, mins, and secs might contain the values 5, 30, and 10; and time2's copies might contain the values 17, 58, and 2. Figure 11–8 is a visual image of the class objects time1 and time2.

(In truth, the C++ compiler does not waste memory by placing duplicate copies of a member function—say, Increment—into both time1 and time2. The compiler generates just one physical copy of Increment, and any class object executes this one copy of the function. Nevertheless, the diagram in Figure 11–8 is a good mental picture of two different class objects.)

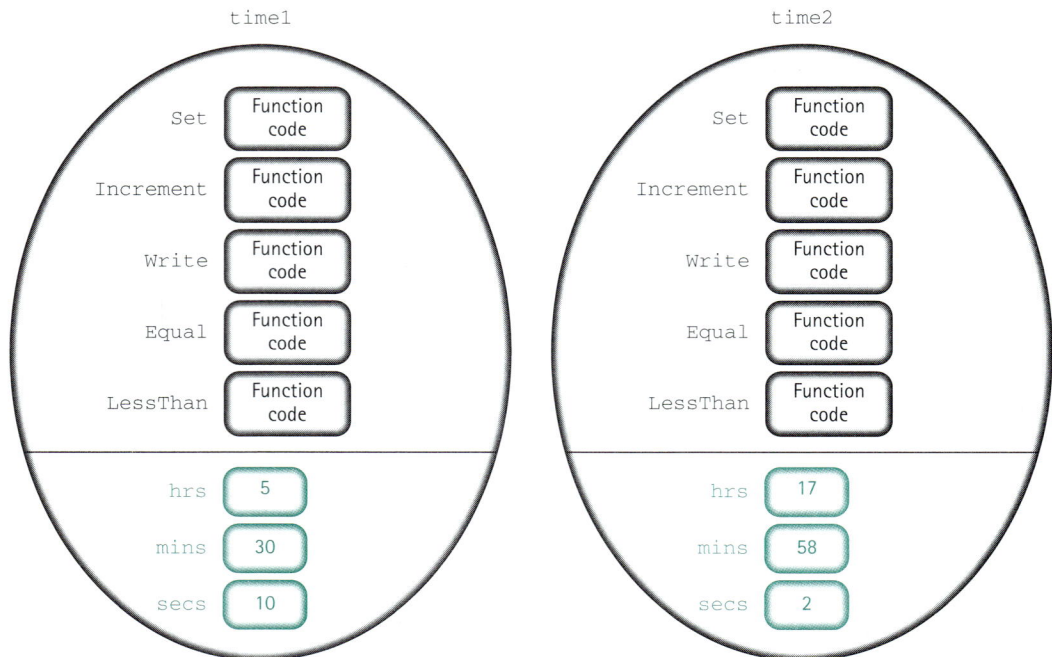

Figure 11–8   *Conceptual View of Two Class Objects*

Be sure you are clear about the difference between the terms *class object* and *class member*. Figure 11–8 depicts two objects of the Time class, and each object has eight members.

Built-in Operations on Class Objects

In many ways, programmer-defined classes are like built-in types. You can declare as many objects of a class as you like. You can pass class objects as arguments to functions and return them as function values. Like any variable, a class object can be automatic (created each time control reaches its declaration and destroyed when control exits its surrounding block) or static (created once when control reaches its declaration and destroyed when the program terminates).

In other ways, C++ treats structs and classes differently from built-in types. Most of the built-in operations do not apply to structs or classes. You cannot use the + operator to add two Time objects, nor can you use the == operator to compare two Time objects for equality.

Two built-in operations that are valid for struct and class objects are member selection (.) and assignment (=). As with structs, you select an individual member of a class by using dot notation. That is, you write the name of the class object, then a dot, then the member name. The statement

```
time1.Increment();
```

invokes the Increment function for the time1 object, presumably to add one second to the time stored in time1. The other built-in operation, assignment, performs aggregate assignment of one class object to another with the following semantics: If x and y are objects of the same class, then the assignment x = y copies the data members of y into x. Below is a fragment of client code that demonstrates member selection and assignment.

```
Time time1;
Time time2;
int   inputHrs;
int   inputMins;
int   inputSecs;

time1.Set(5, 20, 0);
// Assert: time1 corresponds to 5:20:0

cout << "Enter hours, minutes, seconds: ";
cin >> inputHrs >> inputMins >> inputSecs;
time2.Set(inputHrs, inputMins, inputSecs);

if (time1.LessThan(time2))
    DoSomething();
```

```
time2 = time1;                          // Member-by-member assignment
time2.Write();
// Assert: 5:20:0 has been output
```

Earlier we remarked that the `Equal` and `LessThan` functions have only one parameter each, even though they are comparing two `Time` objects. In the If statement of the code segment above, we are comparing `time1` and `time2`. Because `LessThan` is a class member function, we invoke it by giving the name of a class object (`time1`), then a dot, then the function name (`LessThan`). Only one item remains unspecified: the class object with which `time1` should be compared (`time2`). Therefore, the `LessThan` function requires only one parameter, not two. Here is another way of explaining it: If a class member function represents a binary (two-operand) operation, the first operand appears to the left of the dot operator, and the second operand is in the parameter list. (To generalize, an *n*-ary operation has *n* − 1 operands in the parameter list. Thus, a unary operation—such as `Write` or `Increment` in the `Time` class—has an empty parameter list.)

In addition to member selection and assignment, a few other built-in operators are valid for class objects and structs. These operators are used for manipulating memory addresses, and we defer discussing them until later in the book. For now, think of `.` and `=` as the only valid built-in operators.

From the very beginning, you have been working with C++ classes in a particular context: input and output. The standard header file `iostream` contains the declarations of two classes—`istream` and `ostream`—that manage a program's I/O. The C++ standard library declares `cin` and `cout` to be objects of these classes:

```
istream cin;
ostream cout;
```

The `istream` class has many member functions, two of which—the `get` function and the `ignore` function—you already have seen in statements like these:

```
cin.get(someChar);
cin.ignore(200, '\n');
```

As with any C++ class object, we use dot notation to select a particular member function to invoke.

You also have used C++ classes when performing file I/O. The header file `fstream` contains declarations for the `ifstream` and `ofstream` classes. The client code

```
ifstream dataFile;

dataFile.open("input.dat");
```

declares an `ifstream` class object named `dataFile`, then invokes the class member function `open` to try to open a file `input.dat` for input.

We do not examine in detail the `istream`, `ostream`, `ifstream`, and `ofstream` classes and all of their member functions. To study these would be beyond the goals of this book. What is important to recognize is that classes and objects are fundamental to all I/O activity in a C++ program.

Class Scope

We said earlier that member names must be unique within a struct. Additionally, in Chapter 8 we mentioned four kinds of scope in C++: local scope, global scope, namespace scope, and *class scope*. Class scope applies to the member names within structs, unions, and classes. To say that a member name has class scope means that the name is bound to that class (or struct or union). If the same identifier happens to be declared outside the class, the two identifiers are unrelated. Let's look at an example.

The `Time` class has a member function named `Write`. In the same program, another class (say, `SomeClass`) could also have a member function named `Write`. Furthermore, the program might have a global `Write` function that is completely unrelated to any classes. If the program has statements like

```
Time        checkInTime;
SomeClass  someObject;
int         n;
   ⋮
checkInTime.Write();
someObject.Write();
Write(n);
```

then the C++ compiler has no trouble distinguishing among the three `Write` functions. In the first two function calls, the dot notation denotes class member selection. The first statement invokes the `Write` function of the `Time` class, and the second statement invokes the `Write` function of the `SomeClass` class. The final statement does not use dot notation, so the compiler knows that the function being called is the global `Write` function.

Information Hiding

Conceptually, a class object has an invisible wall around it. This wall, called the **abstraction barrier,** protects private data and functions from being accessed by client code. The barrier also prohibits the class object from directly accessing data and functions outside the object. This barrier is a critical characteristic of classes and abstract data types.

> **Abstraction barrier**   The invisible wall around a class object that encapsulates implementation details. The wall can be breached only through the public interface.

For a class object to share information with the outside world (that is, with clients), there must be a gap in the abstraction barrier. This gap is the public interface—the class

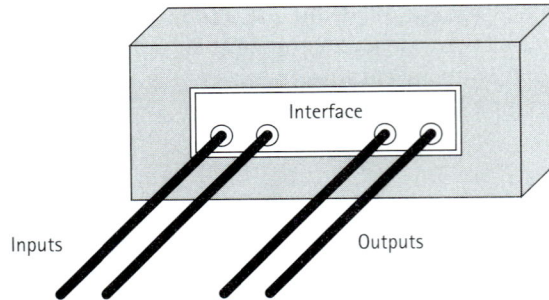

Figure 11-9   *A Black Box*

> **Black box**   An electrical or mechanical device whose inner workings are hidden from view.
>
> **Information hiding**   The encapsulation and hiding of implementation details to keep the user of an abstraction from depending on or incorrectly manipulating these details.

members declared to be `public`. The only way that a client can manipulate the internals of the class object is indirectly—through the operations in the public interface. Engineers have a similar concept called a **black box.** A black box is a module or device whose inner workings are hidden from view. The user of the black box depends only on the written specification of *what* it does, not on *how* it does it. The user connects wires to the interface and assumes that the module works correctly by satisfying the specification (see Figure 11–9).

In software design, the black box concept is referred to as **information hiding.** Information hiding protects the user of a class from having to know all the details of its implementation. Information hiding also assures the class's implementor that the user cannot directly access any private code or data and compromise the correctness of the implementation.

You have been introduced to encapsulation and information hiding before. In Chapter 7, we discussed the possibility of hiding a function's implementation in a separate file. In this chapter, you'll see how to hide the implementations of class member functions by placing them in files that are separate from the client code.

The creator of a C++ class is free to choose which members are private and which are public. However, making data members public (as in a struct) allows the client to inspect and modify the data directly. Because information hiding is so fundamental to data abstraction, most classes exhibit a typical pattern: The private part contains data, and the public part contains the functions that manipulate the data.

The `Time` class exemplifies this organization. The data members `hrs`, `mins`, and `secs` are private, so the compiler prohibits a client from accessing these members directly. The following client statement therefore results in a compile-time error:

```
Time checkInTime;

checkInTime.hrs = 9;    // Prohibited in client code
```

Because only the class's member functions can access the private data, the creator of the class can offer a reliable product, knowing that external access to the private data is impossible. If it is acceptable to let the client *inspect* (but not modify) private data members, a class might provide observer functions. The `Time` class has three such functions: `Write`, `Equal`, and `LessThan`. Because these observer functions are not intended to modify the private data, they are declared with the word `const` following the parameter list:

```
void Write() const;
bool Equal( Time ) const;
bool LessThan( Time ) const;
```

C++ refers to these functions as `const` *member functions*. Within the body of a `const` member function, a compile-time error occurs if any statement tries to modify a private data member. Although not required by the language, it is good practice to declare as `const` those member functions that do not modify private data.

11.7 Specification and Implementation Files

An abstract data type consists of two parts: a specification and an implementation. The specification describes the behavior of the data type without reference to its implementation. The implementation creates an abstraction barrier by hiding the concrete data representation as well as the code for the operations.

The `Time` class declaration serves as the specification of `Time`. This declaration presents the public interface to the user in the form of function prototypes. To implement the `Time` class, we must provide function definitions (declarations with bodies) for all the member functions.

In C++, it is customary (though not required) to package the class declaration and the class implementation into separate files. One file—the *specification file*—is a header (.h) file containing only the class declaration. The second file—the *implementation file*—contains the function definitions for the class member functions. Let's look first at the specification file.

The Specification File

Below is the specification file for the `Time` class. On our computer system, we have named the file `Time.h`. The class declaration is the same as we presented earlier, with one important exception: We include function preconditions and postconditions to specify the semantics of the member functions as unambiguously as possible for the user of the class.

```
//*****************************************************************
// SPECIFICATION FILE (Time.h)
// This file gives the specification
```

```
// of a Time abstract data type
//****************************************************************

class Time
{
public:
    void Set( /* in */ int hours,
              /* in */ int minutes,
              /* in */ int seconds );
        // Precondition:
        //     0 <= hours <= 23  &&  0 <= minutes <= 59
        //   && 0 <= seconds <= 59
        // Postcondition:
        //     Time is set according to the incoming parameters
        // NOTE:
        //     This function MUST be called prior to
        //     any of the other member functions

    void Increment();
        // Precondition:
        //     The Set function has been invoked at least once
        // Postcondition:
        //     Time has been advanced by one second, with
        //     23:59:59 wrapping around to 0:0:0

    void Write() const;
        // Precondition:
        //     The Set function has been invoked at least once
        // Postcondition:
        //     Time has been output in the form HH:MM:SS

    bool Equal( /* in */ Time otherTime ) const;
        // Precondition:
        //     The Set function has been invoked at least once
        //     for both this time and otherTime
        // Postcondition:
        //     Function value == true, if this time equals otherTime
        //                    == false, otherwise

    bool LessThan( /* in */ Time otherTime ) const;
        // Precondition:
        //     The Set function has been invoked at least once
        //     for both this time and otherTime
        //   && This time and otherTime represent times in the
        //     same day
```

```
        // Postcondition:
        //      Function value == true, if this time is earlier
        //                                in the day than otherTime
        //                       == false, otherwise
private:
    int hrs;
    int mins;
    int secs;
};
```

Notice the preconditions for the `Increment`, `Write`, `Equal`, and `LessThan` functions. It is the responsibility of the client to set the time before incrementing, printing, or testing it. If the client fails to set the time, the effect of each of these functions is undefined.

In principle, a specification file should not reveal any implementation details to the user of the class. The file should specify *what* each member function does without disclosing how it does it. However, as you can see in the class declaration, there is one implementation detail that is visible to the user: the concrete data representation of our ADT that is listed in the private part. However, the data representation is still considered hidden information in the sense that the compiler prohibits client code from accessing the data directly.

The Implementation File

The specification (`.h`) file for the `Time` class contains only the class declaration. The implementation file must provide the function definitions for all the class member functions. In the opening comments of the implementation file below, we document the file name as `Time.cpp`. Your system may use a different file name suffix for source code files, perhaps `.c`, `.C`, or `.cxx`.

We recommend that you first skim the C++ code below, not being too concerned about the new language features such as prefixing the name of each function with the symbols

```
Time::
```

Immediately following the program code, we explain the new features.

```
//***********************************************************************
// IMPLEMENTATION FILE (Time.cpp)
// This file implements the Time member functions
//***********************************************************************
#include "Time.h"
#include <iostream>

using namespace std;
```

```cpp
// Private members of class:
//     int hrs;
//     int mins;
//     int secs;

//****************************************************************

void Time::Set( /* in */ int hours,
                /* in */ int minutes,
                /* in */ int seconds )

// Precondition:
//     0 <= hours <= 23   &&   0 <= minutes <= 59
//   && 0 <= seconds <= 59
// Postcondition:
//     hrs == hours  &&  mins == minutes  &&  secs == seconds
// NOTE:
//     This function MUST be called prior to
//     any of the other member functions

{
    hrs = hours;
    mins = minutes;
    secs = seconds;
}

//****************************************************************

void Time::Increment()

// Precondition:
//     The Set function has been invoked at least once
// Postcondition:
//     Time has been advanced by one second, with
//     23:59:59 wrapping around to 0:0:0

{
    secs++;
    if (secs > 59)
    {
        secs = 0;
        mins++;
        if (mins > 59)
        {
            mins = 0;
            hrs++;
```

```cpp
            if (hrs > 23)
                hrs = 0;
        }
    }
}

//******************************************************************

void Time::Write() const

// Precondition:
//     The Set function has been invoked at least once
// Postcondition:
//     Time has been output in the form HH:MM:SS

{
    if (hrs < 10)
        cout << '0';
    cout << hrs << ':';
    if (mins < 10)
        cout << '0';
    cout << mins << ':';
    if (secs < 10)
        cout << '0';
    cout << secs;
}

//******************************************************************

bool Time::Equal( /* in */ Time otherTime ) const

// Precondition:
//     The Set function has been invoked at least once
//     for both this time and otherTime
// Postcondition:
//     Function value == true, if this time equals otherTime
//                    == false, otherwise

{
    return (hrs == otherTime.hrs && mins == otherTime.mins &&
            secs == otherTime.secs);
}

//******************************************************************
```

```
bool Time::LessThan( /* in */ Time otherTime ) const

// Precondition:
//      The Set function has been invoked at least once
//      for both this time and otherTime
//  && This time and otherTime represent times in the
//      same day
// Postcondition:
//      Function value == true, if this time is earlier
//                              in the day than otherTime
//                    == false, otherwise
{
    return (hrs < otherTime.hrs ||
            hrs == otherTime.hrs && mins < otherTime.mins ||
            hrs == otherTime.hrs && mins == otherTime.mins
                                 && secs < otherTime.secs);
}
```

This implementation file demonstrates several important points.

1. The file begins with the preprocessor directive

```
#include "Time.h"
```

Both the implementation file and the client code must #include the specification file. Figure 11–10 pictures this shared access to the specification file. This sharing guarantees that all declarations related to an abstraction are consistent. That is, both client.cpp and Time.cpp must reference the same declaration of the Time class located in Time.h.

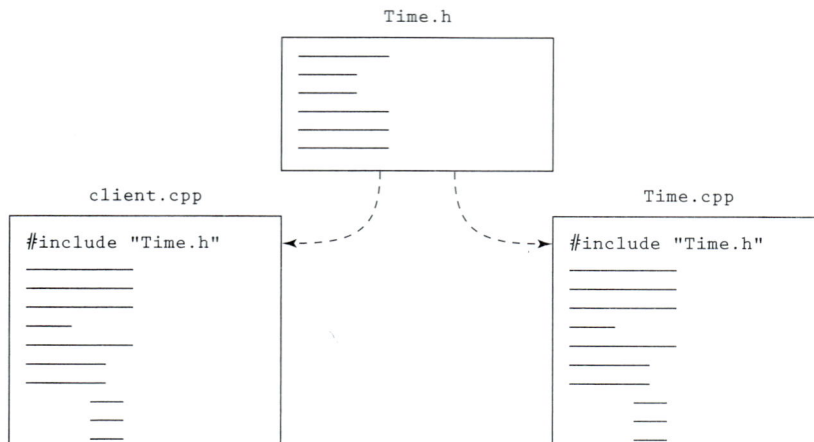

Figure 11–10   *Shared Access to a Specification File*

2. Near the top of the implementation file we have included a comment that restates the private members of the `Time` class.

```
// Private members of class:
//      int hrs;
//      int mins;
//      int secs;
```

This comment reminds the reader that any references to these identifiers are references to the private class members.

3. In the heading of each function definition, the name of the member function is prefixed by the class name (`Time`) and the C++ scope resolution operator (`::`). As we discussed earlier, it is possible for several different classes to have member functions with the same name, say, `Write`. In addition, there may be a global `Write` function that is not a member of any class. The scope resolution operator eliminates any uncertainty about which particular function is being defined.

4. Although clients of a class must use the dot operator to refer to class members (for example, `startTime.Write()`), members of a class refer to each other directly without using dot notation. Looking at the bodies of the `Set` and `Increment` functions, you can see that the statements refer directly to the member variables `hrs`, `mins`, and `secs` without using the dot operator.

   An exception to this rule occurs when a member function manipulates two or more class objects. Consider the `Equal` function. Suppose that the client code has two class objects, `startTime` and `endTime`, and uses the statement

```
if (startTime.Equal(endTime))
    ⋮
```

At execution time, the `startTime` object is the object for which the `Equal` function is invoked. In the body of the `Equal` function, the relational expression

```
hrs == otherTime.hrs
```

refers to class members of two different class objects. The unadorned identifier `hrs` refers to the `hrs` member of the class object for which the function is invoked (that is, `startTime`). The expression `otherTime.hrs` refers to the `hrs` member of the class object that is passed to the parameter, `otherTime`, as a function argument: `endTime`.

5. `Write`, `Equal`, and `LessThan` are observer functions; they do not modify the private data of the class. Because we have declared these to be `const` member functions, the compiler prevents them from assigning new values to the private data. The use of `const` is both an aid to the user of the class (as a visual signal that this function does not modify any private data) and an aid to the class implementor (as a way of preventing accidental modification of the data). Note that the word `const` must appear in both the function prototype (in the class declaration) and the heading of the function definition.

Compiling and Linking a Multifile Program

Now that we have created a specification file and an implementation file for our `Time` class, how do we (or any other programmer) make use of these files in our programs? Let's begin by looking at the notion of *separate compilation* of source code files.

In earlier chapters, we have referred to the concept of a multifile program—a program divided up into several files containing source code. In C++, it is possible to compile each of these files separately and at different times. The compiler translates each source code file into an object code file. Figure 11–11 shows a multifile program consisting of the source code files `myprog.cpp`, `file2.cpp`, and `file3.cpp`. We can compile each of these files independently, yielding object code files `myprog.obj`, `file2.obj`, and `file3.obj`. Although each `.obj` file contains machine language code, it is not yet in executable form. The system's linker program brings the object code together to form an executable program file. (In Figure 11–11, we use the file name suffixes `.cpp`, `.obj`, and `.exe`. Your C++ system may use different file name conventions.)

Files such as `file2.cpp` and `file3.cpp` typically contain function definitions for functions that are called by the code in `myprog.cpp`. An important benefit of separate compilation is that modifying the code in just one file requires recompiling only that file. The new `.obj` file is then relinked with the other existing `.obj` files. Of course, if a modification to one file affects the code in another file—for example, changing a function's interface by altering the number or data types of the function parameters—then the affected files also need to be modified and recompiled.

Returning to our `Time` class, let's assume we have used the system's editor to create the `Time.h` and `Time.cpp` files. Now we can compile `Time.cpp` into object code. If we

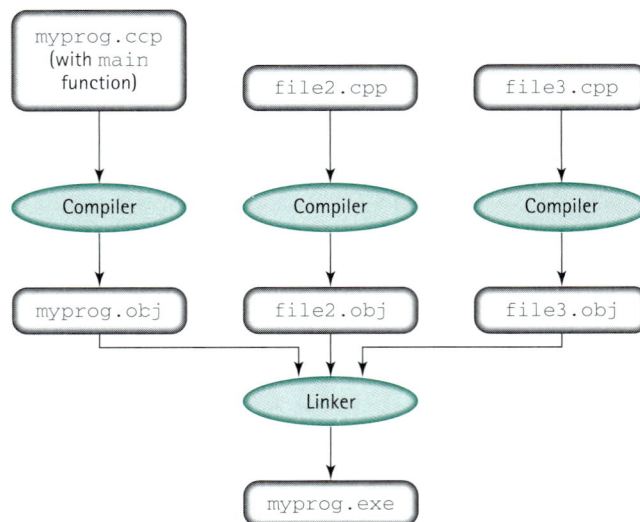

Figure 11–11 *Separate Compilation and Linking*

are working at the operating system's command line, we use a command similar to the following:

```
cc -c Time.cpp
```

In this example, we assume that `cc` is the name of a command that invokes either the C++ compiler or the linker or both, depending on various options given on the command line. The command-line option `-c` means, on many systems, "compile but do not link." In other words, this command produces an object code file, say, `Time.obj`, but does not attempt to link this file with any other file.

A programmer wishing to use the `Time` class will write code that *#includes* the file `Time.h`, then declares and uses `Time` objects:

```
#include "Time.h"
    ⋮
Time appointment;

appointment.Set(15, 30, 0);
appointment.Write();
    ⋮
```

If this client code is in a file named `diary.cpp`, an operating system command like

```
cc diary.cpp Time.obj
```

compiles the client program into object code, links this object code with `Time.obj`, and produces an executable program (see Figure 11–12).

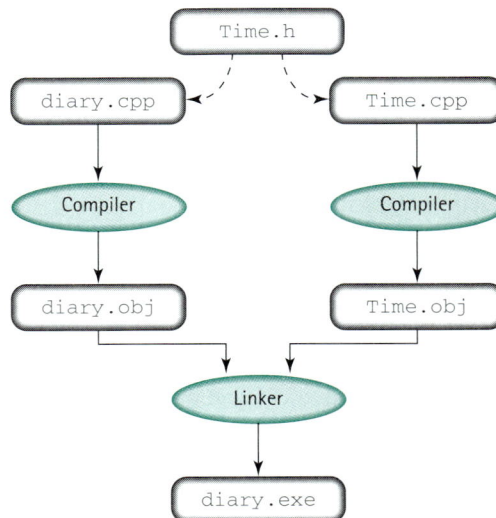

Figure 11–12   *Linking with the `Time` Implementation File*

The mechanics of compiling, linking, and executing vary from one computer system to another. Our examples using the `cc` command assume you are working at the operating system's command line. Many C++ systems provide an *integrated environment*—a program that bundles the editor, the compiler, and the linker into one package. Integrated environments put you back into the editor when a compile-time or link-time error occurs, pinpointing the location of the error. Some integrated environments also manage *project files*. Project files contain information about all the constituent files of a multifile program. With project files, the system automatically recompiles or relinks any files that have become out-of-date because of changes to other files of the program.

Whichever environment you use—the command-line environment or an integrated environment—the overall process is the same: You compile the individual source code files into object code, link the object files into an executable program, then execute the program.

Before leaving the topic of multifile programs, we stress an important point. Referring to Figure 11–12, the files `Time.h` and `Time.obj` must be available to users of the `Time` class. The user needs to examine `Time.h` to see what `Time` objects do and how to use them. The user must also be able to link his or her program with `Time.obj` to produce an executable program. But the user does *not* need to see `Time.cpp`. The implementation of `Time` should be treated as a black box. The main purpose of abstraction is to simplify the programmer's job by reducing complexity. Users of an abstraction should not have to look at its implementation to learn how to use it, nor should they write programs that depend on implementation details. In the latter case, any changes in the implementation could "break" the user's programs. In Chapter 7, the Software Engineering Tip box entitled "Conceptual Versus Physical Hiding of a Function Implementation" discussed the hazards of writing code that relies on implementation details.

11.8 Guaranteed Initialization with Class Constructors

The `Time` class we have been discussing has a weakness. It depends on the client to invoke the `Set` function before calling any other member function. For example, the `Increment` function's precondition is

```
// Precondition:
//      The Set function has been invoked at least once
```

If the client fails to invoke the `Set` function first, this precondition is false and the contract between the client and the function implementation is broken. Because classes nearly always encapsulate data, the creator of a class should not rely on the user to initialize the data. If the user forgets to do so, unpleasant results may occur.

C++ provides a mechanism, called a *class constructor,* to guarantee the initialization of a class object. A constructor is a member function that is implicitly invoked whenever a class object is created.

A constructor function has an unusual name: the name of the class itself. Let's change the Time class by adding two class constructors:

```
class Time
{
public:
    void Set( int, int, int );
    void Increment();
    void Write() const;
    bool Equal( Time ) const;
    bool LessThan( Time ) const;
    Time( int, int, int );          // Constructor
    Time();                         // Constructor
private:
    int hrs;
    int mins;
    int secs;
};
```

This class declaration includes two constructors, differentiated by their parameter lists. The first has three int parameters, which, as we will see, are used to initialize the private data when a class object is created. The second constructor is parameterless and initializes the time to some default value, such as 00:00:00. A parameterless constructor is known in C++ as a *default constructor.*

Constructor declarations are unique in two ways. First, as we have mentioned, the name of the function is the same as the name of the class. Second, the data type of the function is omitted. The reason is that a constructor cannot return a function value. Its purpose is only to initialize a class object's private data.

In the implementation file, the function definitions for the two Time constructors might look like the following:

```
//****************************************************************

Time::Time( /* in */ int initHrs,
            /* in */ int initMins,
            /* in */ int initSecs )
// Constructor

// Precondition:
//      0 <= initHrs <= 23  &&  0 <= initMins <= 59
//   && 0 <= initSecs <= 59
// Postcondition:
//      hrs == initHrs  &&  mins == initMins  &&  secs == initSecs
```

```
{
    hrs = initHrs;
    mins = initMins;
    secs = initSecs;
}

//****************************************************************

Time::Time()

// Default constructor

// Postcondition:
//      hrs == 0  &&  mins == 0  &&  secs == 0

{
    hrs = 0;
    mins = 0;
    secs = 0;
}
```

Invoking a Constructor

Although a constructor is a member of a class, it is never invoked using dot notation. A constructor is automatically invoked whenever a class object is created. The client declaration

```
Time lectureTime(10, 30, 0);
```

includes an argument list to the right of the name of the class object being declared. When this declaration is encountered at execution time, the first (parameterized) constructor is automatically invoked, initializing the private data of lectureTime to the time 10:30:00. The client declaration

```
Time startTime;
```

has no argument list after the identifier startTime. The default (parameterless) constructor is implicitly invoked, initializing startTime's private data to the time 00:00:00.

Remember that a declaration in C++ is a genuine statement and can appear anywhere among executable statements. Placing declarations among executable statements is extremely useful when creating class objects whose initial values are not known until execution time. Here's an example:

```
cout << "Enter appointment time in hours, minutes, and seconds: ";
cin >> hours >> minutes >> seconds;

Time appointmentTime(hours, minutes, seconds);
```

```
cout << "The appointment time is ";
appointmentTime.Write();
    ⋮
```

Revised Specification and Implementation Files for Time

By including constructors for the Time class, we are sure that each class object is initialized before any subsequent calls to the class member functions. One of the constructors allows the client code to specify an initial time; the other creates an initial time of 00:00:00 if the client does not specify a time. Because of these constructors, it is *impossible* for a Time object to be in an uninitialized state after it is created. As a result, we can delete from the Time specification file the warning to call Set before calling any other member functions. Also, we can remove all of the function preconditions that require Set to be called previously. Here is the revised Time specification file:

```
//*********************************************************************
// SPECIFICATION FILE (Time.h)
// This file gives the specification
// of a Time abstract data type
//*********************************************************************

class Time
{
public:
    void Set( /* in */ int hours,
              /* in */ int minutes,
              /* in */ int seconds );
        // Precondition:
        //      0 <= hours <= 23  &&  0 <= minutes <= 59
        //   && 0 <= seconds <= 59
        // Postcondition:
        //      Time is set according to the incoming parameters

    void Increment();
        // Postcondition:
        //      Time has been advanced by one second, with
        //      23:59:59 wrapping around to 00:00:00

    void Write() const;
        // Postcondition:
        //      Time has been output in the form HH:MM:SS

    bool Equal( /* in */ Time otherTime ) const;
```

```
            // Postcondition:
            //     Function value == true,  if this time equals otherTime
            //                    == false, otherwise

        bool LessThan( /* in */ Time otherTime ) const;
            // Precondition:
            //     This time and otherTime represent times in the
            //     same day
            // Postcondition:
            //     Function value == true,  if this time is earlier
            //                                in the day than otherTime
            //                    == false, otherwise

    Time( /* in */ int initHrs,
          /* in */ int initMins,
          /* in */ int initSecs );
            // Precondition:
            //     0 <= initHrs <= 23   &&   0 <= initMins <= 59
            //  && 0 <= initSecs <= 59
            // Postcondition:
            //     Class object is constructed
            //  && Time is set according to the incoming parameters

    Time();
            // Postcondition:
            //     Class object is constructed  &&  Time is 00:00:00
private:
    int hrs;
    int mins;
    int secs;
};
```

To save space, we do not include the revised implementation file here. The only changes are as follows:

1. The inclusion of the function definitions for the two class constructors, which we presented earlier.

2. The deletion of all function preconditions stating that the Set function must be invoked previously.

At this point, you may wonder whether we need the Set function at all. After all, both the Set function and the parameterized constructor seem to do the same thing—set the time according to values passed as arguments—and the implementations of the two functions are essentially identical. The difference is that Set can be invoked for an existing class object whenever and as often as we wish, whereas the parameterized constructor is invoked once only—at the moment a class object is created. Therefore, we retain the Set function to provide maximum flexibility to clients of the class.

The following is a complete client program that invokes all of the `Time` member functions. Observe that the `main` function begins by creating two `Time` objects, one by using the parameterized constructor and the other by using the default constructor. The program's output is shown below the program.

```cpp
//*******************************************************************
// TimeClient program
// This is a very simple client of the Time class
//*******************************************************************
#include <iostream>
#include "Time.h"    // For Time class

using namespace std;

int main()
{
    Time time1(5, 30, 0);
    Time time2;
    int  loopCount;

    cout << "time1: ";
    time1.Write();
    cout << "  time2: ";
    time2.Write();
    cout << endl;
    if (time1.Equal(time2))
        cout << "Times are equal" << endl;
    else
        cout << "Times are NOT equal" << endl;

    time2 = time1;
    cout << "time1: ";
    time1.Write();
    cout << "  time2: ";
    time2.Write();
    cout << endl;

    if (time1.Equal(time2))
        cout << "Times are equal" << endl;
    else
        cout << "Times are NOT equal" << endl;

    time2.Increment();
    cout << "New time2: ";
    time2.Write();
    cout << endl;
```

```
    if (time1.LessThan(time2))
        cout << "time1 is less than time2" << endl;
    else
        cout << "time1 is NOT less than time2" << endl;

    if (time2.LessThan(time1))
        cout << "time2 is less than time1" << endl;
    else
        cout << "time2 is NOT less than time1" << endl;

    time1.Set(23, 59, 55);
    cout << "Incrementing time1 from 23:59:55:" << endl;
    for (loopCount = 1; loopCount <= 10; loopCount++)
    {
        time1.Write();
        cout << ' ';
        time1.Increment();
    }
    cout << endl;
    return 0;
}
```

The output from executing the TimeClient program is as follows.

```
time1: 05:30:00   time2: 00:00:00
Times are NOT equal
time1: 05:30:00   time2: 05:30:00
Times are equal
New time2: 05:30:01
time1 is less than time2
time2 is NOT less than time1
Incrementing time1 from 23:59:55:
23:59:55 23:59:56 23:59:57 23:59:58 23:59:59 00:00:00 00:00:01
00:00:02 00:00:03 00:00:04
```

Guidelines for Using Class Constructors

The class is an essential language feature for creating abstract data types in C++. The class mechanism is a powerful design tool, but along with this power come rules for using classes correctly.

C++ has some very intricate rules about using constructors, many of which relate to language features we have not yet discussed. Below are some guidelines that are pertinent at this point.

1. A constructor cannot return a function value, so the function is declared without a return value type.

2. A class may provide several constructors. When a class object is declared, the compiler chooses the appropriate constructor according to the number and data types of the arguments to the constructor.

3. Arguments to a constructor are passed by placing the argument list immediately after the name of the class object being declared:

```
SomeClass anObject(arg1, arg2);
```

4. If a class object is declared without an argument list, as in the statement

```
SomeClass anObject;
```

then the effect depends upon what constructors (if any) the class provides.

If the class has no constructors at all, memory is allocated for anObject but its private data members are in an uninitialized state.

If the class does have constructors, then the default (parameterless) constructor is invoked if there is one. If the class has constructors but no default constructor, a syntax error occurs.

Before leaving the topic of constructors, we give you a brief preview of another special member function supported by C++: the *class destructor.* Just as a constructor is implicitly invoked when a class object is created, a destructor is implicitly invoked when a class object is destroyed—for example, when control leaves the block in which a local object is declared. A class destructor is named the same as a constructor except that the first character is a tilde (~):

```
class SomeClass
{
public:
    ⋮
    SomeClass();      // Constructor
    ~SomeClass();     // Destructor
private:
    ⋮
};
```

In the next few chapters, we won't be using destructors; the kinds of classes we'll be writing have no need to perform special actions at the moment a class object is destroyed. In Chapter 15, we explore destructors in detail and describe the situations in which you need to use them.

Problem-Solving Case Study

Abstract Data Type Name

In Chapter 4, we displayed a name in different formats. In Chapter 8, the Health Profile program used a name. Adding a name to the BMI and the Mortgage programs would make sense. Names are often necessary pieces of information. Let's stop this duplication of effort and do the job once and for all—let's write the code to support a name as an abstract data type.

The format for this case study is a little different. Because we are developing only one software component—an ADT—and not a complete program, we omit the Input and Output sections. Instead, we include two sections entitled Specification of the ADT and Implementation of the ADT.

PROBLEM Design and implement an abstract data type to represent a name. Make the domain and operations general enough to be used in any program that needs to keep track of a name. The informal specification of the ADT is given below.

TYPE

        Name

DOMAIN

        Each Name is a name in the form of first name, middle name, and last name.

OPERATIONS

        Construct a Name instance

        Set a name

        Read a name

        Inspect the first name

        Inspect the middle name

        Inspect the last name

        Inspect the middle initial

        Compare two names for "before," "same," and "after"

Where did these operations come from? From experience. In Chapter 14, we look at object-oriented design and how to choose the operations, but for the moment assume that these are a good representation. Note that there is no operation to output the name in any particular format. Because we are allowing the user to inspect the parts of the name, the user can combine the parts to suit the user's purpose.

DISCUSSION We create the Name ADT in two stages: specification, followed by implementation. The result of the first stage is a C++ specification (.h) file containing the declaration of a Name class. This file must describe for the user the precise semantics of each ADT operation. The informal specification given above would be unacceptable to the user of the ADT. The descriptions of the operations are too imprecise and ambiguous to be helpful to the user.

The second stage—implementation—requires us to (a) choose a concrete data representation for a name, and (b) implement each of the operations as a C++ function definition. The result is a C++ implementation file containing these function definitions.

SPECIFICATION OF THE ADT   The domain of our ADT is the set of all names made up of a first, middle, and last name. To represent the Name ADT as program code, we use a C++ class named Name. The ADT operations become public member functions of the class. Let's now specify the operations more carefully.

Construct a new Name instance   For this operation, we use a C++ default constructor. The constructor for Time set the hours, seconds, and minutes to zeros. Blanks would be the logical equivalent for class Name.

Set the name   The client must supply three arguments for this operation: first, middle, and last. Although we haven't yet determined a concrete data representation for a name, we must decide what data types the client should use for these arguments. The logical choice is for each value to be represented by a string. After thinking about it, we realize that this operation could be coded as a parameterized constructor. However, what if we want to change a name (set it) after it has already been constructed? Let's provide two operations that take the three parts of the name as parameters: one as a constructor and one as a void function.

Read a name   This operation prompts for and reads the three parts of the name from the standard input device.

Inspect the name's first, middle, and last names   All three of these operations are observer operations. They give the client access, indirectly, to the private data. In the Name class, we represent these operations as value-returning member functions with the following prototypes:

```
string first();
string middle();
string last();
```

Why do we need these observer operations? Why not simply let the data representation of the name be public instead of private so that the client can access the values directly? The answer is that the client should be allowed to inspect *but not modify* these values. If the data were public, a client could change the data, thereby compromising the integrity of an instance.

Inspect the middle initial   This operation requires that the first letter of the middle name be extracted and returned. In Chapter 4, we accessed the middle initial as a one-character string. Should we return it as a string here or as a char variable? It really doesn't matter as long as we are consistent in our code and in our documentation. Let's make this function a char function, just to provide a different example.

Compare two names   This operation compares two names and determines whether the first one comes before the second one, they are the same, or the first one comes after the second one. To indicate the result of the comparison, we define an enumeration type with three values:

```
enum RelationType {BEFORE, SAME, AFTER};
```

Then we can code the comparison operation as a class member function that returns a value of type RelationType. Here is the function prototype:

```
RelationType ComparedTo( /* in */ Name otherName ) const;
```

Because this is a class member function, the name being compared to otherName is the class object for which the member function is invoked. For example, the following client code tests whether name1 comes before name2.

```
Name name1;
Name name2;
  :
if (name1.ComparedTo(name2) == BEFORE)
  DoSomething();
```

We are now almost ready to write the C++ specification file for our Name class. However, the class declaration requires us to include the private part—the private variables that are the concrete data representation of the ADT. Choosing a concrete data representation properly belongs in the ADT implementation phase, not the specification phase. But, to satisfy the C++ class declaration requirement, we now choose a data representation. The simplest representation for a name is three string values—one each for the first, middle, and last. Here, then, is the specification file containing the Name class declaration (along with the declaration of the RelationType enumeration type).

```
//********************************************************************
// SPECIFICATION FILE (Name.h)
// This file gives the specification of the Name abstract
// data type. There are two constructors: one takes the first,
// middle, and last name as parameters and the second sets first,
// middle, and last to blanks
//********************************************************************

#include <iostream>
#include <string>

using namespace std;

enum RelationType{BEFCRE, SAME, AFTER};

class Name
{
public:
    Name();
        // Default constructor
        // Postcondition:
        //      first, middle, and last have been set to blanks
```

```cpp
Name( /* in */ string firstName,
      /* in */ string middleName,
      /* in */ string lastName );
    // Parameterized constructor
    // Postcondition:
    //     first is firstName AND middle is middleName AND
    //     last is lastName

void SetName( /* in */ string firstName,
              /* in */ string middleName,
              /* in */ string lastName );
    // Postcondition:
    //     first is firstName AND middle is middleName AND
    //     last is lastName

void ReadName();
    // Postcondition:
    //     Name is prompted for and read from the standard input
    //     device

string FirstName() const;
    // Postcondition:
    //     Return value is this person's first name

string LastName() const;
    // Postcondition:
    //     Return value is this person's last name

string MiddleName() const;
    // Postcondition:
    //     Return value is this person's middle name

char MiddleInitial() const;
    // Postcondition:
    //     Return value is this person's middle initial

RelationType ComparedTo( /* in */ Name otherName ) const;
    // Postcondition:
    //   Return value is
    //          BEFORE, if this name comes before otherName
    //          SAME, if this name and otherName are the same
    //          AFTER, if this name is after otherName

private:
    string first;            // Person's first name
```

```
        string last;           // Person's last name
        string middle;         // Person's middle name
};
```

IMPLEMENTATION OF THE ADT   We have already chosen a concrete data representation for a name, shown in the specification file as the string variables `first`, `middle`, and `last`. Now we must implement each class member function, placing the function definitions into a C++ implementation file named Name.cpp. As we implement the member functions, we also discuss testing strategies that can help to convince us that the implementations are correct.

The class constructors, FrstName, MiddleName, and LastName.   The implementations of these functions are so straightforward that no discussion is needed.

Name (In: firstName, middleName, lastName)

> Set first to firstName
> Set middle to middleName
> Set last to lastName

Name ()

> Set first to " "
> Set middle to " "
> Set last to " "

SetName (In: firstName, middleName, lastName)

> Set first to firstName
> Set middle to middleName
> Set last to lastName

FirstName ( )
  Out: Function value

> Return first

MiddleName()
Out: Function value

> Return middle

LastName()
Out: Function value

> Return last

ReadName()

> Prompt for first name
> Read first name
> Prompt for middle name
> Read middle name
> Prompt for last name
> Read last name

TESTING   The `FirstName`, `MiddleName`, and `LastName` observer functions can be used to verify that the class constructors, `ReadName`, and `SetName` work correctly. The code

```
Name someName("Susan", "Margaret", "Smith");
cout << someName.FirstName() << ' ' << someName.MiddleName() << ' '
     << someName.LastName() << endl;
Name someName2();
cout << someName2.FirstName() << ' ' << someName2.MiddleName() << ' '
     << someName2.LastName() << endl;
someName2.SetName("Margaret", "Susan", "Smith");
cout << someName2.FirstName() << ' ' << someName2.MiddleName() << ' '
     << someName2.LastName() << endl;
```

should print out three lines: `Susan Margaret Smith`, a line with five blanks, and a line containing `Margaret Susan Smith`.

The Middle Initial function   We need to extract the first character in the middle name. That's easy. We can extract it directly using brackets: `middle[0]`. Remember the first character in a string is in position zero.

The ComparedTo function   If we were to compare two names in our heads, we would look first at the last name. If the last names were different, we would immediately know which name came first. If the last names were the same, we would look at the first names. If the first names were the same, we would have to look at the middle name. As so often happens, we can use this algorithm directly in our function.

ComparedTo (In: otherName)
    Out: Function value

```
IF last < otherName.last
    Return BEFORE
IF last > otherName.last
    Return AFTER

// Last names are equal. Compare first names
IF first < otherName.first
    Return BEFORE
IF first> otherName.first
    Return AFTER

// Last and first names are equal. Compare middle names
IF middle < otherName.middle
    Return BEFORE
IF middle > otherName.middle
    Return AFTER

// Names are equal
Return SAME
```

TESTING In testing this function, we should ensure that each path is taken at least once. Case Study Follow-Up Exercises 2 and 3 ask you to design test data for this function and to write a driver that does the testing.

Here is the implementation file that contains function definitions for all of the ADT operations:

```cpp
//********************************************************************
// IMPLEMENTATION FILE (Name.cpp)
// The file implements the Name member functions
//********************************************************************

#include "Name.h"
#include <iostream>

Name::Name()

// Default constructor
// Postcondition:
//    first, middle, and last have been set to blanks
```

```
{
    first = " ";
    middle = " ";
    last = " ";
}

//*********************************************************************

Name::Name( /* in */ string firstName,      // First name
            /* in */ string middleName,     // Middle name
            /* in */ string lastName )      // Last name

// Parameterized constructor
// Postcondition:
//      firstName has been stored in first; middleName has been
//      stored in middle; lastName has been stored in last

{
    first = firstName;                      // Assign parameters
    last = lastName;
    middle = middleName;
}

//*********************************************************************

void Name::SetName( /* in */ string firstName,      // First name
                    /* in */ string middleName,     // Middle name
                    /* in */ string lastName )      // Last name

// Postcondition:
//      firstName has been stored in first; middleName has been
//      stored in middle; lastName has been stored in last

{
  first = firstName;                        // Assign parameters
  last = lastName;
  middle = middleName;
}

//*********************************************************************

void Name::ReadName()
```

```cpp
// Postcondition:
//      Name  prompted for and read from the standard input device

{
    cout << "Enter first name: ";      // Prompt for first name
    cin >> first;                      // Get first name
    cout << "Enter middle name: ";     // Prompt for middle name
    cin >> middle;                     // Get middle name
    cout << "Enter last name: ";       // Prompt for last name
    cin >> last;                       // Get last name
}

//*********************************************************************

string Name::FirstName() const

// Postcondition:
//    Return value is first

{
    return first;
}


//*********************************************************************

string Name::LastName() const

// Postcondition:
//    Return value is last

{
    return last;
}


//*********************************************************************

string Name::MiddleName() const

// Postcondition:
//    Return value is middle
```

```cpp
{
    return middle;
}


//*************************************************************

char Name::MiddleInitial() const

// Postcondition:
//    Return value is middle initial

{
    return middle[0];
}


//*************************************************************

RelationType Name::ComparedTo( /* in */ Name otherName ) const

// Precondition:
//      Input parameter contains a valid name
// Postcondition:
//      Return value is
//            BEFORE, if this name comes before otherName
//            SAME, if this name and otherName are the same
//            AFTER, if this name is after otherName
{
    if (last < otherName.last)
        return BEFORE;
    else if (otherName.last < last)
        return AFTER;
    else if (first < otherName.first)
        return BEFORE;
    else if (otherName.first < first)
        return AFTER;
    else if (middle < otherName.middle)
        return BEFORE;
    else if (otherName.middle < middle)
        return AFTER;
    else
        return SAME;
}
```

A name is a logical entity for which we now have developed an implementation. We have designed, implemented, and tested a name ADT that we (or any programmer) can use whenever we have a name as part of our program data. If we discover in the future that additional operations on a name would be useful, we can implement, test, and add them to our set of name operations.

We have said that data abstraction is an important principle of software design. What we have done here is an example of data abstraction. From now on, when a problem needs a name, we can stop our decomposition at the logical level. We do not need to worry about implementing a name each time.

Testing and Debugging

Testing and debugging a C++ class amounts to testing and debugging each member function of the class. All of the techniques you have learned about—algorithm walk-throughs, code walk-throughs, hand traces, test drivers, verification of preconditions and postconditions, the system debugger, the `assert` function, and debug outputs—may be brought into play.

Consider how we might test this chapter's `Time` class. Here is the class declaration, abbreviated by leaving out the function preconditions and postconditions:

```cpp
class Time
{
public:
    void Set( /* in */ int hours,
              /* in */ int minutes,
              /* in */ int seconds );
        // Precondition: ...
        // Postcondition: ...

    void Increment();
        // Postcondition: ...

    void Write() const;
        // Postcondition: ...

    bool Equal( /* in */ Time otherTime ) const;
        // Postcondition: ...

    bool LessThan( /* in */ Time otherTime ) const;
        // Precondition: ...
        // Postcondition: ...
```

```
Time( /* in */ int initHrs,
      /* in */ int initMins,
      /* in */ int initSecs );
    // Precondition:  ...
    // Postcondition:  ...

Time();
    // Postcondition:  ...
private:
    int hrs;
    int mins;
    int secs;
};
```

To test this class fully, we must test each of the member functions. Let's step through the process of testing just one of them: the Increment function.

When we implemented the Increment function, we presumably started with a pseudocode algorithm, performed an algorithm walk-through, and translated the pseudocode into the following C++ function:

```
void Time::Increment()

// Postcondition:
//     Time has been advanced by one second, with
//     23:59:59 wrapping around to 00:00:00

{
    secs++;
    if (secs > 59)
    {
        secs = 0;
        mins++;
        if (mins > 59)
        {
            mins = 0;
            hrs++;
            if (hrs > 23)
                hrs = 0;
        }
    }
}
```

Now we perform a code walk-through, verifying that the C++ code faithfully matches the pseudocode algorithm. At this point (or earlier, during the algorithm walk-through), we do a hand trace to confirm that the logic is correct.

For the hand trace we should pick values of hrs, mins, and secs that ensure code coverage. To execute every path through the control flow, we need cases in which the following conditions occur:

1. The first If condition is false.

2. The first If condition is true and the second is false.

3. The first If condition is true, the second is true, and the third is false.

4. The first If condition is true, the second is true, and the third is true.

Below is a table displaying values of hrs, mins, and secs that correspond to these four cases. For each case we also write down what we hope will be the values of the variables after executing the algorithm.

	Initial Values			Expected Results		
Case	hrs	mins	secs	hrs	mins	secs
1	10	5	30	10	5	31
2	4	6	59	4	7	0
3	13	59	59	14	0	0
4	23	59	59	0	0	0

Using the initial values for each case, a hand trace of the code confirms that the algorithm produces the desired results.

Finally, we write a test driver for the Increment function, just to be sure that our understanding of the algorithm logic is the same as the computer's! Here is a possible test driver:

```cpp
#include <iostream>
#include "Time.h"

using namespace std;

int main()
{
    Time time;
    int      hours;
    int      minutes;
    int      seconds;
```

```
cout << "Enter a time (use hours < 0 to quit): ";
cin >> hours >> minutes >> seconds;
while (hours >= 0)
{
    time.Set(hours, minutes, seconds);
    time.Increment();
    cout << "Incremented time is ";
    time.Write();
    cout << endl;
    cout << "Enter a time (use hours < 0 to quit): ";
    cin >> hours >> minutes >> seconds;
}
return 0;
}
```

Now we compile the test driver and `Time.cpp`, link the two object files, and execute the program. For input data, we supply at least the four test cases discussed earlier. The program's output should match the desired results.

Now that we have tested the `Increment` function, we can apply the same steps to the remaining class member functions. We can create a separate test driver for each function, or we can write just one driver that tests all of the functions. The disadvantage of writing just one driver is that devising different combinations of input values to test several functions at once can quickly become complicated.

Before leaving the topic of testing a class, we must emphasize an important point. Even though a class has been tested thoroughly, it is still possible for errors to arise. Let's look at two examples using the `Time` class. The first example is the client statement

```
time.Set(24, 0, 0);
```

The second example is the comparison

```
if (time1.LessThan(time2))
    ⋮
```

where the programmer intends `time1` to be 11:00:00 on a Wednesday and `time2` to be 1:20:00 on a Thursday. (The result of the test is `false`, not `true` as the programmer expects.) Do you see the problem? In each example, the client has violated the function precondition. The precondition of `Set` requires the first argument to have a value from 0 through 23. The precondition of `LessThan` requires the two times to be on the same day, not on two different days.

If a class has been well tested and there are errors when client code uses the class, always check the member function preconditions. You can waste many hours trying to debug a class member function when, in fact, the function is correct. The error may lie in the client code.

Testing and Debugging Hints

1. The declarations of `struct` and `class` types must end with semicolons.

2. Be sure to specify the full member selector when referencing a component of a struct variable or class object.

3. Avoid using anonymous `struct` types.

4. Regarding semicolons, the declarations and definitions of class member functions are treated the same as any C++ function. The member function prototype, located in the class declaration, ends with a semicolon. The function heading—the part of the function definition preceding the body—does not end with a semicolon.

5. When implementing a class member function, don't forget to prefix the function name with the name of the class and the scope resolution operator (`::`).

```
void Time::Increment()
{
    ⋮
}
```

6. For now, the only built-in operations that we apply to struct variables and class objects are member selection (`.`) and assignment (`=`). To perform other operations, such as comparing two struct variables or class objects, you must access the components individually (in the case of struct variables) or write class member functions (in the case of class objects).

7. If a class member function inspects but does not modify the private data, it is a good idea to make it a `const` member function.

8. A class member function does not use dot notation to access private members of the class object for which the function is invoked. In contrast, a member function *must* use dot notation to access the private members of a class object that is passed to it as an argument.

9. To avoid errors caused by uninitialized data, it is good practice to always include a class constructor when designing a class.

10. A class constructor is declared without a return value type and cannot return a function value.

11. If a client of a class has errors that seem to be related to the class, start by checking the preconditions of the class member functions. The errors may be in the client, not the class.

Summary

In addition to being able to create user-defined atomic data types, we can create structured data types. In a structured data type, a name is given to an entire group of components. With many structured types, the group can be accessed as a whole, or each individual component can be accessed separately.

The record is a data structure for grouping together heterogeneous data—data items that are of different types. Individual components of a record are accessed by name. In C++, records are referred to as *structures* or as structs. We can use a struct variable to refer to the struct as a whole, or we can use a member selector to access any individual member (component) of the struct. Entire structs of the same type may be assigned directly to each other, passed as arguments, or returned as function return values. Comparison of structs, however, must be done member by member. Reading and writing of structs must also be done member by member.

Data abstraction is a powerful technique for reducing the complexity and increasing the reliability of programs. Separating the properties of a data type from the details of its implementation frees the user of the type from having to write code that depends on a particular implementation of the type. This separation also assures the implementor of the type that client code cannot accidentally compromise a correct implementation.

An abstract data type (ADT) is a type whose specification is separate from its implementation. The specification announces the abstract properties of the type. The implementation consists of (a) a concrete data representation and (b) the implementations of the ADT operations. In C++, an ADT can be realized by using the class mechanism. Class members can be designated as public or private. Most commonly, the private members are the concrete data representation of the ADT, and the public members are the functions corresponding to the ADT operations.

Among the public member functions of a class, the programmer often includes one or more class constructors—functions that are invoked automatically whenever a class object is created.

Separate compilation of program units is central to the separation of specification from implementation. The declaration of a C++ class is typically placed in a specification (.h) file, and the implementations of the class member functions reside in another file: the implementation file. The client code is compiled separately from the class implementation file, and the two resulting object code files are linked together to form an executable file. Through separate compilation, the user of an ADT can treat the ADT as an off-the-shelf component without ever seeing how it is implemented.

Quick Check

1. How does a C++ union conserve memory space? (pp. 531–533)
2. How do we create an implementation from a specification for an abstract data type? (pp. 533–537)
3. How does the use of a specification file help to provide encapsulation and information hiding for a class? (pp. 547–553)

4. What is contained between the braces of a `struct` definition? (pp. 521–523)
5. What operator is used as the member selector of a `struct`? (pp. 523–524)
6. What do we call a data structure that is implemented by a `struct` that contains other `struct` types? (pp. 529–531)
7. How would you write an expression to access the `hour` member of a `struct` that is itself a member, called `time`, of a `struct` variable called `date`? (pp. 529–531)
8. The members of a `struct`, like a `class`, can include variables, constants, and functions. What default attribute of a member differs between a `class` and a `struct`? (pp. 540–541)
9. Write the declaration of a class object, called `today`, of class `Date`. (pp. 542–543)
10. How would you call member function `GetDay` (which takes no parameters) of an object called `Today` of class `Date`? (pp. 543–545)
11. Where does the `::` scope resolution operator appear in a member function definition within an implementation file? (pp. 549–553)
12. Which file, specification or implementation, omits member function bodies? (pp. 547–549)
13. What distinguishes a class constructor from other member functions? (pp. 556–558)

Answers

1. By allowing a type to have values of different types at different times, avoiding the need to allocate storage for all of the different types at once.   2. By choosing a data representation, and then writing out the operations for the ADT with program instructions.   3. It enables client code to see the formal interface to the class, but none of the implementation details that the creator of the class wishes to hide.   4. A list of the members of the `struct`.   5. The dot (period).   6. A hierarchical record. 7. `date.time.hour`   8. Classes default to private members, structs default to public members. 9. `Date today;`   10. `today.GetDay();`   11. In the heading, between the name of the class and the name of the function.   12. The specification file.   13. Its name is identical to the name of the class, and it is neither void nor does it have a return value type.

Exam Preparation Exercises

1. A `struct` cannot have another `struct` as a member. True or false?
2. A `union` is a `struct` that can hold just one of its members at a time. True or false?
3. Class scope applies to classes, structs, and unions. True or false?
4. Dot notation is used only by class clients to refer to members. Other class members do not need to use dot notation. True or false?
5. Given the following declarations,

```
struct Name
{
    string first;
    string middle;
```

```
      string last;
};
```

```
Name yourName;
Name myName;
```

What are the contents of the two `Name` variables after each of the following statements, assuming they are executed in the order listed?

a. `yourName.first = "George";`
b. `yourName.last = "Smith";`
c. `myName = yourName;`
d. `myName.middle = "Nathaniel";`
e. `yourName.middle = myName.middle[0] + ".";`

6. What are the three aggregate operations allowed on structs?
7. How does a union differ from an enumeration type?
8. Given the declaration of the Name type in Exercise 5, and the following declarations:

```
struct studentRecord
{
    Name studentName;
    Name teacherName;
    int gradeNumber;
    string grades;
}
```

```
studentRecord sally;
```

a. How would you assign the name Sally Ellen Strong to the `studentName` field of variable `sally`?
b. How would you assign the grade number 7 to that field of `sally`?
c. How would you assign the fourth letter from the `grades` field to char variable `spring`?

9. What happens when a struct is passed as an argument to a value parameter of a function? How does this differ from passing it to a reference parameter?
10. Given the following union declaration:

```
union GradeUnion
{
    char gradeLetter;
    int gradeNumber;
}
```

```
GradeUnion grade;
```

What does each of the following statements do, assuming they are executed in the order shown?

    a. `cin >> grade.gradeLetter;`

    b. `if (grade.gradeLetter >= 'A' && grade.gradeLetter <= 'D')`

    c. `grade.gradeNumber =  4 - int(grade.gradeLetter - 'A');`

11. What are the two major properties of an abstract data type that are defined in its specification?

12. How does the data representation differ from the domain of an abstract data type?

13. By default, are class members public or private?

14. Given an object, called `current`, of class `Time`: How would you write the call to its void member function, called `plus`, that adds an integer number of minutes to the current time? The number of minutes to add is in variable `period`.

15. Which kind of operation, constructor, observer, transformer, or iterator is implemented by a function that is declared as `const`?

16. A class may have multiple constructors, all with the same name. How does the compiler decide which one to call?

17. A class called `Calendar` has a default constructor and a constructor that accepts an integer value specifying the year. How would you invoke each of these for an object called `primary`? Use the current year as the argument to the second constructor.

18. How is the name of a class destructor distinguished from a constructor?

Programming Warm-Up Exercises

1. Declare a `struct` type, `Time`, that represents an amount of time, consisting of minutes and seconds.

2. Write statements that assign the time 6 minutes and 54 seconds to a variable, `someTime`, of type `Time`, as declared in Exercise 1.

3. Declare a `struct` type, `Song`, that represents a song entry in an MP-3 library. It should have fields for title, album, artist, playing time in minutes and seconds (use the type declared in Exercise 1), and music category. The music category is represented by an enumeration type called `Category`.

4. Write statements to declare a variable called `mySong` of type `Song`, and assign it a set of values. For the playing time, use the variable `someTime` declared in Exercise 2. Make up values for the other fields. Assume that the enumeration type `Category` includes any song category that you wish to use.

5. Write a statement to output the playing time from `mySong`, as declared in Exercise 4, in the format `mm:ss`.

6. Write a declaration of a `union` type called `Temporal` that can hold a time represented as a string, as an integer, or as a value of type `Time`, as declared in Exercise 1.

7. Write the declaration of a variable called `shift` of type `Temporal`, as declared in Exercise 6, and a statement that assigns the value of `someTime`, as declared in Exercise 2, to `shift`.

8. Programming Problems 3 and 4 in Chapter 10 asked you to develop educational programs for teaching the periods of geologic time. Now that you know how to write classes, you can turn the Period ADT into a class. Write a specification file for the `Period` class that has a private field that's an enumeration type, representing the names of the periods. It should have functions that return the period as a string, that return the period as an `int`, that return the starting date of the period, and that increment the period to the next most recent period (if the period is already QUATERNARY, the increment operation should do nothing). It should have a default constructor that sets the period to PRECAMBRIAN, and a constructor with a parameter of the enumeration type to allow the user to create a Period object containing any period. For ease of reference, the table of the time periods is repeated here from Chapter 10. Be sure to use appropriate documenting comments.

Period Name	Starting Date (millions of years)
Quaternary	2.5
Tertiary	65
Cretaceous	136
Jurassic	192
Triassic	225
Permian	280
Carboniferous	345
Devonian	395
Silurian	435
Ordovician	500
Cambrian	570
Precambrian	4500 or earlier

9. Using the `Period` class as specified in Exercise 8, write a For statement that iterates through the periods of geologic time from earliest to most recent, writing out the name of the period and its starting date.

10. Write the function definitions of the two constructors for the `Period` class as specified in Exercise 8.

11. Write the function definition for the `ToInt` observer of the `Period` class specified in Exercise 8.

12. What would the filename be for the file containing the specification of the `Period` class in Exercise 8?

13. Write the `include` directive that would appear near the beginning of the `Period` class implementation file to include the specification file for the `Period` class as described in Exercise 8.

14. Because of floating point representational errors, monetary amounts that need to be exact should not be stored in floating point types. Code the specification for a class that represents an amount of money as dollars and cents. It should have a default constructor that creates an object with zero dollars and zero cents, an

observer for dollars, an observer for cents, and an observer that returns the amount as a float. It also should have transformers that add and subtract other values of class `Money`. Be sure to use appropriate documenting comments.

15. Write the function definitions of the two constructors for the `Money` class as specified in Exercise 14.

16. What would be the filename for the file containing the specification of the `Money` class in Exercise 14?

17. Write the `include` directive that would appear near the beginning of the `Money` class implementation file to include the specification file for the `Money` class as described in Exercise 14.

18. Write the function definitions for the observer in the `Money` class of Exercise 14 that returns the values as a float.

Programming Problems

1. Programming Problem 3 in Chapter 10 asked you to develop an educational program to teach about geologic time. Rewrite that program using a class to implement an ADT representing a period of geologic time. If you did Programming Warm-Up Exercises 8 through 13, this will be a relatively easy rewrite. The program should let the user enter a range of prehistoric dates (in millions of years), and then output the periods that are included in that range. Each time this is done, the user is asked if they want to continue. The goal of the exercise is for the student to try to figure out when each period began, so that he or she can make a chart of geologic time. See Programming Warm-Up Exercise 8 for a list of the geologic time periods and their starting dates.

2. Programming Problem 4 in Chapter 10 asked you to write a second educational program for learning about geologic time. Rewrite that program using a class to implement an ADT representing a period of geologic time. If you did Programming Warm-Up Exercises 8 through 13, then you've already done some of this rewrite. The ADT in those exercises needs to be enhanced with a constructor that takes a string as an argument and converts the string to the corresponding `Period` value (the constructor should work with any style of capitalization of the period names). In this program, the computer picks a date in geologic time and presents it to the student. The student guesses which period corresponds to the date. The student is allowed to continue guessing until he or she gets the right answer. Then the program asks the student whether he or she wants to try again, and repeats the process if the answer is "yes". You also may want to write a function that returns the period for a given date, however, this does not need to be part of the class.

3. In several chapters since Chapter 4, we have included Programming Problems that ask you to develop or rewrite a program that outputs the user's weight on different planets. Our goal in doing this has been for you to see how the same program can be implemented in different ways. Here we would like you to rewrite the program using a class to represent the planet and its gravity. The class should include a constructor that allows a planet to be specified with a

string, using any capitalization (if the string is not a planet name, then Earth should be assumed). The default constructor for the class will create an object representing Earth. The class has an observer operator that takes a weight on Earth as an argument and returns the weight on the planet. It should have a second observer that returns the name of the planet as a string with proper capitalization.

For ease of reference, the information for the original problem is repeated here. The following table gives the factor by which the weight must be multiplied for each planet. The program should output an error message if the user doesn't type a correct planet name. The prompt and the error message should make it clear to the user how a planet name must be entered. Be sure to use proper formatting and appropriate comments in your code. The output should be clearly labeled and neatly formatted.

Planet	Factor
Mercury	0.4155
Venus	0.8975
Earth	1.0
Moon	0.166
Mars	0.3507
Jupiter	2.5374
Saturn	1.0677
Uranus	0.8947
Neptune	1.1794
Pluto	0.0899

4. Design, implement, and test a `class` that represents an amount of time in minutes and seconds. The class should provide a constructor that sets the time to a specified number of minutes and seconds. The default constructor should create an object for a time of zero minutes and zero seconds. The class should provide observers that return the minutes and the seconds separately, and an observer that returns the total time in seconds (minutes $\times$ 60 + seconds). Boolean comparison observers should be provided that test whether two times are equal, one is greater than the other, or one is less than the other. Transformers should be provided that add one time to another, and that subtract one time from another. The class should not allow negative time (subtraction of more time than is currently stored should result in a time of 0:00).

5. Design, implement and test a class that represents a song on a CD or in an MP-3 library. If you did Programming Warm-Up Exercises 3 through 5, you already know how to represent a song as a `struct`. The goal here is to make the ADT an encapsulated `class`. It should have members for title, album, artist, playing time in minutes and seconds (if you've done Problem 4, you can use that class here), and music category. The music category is represented by an enumeration type called `Category`. Make up an enumeration of your favorite categories. The class should have a constructor that allows all of the data members to be set, and a default constructor that sets them all to appropriate empty values. It should have

an observer operation for each data member, and an observer that returns all of the data for the song as a string. An observer that compares two songs for equality also should be developed. Transformers should be provided to allow each data value to be changed.

6. Design, implement and test a class that represents a phone number. The number should be represented by a country code, an area code, a number, and a type. The first three can be integers. The type member is an enumeration of HOME, OFFICE, FAX, CELL, PAGER. The class should provide a default constructor that sets all of the integer values to zero and the type to HOME. A constructor that enables all of the values to be set also should be provided. You also should provide a constructor that takes just the number and type as arguments, and sets the country and area codes to those of your location. The class will have observers that enable each data member to be retrieved, and transformers that allow each data member to be changed. An additional observer should be provided that compares two phone numbers for equality.

Case Study Follow-Up

1. Classify each of the seven member functions of the `Name` class as a constructor, a transformer, or an observer operation.
2. Write a test plan for testing the `ComparedTo` function of the `Name` class.
3. Write a driver to implement your test plan for the `ComparedTo` function.
4. What happens if the client enters an initial when prompted for the middle name? What happens if the client enters an initial followed by a period when prompted for the middle name?
5. Enhance the `Name` class with a title field and an observer function to return its value. Should the title be used in the `ComparedTo` function? Explain your answer.

Arrays

Goals

Knowledge Goals

- To understand the structure of a one-dimensional array.
- To know how to use a one-dimensional array in solving a problem.
- To understand the structure of arrays of records and class objects.
- To know how index values can be made to have semantic content.
- To understand the structure of a two-dimensional array.
- To understand the structure of a multidimensional array.

Skill Goals

To be able to:

- Declare a one-dimensional array, with and without initialization.
- Perform fundamental operations on one-dimensional arrays.
- Apply subarray processing to a one-dimensional array.
- Declare a two-dimensional array.
- Perform fundamental operations on a two-dimensional array.
- Use arrays as parameters and arguments.
- Declare and process a multi-dimensional array.

Data structures play an important role in the design process. The choice of data structure directly affects the design because it determines the algorithms used to process the data. In Chapter 11, we saw how the record (struct) and the class give us the ability to refer to an entire group of components by one name. This simplifies the design of many programs.

In many problems, however, a data structure has so many components that it is difficult to process them if each one must have a unique member name. For example, the IntList abstract data type (ADT) we proposed briefly in Chapter 11 represents a collection of up to 100 integer values. If we used a struct or a class to hold these values, we would need to invent 100 different member names, write 100 different input statements to read values into the members, and write 100 different output statements to display the values—an incredibly tedious task! An *array*—the fourth of the structured data types supported by C++—is a data type that allows us to program operations of this kind with ease.

In this chapter, we examine array data types as provided by the C++ language; in Chapter 13, we show how to combine classes and arrays to implement an ADT such as IntList.

12.1 One-Dimensional Arrays

If we wanted to input 1000 integer values and print them in reverse order, we could write a program of this form:

```
//****************************
// ReverseNumbers program
//****************************
#include <iostream>

using namespace std;

int main()
{
    int value0;
    int value1;
    int value2;
      ⋮
    int value999;

    cin >> value0;
    cin >> value1;
    cin >> value2;
      ⋮
    cin >> value999;
```

```
        cout << value999 << endl;
        cout << value998 << endl;
        cout << value997 << endl;
           ⋮
        cout << value0 << endl;
        return 0;
}
```

This program is over 3000 lines long, and we have to use 1000 separate variables. Note that all the variables have the same name except for an appended number that distinguishes them. Wouldn't it be convenient if we could put the number into a counter variable and use For loops to go from 0 through 999, and then from 999 back down to 0? For example, if the counter variable were `number`, we could replace the 2000 original input/output statements with the following four lines of code (we enclose `number` in brackets to set it apart from `value`):

```
for (number = 0; number < 1000; number++)
    cin >> value[number];
for (number = 999; number >= 0; number--)
    cout << value[number] << endl;
```

This code fragment is correct in C++ *if* we declare `value` to be a *one-dimensional array*, which is a collection of variables—all of the same type—in which the first part of each variable name is the same, and the last part is an *index value* enclosed in square brackets. In our example, the value stored in `number` is called the *index*.

The declaration of a one-dimensional array is similar to the declaration of a simple variable (a variable of a simple data type), with one exception: You must also declare the size of the array. To do so, you indicate within brackets the number of components in the array:

```
int value[1000];
```

This declaration creates an array with 1000 components, all of type `int`. The first component has index value 0, the second component has index value 1, and the last component has index value 999.

Here is the complete ReverseNumbers program, using array notation. This is certainly much shorter than our first version of the program.

```
//****************************
// ReverseNumbers program
//****************************
#include <iostream>

using namespace std;
```

```
int main()
{
    int value[1000];
    int number;

    for (number = 0; number < 1000; number++)
        cin >> value[number];
    for (number = 999; number >= 0; number--)
        cout << value[number] << endl;
    return 0;
}
```

As a data structure, an array differs from a struct or class in two fundamental ways:

1. An array is a *homogeneous* data structure (all components are of the same data type), whereas structs and classes are heterogeneous types (their components may be of different types).

2. A component of an array is accessed by its *position* in the structure, whereas a component of a struct or class is accessed by an identifier (the member name).

Let's now define arrays formally and look at the rules for accessing individual components.

Declaring Arrays

A **one-dimensional array** is a structured collection of components (often called *array elements*) that can be accessed individually by specifying the position of a component with a single index value. (Later in the chapter, we introduce multidimensional arrays, which are arrays that have more than one index value.)

Here is a syntax template describing the simplest form of a one-dimensional array declaration:

> **One-dimensional array** A structured collection of components, all of the same type, that is given a single name. Each component (array element) is accessed by an index that indicates the component's position within the collection.

ArrayDeclaration

> DataType ArrayName [ConstIntExpression] ;

In the syntax template, DataType describes what is stored in each component of the array. Array components may be of almost any type, but for now we limit our discussion to atomic components. ConstIntExpression is an integer expression composed only of literal or named constants. This expression, which specifies the number of compo-

angle   testScore

```
angle[0]  ▨                   testScore[0]  ▨
angle[1]  ▨                   testScore[1]  ▨
angle[2]  ▨                   testScore[2]  ▨
angle[3]  ▨                   testScore[3]  ▨
                              testScore[4]  ▨
                              testScore[5]  ▨
                              testScore[6]  ▨
                              testScore[7]  ▨
                              testScore[8]  ▨
                              testScore[9]  ▨
```

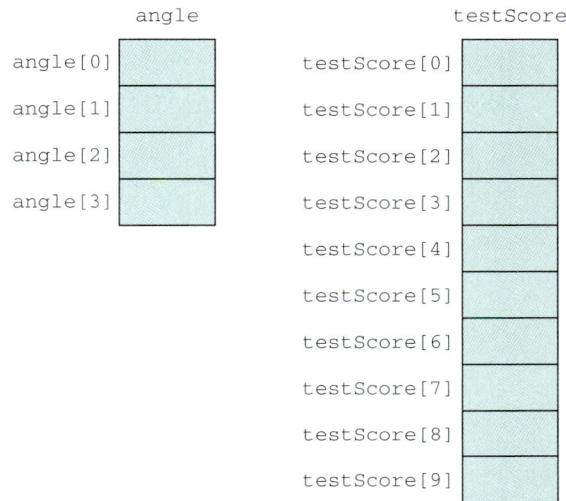

Figure 12–1   *angle* and *testScore* Arrays

nents in the array, must have a value greater than 0. If the value is *n*, the range of index values is 0 through *n* − 1, not 1 through *n*. For example, the declarations

```
float  angle[4];
int    testScore[10];
```

create the arrays shown in Figure 12-1. The `angle` array has four components, each capable of holding one `float` value. The `testScore` array has a total of ten components, all of type `int`.

Accessing Individual Components

Recall that to access an individual component of a struct or class, we use dot notation—the name of the struct variable or class object, followed by a period, followed by the member name. In contrast, to access an individual array component, we write the array name, followed by an expression enclosed in square brackets. The expression specifies which component to access. The syntax template for accessing an array component is

ArrayComponentAccess

```
ArrayName [ IndexExpression ]
```

angle

angle[0]	4.93
angle[1]	-15.2
angle[2]	0.5
angle[3]	1.67

Figure 12-2 *angle Array with Values*

The index expression may be as simple as a constant or a variable name or as complex as a combination of variables, operators, and function calls. Whatever the form of the expression, it must result in an integer value. Index expressions can be of type char, short, int, long, or bool because these are all integral types. Additionally, values of enumeration types can be used as index expressions, with an enumeration value implicitly coerced to an integer.

The simplest form of index expression is a constant. Using our angle array, the sequence of assignment statements

```
angle[0] = 4.93;
angle[1] = -15.2;
angle[2] = 0.5;
angle[3] = 1.67;
```

fills the array components one at a time (see Figure 12-2).

Each array component—angle[2], for instance—can be treated exactly the same as any simple variable of type float. For example, we can do the following to the individual component angle[2]:

```
angle[2] = 9.6;              Assign it a value.
cin >> angle[2];             Read a value into it.
cout << angle[2];           Write its contents.
y = sqrt(angle[2]);         Pass it as an argument.
x = 6.8 * angle[2] + 7.5;   Use it in an arithmetic expression.
```

Let's look at index expressions that are more complicated than constants. Suppose we declare a 1000-element array of int values with the statement

```
int value[1000];
```

and execute the following two statements.

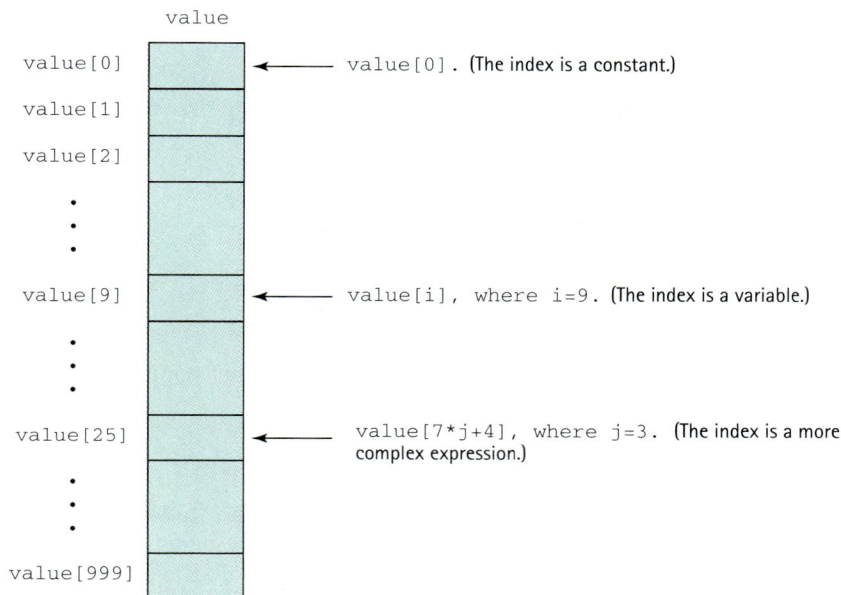

Figure 12–3   *An Index as a Constant, a Variable, and an Arbitrary Expression*

```
value[counter] = 5;
if (value[number+1] % 10 != 0)
    ⋮
```

In the first statement, 5 is stored into an array component. If `counter` is 0, 5 is stored into the first component of the array. If `counter` is 1, 5 is stored into the second place in the array, and so forth.

In the second statement, the expression `number+1` selects an array component. The specific array component accessed is divided by 10 and checked to see if the remainder is nonzero. If `number+1` is 0, we are testing the value in the first component; if `number+1` is 1, we are testing the second place; and so on. Figure 12–3 shows the index expression as a constant, a variable, and a more complex expression.

Note that we have seen the use of square brackets before. In earlier chapters, we said that the `string` class allows you to access an individual character within a string:

```
string aString;

aString = "Hello";
cout << aString[1];     // Prints 'e'
```

Although `string` is a class, not an array, the `string` class was written using the advanced C++ technique of *operator overloading* to give the `[]` operator another meaning (string component selection) in addition to its standard meaning (array element selection). The result is that a `string` object is similar to an array of characters but has special properties.

Out-of-Bounds Array Indexes

Given the declaration

```
float alpha[100];
```

the valid range of index values is 0 through 99. What happens if we execute the statement

```
alpha[i] = 62.4;
```

when `i` is less than 0 or when `i` is greater than 99? The result is that a memory location outside the array is accessed. C++ does not check for invalid (out-of-bounds) array indexes either at compile time or at run time. If `i` happens to be 100 in the statement above, the computer stores 62.4 into the next memory location past the end of the array, destroying whatever value was contained there. It is entirely the programmer's responsibility to make sure that an array index does not step off either end of the array.

> **Out-of-bounds array index** An index value that, in C++, is either less than 0 or greater than the array size minus 1.

Array-processing algorithms often use For loops to step through the array elements one at a time. Here is a loop to zero out our 100-element `alpha` array (`i` is an `int` variable):

```
for (i = 0; i < 100; i++)
    alpha[i] = 0.0;
```

We could also write the first line as

```
for (i = 0; i <= 99; i++)
```

However, C++ programmers commonly use the first version so that the number in the loop test (100) is the same as the array size. With this pattern, it is important to remember to test for *less-than*, not less-than-or-equal.

Initializing Arrays in Declarations

You learned in Chapter 8 that C++ allows you to initialize a variable in its declaration:

```
int delta = 25;
```

The value 25 is called an initializer. You also can initialize an array in its declaration, using a special syntax for the initializer. You specify a list of initial values for the array elements, separate them with commas, and enclose the list within braces:

```
int age[5] = {23, 10, 16, 37, 12};
```

In this declaration, `age[0]` is initialized to 23, `age[1]` is initialized to 10, and so on. There must be at least one initial value between the braces. If you specify too many initial values, you get a syntax error message. If you specify too few, the remaining array elements are initialized to zero.

Arrays follow the same rule as simple variables about the time(s) at which initialization occurs. A static array (one that is either global or declared as `static` within a block) is initialized once only, when control reaches its declaration. An automatic array (one that is local and not declared as `static`) is reinitialized each time control reaches its declaration.

An interesting feature of C++ is that you are allowed to omit the size of an array when you initialize it in a declaration:

```
float temperature[] = {0.0, 112.37, 98.6};
```

The compiler figures out the size of the array (here, 3) according to how many initial values are listed. In general, this feature is not particularly useful. In Chapter 13, though, we'll see that it can be convenient for initializing certain kinds of `char` arrays called C strings.

(Lack of) Aggregate Array Operations

In Chapter 11, we defined an aggregate operation as an operation on a data structure as a whole. Some programming languages allow aggregate operations on arrays, but C++ does not. If x and y are declared as

```
int x[50];
int y[50];
```

there is no aggregate assignment of y to x:

```
x = y;    // Not valid
```

To copy array y into array x, you must do it yourself, element by element:

```
for (index = 0; index < 50; index++)
    x[index] = y[index];
```

Similarly, there is no aggregate comparison of arrays:

```
if (x == y)    // Not valid
```

nor can you perform aggregate I/O of arrays*:

```
cout << x;    // Not valid
```

or aggregate arithmetic on arrays:

```
x = x + y;    // Not valid
```

Finally, it's not possible to return an entire array as the value of a value-returning function:

```
return x;    // Not valid
```

The only thing you can do to an array as a whole is to pass it as an argument to a function:

```
DoSomething(x);
```

Passing an array as an argument gives the function access to the entire array. The following table compares arrays, structs, and classes with respect to aggregate operations.

Aggregate Operation	Arrays	Structs and Classes
I/O	No (except C strings)	No
Assignment	No	Yes
Arithmetic	No	No
Comparison	No	No
Argument passage	By reference only	By value or by reference
Return as a function's return value	No	Yes

Later in the chapter, we look in detail at passing arrays as arguments.

Examples of Declaring and Accessing Arrays

We now look in detail at some specific examples of declaring and accessing arrays. Here are some declarations that a program might use to analyze occupancy rates in an apartment building:

```
const int BUILDING_SIZE = 350;    // Number of apartments

int occupants[BUILDING_SIZE];     // occupants[i] is the number of
                                  //    occupants in apartment i
int totalOccupants;               // Total number of occupants
int counter;                      // Loop control and index variable
```

---

*C++ allows one exception for I/O, which we discuss in Chapter 13. Aggregate I/O is permitted for C strings, which are special kinds of `char` arrays.

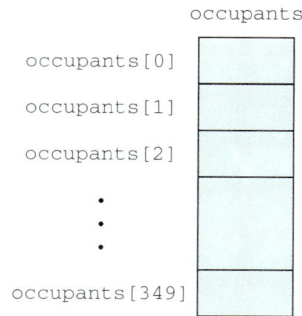

Figure 12-4   *occupants Array*

occupants is a 350-element array of integers (see Figure 12-4). occupants[0] = 3 if the first apartment has three occupants; occupants[1] = 5 if the second apartment has five occupants; and so on. If values have been stored into the array, then the following code totals the number of occupants in the building.

```
totalOccupants = 0;
for (counter = 0; counter < BUILDING_SIZE; counter++)
    totalOccupants = totalOccupants + occupants[counter];
```

The first time through the loop, counter is 0. We add the contents of totalOccupants (that is, 0) to the contents of occupants[0], storing the result into totalOccupants. Next, counter becomes 1 and the loop test occurs. The second loop iteration adds the contents of totalOccupants to the contents of occupants[1], storing the result into totalOccupants. Now counter becomes 2 and the loop test is made. Eventually, the loop adds the contents of occupants[349] to the sum and increments counter to 350. At this point, the loop condition is false, and control exits the loop.

Note how we used the named constant BUILDING_SIZE in both the array declaration and the For loop. When constants are used in this manner, changes are easy to make. If the number of apartments changes from 350 to 400, we need to change only one line: the const declaration of BUILDING_SIZE. If we had used the literal value 350 in place of BUILDING_SIZE, we would need to update several of the statements in the code above, and probably many more throughout the rest of the program.

The following is a complete program that uses the occupants array. The program fills the array with occupant data read from an input file and then lets the user interactively look up the number of occupants in a specific apartment.

```
//*******************************************************************
// Apartment program
// This program allows a building owner to look up how many
// occupants are in a given apartment
// Note: This program is missing code to check for user input errors
//*******************************************************************
#include <iostream>
```

```cpp
#include <fstream>                    // For file I/O

using namespace std;

const int BUILDING_SIZE = 350;        // Number of apartments

int main()
{
    int occupants[BUILDING_SIZE]; // occupants[i] is the number of
                                  //    occupants in apartment i
    int totalOccupants;           // Total number of occupants
    int counter;                  // Loop control and index variable
    int apt;                      // An apartment number
    ifstream inFile;              // File of occupant data (one
                                  //    integer per apartment)

    inFile.open("apt.dat");
    totalOccupants = 0;
    for (counter = 0; counter < BUILDING_SIZE; counter++)
    {
        inFile >> occupants[counter];
        totalOccupants = totalOccupants + occupants[counter];
    }
    cout << "No. of apts. is " << BUILDING_SIZE << endl
         << "Total no. of occupants is " << totalOccupants << endl;

    cout << "Begin apt. lookup..." << endl;
    do
    {
        cout << "Apt. number (1 through " << BUILDING_SIZE
             << ", or 0 to quit): ";
        cin >> apt;
        if (apt > 0)
            cout << "Apt. " << apt << " has " << occupants[apt-1]
                 << " occupants" << endl;
    } while (apt > 0);
    return 0;
}
```

Look closely at the last output statement in the Apartment program. The user enters an apartment number (apt) in the range 1 through BUILDING_SIZE, but the array has indexes 0 through BUILDING_SIZE – 1. Therefore, we must subtract 1 from apt so that we index into the proper place in the array.

Because an array index is an integer value, we access the components by their position in the array—that is, the first, the second, the third, and so on. Using an int index is the most common way of thinking about an array. C++, however, provides more flexibility by allowing an index to be of any integral type or enumeration type. (The index expression still must evaluate to an integer in the range from 0 through one less than the array size.) The next example shows an array in which the indexes are values of an enumeration type.

```
enum Drink {ORANGE, COLA, ROOT_BEER, GINGER_ALE, CHERRY, LEMON};

float salesAmt[6];  // Array of 6 floats, to be indexed by Drink type
Drink flavor;       // Variable of the index type
```

Drink is an enumeration type in which the enumerators ORANGE, COLA, ..., LEMON have internal representations 0 through 5, respectively. salesAmt is a group of six float components representing dollar sales figures for each kind of drink (see Figure 12–5). The following code prints the values in the array (see Chapter 10 to review how to increment values of enumeration types in For loops).

```
for (flavor = ORANGE; flavor <= LEMON; flavor = Drink(flavor + 1))
    cout << salesAmt[flavor] << endl;
```

Here is one last example.

```
const int NUM_STUDENTS = 10;

char grade[NUM_STUDENTS];    // Array of 10 student letter grades
int  idNumber;               // Student ID number (0 through 9)
```

The grade array is pictured in Figure 12–6. Values are shown in the components, which implies that some processing of the array has already occurred. Following are some simple examples showing how the array might be used.

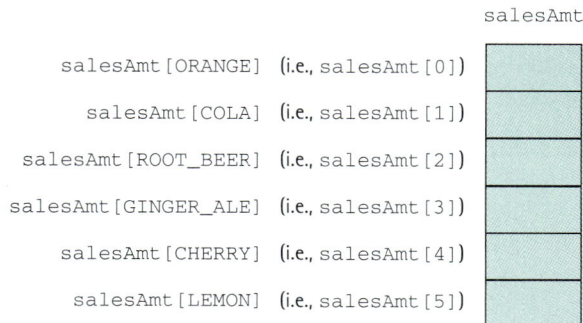

		salesAmt
salesAmt[ORANGE]	(i.e., salesAmt[0])	
salesAmt[COLA]	(i.e., salesAmt[1])	
salesAmt[ROOT_BEER]	(i.e., salesAmt[2])	
salesAmt[GINGER_ALE]	(i.e., salesAmt[3])	
salesAmt[CHERRY]	(i.e., salesAmt[4])	
salesAmt[LEMON]	(i.e., salesAmt[5])	

Figure 12–5 *salesAmt Array*

grade

Figure 12–6   *grade Array with Values*

`cin >> grade[2];`	Reads the next nonwhitespace character from the input stream and stores it into the component in grade indexed by 2.
`grade[3] = 'A';`	Assigns the character 'A' to the component in grade indexed by 3.
`idNumber = 5;`	Assigns 5 to the index variable idNumber.
`grade[idNumber] = 'C';`	Assigns the character 'C' to the component of grade indexed by idNumber (that is, by 5).

`for (idNumber = 0; idNumber < NUM_STUDENTS;`
`    idNumber++)`
`    cout << grade[idNumber];`
	Loops through the grade array, printing each component. For this loop, the output would be FBCAFCAACB.

`for (idNumber = 0; idNumber < NUM_STUDENTS;`
`    idNumber++)`
`    cout << "Student " << idNumber`
`        << " Grade " << grade[idNumber]`
`        << endl;`
	Loops through grade, printing each component in a more readable form.

In the last example, idNumber is used as the index, but it also has semantic content—it is the student's identification number. The output would be

```
Student 0 Grade F
Student 1 Grade B
   ⋮
Student 9 Grade B
```

Passing Arrays as Arguments

In Chapter 8, we said that if a variable is passed to a function and it is not to be changed by the function, then the variable should be passed by value instead of by reference. We specifically excluded stream variables (such as those representing data files) from this rule and said that there would be one more exception. Arrays are this exception.

By default, C++ simple variables are always passed by value. To pass a simple variable by reference, you must append an ampersand (&) to the data type name in the function's parameter list:

```
int SomeFunc( float param1,    // Pass-by-value
              char& param2 )   // Pass-by-reference
{
    ⋮
}
```

It is impossible to pass a C++ array by value; arrays are *always* passed by reference. Therefore, you never use & when declaring an array as a parameter. When an array is passed as an argument, its **base address**—the memory address of the first element of the array—is sent to the function. The function then knows where the caller's actual array is located and can access any element of the array.

> **Base address**   The memory address of the first element of an array.

Here is a C++ function that will zero out a one-dimensional `float` array of any size:

```
void ZeroOut( /* out */ float arr[],
              /* in */  int   numElements )
{
    int i;

    for (i = 0; i < numElements; i++)
        arr[i] = 0.0;
}
```

In the parameter list, the declaration of `arr` does not include a size within the brackets. If you include a size, the compiler ignores it. The compiler only wants to know that it is a `float` array, not a `float` array of any particular size. Therefore, in the `ZeroOut` function you must include a second parameter—the number of array elements—in order for the For loop to work correctly.

The calling code can invoke the `ZeroOut` function for a `float` array of any size. The following code fragment makes function calls to zero out two arrays of different sizes. Notice how an array parameter is declared in a function prototype.

```
void ZeroOut( float[], int );    // Function prototype
 ⋮
int main()
{
    float velocity[30];
    float refractionAngle[9000];
     ⋮
    ZeroOut(velocity, 30);
    ZeroOut(refractionAngle, 9000);
     ⋮
}
```

With simple variables, passing by value prevents a function from modifying the caller's argument. Although you cannot pass arrays by value in C++, you can still prevent the function from modifying the caller's array. To do so, you use the reserved word const in the declaration of the parameter. Below is a function that copies one int array into another. The first parameter—the destination array—is expected to be modified, but the second array is not.

```
void Copy( /* out */        int destination[],
           /* in */   const int source[],
           /* in */        int size            )
{
    int i;

    for (i = 0; i < size; i++)
        destination[i] = source[i];
}
```

The word const guarantees that any attempt to modify the source array within the Copy function results in a compile-time error.

Here's a table that summarizes argument passage for simple variables and one-dimensional arrays:

Argument	Parameter Declaration for a Pass by Value	Parameter Declaration for a Pass by Reference
Simple variable	int cost	int& price
Array	Impossible*	int arr[]

*However, prefixing the array declaration with the word const prevents the function from modifying the parameter.

One final remark about argument passage: It is a common mistake to pass an array *element* to a function when passing the entire array was intended. For example, our

ZeroOut function expects the base address of a `float` array to be sent as the first argument. In the following code fragment, the function call is an error.

```
float velocity[30];
   ⋮
ZeroOut(velocity[30], 30);    // Error
```

First of all, `velocity[30]` denotes a single array element—one floating-point number—and not an entire array. Furthermore, there is no array element with an index of 30. The indexes for the `velocity` array run from 0 through 29.

Background Information

C, C++, and Arrays as Arguments

Some programming languages allow arrays to be passed either by value or by reference. Remember that with passing by value, a copy of the argument is sent to the function. When an array is passed by value, the entire array is copied. Not only is extra space required in the function to hold the copy, but the copying itself takes time. Passing by reference requires only that the address of the argument be passed to the function, so when an array is passed by reference, just the address of the first array component is passed. Thus, passing large arrays by reference saves both memory and time.

The C programming language—the direct predecessor of C++—was designed to be a system programming language. System programs, such as compilers, assemblers, linkers, and operating systems, must be both fast and economical with memory space. In the design of the C language, passing arrays by value was judged to be an unnecessary language feature. Serious system programmers never used a pass by value when working with arrays. Therefore, both C and C++ pass arrays only by reference.

Of course, using a reference parameter can lead to inadvertent errors if the values are changed within the function. In early versions of the C language, there was no way to protect the caller's array from being modified by the function.

C++ (and recent versions of C) added the ability to declare an array parameter as `const`. By declaring the array as `const`, a compile-time error occurs if the function attempts to modify the array. As a result, C++ supports the efficiency of passing arrays by reference yet also provides the protection (through `const`) of passing by value.

Whenever your design of a function's interface identifies an array parameter as incoming-only (to be inspected but not modified by the function), declare the array as `const` to obtain the same protection as passing by value.

Assertions About Arrays

In assertions written as comments, we often need to refer to a range of array elements:

```
// Assert: alpha[i] through alpha[j] have been printed
```

To specify such ranges, it is more convenient to use an abbreviated notation consisting of two dots:

```
// Assert: alpha[i]..alpha[j] have been printed
```

or, more briefly:

```
// Assert: alpha[i..j] have been printed
```

Note that this dot-dot notation is not valid syntax in C++ language statements. We are talking only about comments in a program.

As an example of the use of this notation, here is how we would write the precondition and postcondition for our ZeroOut function:

```
void ZeroOut( /* out */ float arr[],
              /* in */  int   numElements )

// Precondition:
//     numElements is assigned
// Postcondition:
//     arr[0..numElements-1] == 0.0

{
    int i;

    for (i = 0; i < numElements; i++)
        arr[i] = 0.0;
}
```

Using Typedef with Arrays

In Chapter 10, we discussed the Typedef statement as a way of giving an additional name to an existing data type. We said that before bool became a built-in type in C++, programmers often used a Typedef statement such as the following:

```
typedef int Boolean;
```

We can also use Typedef to give a name to an array type. Here's an example:

```
typedef float FloatArr[100];
```

This statement says that the type `FloatArr` is the same as the type "100-element array of `float`." (Notice that the array size in brackets comes at the very end of the statement.) We can now declare variables to be of type `FloatArr`:

```
FloatArr angle;
FloatArr velocity;
```

The compiler essentially translates these declarations into

```
float angle[100];
float velocity[100];
```

In this book, we don't often use Typedefs to give names to one-dimensional array types. However, when we discuss multidimensional arrays later in the chapter, we'll see that the technique can come in handy.

12.2 Arrays of Records and Class Objects

Although arrays with atomic components are very common, many applications require a collection of records or class objects. For example, a business needs a list of parts records, and a teacher needs a list of students in a class. Arrays are ideal for these applications. We simply define an array whose components are records or class objects.

Arrays of Records

Let's define a grade book to be a collection of student records as follows:

```
const int MAX_STUDENTS = 150;

enum GradeType {A, B, C, D, F};

struct StudentRec
{
    string    stuName;
    float     gpa;
    int       examScore[4];
    GradeType courseGrade;
};


StudentRec gradeBook[MAX_STUDENTS];
int        count;
```

This data structure can be visualized as shown in Figure 12–7.

gradeBook

Figure 12–7   *gradeBook Array with Records as Elements*

An element of gradeBook is selected by an index. For example, gradeBook[2] is the third component in the array gradeBook. Each component of gradeBook is a record of type StudentRec. To access the course grade of the third student, we use the following expression:

gradeBook[2].courseGrade

Specifies third record in array gradeBook

Specifies courseGrade member in record gradeBook[2]

The record component gradeBook[2].examScore is an array. We can access the individual elements in this component just as we would access the elements of any other array: We give the name of the array followed by the index, which is enclosed in brackets.

gradeBook[2].examScore[0]

Specifies third record in array gradeBook

Specifies examScore member (an array)

Specifies first score in examScore member

The following code fragment prints the name of each student in the class:

```
for (count = 0; count < MAX_STUDENTS; count++)
    cout << gradeBook[count].stuName << endl;
```

Arrays of Class Objects

The syntax for declaring and using arrays of class objects is the same as for arrays of structs. Given the `Time` class of Chapter 11, we can maintain a collection of ten appointment times by starting with the declaration

```
Time appointment[10];
```

This statement creates a ten-element array named `appointment`, in which each element is a `TimeType` object. The following statements set the first two appointment times to 8:45:00 and 10:00:00.

```
appointment[0].Set(8, 45, 0);
appointment[1].Set(10, 0, 0);
```

To output all ten appointment times, we would write

```
for (index = 0; index < 10; index++)
{
    appointment[index].Write();
    cout << endl;
}
```

Recall that the `Time` class has two constructors defined for it. One is the default (parameterless) constructor, which sets the time for a newly created object to 00:00:00. The other is a parameterized constructor with which the client code can specify an initial time when the class object is created. How are constructors handled when you declare an array of class objects? Here is the rule in C++:

If a class has at least one constructor, and an array of class objects is declared:

```
SomeClass arr[50];
```

then one of the constructors *must* be the default (parameterless) constructor. This constructor is invoked for each element of the array.

Therefore, with our declaration of the `appointment` array

```
Time appointment[10];
```

the default constructor is called for all ten array elements, setting each time to an initial value of 00:00:00.

12.3 Special Kinds of Array Processing

Two types of array processing occur especially often: using only part of the declared array (a subarray) and using index values that have specific meaning within the problem (indexes with semantic content). We describe both of these methods briefly here and give further examples in the remainder of the chapter.

Subarray Processing

The *size* of an array—the declared number of array components—is established at compile time. We have to declare it to be as big as it would ever need to be. Because the exact number of values to be put into the array often depends on the data itself, however, we may not fill all of the array components with values. The problem is that to avoid processing empty ones, we must keep track of how many components are actually filled.

As values are put into the array, we keep a count of how many components are filled. We then use this count to process only components that have values stored in them. Any remaining places are not processed. For example, if there are 250 students in a class, a program to analyze test grades would set aside 250 locations for the grades. However, some students may be absent on the day of the test. So the number of test grades must be counted, and that number, rather than 250, is used to control the processing of the array.

If the number of data items actually stored in an array is less than its declared size, functions that receive array parameters must also receive the number of data items as a parameter. For example,

```
void Print( /* in */ const char grade[],        // Array for up to
                                                 //    250 students
               /* in */        int  numGrades )  // Number of grades
                                                 //    actually in array
```

Indexes with Semantic Content

In some problems, an array index has meaning beyond simple position; that is, the index has *semantic content*. An example is the `salesAmt` array we showed earlier. This array is indexed by a value of enumeration type `Drink`. The index of a specific sales amount is the kind of soft drink sold; for example, `salesAmt[ROOT_BEER]` is the dollar sales figure for root beer.

The next section gives additional examples of indexes with semantic content.

12.4 Two-Dimensional Arrays

A one-dimensional array is used to represent items in a list or sequence of values. In many problems, however, the relationships between data items are more complex than a simple list. A **two-dimensional array** is used to represent items in a table with rows and columns, provided each item in the table is of the same data type. Two-dimensional arrays are useful for representing board games, such as chess, tic-tac-toe, or Scrabble, and in computer graphics, where the screen is thought of as a two-dimensional array. A component in

> **Two-dimensional array**   A collection of components, all of the same type, structured in two dimensions. Each component is accessed by a pair of indexes that represent the component's position in each dimension.

a two-dimensional array is accessed by specifying the row and column indexes of the item in the array. This is a familiar task. For example, if you want to find a street on a map, you look up the street name on the back of the map to find the coordinates of the street, usually a letter and a number. The letter specifies a column to look on, and the number specifies a row. You find the street where the row and column meet.

Figure 12–8 shows a two-dimensional array with 100 rows and 9 columns. The rows are accessed by an integer ranging from 0 through 99; the columns are accessed by an integer ranging from 0 through 8. Each component is accessed by a row-column pair—for example, 0, 5.

A two-dimensional array is declared in exactly the same way as a one-dimensional array, except that sizes must be specified for two dimensions. On the next page is the syntax template for declaring an array with more than one dimension, along with an example.

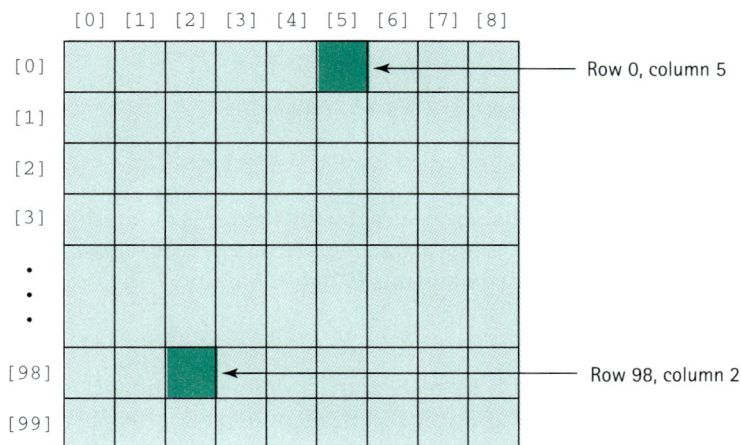

Figure 12–8   *A Two-Dimensional Array*

ArrayDeclaration

DataType ArrayName [ConstIntExpression] [ConstIntExpression] ... ;

```
const int NUM_ROWS = 100;
const int NUM_COLS = 9;
  ⋮
float alpha[NUM_ROWS][NUM_COLS];
```

First
dimension

Second
dimension

This example declares `alpha` to be a two-dimensional array, all of whose components are `float` values. The declaration creates the array that is pictured in Figure 12–8.

To access an individual component of the `alpha` array, two expressions (one for each dimension) are used to specify its position. Each expression is in its own pair of brackets next to the name of the array:

```
alpha[0][5] = 36.4;
```

Row
number

Column
number

The syntax template for accessing an array component is

ArrayComponentAccess

ArrayName [IndexExpression] [IndexExpression] ...

As with one-dimensional arrays, each index expression must result in an integer value.

Let's look now at some examples. Here is the declaration of a two-dimensional array with 364 integer components ($52 \times 7 = 364$):

```
int hiTemp[52][7];
```

`hiTemp` is an array with 52 rows and 7 columns. Each place in the array (each component) can contain any `int` value. Our intention is that the array contains high temperatures for each day in a year. Each row represents one of the 52 weeks in a year, and each column represents one of the 7 days in a week. (To keep the example simple, we

hiTemp

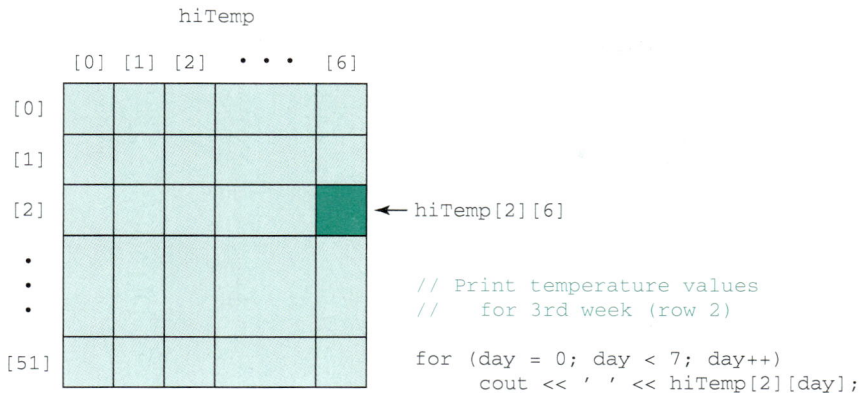

Figure 12–9   *hiTemp Array*

ignore the fact that there are 365—and sometimes 366—days in a year.) The expression
hiTemp[2][6] refers to the int value in the third row (row 2) and the seventh column
(column 6). Semantically, hiTemp[2][6] is the temperature for the seventh day of the
third week. The code fragment shown in Figure 12–9 would print the temperature values
for the third week.

Another representation of the same data might be as follows:

```
enum DayType
{
    MONDAY, TUESDAY, WEDNESDAY, THURSDAY, FRIDAY, SATURDAY, SUNDAY
};


int hiTemp[52][7];
```

Here, hiTemp is declared the same as before, but we can use an expression of type
DayType for the column index. hiTemp[2][SUNDAY] corresponds to the same component as hiTemp[2][6] in the first example. (Recall that enumerators such as MONDAY,
TUESDAY,... are represented internally as the integers 0, 1, 2, ...) If day is of type
DayType and week is of type int, the code fragment shown in Figure 12–10 sets the
entire array to 0. (Notice that by using DayType, the temperature values in the array
begin with the first Monday of the year, not necessarily with January 1.)

Another way of looking at a two-dimensional array is to see it as a structure in
which each component has two features. For example, in the following code,

```
enum Colors {RED, ORANGE, YELLOW, GREEN, BLUE, INDIGO, VIOLET};
enum Makes
{
    FORD, TOYOTA, HYUNDAI, JAGUAR, CITROEN, BMW, FIAT, SAAB
};
```

hiTemp

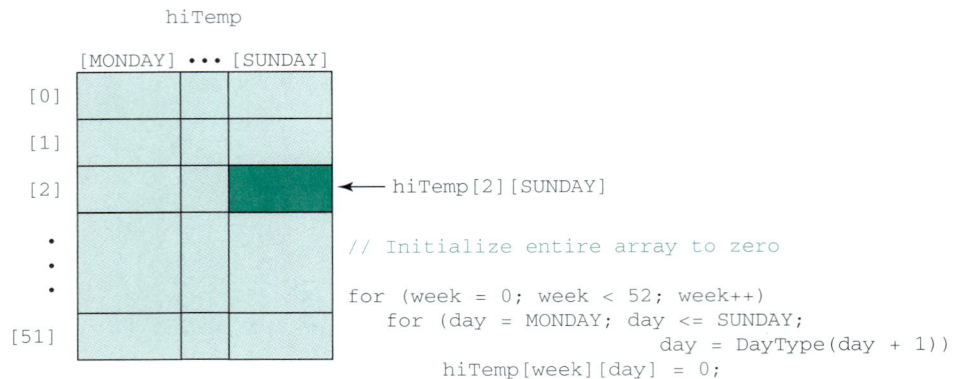

```
// Initialize entire array to zero

for (week = 0; week < 52; week++)
    for (day = MONDAY; day <= SUNDAY;
                day = DayType(day + 1))
        hiTemp[week][day] = 0;
```

Figure 12–10   *hiTemp Array (Alternate Form)*

```
const int NUM_COLORS = 7;
const int NUM_MAKES = 8;

float crashRating[NUM_COLORS][NUM_MAKES];   // Array of crash
                                            // likelihoods by color
                                            // and make
    ⋮
crashRating[BLUE][JAGUAR] = 0.83;           // Blue Jaguars have a crash
                                            //    likelihood of 0.83
crashRating[RED][FORD] = 0.19;              // Red Fords have a crash
                                            //    likelihood of 0.19
```

the data structure uses one dimension to represent the color and the other to represent the make of automobile. In other words, both indexes have semantic content—a concept we discussed in the previous section.

12.5 Processing Two-Dimensional Arrays

Processing data in a two-dimensional array generally means accessing the array in one of four patterns: randomly, along rows, along columns, or throughout the entire array. Each of these may also involve subarray processing.

The simplest way to access a component is to look directly in a given location. For example, a user enters map coordinates that we use as indexes into an array of street names to access the desired name at those coordinates. This process is referred to as *random access* because the user may enter any set of coordinates at random.

There are many cases in which we might wish to perform an operation on all the elements of a particular row or column in an array. Consider the `hiTemp` array defined previously, in which the rows represent weeks of the year and the columns represent days of the week. If we wanted the average high temperature for a given week, we would sum the values in that row and divide by 7. If we wanted the average for a given day of the week, we would sum the values in that column and divide by 52. The former case is access by row; the latter case is access by column.

Now suppose that we wish to determine the average for the year. We must access every element in the array, sum them, and divide by 364. In this case, the order of access—by row or by column—is not important. (The same is true when we initialize every element of an array to zero.) This is access throughout the array.

There are times when we must access every array element in a particular order, either by rows or by columns. For example, if we wanted the average for every week, we would run through the entire array, taking each row in turn. However, if we wanted the average for each day of the week, we would run through the array a column at a time.

Let's take a closer look at these patterns of access by considering four common examples of array processing.

1. Sum the rows.
2. Sum the columns.
3. Initialize the array to all zeros (or some special value).
4. Print the array.

First, let's define some constants and variables using general identifiers, such as `row` and `col`, rather than problem-dependent identifiers. Then let's look at each algorithm in terms of generalized two-dimensional array processing.

```
const int NUM_ROWS = 50;
const int NUM_COLS = 50;

int arr[NUM_ROWS][NUM_COLS];      // A two-dimensional array
int row;                          // A row index
int col;                          // A column index
int total;                        // A variable for summing
```

Sum the Rows

Suppose we want to sum row number 3 (the fourth row) in the array and print the result. We can do this easily with a For loop:

```
total = 0;
for (col = 0; col < NUM_COLS; col++)
    total = total + arr[3][col];
cout << "Row sum: " << total << endl;
```

This For loop runs through each column of `arr`, while keeping the row index fixed at 3. Every value in row 3 is added to `total`.

Now suppose we want to sum and print two rows—row 2 and row 3. We can use a nested loop and make the row index a variable:

```
for (row = 2; row < 4; row++)
{
    total = 0;
    for (col = 0; col < NUM_COLS; col++)
        total = total + arr[row][col];
    cout << "Row sum: " << total << endl;
}
```

The outer loop controls the rows, and the inner loop controls the columns. For each value of `row`, every column is processed; then the outer loop moves to the next row. In the first iteration of the outer loop, `row` is held at 2 and `col` goes from 0 through `NUM_COLS-1`. Therefore, the array is accessed in the following order:

```
arr[2][0]    [2][1]    [2][2]    [2][3]  . . .    [2][NUM_COLS-1]
```

In the second iteration of the outer loop, `row` is incremented to 3, and the array is accessed as follows:

```
arr[3][0]    [3][1]    [3][2]    [3][3]  . . .    [3][NUM_COLS-1]
```

We can generalize this row processing to run through every row of the array by having the outer loop run from 0 through `NUM_ROWS-1`. However, if we want to access only part of the array (subarray processing), given variables declared as

```
int rowsFilled;    // Data is in 0..rowsFilled-1
int colsFilled;    // Data is in 0..colsFilled-1
```

then we write the code fragment as follows:

```
for (row = 0; row < rowsFilled; row++)
{
    total = 0;
    for (col = 0; col < colsFilled; col++)
        total = total + arr[row][col];
    cout << "Row sum: " << total << endl;
}
```

Figure 12–11 illustrates subarray processing by row.

arr

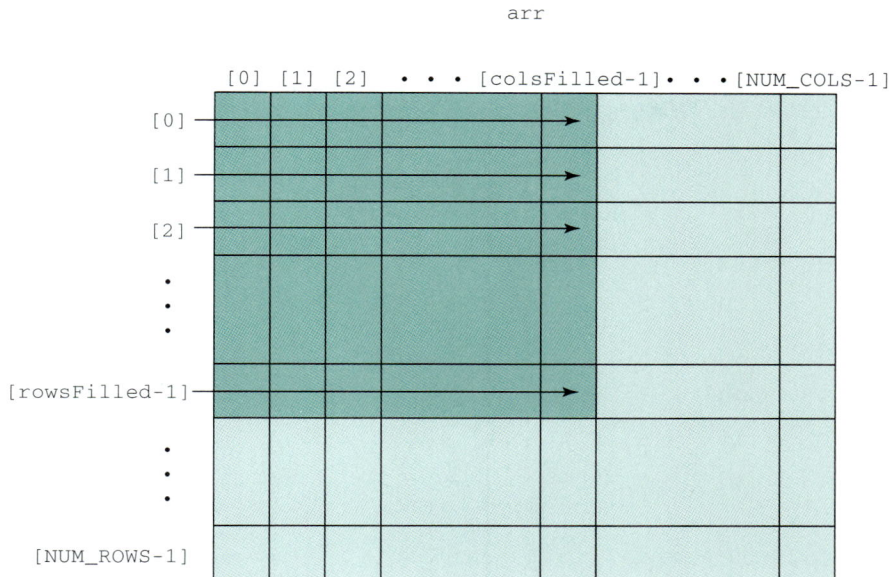

Figure 12-11   *Partial Array Processing by Row*

Sum the Columns

Suppose we want to sum and print each column. The code to perform this task follows. Again, we have generalized the code to sum only the portion of the array that contains valid data.

```
for (col = 0; col < colsFilled; col++)
{
    total = 0;
    for (row = 0; row < rowsFilled; row++)
        total = total + arr[row][col];
    cout << "Column sum: " << total << endl;
}
```

In this case, the outer loop controls the column, and the inner loop controls the row. All the components in the first column are accessed and summed before the outer loop index changes and the components in the second column are accessed. Figure 12–12 illustrates subarray processing by column.

arr

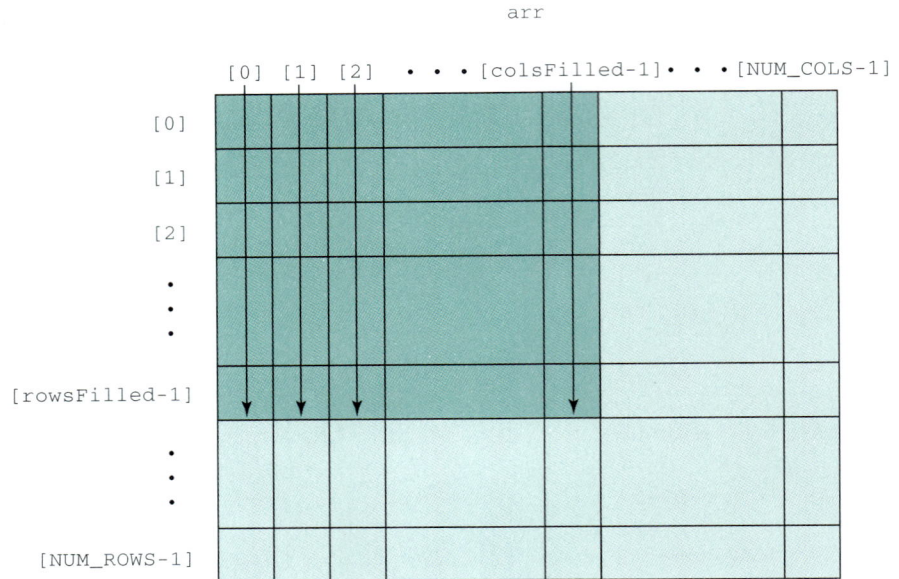

Figure 12–12   *Partial Array Processing by Column*

Initialize the Array

As with one-dimensional arrays, we can initialize a two-dimensional array either by initializing it in its declaration or by using assignment statements. If the array is small, it is simplest to initialize it in its declaration. To initialize a two-row by three-column array to look like this:

```
14    3   -5
 0   46    7
```

we can use the following declaration.

```
int arr[2][3] =
{
    {14, 3, -5},
    {0, 46, 7}
};
```

In this declaration, the initializer list consists of two items, each of which is itself an initializer list. The first inner initializer list stores 14, 3, and –5 into row 0 of the array; the second stores 0, 46, and 7 into row 1. The use of two initializer lists makes sense if you think of each row of the two-dimensional array as a one-dimensional array of three ints. The first initializer list initializes the first array (the first row), and the second list initializes the second array (the second row). Later in the chapter, we revisit this notion of viewing a two-dimensional array as an array of arrays.

Initializing an array in its declaration is impractical if the array is large. For a 100-row by 100-column array, you don't want to list 10,000 values. If the values are all different, you should store them into a file and input them into the array at run time. If the values are all the same, the usual approach is to use nested For loops and an assignment statement. Here is a general-purpose code segment that zeros out an array with NUM_ROWS rows and NUM_COLS columns:

```
for (row = 0; row < NUM_ROWS; row++)
    for (col = 0; col < NUM_COLS; col++)
        arr[row][col] = 0;
```

In this case, we initialized the array a row at a time, but we could just as easily have run through each column instead. The order doesn't matter as long as we access every element.

Print the Array

If we wish to print out an array with one row per line, then we have another case of row processing:

```
#include <iomanip>    // For setw()
   ⋮
for (row = 0; row < NUM_ROWS; row++)
{
    for (col = 0; col < NUM_COLS; col++)
        cout << setw(15) << arr[row][col];
    cout << endl;
}
```

This code fragment prints the values of the array in columns that are 15 characters wide. As a matter of proper style, this fragment should be preceded by code that prints headings over the columns to identify their contents.

There's no rule that we have to print each row on a line. We could turn the array sideways and print each column on one line simply by exchanging the two For loops. When you are printing a two-dimensional array, you must consider which order of presentation makes the most sense and how the array fits on the page. For example, an array with 6 columns and 100 rows would be best printed as 6 columns, 100 lines long.

Almost all processing of data stored in a two-dimensional array involves either processing by row or processing by column. In most of our examples the index type has been int, but the pattern of operation of the loops is the same no matter what types the indexes are.

The looping patterns for row processing and column processing are so useful that we summarize them below. To make them more general, we use minRow for the first row number and minCol for the first column number. Remember that row processing has the row index in the outer loop, and column processing has the column index in the outer loop.

Row Processing

```
for (row = minRow; row < rowsFilled; row++)
    for (col = minCol; col < colsFilled; col++)
        ⋮              // Whatever processing is required
```

Column Processing

```
for (col = minCol; col < colsFilled; col++)
    for (row = minRow; row < rowsFilled; row++)
        ⋮              // Whatever processing is required
```

12.6 Passing Two-Dimensional Arrays as Arguments

Earlier in the chapter, we said that when one-dimensional arrays are declared as parameters in a function, the size of the array usually is omitted from the square brackets:

```
void SomeFunc( /* inout */ float alpha[],
               /* in */    int   size   )
{
    ⋮
}
```

If you include a size in the brackets, the compiler ignores it. As you learned, the base address of the caller's argument (the memory address of the first array element) is passed to the function. The function works for an argument of any size. Because the function cannot know the size of the caller's array, we either pass the size as an argument—as in SomeFunc above—or use a named constant if the function always operates on an array of a certain size.

When a two-dimensional array is passed as an argument, again the base address of the caller's array is sent to the function. But you cannot leave off the sizes of both of the array dimensions. You can omit the size of the first dimension (the number of rows) but not the second (the number of columns). Here is the reason.

In the computer's memory, C++ stores two-dimensional arrays in row order. Thinking of memory as one long line of memory cells, the first row of the array is followed by the second row, which is followed by the third, and so on (see Figure 12–13). To locate beta[1][0] in this figure, a function that receives beta's base address must be able to know that there are four elements in each row—that is, that the array consists of four columns. Therefore, the declaration of a parameter must always state the number of columns:

```
void AnotherFunc( /* inout */ int beta[][4] )
{
    ⋮
}
```

MEMORY

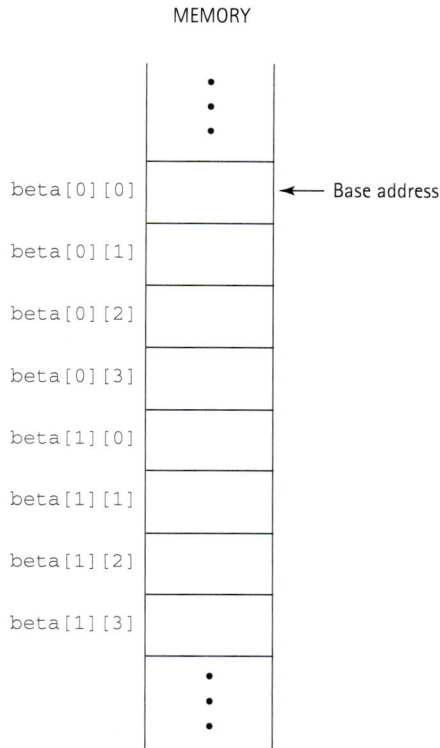

Figure 12–13 *Memory Layout for a Two-Row by Four-Column Array*

Furthermore, the number of columns declared for the parameter must be *exactly* the same as the number of columns in the caller's array. As you can tell from Figure 12–13, if there is any discrepancy in the number of columns, the function will access the wrong array element in memory.

Our AnotherFunc function works for a two-dimensional array of any number of rows, as long as it has exactly four columns. In practice, we seldom write programs that use arrays with a varying number of rows but the same number of columns. To avoid problems with mismatches in argument and parameter sizes, it's practical to use a Typedef statement to define a two-dimensional array type and then declare both the argument and the parameter to be of that type. For example, we might make the declarations

```
const int NUM_ROWS = 10;
const int NUM_COLS = 20;
typedef int ArrayType[NUM_ROWS][NUM_COLS];
```

and then write the following general-purpose function that initializes all elements of an array to a specified value:

```cpp
void Initialize( /* out */ ArrayType arr,      // Array to initialize
                 /* in */  int        initVal) // Initial value

// Initializes each element of arr to initVal

// Precondition:
//     initVal is assigned
// Postcondition:
//     arr[0..NUM_ROWS-1][0..NUM_COLS-1] == initVal

{
    int row;
    int col;

    for (row = 0; row < NUM_ROWS; row++)
        for (col = 0; col < NUM_COLS; col++)
            arr[row][col] = initVal;
}
```

The calling code could then declare and initialize one or more arrays of type ArrayType by making calls to the Initialize function. For example,

```cpp
ArrayType delta;
ArrayType gamma;

Initialize(delta, 0);
Initialize(gamma, -1);
    ⋮
```

12.7 Another Way of Defining Two-Dimensional Arrays

We hinted earlier that a two-dimensional array can be viewed as an array of arrays. This view is supported by C++ in the sense that the components of a one-dimensional array do not have to be atomic. The components can themselves be structured—structs, class objects, even arrays. For example, our hiTemp array could be declared as follows.

```cpp
typedef int WeekType[7];    // Array type for 7 temperature readings

WeekType hiTemp[52];        // Array of 52 WeekType arrays
```

With this declaration, the 52 components of the hiTemp array are one-dimensional arrays of type WeekType. In other words, hiTemp has two dimensions. We can refer to each row as an entity: hiTemp[2] refers to the array of temperatures for week 2. We can also access each individual component of hiTemp by specifying both indexes: hiTemp[2][0] accesses the temperature on the first day of week 2.

Does it matter which way we declare a two-dimensional array? Not to C++. The choice should be based on readability and understandability. Sometimes the features of the data are shown more clearly if both indexes are specified in a single declaration. At other times, the code is clearer if one dimension is defined first as a one-dimensional array type.

Here is an example of when it is advantageous to define a two-dimensional array as an array of arrays. If the rows have been defined first as a one-dimensional array type, each row can be passed to a function whose parameter is a one-dimensional array of the same type. For example, the following function calculates and returns the maximum value in an array of type WeekType.

```
int Maximum( /* in */ const WeekType data )   // Array to be examined

// Precondition:
//      data[0..6] are assigned
// Postcondition:
//      Function value == maximum value in data[0..6]

{
    int max;        // Temporary max. value
    int index;      // Loop control and index variable

    max = data[0];
    for (index = 1; index < 7; index++)
        if (data[index] > max)
            max = data[index];
    return max;
}
```

Our two-part declaration of hiTemp permits us to call Maximum using a component of hiTemp as follows.

```
highest = Maximum(hiTemp[20]);
```

Row 20 of hiTemp is passed to Maximum, which treats it like any other one-dimensional array of type WeekType (see Figure 12–14). It makes sense to pass the row as an argument because both it and the function parameter are of the same named type, Week-Type.

hiTemp

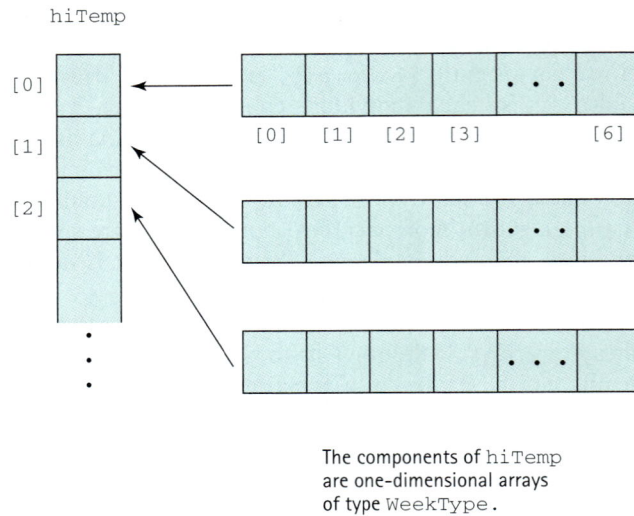

The components of hiTemp
are one-dimensional arrays
of type WeekType.

Figure 12–14   *A One-Dimensional Array of One-Dimensional Arrays*

With hiTemp declared as an array of arrays, we can output the maximum temperature of each week of the year with the following code:

```
cout << " Week   Maximum" << endl
     << "Number Temperature" << endl;
for (week = 0; week < 52; week++)
     cout << setw(6) << week
          << setw(9) << Maximum(hiTemp[week]) << endl;
```

12.8 Multidimensional Arrays

C++ does not place a limit on the number of dimensions that an array can have. We can generalize our definition of an array to cover all cases.

> **Array** A collection of components, all of the same type, ordered on *N* dimensions (*N* ≥ 1). Each component is accessed by *N* indexes, each of which represents the component's position within that dimension.

You might have guessed from the syntax templates that you can have as many dimensions as you want. How many should you have in a particular case? Use as many as there are features that describe the components in the array.

Take, for example, a chain of department stores. Monthly sales figures must be kept for each item by store. There are three important pieces of information about each item: the month in which it was sold, the store from which it was purchased, and the item number. We can define an array type to summarize this data as follows:

```
const int NUM_ITEMS = 100;
const int NUM_STORES = 10;
```

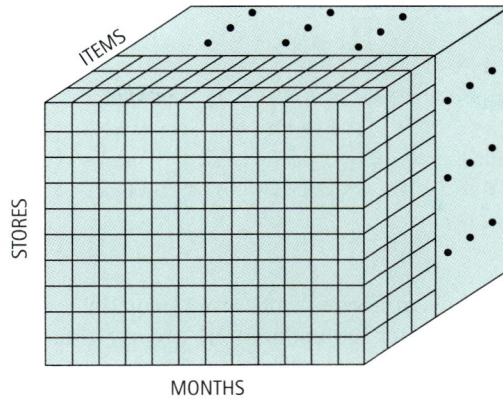

Figure 12-15   *Graphical Representation of* `sales` *Array*

```
typedef int SalesType[NUM_STORES][12][NUM_ITEMS];

SalesType sales;    // Array of sales figures
int       item;
int       store;
int       month;
int       numberSold;
int       currentMonth;
```

A graphic representation of the `sales` array is shown in Figure 12-15.

The number of components in `sales` is 12,000 (10 × 12 × 100). If sales figures are available only for January through June, then half the array is empty. If we want to process the data in the array, we must use subarray processing. The following program fragment sums and prints the total number of each item sold this year to date by all stores.

```
for (item = 0; item < NUM_ITEMS; item++)
{
    numberSold = 0;
    for (store = 0; store < NUM_STORES; store++)
        for (month = 0; month <= currentMonth; month++)
            numberSold = numberSold + sales[store][month][item];
    cout << "Item #" << item << " Sales to date = " << numberSold
        << endl;
}
```

Because `item` controls the outer For loop, we are summing each item's sales by `month` and `store`. If we want to find the total sales for each store, we use `store` to control the outer For loop, summing its sales by `month` and `item` with the inner loops.

```
for (store = 0; store < NUM_STORES; store++)
{
    numberSold = 0;
    for (item = 0; item < NUM_ITEMS; item++)
        for (month = 0; month <= currentMonth; month++)
            numberSold = numberSold + sales[store][month][item];
    cout << "Store #" << store << " Sales to date = " << numberSold
        << endl;
}
```

It takes two loops to access each component in a two-dimensional array; it takes three loops to access each component in a three-dimensional array. The task to be accomplished determines which index controls the outer loop, the middle loop, and the inner loop. If we want to calculate monthly sales by store, `month` controls the outer loop and `store` controls the middle loop. If we want to calculate monthly sales by item, `month` controls the outer loop and `item` controls the middle loop.

If we want to keep track of the departments that sell each item, we can add a fourth dimension.

```
enum Departments {A, B, C, D, E, F, G};
const int NUM_DEPTS = 7;
typedef int SalesType[NUM_STORES][12][NUM_ITEMS][NUM_DEPTS];
```

How would we visualize this new structure? Not very easily! Fortunately, we do not have to visualize a structure in order to use it. If we want the number of sales in store 1 during June for item number 4 in department C, we simply access the array element

```
sales[1][5][4][C]
```

When a multidimensional array is declared as a parameter in a function, C++ requires you to state the sizes of all dimensions except the first. For our four-dimensional version of `SalesType`, a function heading would look either like this:

```
void DoSomething( /* inout */ int arr[][12][NUM_ITEMS][NUM_DEPTS] )
```

or, better yet, like this:

```
void DoSomething( /* inout */ Sales arr )
```

The second version is the safest (and the most uncluttered to look at). It ensures that the sizes of all dimensions of the parameter match those of the argument exactly. With the first version, the reason that you must declare the sizes of all but the first dimension is the same as we discussed earlier for two-dimensional arrays. Because arrays are stored linearly in memory (one array element after another), the compiler must use this size information to locate correctly an element that lies within the array.

Problem–Solving Case Study

Calculating Exam Statistics

PROBLEM   You are the grader in your Government class. The teacher has asked you to prepare the following statistics for the last exam: average grade, maximum grade, minimum grade, number of grades above the average, and number of grades below the average. Because this is the first exam, you decide to write a program to calculate these statistics so you can use the program for the remaining exams as well.

DISCUSSION   Let's abstract this problem from the given context and look at the tasks in isolation. There are three separate things to be done in this problem: compute an average of values on a file, find the minimum value and maximum value in a file, and compare each value to the average. There are several approaches to the solution to this problem. In the next chapter, we will look at an entirely different solution technique; however, here we base our solution on the fact that the values in the list are between 0 and 100. We use an array where the indexes have semantic content: Each index represents a grade.

The by-hand analogy is to mark off 101 lines on a sheet of paper and number (or label) the lines from 0 to 100. Each line number represents a possible grade. As you read a grade, make a hash mark on the line whose number is the same as the grade. When you have finished recording each grade in this fashion, you compute the sum of the grades by summing the products of each grade (line number) times the number of hash marks on that line. The number of grades can be calculated either when they are read or when the sum is calculated.

To calculate the lowest grade, start looking at line number 0 and look forward; the line number of the first line with a hash mark is the lowest grade. To calculate the highest grade, start looking backward from line number 100, and the line number of the first line to contain a hash mark is the highest grade. To determine how many grades are above the average, start at the line whose number is the average grade plus 1 and count the hash marks on the lines from there through line 100. To determine how many grades are below the average, sum the hash marks from the line whose number is the truncated average through line 0.

The data structure equivalent of your sheet of paper is an integer array declared to be of size 101. The index is the line number; the component corresponds to where you make hash marks (increment the component) each time the grade corresponding to the index occurs.

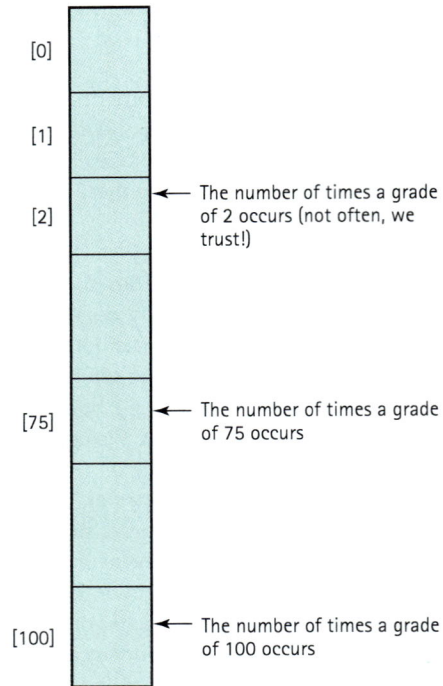

The number of times a grade of 2 occurs (not often, we trust!)

The number of times a grade of 75 occurs

The number of times a grade of 100 occurs

Figure 12–16

INPUT A file, whose name is input from the keyboard, containing test grades.

OUTPUT A file, whose name is input from the keyboard, showing the following statistics properly labeled.

Number of grades
Average grade
Lowest grade
Highest grade
Number of grades above the average
Number of grades below the average

Main	Level 0

```
Open files
Input grades
Calculate average
Calculate highest
Calculate lowest
Calculate above average
Calculate below average
Close files
```

We can use the same open files function we have used in several other programs. However, the heading that is printed on the output needs to be changed.

Input Grades	Level 1

This function must have the file name and the array as parameters. The program needs to know the number of grades. As we said, this value can be calculated as the grades are read or calculated as the grades are summed to get the average. Let's calculate it here and pass it as an argument to the function that computes the average.

(Inout: inData, grades, numGrades)

```
Set grades to all zero
Set numGrades to 0
Read grade
WHILE NOT eof
    Increment grades[grade]
    Increment numGrades
    Read grade
```

CalculateAverage(In: grades, numGrades)
Out: Function value

```
Set sum to 0
FOR index going from 0 through 100
    Set sum to sum + grades[index] * index;
Return float(sum) / float(numGrades);
```

CalculateHighest(In: grades)
Out: Function value

```
Set highGrade to 100;
 WHILE grades[highGrade] equal to 0
     Decrement highGrade
 Return highGrade;
```

CalculateLowest(In: grades)
Out: Function value

```
Set lowGrade to 0
WHILE grades[lowGrade] equal to 0
    Increment lowGrade
Return lowGrade
```

CalculateAboveAverage(In: grades, average)
Out: Function value

```
Set averagePlus to int(average) + 1
Set number to zero
FOR index going averagePlus to 100
    Set number to number + grades[index]
Return number
```

CalculateBelowAverage(In: grades, average)
Out: Function value

```
Set truncatedAverage to (int) average
Set number to zero
FOR index going from 0 to truncatedAverage
    Set number to number + grades[index]
Return number
```

PrintResults(Inout: outData; In: numGrades, average, highest,
   lowest, numberAbove, numberBelow)

> Print on outdata "The number of grades is " numGrades
> Print on outData "The average grade is " average
> Print on outData "The highest grade is " highest
> Print on outData "The lowest grade is " lowest
> Print on outData "The number of grades above the average is "
>   aboveAverage
> Print on outData "The number of grades below the average is "
>   belowAverage

MODULE STRUCTURE CHART

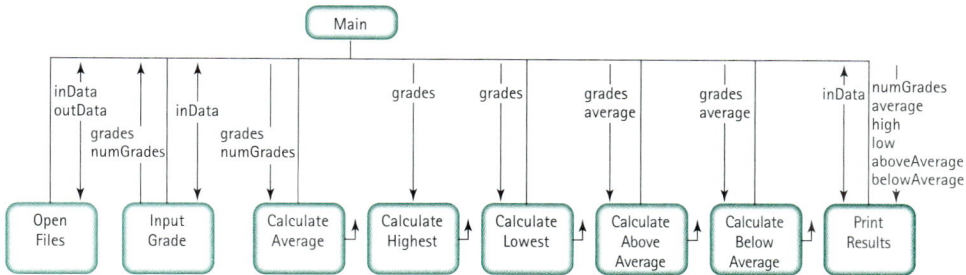

```
//****************************************************************
// Statistics Program
// This program calculates the average, high score, low score,
// number above the average, and number below the average for
// a file of test scores.
// To save space, we omit from each function the precondition
// comments that document the assumptions made about valid input
// parameter data. These would be included in a program intended
// for actual use.
// Assumption: File contains at least one non-zero value
//****************************************************************

#include <iostream>
#include <fstream>
#include <iomanip>
```

```cpp
using namespace std;

// Declare function prototypes
void OpenFiles(ifstream& inData, ofstream& outData);
void InputGrades(int grades[], int& numGrades, ifstream& inData);
float CalculateAverage(int const grades[], int numGrades);
int CalculateHighest(int const grades[]);
int CalculateLowest(int const grades[]);
int CalculateAboveAverage(int const grades[], float average);
int CalculateBelowAverage(int const grades[], float average);
void PrintResults(ofstream& outData, int numGrades, float average,
    int highest, int lowest, int aboveAverage, int belowAverage);

int main()
{
    int grades[101];        // Array of counters for each grade
    int numGrades;          // Number of grades
    float average;          // Average grade
    int highest;            // Highest grade
    int lowest;             // Lowest grade
    int aboveAverage;       // Number of grades above the average
    int belowAverage;       // Number of grades below the average

    // Declare and open files
    ifstream inData;
    ofstream outData;
    OpenFiles(inData, outData);
    if ( !inData || !outData )
    {
        cout << "Files not opened successfully." << endl;
        return 1;
    }

    // Read and process grades
    InputGrades(grades, numGrades, inData);
    average = CalculateAverage(grades, numGrades);
    highest = CalculateHighest(grades);
    lowest = CalculateLowest(grades);
    aboveAverage = CalculateAboveAverage(grades, average);
    belowAverage = CalculateBelowAverage(grades, average);
    PrintResults(outData, numGrades, average, highest, lowest,
        aboveAverage, belowAverage);

    inData.close();
    outData.close();
    return 0;
}
```

```
//*****************************************************************

void OpenFiles( /* inout */ ifstream& text,
                /* inout */ ofstream& outFile )

// Function OpenFiles reads in the names of the input file and
// the output file and opens them for processing
// Postcondition:
//     Files have been opened AND a label has been written on
//     the output file

{
    string inFileName;
    string outFileName;
    cout << "Enter the name of the file to be processed"
        << endl;
    cin >> inFileName;
    text.open(inFileName.c_str());
    cout << "Enter the name of the output file" << endl;
    cin >> outFileName;
    outFile.open(outFileName.c_str());
    outFile << "Analysis of exams on file " << inFileName
        << endl << endl;
}


//*****************************************************************

float CalculateAverage
    ( /* inout */ int const grades[], // Grade structure
      /* in */      int numGrades )    // Number of grades

// This function calculates the average test score
// Postcondition:
//     Return value is the average grade

{
    int sum = 0;
    // Sum number of grades times index
    for (int index = 0; index <= 100; index++)
        sum = sum + grades[index] * index;

    return float(sum) / float(numGrades);
}
```

```
//************************************************************************

void InputGrades
    ( /* inout */ int grades[],      // Grade structure
      /* inout */ int& numGrades,    // Number of grades
      /* inout */ ifstream& inData) // Input file

// Grades are input from file inData. Each slot in grades is set
// to zero. As each grade is read in, the grade is used as an
// index and that slot is incremented.
// Precondition:
//      File is not empty
// Postcondition:
//      For each grade in the file, grades, indexed by the grade,
//      has been incremented

{
    int grade;
    // Zero out the array of counters
    for (int index = 0; index <= 100; index++)
        grades[index] = 0;
    numGrades = 0;

    inData >> grade;                        // Read a character

    // Increment counters for grades
    while (inData)
    { // Process data
        grades[grade]++;
        numGrades++;
        inData >> grade;
    }
}


//************************************************************************

int CalculateHighest
    ( /* in */ int const grades[] ) // Grade structure

// This function calculates the highest grade by beginning at index
// 100 and working backward until a nonzero slot is found. The
// index of this slot is the highest grade.
// Postcondition:
//      Return value is the highest grade
```

```
{
    int highGrade = 100;
    // Index of first nonzero grade is the high grade
    while (grades[highGrade] == 0)
        highGrade--;
    return highGrade;
}
```

```
//****************************************************************

int CalculateLowest
    ( /* in */ int const grades[] )  // Grade structure

// This function calculates the lowest grade by beginning at index
// 0 and working forward until a nonzero slot is found. The index
// of this slot is the lowest grade.
// Postcondition:
//     Return value is the lowest grade

{
    // Index of first nonzero grade is the low grade
    int lowGrade = 0;
    while (grades[lowGrade] == 0)
        lowGrade++;
    return lowGrade;
}
```

```
//****************************************************************

int CalculateAboveAverage
    ( /* in */ int const grades[],        // Grade structure
      /* inout */  float average )         // Average grade

// This function calculates the number of grades above the average
// by counting the numbers in the array from the rounded
// average to the 100th slot.
// Postcondition:
//     Return value is the number of grades above average
{
    int averagePlus = (int)(average) + 1;
    int index;
    int number = 0;
    for (index = averagePlus; index <= 100; index++)
        number = number + grades[index];
    return number;
}
```

```
//**********************************************************************

int CalculateBelowAverage
    ( /* in */ int const grades[],        // Grade structure
      /* inout */  float average )         // Average grade

// This function calculates the number of grades below the average
// by counting the numbers in the array from index 0 to index
// truncated average.
// Postcondition:
//      Return value is the number of grades below average

{
    int truncatedAverage = (int) (average);
    int index;
    int number = 0;
    // Sum number of grades below average
    for (index = 0; index <= truncatedAverage; index++)
        number = number + grades[index];
    return number;
}

//**********************************************************************

void PrintResults
        ( /* inout */ ofstream& outData,  // Output file
          /* in */      int numGrades,     // Number of grades
          /* in */      float average,     // Average
          /* in */      int highest,       // Max grade
          /* in */      int lowest,        // Min grade
          /* in */      int aboveAverage,  // Number above
          /* in */      int belowAverage)  // Number below

// Statistics are printed on file outData
// Precondition:
//      Output file has been successfully opened
// Postcondition:
//      Statistics have been written on outData, appropriately
//      labeled

{
    outData << "The number of grades is " << numGrades << endl;
    outData << fixed << setprecision(2)
            << "The average grade is " << average << endl;
```

```
outData << "The highest grade is " << highest << endl;
outData << "The lowest grade is " << lowest << endl;
outData << "The number of grades above the average is "
        << aboveAverage  << endl;
outData << "The number of grades below the average is "
        << belowAverage << endl;
}
```

TESTING   When testing this program, it is the values of grades, not the size of the file, that determines the test cases. The test cases must include values of MinGrade, MaxGrade, and values in between. Here is a sample data set that meets this criterion. The output is shown below.

```
88
87
88
66
55
56
75
75
78
80
80
90
99
87
44
34
0
100
```

```
testResults2 - Notepad

File  Edit  Format  View  Help

Analysis of exams on file testScores2

The number of grades is 18
The average grade is 71.22
The highest grade is 100
The lowest grade is 0
The number of grades above the average is 12
The number of grades below the average is 6
```

Problem-Solving Case Study

Favorite Rock Group

PROBLEM   At a small college, four campus rock groups have organized a fund-raising project, in which there is going to be a play-off among the groups. Each student gets to vote for his or her favorite and there are two prizes: the best group gets a prize and the class with the best participation gets a prize.

INPUT   An arbitrary number of votes in a file `voteFile`, with each vote represented as a pair of numbers: a class number (1 through 4) and a rock group number (1 through 4); and group names, entered from the keyboard (to be used for printing the output).

OUTPUT   The following three items, written to a file `reportFile`: a tabular report showing how many votes each rock group received in each class, the total number of votes for each rock group, and the total number of votes cast by each class.

DISCUSSION   The data consists of a pair of numbers for each vote. The first number is the class number; the second number is the rock group number.

   If we were doing the analysis by hand, our first task would be to go through the data, counting how many people in each class voted for each group. We would probably create a table with classes down the side and rock group names across the top. Each vote would be recorded as a hash mark in the appropriate row and column (see Figure 12–17).

	Fish	Snake	Sharks	Leopards
1	ᵗʰᵗʰ //	//	ᵗʰᵗʰ ᵗʰᵗʰ //	ᵗʰᵗʰ
2	ᵗʰᵗʰ ᵗʰᵗʰ	//	ᵗʰᵗʰ	///
3	//	ᵗʰᵗʰ ///	ᵗʰᵗʰ ᵗʰᵗʰ ᵗʰᵗʰ	///
4	ᵗʰᵗʰ	ᵗʰᵗʰ ///	ᵗʰᵗʰ ᵗʰᵗʰ	//

Figure 12–17   *Vote-Counting Table*

   When all of the votes had been recorded, a sum of each column would tell us how many votes each group received. A sum of each row would tell us how many people voted in each class.

   As is so often the case, we can use this by-hand algorithm directly in our program. We can create a two-dimensional array in which each component is a counter for the number of votes for a particular group in each class; for example, the value indexed by `[2] [1]` would be the counter for the votes in class 2 (sophomore) for group 1. Well, not quite. C++ arrays are indexed beginning at 0, so the correct array component would be indexed by `[1] [0]`. When we input a class number and group number, we must remember to subtract 1 from each before indexing into the array. Likewise, we must add 1 to an array index that represents a class number or group number before printing it out.

DATA STRUCTURES A two-dimensional array named `votes`, where the rows represent classes and the columns represent groups.

A one-dimensional array of strings containing the names of the groups, to be used for printing (see Figure 12–18).

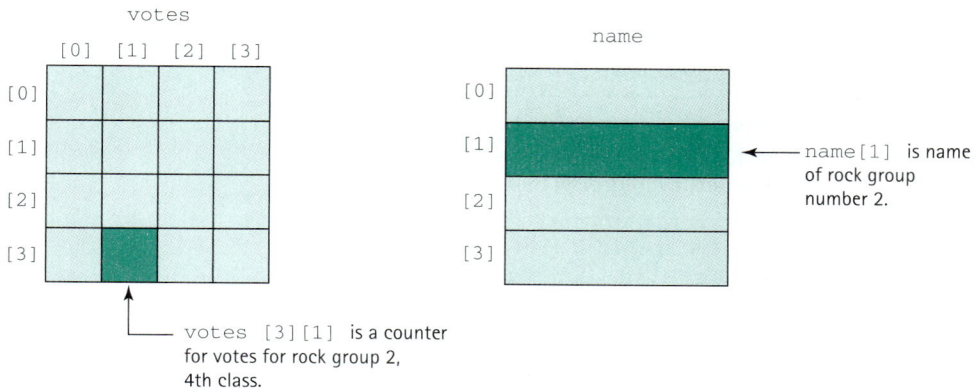

Figure 12–18 *Data Structures for Election Program*

In our discussion we have used the word "class" to represent freshmen, sophomore, junior, or senior. However, we need to be careful. We cannot use the word "class" in our program because it is a reserved word. Let's make the switch here and use the word "level" instead. In the design that follows, we use the named constants NUM_LEVELS and NUM_ROCK_GROUPS in place of the literal constants 4 and 4.

Main	Level 0

Open files
Get group names
Set votes array to 0
Read level, group from voteFile
WHILE NOT EOF on voteFile
    Increment votes[level–1][group–1] by 1
    Read level, rockGroup from voteFile
Write report to reportFile
Write totals per group to reportFile
Write totals per level to reportFile

Get RockGroup Names (Out: name)   Level 1

> Print "Enter the names of the rock groups, one per line,
>   in the order they appear on the ballot."
> FOR rockGroup going from 0 through NUM_ROCK_GROUPS – 1
>   Read name[rockGroup]

Note that each rock group's name is stored in the slot in the name array corresponding to its group's number (minus 1). These names are useful when the totals are printed.

Set Votes to Zero (Out: votes)

> FOR each level
>   FOR each group
>   Set votes[level][group] to 0

Write Report (In: votes, name; Inout: reportFile)

> FOR each rockGroup   // Set up headings
>   Write name[rockGroup] to reportFile
> FOR each level   // Print array by row
>   FOR each rockGroup
>   Write votes[level][rockGroup] to reportFile

Write Totals per RockGroup (In: votes, name; Inout: reportFile)

> FOR each rockGroup
>   Set total = 0
> FOR each level   // Compute column sum
>   Add votes[level][rockGroup] to total
>   Write "Total votes for", name[rockGroup], total to reportFile

Write Totals per Level (In: votes; Inout: reportFile)

> FOR each level
>   Set total = 0
>   FOR each rockGroup   // Compute row sum
>   Add votes[level][rockGroup] to total
>   Write "Total votes for level", level, ':', total to reportFile

MODULE STRUCTURE CHART

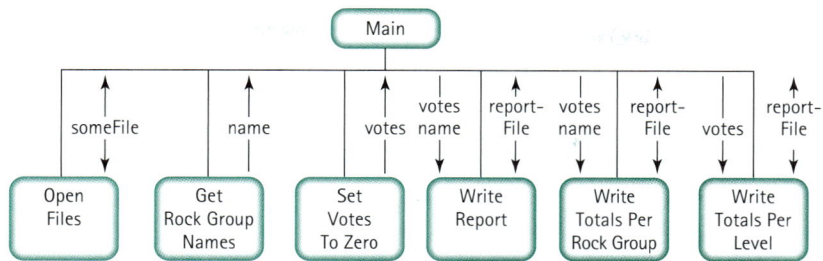

```
//*****************************************************************
// Favorite Rock Group program
// This program reads votes represented by level number and
// rock group number from a data file, calculates the sums per
// level and per rock group, and writes all totals to an
// output file
//*****************************************************************
#include <iostream>
#include <iomanip>      // For setw()
#include <fstream>      // For file I/O
#include <string>       // For string level

using namespace std;

const int NUM_LEVELS = 4;
const int NUM_ROCK_GROUPS = 4;
typedef int VoteArray[NUM_LEVELS][NUM_ROCK_GROUPS];
                                // 2-dimensional array type
                                //   for votes
void GetNames( string[] );
void OpenFiles( ifstream&, ofstream& );
void WritePerRockGroup( const VoteArray, const string[],
                        ofstream& );
void WritePerLevel( const VoteArray, ofstream& );
void WriteReport( const VoteArray, const string[], ofstream& );
void ZeroVotes( VoteArray );

int main()
{
    string    name[NUM_ROCK_GROUPS];  // Array of rockGroup names
    VoteArray votes;            // Totals for level vs. rockGroups
    int       rockGroup;        // rockGroup number input from voteFile
```

```cpp
    int       level;      // level number input from voteFile
    ifstream  voteFile;   // Input file of level, rockGroups
    ofstream  reportFile; // Output file receiving summaries

    OpenFiles(voteFile, reportFile);
    if ( !voteFile || !reportFile )
    {
        cout << "Files did not open successfully." << endl;
        return 1;
    }


    GetNames(name);
    ZeroVotes(votes);

    // Read and tally votes

    voteFile >> level >> rockGroup;
    while (voteFile)
    {
        votes[level-1][rockGroup-1]++;
        voteFile >> level >> rockGroup;
    }

    // Write results to report file

    WriteReport(votes, name, reportFile);
    WritePerRockGroup(votes, name, reportFile);
    WritePerLevel(votes, reportFile);

    return 0;
}
//*********************************************************************


void OpenFiles( /* inout */ ifstream& text,
                /* inout */ ofstream& outFile )

// Function OpenFiles reads in the names of the input file and
// the output file and opens them for processing
// Postcondition:
//     Files have been opened AND a label has been written on
//     the output file

{
    string inFileName;
    string outFileName;
```

```
        cout << "Enter the name of the file to be processed"
                  << endl;
        cin >> inFileName;
        text.open(inFileName.c_str());
        cout << "Enter the name of the output file" << endl;
        cin >> outFileName;
        outFile.open(outFileName.c_str());
        outFile << "Analysis of Favorite Rock Groups " << inFileName
                << endl << endl;
}

//*******************************************************************

void GetNames( /* out */ string name[] )      // Array of rockGroup
                                              //    names
// Reads the rockGroup names from standard input

// Postcondition:
//      The user has been prompted to enter the rockGroup names
//      && name[0..NUM_ROCKGROUPS-1] contain the input names,
//      truncated to 10 characters each

{
    string inputStr;        // An input string
    int    rockGroup;       // Loop counter

    cout << "Enter the names of the rockGroups, one per line,"
         << endl << "in the order they appear on the ballot."
         << endl;
    for (rockGroup = 0; rockGroup < NUM_ROCK_GROUPS; rockGroup++)
    {
        cin >> inputStr;
        name[rockGroup] = inputStr.substr(0, 10);
    }
}

//*******************************************************************

void ZeroVotes( /* out */ VoteArray votes )   // Array of vote totals

// Zeros out the votes array

// Postcondition:
//      All votes[0..NUM_LEVELS-1][0..NUM_ROCKGROUPS-1] == 0
```

```cpp
{
    int level;          // Loop counter
    int rockGroup;      // Loop counter

    for (level = 0; level < NUM_LEVELS; level++)
        for (rockGroup = 0; rockGroup < NUM_ROCK_GROUPS; rockGroup++)
            votes[level][rockGroup] = 0;
}

//*******************************************************************

void WriteReport(
        /* in */      const VoteArray votes,      // Total votes
        /* in */      const string    name[],     // rockGroup names
        /* inout */        ofstream& reportFile )  // Output file

// Writes the vote totals in tabular form to the report file

// Precondition:
//      votes[0..NUM_LEVELS-1][0..NUM_ROCKGROUPS] are assigned
//   && name[0..NUM_ROCKGROUPS-1] are assigned
// Postcondition:
//      The name array has been output across one line, followed by
//      the votes array, one row per line

{
    int level;          // Loop counter
    int rockGroup;      // Loop counter
    // Set up headings

    reportFile << "                ";
    for (rockGroup = 0; rockGroup < NUM_ROCK_GROUPS; rockGroup++)
        reportFile << setw(12) << name[rockGroup];
    reportFile << endl;

    // Print array by row

    for (level = 0; level < NUM_LEVELS; level++)
    {
        reportFile << "level" << setw(4) << level + 1;
        for (rockGroup = 0; rockGroup < NUM_ROCK_GROUPS; rockGroup++)
            reportFile << setw(12) << votes[level][rockGroup];
        reportFile << endl;
    }
```

```
        reportFile << endl;
}

//*******************************************************************

void WritePerRockGroup(
        /* in */     const VoteArray  votes,      // Total votes
        /* in */     const string     name[],     // rockGroup names
        /* inout */        ofstream&   reportFile )   // Output file

// Sums the votes per person and writes the totals to the
// report file

// Precondition:
//      votes[0..NUM_LEVELS-1][0..NUM_ROCKGROUPS] are assigned
//   && name[0..NUM_ROCKGROUPS-1] are assigned
// Postcondition:
//      For each person i, name[i] has been output,
//      followed by the sum
//      votes[0][i] + votes[1][i] + ...  + votes[NUM_LEVELS-1][i]

{
    int level;          // Loop counter
    int rockGroup;      // Loop counter
    int total;          // Total votes for a rockGroup

    for (rockGroup = 0; rockGroup < NUM_ROCK_GROUPS; rockGroup++)
    {
        total = 0;
        // Compute column sum

        for (level = 0; level < NUM_LEVELS; level++)
            total = total + votes[level][rockGroup];

        reportFile << "Total votes for"
                   << setw(10) << name[rockGroup] << ":"
                   << setw(3) << total << endl;
    }
    reportFile << endl;
}

//*******************************************************************
```

```
void WritePerLevel(
        /* in */      const VoteArray votes,         // Total votes
        /* inout */        ofstream& reportFile )    // Output file

// Sums the votes per level and writes the totals to the
// report file

// Precondition:
//     votes[0..NUM_LEVELS-1][0..NUM_ROCKGROUPS] are assigned
// Postcondition:
//     For each level i, the value i+1 has been output,
//     followed by the sum
//     votes[i][0] + votes[i][1] + ...  + votes[i][NUM_ROCKGROUPS-1]


{
    int level;         // Loop counter
    int rockGroup;     // Loop counter
    int total;         // Total votes for a level

    for (level = 0; level < NUM_LEVELS; level++)
    {
        total = 0;

        // Compute row sum

        for (rockGroup = 0; rockGroup < NUM_ROCK_GROUPS; rockGroup++)
            total = total + votes[level][rockGroup];

        reportFile << "Total votes for level"
                << setw(3) << level + 1 << ':'
                << setw(3) << total << endl;
    }
}
```

TESTING   This program was executed with the data listed on the next page. (We list the data in three columns to save space.) The names of the groups entered from the keyboard were Fish, Snake, Sharks, and Leopards. In this data set, there is at least one vote for each group in each class. Case Study Follow-Up Exercise 7 asks you to outline a complete testing strategy for this program.

Input Data

```
1 1      3 1      3 3
1 1      4 3      4 4
1 2      3 4      4 4
1 2      3 2      4 3
1 3      3 3      4 4
1 4      2 1      4 4
2 2      2 3      4 1
2 2      4 3      4 2
2 3      4 4      2 4
2 1      3 2      4 4
```

```
Report.out - Notepad
File  Edit  Format  View  Help

Analysis of Favorite Rock Groups Votes.in

                    Fish      Snake     Sharks    Leopards
level   1           2         2         1         1
level   2           2         2         2         1
level   3           1         2         2         1
level   4           1         1         3         6

Total votes for       Fish:   6
Total votes for      Snake:   7
Total votes for     Sharks:   8
Total votes for   Leopards:   9

Total votes for level  1:   6
Total votes for level  2:   7
Total votes for level  3:   6
Total votes for level  4:  11
```

Testing and Debugging

One-Dimensional Arrays

The most common error in processing arrays is an out-of-bounds array index. That is, the program attempts to access a component using an index that is either less than 0 or greater than the array size minus 1. For example, given the declarations

```
char line[100];
int  counter;
```

the following For statement would print the 100 elements of the `line` array and then print a 101st value—the value that resides in memory immediately beyond the end of the array.

```
for (counter = 0; counter <= 100; counter++)
    cout << line[counter];
```

This error is easy to detect because 101 characters get printed instead of 100. The loop test should be `counter < 100`. But you won't always use a simple For statement when accessing arrays. Suppose we read data into the `line` array in another part of the program. Let's use a While statement that reads to the newline character:

```
counter = 0;
cin.get(ch);
while (ch != '\n')
{
    line[counter] = ch;
    counter++;
    cin.get(ch);
}
```

This code seems reasonable enough, but what if the input line has more than 100 characters? After the hundredth character is read and stored into the array, the loop continues to execute with the array index out of bounds. Characters are stored into memory locations past the end of the array, wiping out other data values (or even machine language instructions in the program!).

The moral is: When processing arrays, give special attention to the design of loop termination conditions. Always ask yourself if the loop could possibly keep running after the last array component has been processed.

Whenever an array index goes out of bounds, the first suspicion should be a loop that fails to terminate properly. The second thing to check is any array access involving an index that is based on input data or a calculation. When an array index is input as data, a data validation check is an absolute necessity.

Complex Structures

As we have demonstrated in many examples in this chapter and the last, it is possible to combine data structures in various ways: structs whose components are structs, structs whose components are arrays, arrays whose components are structs or class objects, arrays whose components are arrays (multidimensional arrays), and so forth. When arrays, structs, and class objects are combined, there can be confusion about precisely where to place the operators for array element selection (`[]`) and struct or class member selection (`.`).

To summarize the correct placement of these operators, let's use the `StudentRec` type we introduced in this chapter:

```
struct StudentRec
{
    string    stuName;
    float     gpa;
    int       examScore[4];
    GradeType courseGrade;
};
```

If we declare a variable of type `StudentRec`,

```
StudentRec student;
```

then what is the syntax for selecting the first exam score of the student (that is, for selecting element 0 of the `examScore` member of `student`)? The dot operator is a binary (two-operand) operator; its left operand denotes a struct variable, and its right operand is a member name:

StructVariable . MemberName

The `[]` operator is a unary (one-operand) operator; it comes immediately after an expression denoting an array:

Array [IndexExpression]

Therefore, the expression

```
student
```

denotes a struct variable, the expression

```
student.examScore
```

denotes an array, and the expression

```
student.examScore[0]
```

denotes an integer—the integer located in element 0 of the `student.examScore` array.

With arrays of structs or class objects, again you have to be sure that the `[]` and `.` operators are in the proper positions. Given the declaration

```
StudentRec gradeBook[150];
```

we can access the `gpa` member of the first element of the `gradeBook` array with the expression

```
gradeBook[0].gpa
```

The index `[0]` is correctly attached to the identifier `gradeBook` because `gradeBook` is the name of an array. Furthermore, the expression

```
gradeBook[0]
```

denotes a struct, so the dot operator selects the `gpa` member of this struct.

Multidimensional Arrays

Errors with multidimensional arrays usually fall into two major categories: index expressions that are out of order and index range errors.

Suppose we were to expand the rock group program to accommodate ten rock groups and four levels. Let's declare the `votes` array as

```
int votes[4][10];
```

The first dimension represents the levels, and the second represents the rock groups. An example of the first kind of error—incorrect order of the index expressions—would be to print out the `votes` array as follows.

```
for (level = 0; level < 4; level++)
{
    for (rockgroup = 0; rockgroup < 10; rockgroup++)
        cout << setw(4) << votes[rockgroup][level];
    cout << endl;
}
```

The output statement specifies the array indexes in the wrong order. The loops march through the array with the first index ranging from 0 through 9 (instead of 0 through 3) and the second index ranging from 0 through 3 (instead of 0 through 9). The effect of executing this code may vary from system to system. The program may output the wrong array components and continue executing, or the program may crash with a memory access error.

An example of the second kind of error—an incorrect index range in an otherwise correct loop—can be seen in this code:

```
for (level = 0; level < 10; level++)
{
    for (rockgroup = 0; rockgroup < 4; rockgroup++)
        cout << setw(4) << votes[level][rockgroup];
    cout << endl;
}
```

Here, the output statement correctly uses `level` for the first index and `rockgroup` for the second. However, the For statements use incorrect upper limits for the index variables. As with the preceding example, the effect of executing this code is undefined but is certainly wrong. A valuable way to prevent this kind of error is to use named constants instead of the literals 10 and 4. In the case study, we used NUM_LEVELS and NUM_ROCK_GROUPS. You are much more likely to spot an error (or to avoid making an error in the first place) if you write something like this:

```
for (level = 0; level < NUM_LEVELS; level++)
```

than if you use a literal constant as the upper limit for the index variable.

Testing and Debugging Hints

1. When an individual component of a one-dimensional array is accessed, the index must be within the range 0 through the array size minus 1. Attempting to use an index value outside this range causes your program to access memory locations outside the array.

2. The individual components of an array are themselves variables of the component type. When values are stored into an array, they should either be of the component type or be explicitly converted to the component type; otherwise, implicit type coercion occurs.

3. C++ does not allow aggregate operations on arrays. There is no aggregate assignment, aggregate comparison, aggregate I/O, or aggregate arithmetic. You must write code to do all of these operations, one array element at a time.

4. Omitting the size of a one-dimensional array in its declaration is permitted only in two cases: (1) when an array is declared as a parameter in a function heading and (2) when an array is initialized in its declaration. In all other declarations, you *must* specify the size of the array with a constant integer expression.

5. If an array parameter is incoming-only, declare the parameter as `const` to prevent the function from modifying the caller's argument accidentally.

6. Don't pass an individual array component as an argument when the function expects to receive the base address of an entire array.

7. The size of an array is fixed at compile time, but the number of values actually stored there is determined at run time. Therefore, an array must be declared to be as large as it could ever be for the particular problem. Subarray processing is used to process only the components that have data in them.

8. When functions perform subarray processing on a one-dimensional array, pass both the array name and the number of data items actually stored in the array.

9. With multidimensional arrays, use the proper number of indexes when referencing an array component, and make sure the indexes are in the correct order.

10. In loops that process multidimensional arrays, double-check the upper and lower bounds on each index variable to be sure they are correct for that dimension of the array.

11. When declaring a multidimensional array as a parameter, you must state the sizes of all but the first dimension. Also, these sizes must agree exactly with the sizes of the caller's argument.

12. To eliminate the chances of the size mismatches referred to in item 11, use a Typedef statement to define a multidimensional array type. Declare both the argument and the parameter to be of this type.

Summary

The one-dimensional array is a homogeneous data structure that gives a name to a sequential group of like components. Each component is accessed by its relative position within the group (rather than by name, as in a struct or class), and each component is a variable of the component type. To access a particular component, we give the name of the array and an index that specifies which component of the group we want. The index can be an expression of any integral type, as long as it evaluates to an integer from 0 through the array size minus 1. Array components can be accessed in random order directly, or they can be accessed sequentially by stepping through the index values one at a time.

Two-dimensional arrays are useful for processing information that is represented naturally in tabular form. Processing data in two-dimensional arrays usually takes one of two forms: processing by row or processing by column. An array of arrays, which is useful if rows of the array must be passed as arguments, is an alternative way of defining a two-dimensional array.

A multidimensional array is a collection of like components that are ordered on more than one dimension. Each component is accessed by a set of indexes, one for each dimension, that represents the component's position on the various dimensions. Each index may be thought of as describing a feature of a given array component.

Quick Check

1. Why do we say that an array is a homogeneous data structure? (pp. 590–591)
2. You are solving a problem that requires you to store 24 temperature readings. Which structure would be most appropriate for this: a record, a union, a class or an array? (pp. 588–590)
3. How would you access the 3rd letter in a string data member (called `street`) of a class variable that is the 12th element of an array called `mailList`? (pp. 605–607)
4. Explain how the index of an array of 24 hourly temperature readings has semantic content, if the index is an integer ranging from 0 through 23. (p. 608)
5. How does a two-dimensional array differ syntactically from a one-dimensional array? (pp. 609–612)

6. What aspect of a problem would lead you to consider using a multidimensional array as the representation of its data structure? (pp. 622–624)

7. Write a declaration of an array variable called `temps` that holds 24 values of type `float`. (pp. 590–591)

8. Write a For loop that fills every element of the `temps` array declared in Exercise 7 with the value 32.0. (pp. 616–617)

9. Write a loop that reads values from file `indata` into the `temps` array of Exercise 7, until either end-of-file or 24 values are input. It should keep track of the number of values in the array in an `int` variable called `count`. (pp. 596–600)

10. Write the declaration for a two-dimensional array, called `allTemps`, that holds the 24 hourly readings for each day of a year (up to 366 days). (pp. 609–612)

11. Write a nested For loop that outputs the contents of the `allTemps` array declared in Exercise 7, with the 24 temperatures for a day on a line and 366 lines of days. (pp. 612–618)

12. Write the heading for a function that accepts the `temps` array of Exercise 7 and its length as parameters. Call the function `Quick`, and have it be a `void` function. (pp. 618–620)

13. Write a declaration for a multidimensional array that stores 24 hourly temperatures for each day of a year for a decade. Call the array `decadeTemps`. (pp. 622–624)

Answers

1. Because its elements are all of the same type. 2. An array. 3. `mailList[12].street[2]`
4. The index represents the hour during which the reading was taken, based on a 24-hour clock.
5. It is declared and accessed with two index values instead of one. 6. If the problem has a homogeneous collection of data that is ordered by more than two indexes.

7. `float temps[24];`

8.
```
for (int count = 0; count <=23; count++)
    temps[count] = 32.0;
```

9.
```
count = 0;
cin >> inTemp;
while (indata && count <= 24)
{
    count++;
    temps[count - 1] = inTemp;
    cin >> inTemp;
}
```

10. `float allTemps[24][366];`

11.
```
for (day = 0; day <= 365; day++)
{
    for (hour = 0; hour <= 23; hour++)
        cout << allTemps[hour][day];
    cout << endl;
}
```

12.
```
void Quick (/* inout */ float arr[],
            /* in */ int numElements)
```

13. `float decadeTemps[24][366][10]`

Exam Preparation Exercises

1. The components of an array can be of different types. True or false?
2. Arrays can have any type for their components. True or false?
3. Multidimensional arrays are limited to no more than four dimensions. True or false?
4. In declaring a one-dimensional array, its size must be specified with an integer. True or false?
5. The type of an index expression can be any of the integral types or an enumeration type. True or false?
6. What happens if a program tries to access an array using an index of –1?
7. What aggregate operation(s) are allowed on arrays?
8. To what does the term "base address of an array" refer, and how is it used in a function call?
9. What special type of array can be returned by a value-returning function?
10. If you want to use a nested loop to process a two-dimensional array row-by-row, which dimension's index (row or column) would you increment in the inner loop, and which would you increment in the outer loop?
11. How many elements are there in each of the following arrays?
    a. `int x[27];`
    b. `const int base = 10;`
       `int y[base + 5];`
    c. `int z[100][100][100][100];`
12. What's wrong with the following code segment?

```
int prep[100];
for (int index = 1; index <= 100; index++)
   prep[index] = 0;
```

13. What's wrong with the following code segment?

```
const int limit = 100;
int eprep[limit];
int examp[limit];
for (int index = 0; index <= limit - 1; index++)
{
   eprep[index] = 0;
   examp[index] = 0;
}
if (eprep == examp)
   cout << "Equal";
```

14. What's wrong with the following code segment?

```
typedef int Exrep[50];

Exrep Init(/* in */ Exrep); // Prototype
```

15. What's wrong with the following code segment?

```
int prepex[3][4] =
{
    {1, 2, 3},
    {4, 5, 6},
    {7, 8, 9},
    {0, -1, -2}
};
```

16. What's the potential danger in the following code segment?

```
int index;
int value;
int xeperp[100];
cin >> index >> value;
xeperp[index] = value;
```

17. What is the side effect of the following function?

```
int Max (/* in */ int trio[3])
{
    int temp;
    if (trio[0] > trio[1])
    {
        temp = trio[1];
        trio[1] = trio[0];
        trio[0] = temp;
    }
    if (trio[1] > trio[2])
    {
        temp = trio[2];
        trio[2] = trio[1];
        trio[1] = temp;
    }
    return trio[2];
}
```

18. What does the following code segment output?

```
char pattern[5][5] =
{
    {'*', ' ', '*', ' ', '*'},
    {' ', '*', ' ', '*', ' '},
    {'*', ' ', '*', ' ', '*'},
    {' ', '*', ' ', '*', ' '},
    {'*', ' ', '*', ' ', '*'}
}
```

```
for (int outer = 0; outer < 5; outer++)
{
   for (int inner = 1; inner <= 5; inner++)
     cout << pattern[outer][inner % 5];
   cout << endl;
}
```

19. Given the declaration of pattern in Exercise 18, what does the following loop output?

```
for (int index = 0; index < 5; index++)
  cout << pattern[index][(index+2) % 5];
```

20. Given the declaration of pattern in Exercise 18, what does the following loop output?

```
for (int outer = 0; outer < 5; outer++)
{
   for (int inner = 0; inner < 5; inner++)
     cout << pattern[inner][outer];
   cout << endl;
}
```

21. Given the following declaration:

```
int examPrep [12][15];
```

   a. Write a loop to print the first row of the array on one line on cout.
   b. Write a loop to print the first column of the array on one line on cout.
   c. Write a loop to print the first seven rows of the array, each on a single line.
   d. Write a loop to print the entire array backwards and upside down, so that the last line appears first, with last column on the left.

Programming Warm-Up Exercises

1. Write the following declarations.
   a. An array called topTenList, of 10 values of type string.
   b. An enumeration type of the seven major colors of the spectrum, and a matching array declaration that can be indexed by the spectrum type. The array should be called colorMix, and contain values of type float.
   c. A two-dimensional array representing the days on a calendar page with up to 6 weeks. Call the array month, and declare an enumeration type consisting of the names of the days, that can be used to index the array columns. The weeks should be indexed by an int. For the component type of the array, declare a struct consisting of an int field called day, and a string field called activity.

2. Write a declaration of a named array type, and then declare three arrays of that type. The array type should be called `DataSet`, and the three arrays should be called `input`, `output`, and `working`. Each array should hold five `float` values.

3. Using the `DataSet` type declared in Exercise 2, declare an array of three data sets, called `set`.

4. Using the `set` array declared in Exercise 3, write a nested For loop that initializes all of the values of the three data sets to 0.0.

5. Write a function heading for a function called `Equals` that takes two arrays of the `DataSet` type declared in Exercise 2, and returns a `bool` result. The array parameters should be `const`, as they are input-only parameters to the function.

6. Write the body of the `Equals` function described in Exercise 5. It should return `true` if each element of the first array is equal to its corresponding element in the second array.

7. A gallery needs to keep track of its paintings and photographs. It keeps at most 120 art works on its walls. Each one is described by the following information:

   Artist (string)
   Title (string)
   Medium (oil, watercolor, pastel, acrylic, print, color photo, black and white
           photo)
   Size (struct)
      Height (int)
      Width (int)
   Room where it is hung (main, green, blue, north, south, entry, balcony)
   Price (float)

   Write a declaration for a `struct` that represents a piece of art. Declare `struct` and enumeration types as needed to make up the fields of the `ArtWork` type. Write an additional declaration of a named array type that holds the list of all the art works in the gallery. Lastly, declare an array of this type called `currentList` and an `int` variable `numPieces`. The `numPieces` variable contains the number of pieces represented in the array.

8. Write expressions that retrieve the following values from the array declared in Exercise 7.
   a. The 37th work of art.
   b. The title of the 12th work of art.
   c. The width of the 85th work of art.
   d. The room for the 120th work of art.
   e. The first letter of the artist's name for the 78th work of art.

9. Write a For loop that prints a list of the artist, title, and price for every work in the `currentList` array defined in Exercise 7.

10. Write a code segment that sums the prices of the works in the gallery described in Exercise 7.

11. Write a code segment that outputs the titles of the works in the blue room of the gallery described in Exercise 7.

12. Write a code segment that sums the prices of the oil paintings in the gallery described in Exercise 7 that are larger than 400 square inches in size.

13. A piano is tuned in a scale that is slightly unequal (called a well-tempered scale), rather than a perfectly scientific scale in which each note sounds at twice the frequency of the same note an octave below (called a "just scale"). For this reason, we can't simply calculate the frequency of a note, but must keep it in a table. Declare a two-dimensional array (`scale`) to hold the frequencies of the well-tempered scale. A frequency is represented by a `float` value. The row dimension is indexed by an `int` value representing the octave (there are 8 octaves, numbered 0 through 7), and the other should be indexed by an enumeration type (`Notes`) consisting of the names of the notes. When you write the declaration of the enumeration type, use only sharps (no flats). Thus, the note names of an octave are: C, CSHARP, D, DSHARP, E, F, FSHARP, G, GSHARP, A, ASHARP, and B, in that order.

14. Write a code segment that reads a table of frequencies into the `scale` array declared in Exercise 13 from a file called `frequencies.dat`. The frequency values are arranged one per line on the file.

15. Write a code segment that outputs the frequencies of the notes in the fourth octave of the `scale` array declared in Exercise 13.

16. Write a code segment that outputs the frequencies of all the C notes in the `scale` array declared in Exercise 13.

17. Write a declaration for a four-dimensional array that is indexed by 10 years (0 – 9), 52 weeks (0–51), the 50 states (0–49), and an enumeration type consisting of MAX, MIN, and AVERAGE, called `Type`. The array holds humidity measurements (each component is a `float`).

18. Write a C++ function called `Reset`, that sets all of the components to zero in the array declared in exercise 17.

19. Write a declaration of a `struct` type called `TimePlace` that has three fields, one for each for the first three index values (year, week, state) in the `humidity` array declared in Exercise 17. `TimePlace` should have a fourth field called `difference`, which is a `float`. Then write a C++ function called `MaxSpread` that takes the `humidity` array as a parameter, and scans through it to find the year, week, and state with the greatest difference in humidity, and returns these values as a `TimePlace struct`. If there is more than one week with the greatest difference, then the first one should be returned.

20. Write a code segment that outputs the AVERAGE component of the `humidity` array of Exercise 17, for all the weeks in the last 5 years for the 23rd state.

Programming Problems

1. Write a program to play a game in which you try to sink a fleet of five navy vessels by guessing their locations on a grid. The program uses random numbers

to position its ships on a 15 × 15 grid. The ships are of different lengths as follows:

Frigate: 2 locations
Tender: 2 locations
Destroyer: 3 locations
Cruiser: 3 locations
Carrier: 4 locations

The program must pick one square as the starting location, then pick the direction of the ship on the board, and mark off the number of squares in that direction to represent the size of the ship. It must not allow a ship to overlap with another ship, or to run off the board.

The user enters coordinates in the range of 1 through 15 for the rows and A through O for the columns. The program checks this location, and reports whether it is a hit or a miss. If it is a hit, the program also checks whether the ship has been hit in every location that it occupies. If so, the ship is reported as sunk, and the program identifies which ship it is.

The user gets 60 shots to attempt to sink the fleet. If the user sinks all of the ships before using all 60 shots, then he or she wins the game. At the end of the game, the program should output the grid, so that the user can see where the ships are located.

2. Programming Warm-Up Exercises 7 to 12 deal with an array representing the inventory for an art gallery. Using the same representation, write a C++ program that reads the gallery's inventory from a file called `art.dat` into the array. Then allow the user to look up the art by specifying any field in the record. As a reminder, here are the fields:

Artist (string)
Title (string)
Medium (oil, watercolor, pastel, acrylic, print, color photo, black and white photo)
Size (struct)
    Height (int)
    Width (int)
Room where it is hung (main, green, blue, north, south, entry, balcony)
Price (float)

Thus, the user should be able to specify a field, and a value for that field, and the program returns all works that match. For example, the user may specify Artist and Smithely, and the program will output all of the information concerning every work in the gallery by that artist.

3. Programming Problem 1 in Chapter 9 asked you to write a program that inputs a string and then outputs the corresponding words in the International Civil Aviation Organization alphabet that would be used to spell it out phonetically. For

that program, you should have used a large Switch statement. Rewrite that program using an array of strings to hold the words of the alphabet, and index the array by the positions of the letters of the alphabet. By using an index with semantic content, you can avoid the need for the case statement. Be sure that you don't try to index into the array using non-alphabetic characters, as that will result in an out-of-bounds access. For ease of reference, the ICAO alphabet is repeated here from Chapter 9:

A   Alpha
B   Bravo
C   Charlie
D   Delta
E   Echo
F   Foxtrot
G   Golf
H   Hotel
I   India
J   Juliet
K   Kilo
L   Lima
M   Mike
N   November
O   Oscar
P   Papa
Q   Quebec
R   Romeo
S   Sierra
T   Tango
U   Uniform
V   Victor
W   Whiskey
X   X-ray
Y   Yankee
Z   Zulu

Be sure to use proper formatting and appropriate comments in your code. Provide appropriate prompts to the user. The output should be clearly labeled and neatly formatted.

4. Programming Problem 4 in Chapter 6 asked you to write a program to check whether an input line is a palindrome (a word or phrase that is the same backwards and forwards). At that time, we needed to use the substring function to extract individual characters from a string. Because this is a cumbersome way to work with a string, we limited our definition of palindromes to just perfect

palindromes—every letter and blank exactly the same in both forward and backward versions. Now that we know how to use arrays, we can expand the definition to ignore blanks, punctuation, and letter case. Thus

```
madam I'm adam
```

becomes

```
madamimadam
```

which is now a palindrome. Write a C++ program that reads a line of input and checks whether it is a palindrome on the basis of this less restrictive definition. Output the reversed line, with all blanks and punctuation removed, and all letters converted to lowercase along with the program's decision.

5. In Chapter 5, Programming Problem 5 asked you to create a class representing a song on a CD or in an MP-3 library. Write a C++ program using that class, which allows the user to specify the name of a data file containing songs (assume there are fewer than 200 songs on the file), and then reads the song data from the file into an array of song objects. The user should then be allowed to enter the name of an artist, and the program will output all of the songs by that artist, along with any other information about the song that is in the array.

Case Study Follow-Up

1. There is no error checking in the Calculating Exam Statistics program. List at least two errors that could easily be checked.
2. All of the functions except `OpenFiles`, `InputGrades`, and `PrintResults` are value-returning functions. Rather than calculating and storing the values they calculate, could they be calculated as they are being printed in `PrintResult`? If so, would it be a good idea to do it?
3. This solution makes use of a technique called indexes with semantic content. Explain what this means in relation to this problem.
4. The heading for the output is coded directly in the `OpenFiles` function. Remove this statement, prompt the user to enter a heading, and write this heading on the output file.
5. Exercise 4 had the heading written in the `OpenFiles` function. Would it be better to have the `PrintResults` function prompt for the heading?
6. Rewrite the Favorite Rock Group program using an enumerated type for class (or level). Which code is more readable and self-documenting?
7. Design a complete testing strategy for the Favorite Rock Group program.

Array-Based Lists

Knowledge Goals

- *To understand the structure of a list ADT.*
- *To know the basic operations associated with a list ADT.*
- *To know how a linear search algorithm works.*
- *To understand the properties of a sorted list ADT.*
- *To know how an insertion sort works.*
- *To know how the binary search algorithm works.*

Skill Goals

To be able to:

- *Represent a list ADT using a C++ class.*
- *Insert and delete list values.*
- *Represent a sorted list ADT using a C++ class.*
- *Implement an insertion sort.*
- *Implement a binary search on a sorted list.*

Chapter 12 introduced the array, a data structure that is a collection of components of the same type given a single name. In general, a one-dimensional array is a structure used to hold a list of items. In this chapter, we examine algorithms that build and manipulate data stored as a list in a one-dimensional array. These algorithms are implemented as general-purpose functions that can be modified easily to work with many kinds of lists.

We also consider the C *string*, a special kind of built-in one-dimensional array that is used for storing character strings. We conclude with a case study that uses an array as the main data structure.

13.1 The List as an Abstract Data Type

As defined in Chapter 12, a one-dimensional array is a built-in data structure that consists of a fixed number of homogeneous components. One use for an array is to store a list of values. A list may contain fewer values than the number of places reserved in the array.

For example, given an array `firstList` with 500 places, only the first `length-1` components might contain valid data. In Figure 13–1, you can see that the *array* goes from `firstList[0]` through `firstList[499]`, but the *list* stored in the array goes from `firstList[0]` through `firstList[length-1]`. The number of places in the array is fixed, but the number of values in the list stored there may vary.

For a moment, let's think of the concept of a list not in terms of arrays but as a separate data type. We can define a list as a varying-length, linear collection of homogeneous components. That's quite a mouthful. By *linear* we mean that each component (except the first) has a unique component that comes before it and each component (except the last) has a unique component that comes after it. The length of a list—the number of values currently stored in the list—can vary during the execution of the program.

> **List** A variable-length, linear collection of homogeneous components.
>
> **Length** The number of values currently stored in a list.

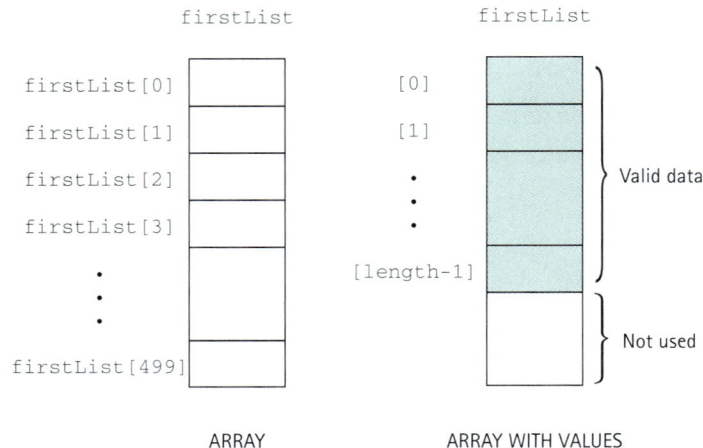

Figure 13–1 *firstList array*

Like any data type, a list must have associated with it a set of allowable operations. What kinds of operations would we want to define for a list? Here are some possibilities: create a list, add an item to a list, delete an item from a list, print a list, search a list for a particular value, sort a list into alphabetical or numerical order, and so on. When we define a data type formally—by specifying its properties and the operations that preserve those properties—we are creating an abstract data type (ADT). In fact, in Chapter 11 we proposed an ADT named IntList, a data type for a list of up to 100 integer values. At the time, we did not implement this ADT because we did not have at our disposal a suitable concrete data representation. Now that we are familiar with the idea of using a one-dimensional array to represent a list, we can combine C++ classes and arrays to implement list ADTs.

Let's generalize the IntList ADT by (a) allowing the components to be of *any* simple type or of type string, (b) replacing the maximum length of 100 with a maximum of MAX_LENGTH, a defined constant, and (c) including a wider variety of allowable operations. Here is the specification of the more general ADT:

TYPE
  List
DOMAIN
  Each instance of type List is a collection of up to MAX_LENGTH components,
     each of type ItemType.
OPERATIONS
  Create an initially empty list.
  Report whether the list is empty (true or false).
  Report whether the list is full (true or false).
  Return the current length of the list.
  Insert an item into the list.
  Delete an item from the list.
  Search for a specified item, returning true or false according to whether the
     item is present in the list.
  Sort the list into ascending order.
  Iterate through the list, returning each item in turn.

We can use a C++ class named List to represent the List ADT in our programs. For the concrete data representation, we use two items: a one-dimensional array to hold the list items, and an int variable that stores the current length of the list. When we compile the List class, we need to supply definitions for MAX_LENGTH and ItemType:

```
const int MAX_LENGTH = _____;   // Maximum possible number of
                                   //   components needed
typedef _____ ItemType;         // Type of each component
                                   //   (a simple type or the
                                   //   string class)
```

Here is the specification file for our List ADT. Notice that we use 50 for MAX_LENGTH and int for ItemType. Notice also that the abstract operation *Create an initially empty list* is implemented as the class constructor List().

```
//*************************************************************
// SPECIFICATION FILE (list.h)
// This file gives the specification of a list abstract data type.
// The list components are not assumed to be in order by value.
// To save space, we omit from each function the precondition
// comments that document the assumptions made about valid input
// parameter data. These would be included in a program intended
// for actual use.
//*************************************************************

const int MAX_LENGTH =100;      // Maximum possible number of
                                //    components needed
typedef int ItemType;           // Type of each component
                                //    (a simple type or string class)

class List
{
public:
    bool IsEmpty() const;

        // Postcondition:
        //      Return value == true, if list is empty
        //                   == false, otherwise

    bool IsFull() const;

        // Postcondition:
        //      Return value == true, if list is full
        //                   == false, otherwise

    int Length() const;

        // Postcondition:
        //      Return value == length of list

    void Insert( /* in */ ItemType item );

        // Precondition:
        //      NOT IsFull()
        // Postcondition:
        //      item is in list
        //   && Length() == Length()@entry + 1

    void Delete( /* in */ ItemType item );

        // Precondition:
        //      NOT IsEmpty()
        // Postcondition:
```

```
//      IF item is in list at entry
//          First occurrence of item is no longer in list
//          && Length() == Length()@entry - 1
//      ELSE
//          List is unchanged

bool IsPresent( /* in */ ItemType item ) const;

// Postcondition:
//      Return value == true, if item is in list
//                   == false, otherwise

void Reset();

// Postcondition:
//      Iteration is initialized

ItemType GetNextItem();

// Precondition:
//      Iteration has been initialized by call to Reset;
//      No transformers have been invoked since last call
// Postcondition:
//      Return value is the item at the current position
//      in the list on entry;
//      If last item has been returned, the next call will
//      return the first item.

void SelSort();

// Postcondition:
//      List components are in ascending order of value

List();

// Constructor
// Postcondition:
//      Empty list is created
private:
    int     length;
    int     currentPos;
    ItemType data[MAX_LENGTH];
};
```

In Chapter 11, we classified ADT operations as constructors, transformers, observers, and iterators. IsEmpty, IsFull, Length, and IsPresent, are observers. Reset, Insert, Delete, and SelSort are transformers. GetNextItem is an iterator. The class constructor is an ADT constructor operation.

The private part of the class declaration shows our data representation of a list: two `int` variables and an array (see Figure 13–2). However, notice that the preconditions and post-conditions of the member functions mention nothing about an array. The abstraction is a list, not an array. The user of the class is interested only in manipulating lists of items and does not care how we implement a list. If we change to a different data representation (as we do in Chapter 15), neither the public interface nor the client code needs to be changed.

Let's look at an example of a client program. A data file contains a weather station's daily maximum temperature readings for one month, one integer value per day. Unfortunately, the temperature sensor is faulty and occasionally registers a temperature of 200 degrees. The following program uses the `List` class to store the temperature readings, delete any spurious readings of 200 degrees, and output the remaining readings in sorted order. Presumably, the data file contains no more than 31 integers for the month, which should be well under the `List` class's `MAX_LENGTH` of 50. However, just in case the file erroneously contains more than `MAX_LENGTH` values, the reading loop in the following program terminates not only if end-of-file is encountered but also if the list becomes full (`IsFull`). Another reason to use the `IsFull` operation in this loop can be found by looking at the function specifications in file `list.h`—namely, we must guarantee `Insert`'s precondition that the list is not full. Similarly, in the loop that deletes the spurious readings of 200 degrees, we must use the `IsEmpty` operation to guarantee `Delete`'s precondition that the list is not empty.

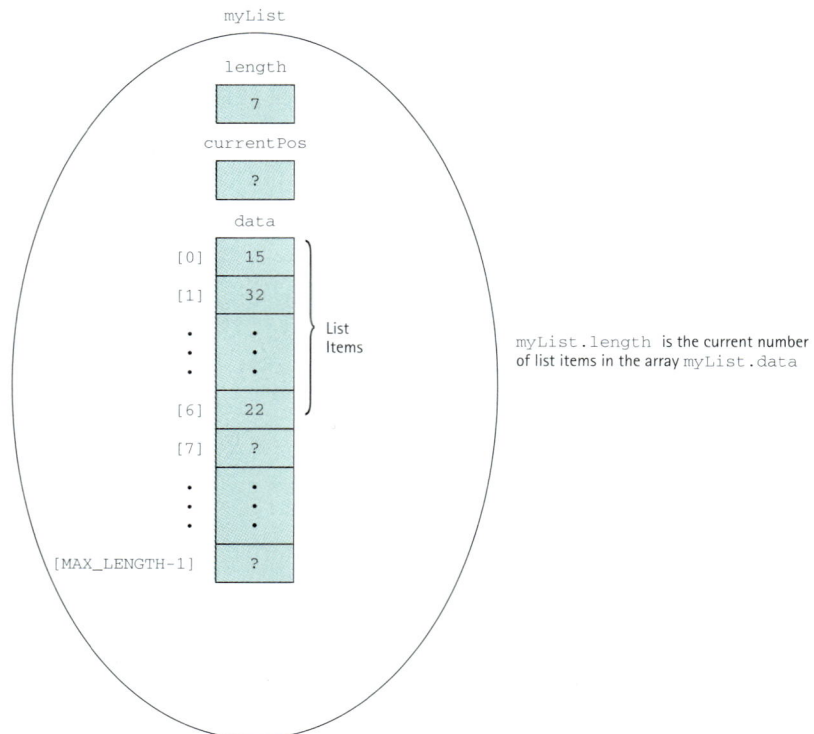

Figure 13–2 *myList, a Class Object of Type* `List`

```
//*******************************************************************
// Temperatures program
// This program inputs one month's temperature readings from a file,
// deletes spurious readings of 200 degrees from a faulty sensor,
// and outputs the values in sorted order
//*******************************************************************
#include <fstream>      // For file I/O
#include "list.h"       // For List class

using namespace std;

int main()
{
    List temps;         // List of temperature readings
    int  oneTemp;       // One temperature reading
    ifstream inData;    // File of temperature readings
    int limit;          // The number of readings
    ofstream outData;   // Output file

    inData.open("temps.dat");
    if ( !inData )
    {
        outData << "Can't open file temps.dat" << endl;
        return 1;
    }

    outData.open("temps.ans");

    // Get temperature readings from file

    inData >> oneTemp;
    while (inData && !temps.IsFull())
    {
        temps.Insert(oneTemp);
        inData >> oneTemp;
    }

    // Output original list

    temps.Reset();                          // Set up for an iteration
    limit = temps.Length();                 // Get number of items
    outData << "No. of readings: " << limit << endl;
    outData << "Original list:" << endl;

    for (int count = 0; count < limit; count++)
    {
```

```
        oneTemp = temps.GetNextItem();
        outData << oneTemp << endl;
    }

    // Discard spurious readings of 200 degrees

    while ( !temps.IsEmpty() && temps.IsPresent(200))
        temps.Delete(200);

    temps.SelSort();                        // Sort list

    // Output sorted list

    temps.Reset();                          // Set up for an iteration
    limit = temps.Length();                 // Get number of items
    outData << "No. of valid readings: " << limit << endl;
    outData << "Sorted list:" << endl;

    for (int count = 0; count < limit; count++)
    {
        oneTemp = temps.GetNextItem();
        outData << oneTemp << endl;
    }
    inData.close();
    outData.close();
    return 0;
}
```

The following output file is shown in two columns rather than one.

No. of readings: 30	No. of valid readings: 21
Original list:	Sorted list:
70	61
68	65
69	66
68	67
68	68
72	68
200	68
69	68
87	69
200	69
82	69
200	70
200	71

Output file continued:

```
No. of readings: 30        No. of valid readings: 21
Original list:             Sorted list:
81                         72
200                        75
75                         77
78                         78
68                         78
67                         81
200                        82
65                         87
66
200
61
71
200
200
77
78
69
```

We now consider how to implement each of the ADT operations, given that the list items are stored in an array. Before we do so, however, we must distinguish between lists whose components must always be kept in alphabetical or numerical order (*sorted lists*) and lists in which the components are not arranged in any particular order (*unsorted lists*). We begin with unsorted lists.

13.2 Unsorted Lists

Basic Operations

As we discussed in Chapter 11, an ADT is typically implemented in C++ by using a pair of files: the specification file (such as the preceding list.h file) and the implementation file, which contains the implementations of the class member functions. Here is how the implementation file list.cpp starts out:

```
//************************************************************
// IMPLEMENTATION FILE (list.cpp)
// This file implements the List class member functions
// List representation: a one-dimensional array and a length
//                      variable
//************************************************************
#include "list.h"
#include <iostream>

using namespace std;
```

```
// Private members of class:
//      int        length;               Length of the list
//      int        currentPos;           Current position during iteration
//      ItemType data[MAX_LENGTH];       Array holding the list
```

Let's look now at the implementations of the basic list operations.

Creating an Empty List   As Figure 13–2 shows, the list exists in the array elements `data[0]` through `data[length-1]`. To create an empty list, it is sufficient to set the `length` member to 0. We do not need to store any special values into the `data` array to make the list empty, because only those values in `data[0]` through `data[length-1]` are processed by the list algorithms.

In the `List` class, the appropriate place to initialize the list to be empty is the class constructor:

```
List::List()

// Constructor

// Postcondition:
//      length == 0


{
    length = 0;
}
```

One thing you will notice as we go through the `List` member functions is that the *implementation assertions* (the preconditions and postconditions appearing in the implementation file) are often stated differently from the *abstract assertions* (those located in the specification file). Abstract assertions are written in terms that are meaningful to the user of the ADT; implementation details should not be mentioned. In contrast, implementation assertions can be made more precise by referring directly to variables and algorithms in the implementation code. In the case of the `List` class constructor, the abstract postcondition is simply that an empty list has been created. On the other hand, the implementation postcondition

```
// Postcondition:
//      length == 0
```

is phrased in terms of our private data representation.

The IsEmpty Operation   This operation returns `true` if the list is empty and `false` if the list is not empty. Using our convention that `length` equals 0 if the list is empty, the implementation of this operation is straightforward.

```
bool List::IsEmpty() const

// Reports whether list is empty

// Postcondition:
//     Return value == true, if length == 0
//                  == false, otherwise

{
    return (length == 0);
}
```

The IsFull Operation   The list is full if there is no more room in the array holding the list items—that is, if the list length equals MAX_LENGTH.

```
bool List::IsFull() const

// Reports whether list is full

// Postcondition:
//     Return value == true, if length == MAX_LENGTH
//                  == false, otherwise

{
    return (length == MAX_LENGTH);
}
```

The Length Operation   This operation simply returns to the client the current length of the list.

```
int List::Length() const

// Returns current length of list

// Postcondition:
//     Return value == length

{
    return length;
}
```

Insertion and Deletion

To devise an algorithm for inserting a new item into the list, we first observe that we are working with an unsorted list and that the values do not have to be maintained in any particular order. Therefore, we can store a new value into the next available position in the array—data[length]—and then increment length. This algorithm brings up a question: Do we need to check that there is room in the list for the new item? We have two choices. The Insert function can test length against MAX_LENGTH and return an error flag if there isn't any room, or we can let the client code make the test before calling Insert (that is, make it a precondition that the list is not full). If you look back at the List class declaration in list.h, you can see that we have chosen the second approach. The client can use the IsFull operation to make sure the precondition is true. If the client fails to satisfy the precondition, the contract between client and function is broken, and the function is not required to satisfy the postcondition.

```
void List::Insert( /* in */ ItemType item )

// Inserts item into the list

// Precondition:
//      length < MAX_LENGTH
// Postcondition:
//       data[length@entry] == item
//    && length == length@entry+1

{
    data[length] = item;
    length++;
}
```

Deleting a component from a list consists of two parts: finding the component and removing it from the list. Before we can write the algorithm, we must know what to do if the component is not there. *Delete* can mean "Delete, if it's there" or "Delete, it *is* there." According to the List class declaration in list.h, we assume the first meaning; the code for the first definition works for the second as well but is not as efficient. We must start at the beginning of the list and search for the value to be deleted. If we find it, how do we remove it? We take the last value in the list (the one stored in data[length-1]), put it where the item to be deleted is located, and then decrement length. Moving the last item from its original position is appropriate only for an unsorted list because we don't need to preserve the order of the items in the list.

The definition "Delete, if it's there" requires a searching loop with a compound condition. We examine each component in turn and stop looking when we find the item to be deleted or when we have looked at all the items and know that it is not there.

```
void List::Delete( /* in */ ItemType item )

// Deletes item from the list, if it is there

// Precondition:
//      length > 0
```

```
// Postcondition:
//     IF item is in data array at entry
//          First occurrence of item is no longer in array
//       && length == length@entry - 1
//     ELSE
//          length and data array are unchanged

{
    int index = 0;     // Index variable

    while (index < length && item != data[index])
        index++;

    if (index < length)
    {                                          // Remove item
        data[index] = data[length-1];
        length--;
    }
}
```

To see how the While loop and the subsequent If statement work, let's look at the two possibilities: Either item is in the list or it is not. If item is in the list, the loop terminates when the expression index < length is true and the expression item != data[index] is false. After the loop exit, the If statement finds the expression index < length to be true and removes the item. On the other hand, if item is not in the list, the loop terminates when the expression index < length is false—that is, when index becomes equal to length. Subsequently, the If condition is false, and the function returns without changing anything.

Sequential Search

In the Delete function, the algorithm we used to search for the item to be deleted is known as a *sequential* or *linear search* in an unsorted list. We use the same algorithm to implement the IsPresent function of the List class.

```
bool List::IsPresent( /* in */ ItemType item ) const

// Searches the list for item, reporting whether it was found

// Postcondition:
//     Return value == true, if item is in data[0..length-1]
//                  == false, otherwise

{
    int index = 0;     // Index variable

    while (index < length && item != data[index])
```

```
        index++;

    return (index < length);
}
```

This algorithm is called a sequential search because we start at the beginning of the list and look at each item in sequence. We stop the search as soon as we find the item we are looking for (or when we reach the end of the list, concluding that the desired item is not present in the list).

We can use this algorithm in any program requiring a list search. In the form shown, it searches a list of `ItemType` components, provided that `ItemType` is an integral type or the `string` class. To use the function with a list of floating-point values, we must modify it so that the While statement tests for near equality rather than exact equality (for the reasons discussed in Chapter 10). In the following statement, we assume that `EPSILON` is defined as a global constant.

```
while (index < length && fabs(item - data[index]) >= EPSILON)
    index++;
```

The sequential search algorithm finds the first occurrence of the searched-for item. How would we modify it to find the last occurrence? We would initialize `index` to `length-1` and decrement `index` each time through the loop, stopping when we found the item we wanted or when `index` became −1.

Before we leave this search algorithm, let's introduce a variation that makes the program more efficient, although a little more complex. The While loop contains a compound condition: It stops when it either finds `item` or reaches the end of the list. We can insert a copy of `item` into `data[length]`—that is, into the array component beyond the end of the list—as a sentinel. By doing so, we are guaranteed to find `item` in the list. Then we can eliminate the condition that checks for the end of the list (`index < length`) (see Figure 13–3). Eliminating a condition saves the computer the time that would be required to test it. In this case, we save time during every iteration of the loop, so the savings add up quickly. Note, however, that we are gaining efficiency at the expense of space. We must declare the array size to be 1 larger than `MAX_LENGTH` to hold the sentinel value if the list becomes full. That is, we must change the private part of the class declaration as follows:

```
class List
{
    ⋮
private:
    int       length;
    int       currentPos;
    ItemType  data[MAX_LENGTH+1];
};
```

Figure 13–3 reflects this change. The last array element shows an index of `MAX_LENGTH` rather than `MAX_LENGTH-1`, as in Figure 13–2.

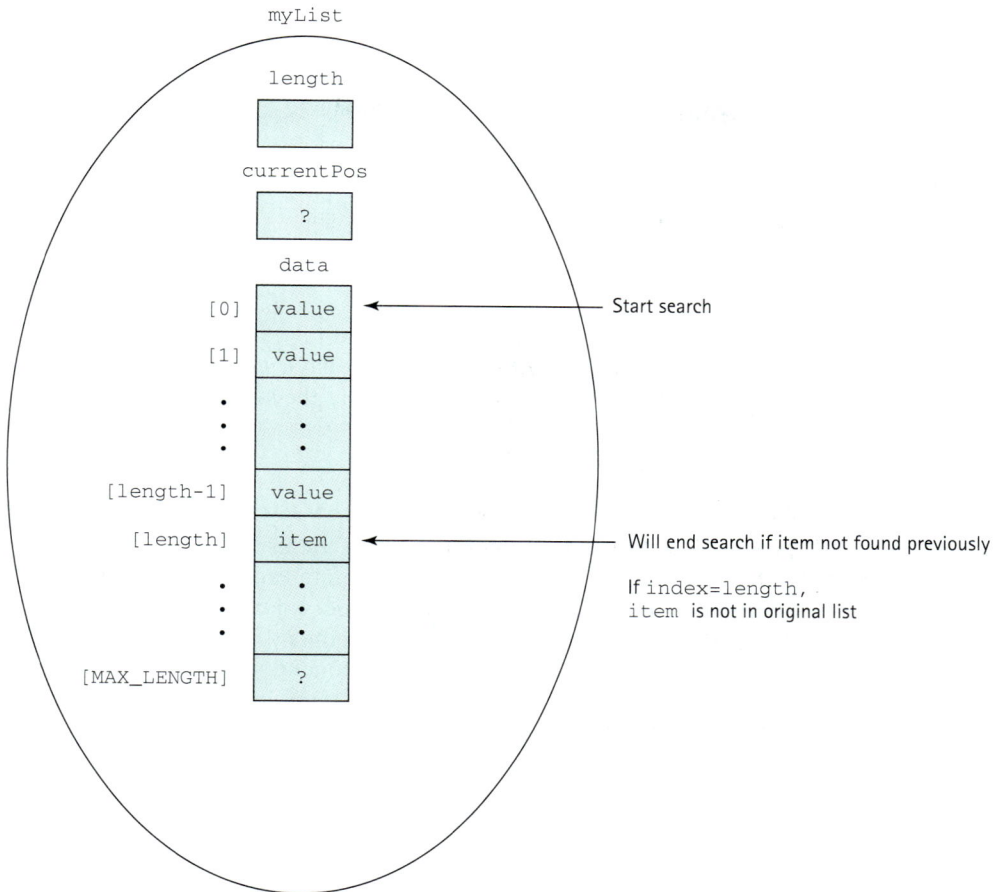

Figure 13–3   *Sequential Search with Copy of `item` in `data[length]`*

The following function, `IsPresent2`, implements this new algorithm. After the search loop terminates, the function returns `true` if `index` is less than `length`; otherwise, it returns `false`.

```
bool List::IsPresent2( /* in */ ItemType item ) const

// Searches the list for item, reporting whether it was found

// Postcondition:
//     data[0..length-1] are the same as at entry
//  && data[length] is overwritten to aid in the search
//  && Return value == true, if item is in data[0..length-1]
//                  == false, otherwise
```

```
{
    int index = 0;                      // Index variable

    data[length] = item;                // Store item at position beyond
                                        //    end of list
    while (item != data[index])
        index++;

    return (index < length);
}
```

Note that the declaration of our List class in the file list.h includes the member function IsPresent but not IsPresent2. We have presented IsPresent2 only to show you an alternative approach to implementing the search operation.

Iterators

Iterators are used with composite types to allow the user to process an entire structure component by component. To give the user access to each item in sequence, we provide two operations: one to initialize the iteration process (analogous to Reset or Open with a file) and one to return a copy of the "next component" each time it is called. The user can then set up a loop that processes each component. We call these operations Reset and GetNextItem. Note that Reset is not an iterator itself, but is an auxiliary transformer that supports the iteration. Another type of iterator is one that takes an operation and applies it to every element in the list.

The Reset function is analogous to the open operation for a file in which the file pointer is positioned at the beginning of the file so that the first input operation accesses the first component of the file. Each successive call to an input operation gets the next item in the file. Therefore, we need a variable that keeps track of the next item to be returned from an iteration. We call that variable currentPos. Reset must initialize currentPos to point to the first item in the list.

The GetNextItem operation is analogous to an input operation; it accesses the next item, the one at currentPos, increments currentPos, and returns the item it accessed. What happens if the last item has been accessed? Let's put currentPos back to the first item. This way, the program may get the wrong answer, but it won't access data outside the list.

Reset

Initialize currentPos to first item

GetNextItem

```
Set item to data[currentPos]
IF currentPos is length - 1
    Set currentPos to 0
ELSE
    Increment currentPos
Return item
```

currentPos is undefined until it is initialized by Reset. After the first call to GetNextItem, currentPos is the location of the next item to be accessed by GetNextItem. Therefore, to implement this algorithm in an array-based list in C++, currentPos must be initialized to 0. These operations are coded as follows.

```
void List::Reset()
// Post: currentPos has been initialized.
{
    currentPos = 0;
}
```

What would happen if a transformer operation is executed between calls to Get-NextItem? The iteration would be invalid. That is why there is a precondition to prevent this from happening.

```
Itemtype List::GetNextItem()

// Precondition:
//     No transformer has been executed since last
//     call
// Postcondition:
//     Return value is currentPos@entry
//     && current position has been updated
//     If last item has been returned, the next call
//     returns the first item

{
    ItemType item;
    item = data[currentPos];
    if (currentPos == length - 1)
        currentPos = 0;
    else
        currentPos++;
    return item;
}
```

Reset and GetNextItem are designed to be used in a loop in the client program that iterates through all of the items in the list. The precondition in the specifications for GetNextItem protects against trying to access an array element that is not in the list. Look back at the Temperature program. Reset and GetNextItem were used twice: once to print the original list and once to print the corrected sorted list.

Sorting

Although we are implementing an unsorted list ADT, there are times when the user of the List class may want to rearrange the list components into a certain order just before calling the Print function. For example, the user might want to put a list of stock numbers into either ascending or descending order, or the user might want to put a list of words into alphabetical order. In software development, arranging list items into order is a very common operation and is known as **sorting**.

> **Sorting** Arranging the components of a list into order (for instance, words into alphabetical order or numbers into ascending or descending order).

If you were given a sheet of paper with a column of 20 numbers on it and were asked to write the numbers in ascending order, you would probably do the following:

1. Make a pass through the list, looking for the smallest number.
2. Write it on the paper in a second column.
3. Cross the number off the original list.
4. Repeat the process, always looking for the smallest number remaining in the original list.
5. Stop when all the numbers have been crossed off.

We can implement this algorithm directly in C++, but we need two arrays—one for the original list and a second for the sorted list. If the list is large, we might not have enough memory for two copies of it. Also, how do we "cross off" an array component? We could simulate crossing off a value by replacing it with some dummy value like INT_MAX. That is, we would set the value of the crossed-off variable to something that would not interfere with the processing of the rest of the components. However, a slight variation of our hand-done algorithm allows us to sort the components *in place*. We do not have to use a second array; we can put a value into its proper place in the list by having it swap places with the component currently in that position.

We can state the algorithm as follows. We search for the smallest value in the list and exchange it with the component in the first position in the list. We search for the next-smallest value in the list and exchange it with the component in the second position in the list. This process continues until all the components are in their proper places.

```
FOR count going from 0 through length–2
    Find minimum value in data[count .. length–1]
    Swap minimum value with data[count]
```

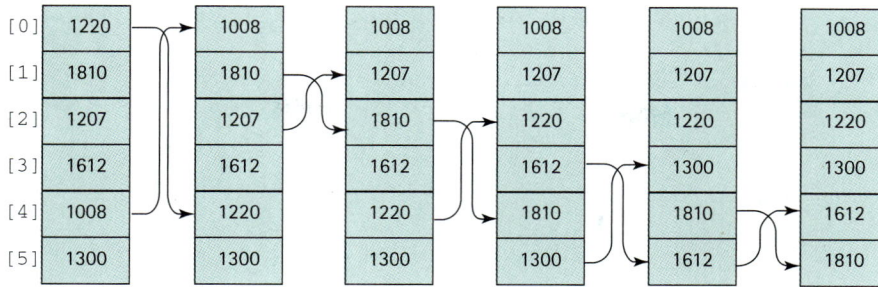

Figure 13-4 *Straight Selection Sort*

Figure 13–4 illustrates how this algorithm works.

Observe that we perform `length-1` passes through the list because `count` runs from 0 through `length-2`. The loop does not need to be executed when `count` equals `length-1` because the last value, `data[length-1]`, is in its proper place after the preceding components have been sorted.

This sort, known as the *straight selection sort,* belongs to a class of sorts called selection sorts. There are many types of sorting algorithms. Selection sorts are characterized by finding the smallest (or largest) value left in the unsorted portion at each iteration and swapping it with the value indexed by the iteration counter. Swapping the contents of two variables requires a temporary variable so that no values are lost (see Figure 13–5).

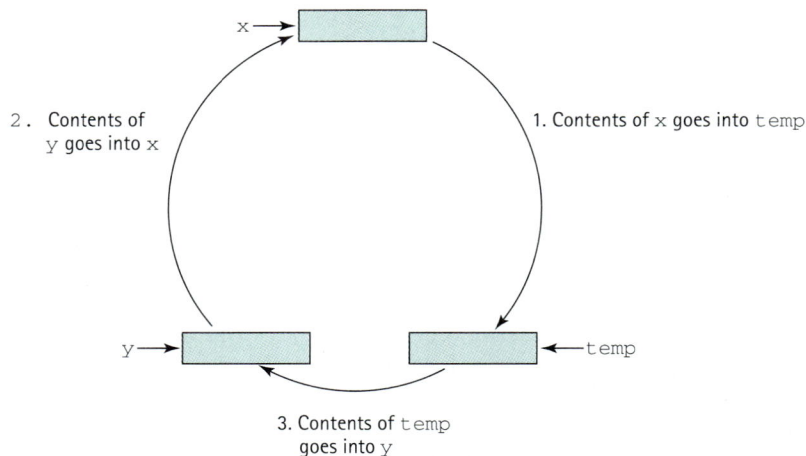

Figure 13-5 *Swapping the Contents of Two Variables, x and y*

Here is the code for the sorting operation of the `List` class:

```
void List::SelSort()

// Sorts list into ascending order

// Postcondition:
//     data array contains the same values as data@entry, rearranged
//     into ascending order

{
    ItemType temp;              // Temporary variable
    int      passCount;         // Loop control variable
    int      searchIndx;        // Loop control variable
    int      minIndx;           // Index of minimum so far

    for (passCount = 0; passCount < length - 1; passCount++)
    {
        minIndx = passCount;

        // Find the index of the smallest component
        // in data[passCount..length-1]

        for (searchIndx = passCount + 1; searchIndx < length;
                                              searchIndx++)
            if (data[searchIndx] < data[minIndx])
                minIndx = searchIndx;

        // Swap data[minIndx] and data[passCount]

        temp = data[minIndx];
        data[minIndx] = data[passCount];
        data[passCount] = temp;
    }
}
```

Note that with each pass through the outer loop, we are looking for the minimum value in the rest of the list (`data[passCount]` through `data[length-1]`). Therefore, `minIndx` is initialized to `passCount` and the inner loop runs from `searchIndx` equal to `passCount+1` through `length-1`. Upon exit from the inner loop, `minIndx` contains the position of the smallest value. (Note that the If statement is the only statement in the loop.)

Note also that we may swap a component with itself, which occurs if no value in the remaining list is smaller than `data[passCount]`. We could avoid this unnecessary swap by checking to see if `minIndx` is equal to `passCount`. Because this comparison would be made during each iteration of the outer loop, it is more efficient not to check for this possibility and just to swap something with itself occasionally. If the components we are sorting are much more complex than simple numbers, we might reconsider this decision.

This algorithm sorts the components into ascending order. To sort them into descending order, we would scan for the maximum value instead of the minimum value. To do so, we would simply change the relational operator in the inner loop from < to >. Of course, `minIndx` would no longer be an appropriate identifier and should be changed to `maxIndx`.

By providing the user of the `List` class with a sorting operation, we have not turned our unsorted list ADT into a sorted list ADT. The `Insert` and `Delete` algorithms we wrote do not preserve ordering by value. `Insert` places a new item at the end of the list, regardless of its value, and `Delete` moves the last item to a different position in the list. After `SelSort` has executed, the list items remain in sorted order only until the next insertion or deletion takes place. We now look at a sorted list ADT in which all the list operations cooperate to preserve the sorted order of the list components.

13.3 Sorted Lists

In the `List` class, the `IsPresent` and `IsPresent2` algorithms both assume that the list to be searched is unsorted. A drawback to searching an unsorted list is that we must scan the entire list to discover that the search item is not there. Think what it would be like if your city telephone book contained people's names in random rather than alphabetical order. To look up Mary Anthony's phone number, you would have to start with the first name in the phone book and scan sequentially, page after page, until you found it. In the worst case, you might have to examine tens of thousands of names only to find out that Mary's name is not in the book.

Of course, telephone books *are* alphabetized, and the alphabetical ordering makes searching easier. If Mary Anthony's name is not in the book, you discover this fact quickly by starting with the A's and stopping the search as soon as you have passed the place where her name should be.

Let's define a sorted list ADT in which the components always remain in order by value, no matter what operations are applied. Below is the `slist.h` file that contains the declaration of a `SortedList` class.

```
//*****************************************************************
// SPECIFICATION FILE (SortedList.h)
// This file gives the specification of a SortedList abstract data
// type. The components are assumed to be in order by value.
// To save space, we omit from each function the precondition
// comments that document the assumptions made about valid input
// parameter data. These would be included in a program intended
// for actual use.
//*****************************************************************
```

```cpp
const int MAX_LENGTH =100;      // Maximum possible number of
                                //    components needed
typedef int ItemType;           // Type of each component
                                //    (a simple type or string class)


class SortedList
{
public:
    bool IsEmpty() const;

        // Postcondition:
        //      Return value == true, if SortedList is empty
        //                   == false, otherwise


    bool IsFull() const;

        // Postcondition:
        //      Return value == true, if SortedList is full
        //                   == false, otherwise


    int Length() const;

        // Postcondition:
        //      Return value == length of SortedList


    void Insert( /* in */ ItemType& item );

        // Inserts item into the SortedList

        // Precondition:
        //      length < MAX_LENGTH
        //   && data[0..length-1] are in ascending order
        // Postcondition:
        //      item is in the SortedList
        //   && length == length@entry + 1
        //   && data[0..length-1] are in ascending order


    void Delete( /* in */ ItemType item );

        // Precondition:
        //      NOT IsEmpty()
        // Postcondition:
        //      IF item is in SortedSortedList at entry
        //          First occurrence of item is no longer
        //          in SortedList
```

```
//              && Length() == Length()@entry - 1
//        ELSE
//            SortedList is unchanged

    bool IsPresent( /* in */ ItemType item ) const;

        // Precondition:
        // Postcondition:
        //      Return value == true, if item is in SortedList
        //                   == false, otherwise

    void Reset();

        // Postcondition:
        //      Iteration is initialized

    ItemType GetNextItem();

        // Precondition:
        // Iteration has been initialized by call to Reset;
        //      No transformers have been invoked since last call
        // Postcondition:
        //      Returns item at the current position in the
        //      SortedList

    SortedList();

        // Constructor
        // Postcondition:
        //      Empty SortedList is created
private:
    int      length;
    int      currentPos;
    ItemType data[MAX_LENGTH];
    void BinSearch( ItemType, bool&, int& ) const;
};
```

How does the declaration of SortedList differ from the declaration of our original List class? Apart from a few changes in the documentation comments, there are only two differences:

1. The SortedList class does not supply a sorting operation to the client. Such an operation is needless, because the list components are assumed to be kept in sorted order at all times.

2. The SortedList class has an additional class member in the private part: a BinSearch function. This function is an auxiliary ("helper") function that is used only by other class member functions and is inaccessible to clients. We discuss its purpose when we examine the class implementation.

Let's look at what changes, if any, are required in the algorithms for the ADT operations, given that we are now working with a sorted list instead of an unsorted list.

Basic Operations

The algorithms for the class constructor, `IsEmpty`, `IsFull`, `Length`, `Reset` and `GetNextItem` are identical to those in the `List` class. The constructor sets the private data member `length` to 0, `IsEmpty` reports whether `length` equals 0, `IsFull` reports whether `length` equals `MAX_LENGTH`, `Length` returns the value of `length`, and `Print` outputs the list items from first to last.

Insertion

To add a new value to an already sorted list, we could store the new value at `data[length]`, increment `length`, and sort the array again. However, such a solution is *not* an efficient way of solving the problem. Inserting five new items results in five separate sorting operations.

If we were to insert a value by hand into a sorted list, we would write the new value out to the side and draw a line showing where it belongs. To find this position, we start at the top and scan the list until we find a value greater than the one we are inserting. The new value goes in the list just before that point.

We can use a similar process in our `Insert` function. We find the proper place in the list using the by-hand algorithm. Instead of writing the value to the side, we shift all the values larger than the new one down one place to make room for it. The main algorithm is expressed as follows, where `item` is the value being inserted.

```
WHILE place not found AND more places to look
    IF item > current component in list
        Increment current position
    ELSE
        Place found
Shift remainder of list down
Insert item
Increment length
```

Assuming that `index` is the place where `item` is to be inserted, the algorithm for Shift List Down is

```
Set data[length]    = data[length–1]
Set data[length–1] = data[length–2]
      ⋮                    ⋮
Set data[index+1]  = data[index]
```

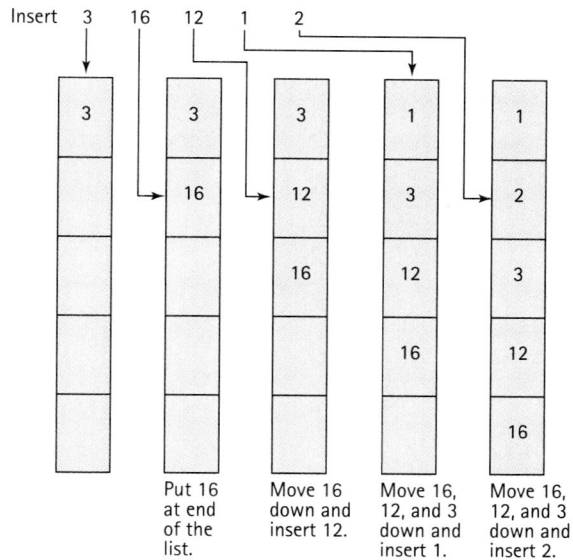

Figure 13–6   *Inserting into a Sorted List*

This algorithm is illustrated in Figure 13–6.

This algorithm is based on how we would accomplish the task by hand. Often, such an adaptation is the best way to solve a problem. However, in this case, further thought reveals a slightly better way. Notice that we search from the front of the list (people always do), and we shift down from the end of the list upward. We can combine the searching and shifting by beginning at the *end* of the list.

If `item` is the new item to be inserted, compare `item` to the value in `data[length-1]`. If `item` is *less*, put `data[length-1]` into `data[length]` and compare `item` to the value in `data[length-2]`. This process continues until you find the place where `item` is greater than or equal to the item in the list. Store `item` directly below it. Here is the algorithm:

```
Set index = length – 1
WHILE index ≥ 0 AND item < data[index]
    Set data[index + 1] = data[index]
    Decrement index
Set data[index + 1] = item
Increment length
```

What about duplicates? The algorithm continues until an item is found that is less than the one we are inserting. Therefore, the new item is inserted below a duplicate value (if one is there). Here is the code:

```
void SortedList::Insert( /* in */ ItemType item )

// Inserts item into the list

// Precondition:
//      length < MAX_LENGTH
// Postcondition:
//      item is in the list

{
    int index;      // Index and loop control variable

    index = length - 1;
    while (index >= 0 && item < data[index])
    {
        data[index+1] = data[index];
        index--;
    }
    data[index+1] = item;           // Insert item
    length++;
}
```

Notice that this algorithm works even if the list is empty. When the list is empty, length is 0 and the body of the While loop is not entered. So item is stored into data[0], and length is incremented to 1. Does the algorithm work if item is the smallest? The largest? Let's see. If item is the smallest, the loop body is executed length times, and index is −1. Thus, item is stored into position 0, where it belongs. If item is the largest, the loop body is not entered. The value of index is still length − 1, so item is stored into data[length], where it belongs.

Are you surprised that the general case also takes care of the special cases? This situation does not happen all the time, but it occurs often enough that it is good programming practice to start with the general case. If we begin with the special cases, we usually generate a correct solution, but we may not realize that we don't need to handle the special cases separately. So begin with the general case, then treat as special cases only those situations that the general case does not handle correctly.

This algorithm is the basis for another general-purpose sorting algorithm—an *insertion sort*. In an insertion sort, values are inserted one at a time into a list that was originally empty. An insertion sort is often used when input data must be sorted; each value is put into its proper place as it is read. We use this technique in the Problem-Solving Case Study at the end of this chapter.

Sequential Search

When we search for an item in an unsorted list, we won't discover that the item is missing until we reach the end of the list. If the list is already sorted, we know that an item is missing when we pass the place where it should be in the list. For example, if a list contains the values

```
  7
 11
 13
 76
 98
102
```

and we are looking for 12, we need only compare 12 with 7, 11, and 13 to know that 12 is not in the list.

If the search item is greater than the current list component, we move on to the next component. If the item is equal to the current component, we have found what we are looking for. If the item is less than the current component, then we know that it is not in the list. In either of the last two cases, we stop looking. We can restate this algorithmically with the following code, in which found is set to true if the search item was found.

```
// Sequential search in a sorted list

index = 0;
while (index < length && item > data[index])
    index++;

found = (index < length && item == data[index]);
```

On average, searching a sorted list in this way takes the same number of iterations to find an item as searching an unsorted list. The advantage of this new algorithm is that we find out sooner if an item is missing. Thus, it is slightly more efficient; however, it works only on a sorted list.

We do not use this algorithm to implement the SortedList::IsPresent function. There is a better algorithm, which we look at next.

Binary Search

There is a second search algorithm on a sorted list that is considerably faster both for finding an item and for discovering that an item is missing. This algorithm is called a *binary search*. A binary search is based on the principle of successive approximation. The algorithm divides the list in half (divides by 2—that's why it's called *binary* search) and decides which half to look in next. Division of the selected portion of the list is repeated until the item is found or it is determined that the item is not in the list.

This method is analogous to the way in which we look up a word in a dictionary. We open the dictionary in the middle and compare the word with one on the page that we turned to. If the word we're looking for comes before this word, we continue our search in the left-hand section of the dictionary. Otherwise, we continue in the right-hand section of the dictionary. We repeat this process until we find the word. If it is not there, we realize that either we have misspelled the word or our dictionary isn't complete.

The algorithm for a binary search is given below. The list of values is in the array `data`, and the value being looked for is `item` (see Figure 13-7).

1. Compare `item` to `data[middle]`. If `item = data[middle]`, then we have found it. If `item < data[middle]`, then look in the first half of `data`. If `item > data[middle]`, then look in the second half of `data`.

2. Redefine `data` to be the half of `data` that we search next, and repeat step 1.

3. Stop when we have found `item` or know it is missing. We know it's missing when there is nowhere else to look and we still have not found it.

This algorithm should make sense. With each comparison, at best, we find the item for which we are searching; at worst, we eliminate half of the remaining list from consideration.

We need to keep track of the first possible place to look (`first`) and the last possible place to look (`last`). At any one time, we are looking only in `data[first]` through `data[last]`. When the function begins, `first` is set to 0 and `last` is set to `length-1` to encompass the entire list.

Our three previous search algorithms have been Boolean observer operations. They just answer the question, Is this item in the list? Let's code the binary search as a void function that not only asks if the item is in the list but also asks which one it is (if it's there). To do so, we need to add two parameters to the parameter list: a Boolean flag `found` (to tell us whether the item is in the list) and an integer variable `position` (to tell us which item it is). If `found` is `false`, `position` is undefined.

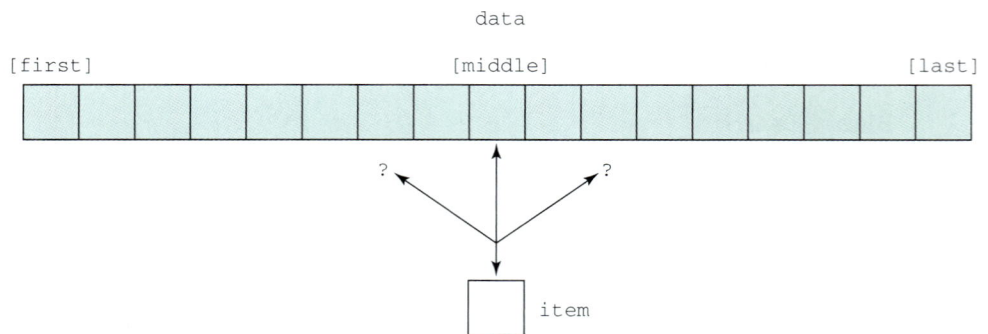

Figure 13-7   *Binary Search*

```
void SortedList::BinSearch(
        /* in */   ItemType item,          // Item to be found
        /* out */  bool&     found,         // True if item is found
        /* out */  int&      position ) const    // Location if found

// Searches list for item, returning the index
// of item if item was found.

// Precondition:
//      length <= INT_MAX / 2
// Postcondition:
//      IF item is in the list
//          found == true  &&  data[position] contains item
//      ELSE
//          found == false  &&  position is undefined

{
    int first = 0;              // Lower bound on list
    int last = length - 1;      // Upper bound on list
    int middle;                 // Middle index

    found = false;
    while (last >= first && !found)
    {
        middle = (first + last) / 2;
        if (item < data[middle])
            // Assert: item is not in data[middle..last]
            last = middle - 1;
        else if (item > data[middle])
            // Assert: item is not in data[first..middle]
            first = middle + 1;
        else
            // Assert: item == data[middle]
            found = true;
    }
    if (found)
        position = middle;
}
```

Should `BinSearch` be a public member of the `SortedList` class? No. The function returns the index of the array element where the item was found. An array index is useless to a client of `SortedList`. The array containing the list items is encapsulated within the private part of the class and is inaccessible to clients. If you review the `SortedList` class declaration, you'll see that `BinSearch` is a *private*, not public, class member. We intend to use it as a helper function when we implement the public operations `IsPresent` and `Delete`.

Let's do a code walk-through of the binary search algorithm. The value being searched for is 24. Figure 13-8a shows the values of `first`, `last`, and `middle` during the first iteration. In this iteration, 24 is compared with 103, the value in `data[middle]`. Because 24 is less than 103, `last` becomes `middle-1` and `first` stays the same. Figure 13-8b shows the situation during the second iteration. This time, 24 is compared with 72, the value in `data[middle]`. Because 24 is less than 72, `last` becomes `middle-1` and `first` again stays the same.

In the third iteration (Figure 13-8c), `middle` and `first` are both 0. The value 24 is compared with 12, the value in `data[middle]`. Because 24 is greater than 12, `first` becomes `middle+1`. In the fourth iteration (Figure 13-8d), `first`, `last`, and `middle` are all the same. Again, 24 is compared with the value in `data[middle]`. Because 24 is less than 64, `last` becomes `middle-1`. Now that `last` is less than `first`, the process stops; `found` is `false`.

The binary search is the most complex algorithm that we have examined so far. The following table shows `first`, `last`, `middle`, and `data[middle]` for searches of the values 106, 400, and 406, using the same data as in the previous example. Examine the results in this table carefully.

item	first	last	middle	data[middle]	Termination of Loop
106	0	10	5	103	
	6	10	8	200	
	6	7	6	106	found = true
400	0	10	5	103	
	6	10	8	200	
	9	10	9	300	
	10	10	10	400	found = true
406	0	10	5	103	
	6	10	8	200	
	9	10	9	300	
	10	10	10	400	
	11	10			last < first
					found = false

The calculation

```
middle = (first + last) / 2;
```

explains why the function precondition restricts the value of `length` to `INT_MAX/2`. If the item being searched for happens to reside in the last position of the list (for example, when `item` equals 400 in our sample list), then `first + last` equals `length + length`. If `length` is greater than `INT_MAX/2`, the sum `length + length` would produce an integer overflow.

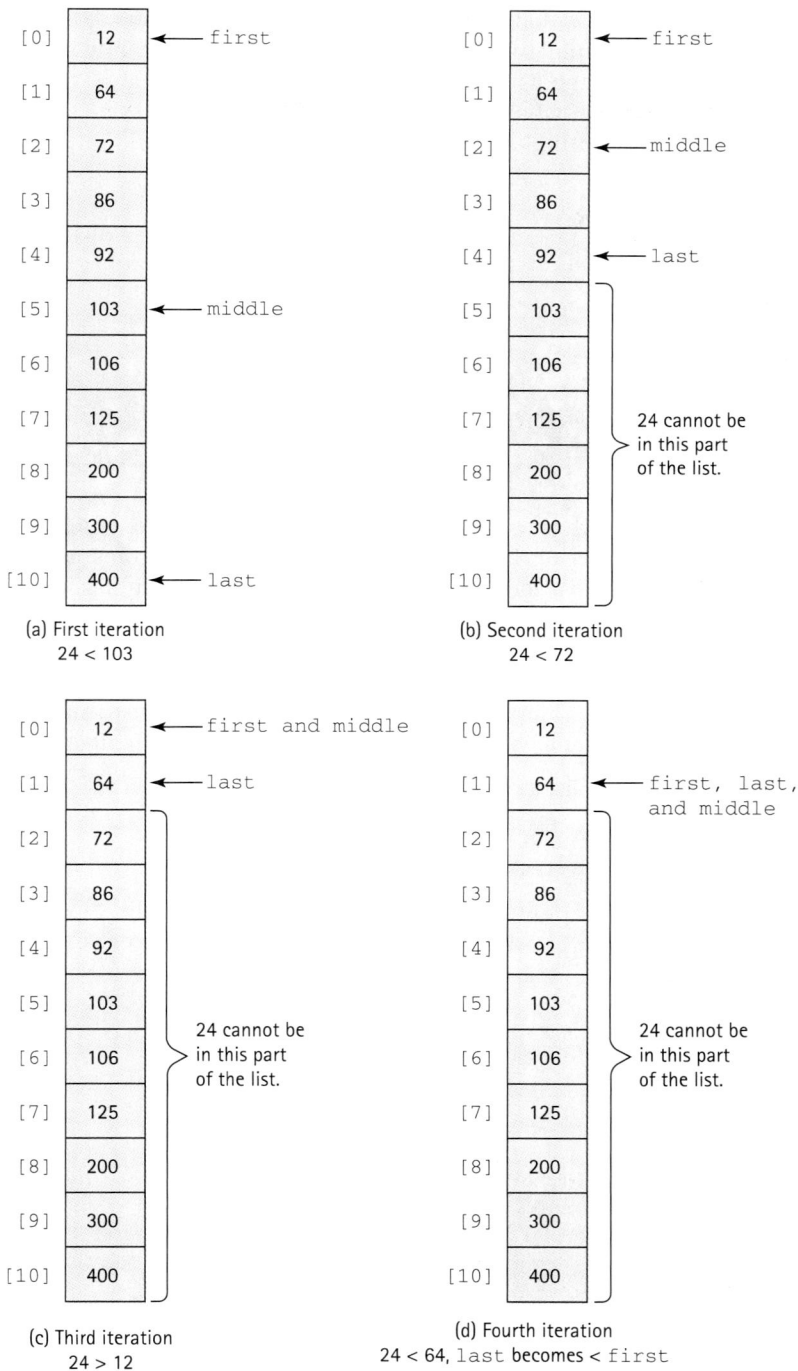

Figure 13–8   *Code Walk-Through of* BinSearch *Function (Search Item Is 24)*

Notice in the table that whether we searched for 106, 400, or 406, the loop never executed more than four times. It never executes more than four times in a list of 11 components because the list is being cut in half each time through the loop. The table below compares a sequential search and a binary search in terms of the average number of iterations needed to find an item.

	Average Number of Iterations	
Length of List	Sequential Search	Binary Search
10	5.5	2.9
100	50.5	5.8
1000	500.5	9.0
10,000	5000.5	12.4

If the binary search is so much faster, why not use it all the time? It certainly is faster in terms of the number of times through the loop, but more computations are performed within the binary search loop than in the other search algorithms. So if the number of components in the list is small (say, less than 20), the sequential search algorithms are faster because they perform less work at each iteration. As the number of components in the list increases, the binary search algorithm becomes relatively more efficient. Remember, however, that the binary search requires the list to be sorted, and sorting takes time. Keep three factors in mind when you are deciding which search algorithm to use:

1. The length of the list to be searched

2. Whether or not the list is already sorted

3. The number of times the list is to be searched

Given the `BinSearch` function (a private member of the `SortedList` class), it's easy to implement the `IsPresent` function (a public member of the class).

```
bool SortedList::IsPresent( /* in */ ItemType item ) const

// Searches the list for item, reporting whether it was found

// Precondition:
//      length <= INT_MAX / 2
// Postcondition:
//      Return value == true, if item is in data[0..length-1]
//                   == false, otherwise

{
    bool found;        // True if item is found
    int position;      // Required (but unused) argument for
                       //    the call to BinSearch
```

```
    BinSearch(item, found, position);
    return found;
}
```

The body of IsPresent calls BinSearch, obtaining the result of the search in the variables found and position. Like the children's game of Pass It On, IsPresent receives the value of found from BinSearch and simply passes it on to the client (via the return statement). The body of IsPresent is not interested in where the item was found, so it ignores the value returned in the position argument. Why did we include this third argument when we designed BinSearch? The answer is that the Delete operation, which we look at next, calls BinSearch and *does* use the position argument.

Deletion

In the List::Delete function, we deleted an item by moving up the last component in the list to fill the deleted item's position. Although this algorithm is fine for unsorted lists, it won't work for sorted lists. Moving the last component to an arbitrary position in the list is almost certain to disturb the sorted order of the components. We need a new algorithm for sorted lists.

Let's call BinSearch to tell us the position of the item to be deleted. Then we can "squeeze out" the deleted item by shifting up all the remaining array elements by one position:

```
BinSearch(item, found, position)
IF found
     Shift remainder of list up
     Decrement length
```

The algorithm for Shift List Up is

```
Set data[position]     =  data[position+1]
Set data[position+1] =  data[position+2]
     ⋮                        ⋮
Set data[length–2]     =  data[length–1]
```

Here is the coded version of this algorithm:

```
void SortedList::Delete( /* in */ ItemType item )

// Deletes item from the list, if it is there

// Precondition:
//      0 < length <= INT_MAX/2
// Postcondition:
//      IF item is in data array at entry
//              First occurrence of item is no longer in array
```

```
//          && length == length@entry - 1
//          && data[0..length-1] are in ascending order
//      ELSE
//          length and data array are unchanged

{
    bool found;         // True if item is found
    int position;       // Position of item, if found
    int index;          // Index and loop control variable

    BinSearch(item, found, position);
    if (found)
    {
        // Shift data[position..length-1] up one position

        for (index = position; index < length - 1; index++)
            data[index] = data[index+1];
        length--;
    }
}
```

Theoretical Foundations

Complexity of Searching and Sorting

We introduced Big-O notation in Chapter 6 as a way of comparing the work done by different algorithms. Let's apply it to the algorithms that we've developed in this chapter and see how they compare with each other. In each algorithm, we start with a list containing some number of values, N.

In the worst case, our `List::IsPresent` function scans all N values to locate an item. Thus, it requires N steps to execute. On average, `List::IsPresent` takes roughly $N/2$ steps to find an item; however, recall that in Big-O notation, we ignore constant factors (as well as lower-order terms). Thus, function `List::IsPresent` is an order N—that is, an $O(N)$—algorithm.

`List::IsPresent2` is also an $O(N)$ algorithm because even though we saved a comparison on each loop iteration, the same number of iterations are performed. However, making the loop more efficient without changing the number of iterations decreases the constant (the number of steps) that N is multiplied by in the algorithm's work formula. Thus, function `List::IsPresent2` is said to be a constant factor faster than `List::IsPresent`.

What about the algorithm we presented for a sequential search in a sorted list? The number of iterations is decreased for the case in which the item is missing from the list. However, all we have done is take a case that would require N steps and reduce its time, on average, to $N/2$ steps. Therefore, this algorithm is also $O(N)$.

(continued) ▼

Complexity of Searching and Sorting

Now consider `BinSearch`. In the worst case, it eliminates half of the remaining list components on each iteration. Thus, the worst-case number of iterations is equal to the number of times N must be divided by 2 to eliminate all but one value. This number is computed by taking the logarithm, base 2, of N (written $\log_2 N$). Here are some examples of $\log_2 N$ for different values of N:

N	Log$_2$N
2	1
4	2
8	3
16	4
32	5
1024	10
32,768	15
1,048,576	20
33,554,432	25
1,073,741,824	30

As you can see, for a list of over 1 billion values, `BinSearch` takes only 30 iterations. It is definitely the best choice for searching large lists. Algorithms such as `BinSearch` are said to be of *logarithmic order*.

Now let's turn to sorting. Function `SelSort` contains nested For loops. The total number of iterations is the product of the iterations performed by the two loops. The outer loop executes $N - 1$ times. The inner loop also starts out executing $N - 1$ times, but steadily decreases until it performs just one iteration: The inner loop executes $N/2$ iterations. The total number of iterations is thus

$$\frac{(N-1) \times N}{2}$$

Ignoring the constant factor and lower-order term, this is N^2 iterations, and `SelSort` is an $O(N^2)$ algorithm. Whereas `BinSearch` takes only 30 iterations to search a sorted array of 1 billion values, putting the array into order takes `SelSort` approximately 1 billion times 1 billion iterations!

We mentioned that the `SortedList::Insert` algorithm forms the basis for an insertion sort, in which values are inserted into a sorted list as they are input. On average, `SortedList::Insert` must shift down half of the values ($N/2$) in the list; thus, it is an $O(N)$ algorithm. If

(continued) ▼

> ### Complexity of Searching and Sorting
>
> `SortedList::Insert` is called for each input value, we are executing an $O(N)$ algorithm N times; therefore, an insertion sort is an $O(N^2)$ algorithm.
>
> Is every sorting algorithm $O(N^2)$? Most of the simpler ones are, but $O(N \times \log_2 N)$ sorting algorithms exist. Algorithms that are $O(N \times \log_2 N)$ are much closer in performance to $O(N)$ algorithms than are $O(N^2)$ algorithms. For example, if N is 1 million, then an $O(N^2)$ algorithm takes a million times a million (1 trillion) iterations, but an $O(N \times \log_2 N)$ algorithm takes only 20 million iterations—that is, it is 20 times slower than the $O(N)$ algorithm but 50,000 times faster than the $O(N^2)$ algorithm.

Now let's turn our attention to another example of array-based lists—a special kind of array that is useful when working with alphanumeric character data.

13.4 Understanding Character Strings

Ever since Chapter 2, we have been using the `string` class to store and manipulate character strings.

```
string name;

name = "James Smith";
len = name.length();
   ⋮
```

In some contexts, we think of a string as a single unit of data. In other contexts, we treat it as a group of individually accessible characters. In particular, we think of a string as a variable-length, linear collection of homogeneous components (of type `char`). Does this sound familiar? It should. As an abstraction, a string is a list of characters that, at any moment in time, has a length associated with it.

C string In C and C++, a null-terminated sequence of characters stored in a `char` array.

Thinking of a string as an ADT, how would we implement the ADT? There are many ways to implement strings. Programmers have specified and implemented their own string classes—the `string` class from the standard library, for instance. And the C++ language has its own built-in notion of a string: the **C string**. In C++, a string constant (or string literal, or literal string) is a sequence of characters enclosed by double quotes:

```
"Hi"
```

A string constant is stored as a `char` array with enough components to hold each specified character plus one more—the *null character*. The null character, which is the first character in both the ASCII and EBCDIC character sets, has internal representation 0. In C++, the escape sequence \0 stands for the null character. When the compiler encounters the string "Hi" in a program, it stores the three characters 'H', 'i', and '\0' into a three-element, anonymous (unnamed) `char` array as follows:

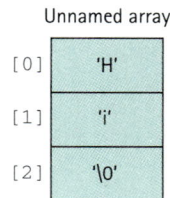

Unnamed array

[0]	'H'
[1]	'i'
[2]	'\0'

The C string is the only kind of C++ array for which there exists an aggregate constant—the string constant. Notice that in a C++ program, the symbols 'A' denote a single character, whereas the symbols "A" denote two: the character 'A' and the null character.*

In addition to C string constants, we can create C string *variables*. To do so, we explicitly declare a `char` array and store into it whatever characters we want to, finishing with the null character. Here's an example:

```
char myStr[8];     // Room for 7 significant characters plus '\0'

myStr[0] = 'H';
myStr[1] = 'i';
myStr[2] = '\0';
```

In C++, all C strings (constants or variables) are assumed to be null-terminated. This convention is agreed upon by all C++ programmers and standard library functions. The null character serves as a sentinel value; it allows algorithms to locate the end of the string. For example, here is a function that determines the length of any C string, not counting the terminating null character:

```
int StrLength( /* in */ const char str[] )

// Precondition:
//      str holds a null-terminated string
// Postcondition:
//      Function value == number of characters in str (excluding '\0')
```

---

*C *string* is not an official term used in C++ language manuals. Such manuals typically use the term *string*. However, we use C *string* to distinguish between the general concept of a string and the built-in array representation defined by the C and C++ languages.

```
{
    int i = 0;    // Index variable

    while (str[i] != '\0')
        i++;
    return i;
}
```

The value of `i` is the correct value for this function to return. If the array being examined is

then `i` equals 2 at loop exit. The string length is therefore 2.

The argument to the `StrLength` function can be a C string variable, as in the function call

```
cout << StrLength(myStr);
```

or it can be a string constant:

```
cout << StrLength("Hello");
```

In the first case, the base address of the `myStr` array is sent to the function, as we discussed in Chapter 12. In the second case, a base address is also sent to the function—the base address of the unnamed array that the compiler has set aside for the string constant.

There is one more thing we should say about our `StrLength` function. A C++ programmer would not actually write this function. The standard library supplies several string-processing functions, one of which is named `strlen` and does exactly what our `StrLength` function does. Later in the chapter, we look at `strlen` and other library functions.

Initializing C Strings

In Chapter 12, we showed how to initialize an array in its declaration by specifying a list of initial values within braces, like this:

```cpp
int delta[5] = {25, -3, 7, 13, 4};
```

To initialize a C string variable in its declaration, you could use the same technique:

```cpp
char message[8] = {'W', 'h', 'o', 'o', 'p', 's', '!', '\0'};
```

However, C++ allows a more convenient way to initialize a C string. You can simply initialize the array by using a string constant:

```cpp
char message[8] = "Whoops!";
```

This shorthand notation is unique to C strings because there is no other kind of array for which there are aggregate constants.

We said in Chapter 12 that you can omit the size of an array when you initialize it in its declaration (in which case, the compiler determines its size). This feature is often used with C strings because it keeps you from having to count the number of characters. For example,

```cpp
char promptMsg[] = "Enter a positive number:";   // Size is 25
char errMsg[] = "Value must be positive.";       // Size is 24
```

Be very careful about one thing: C++ treats initialization (in a declaration) and assignment (in an assignment statement) as two distinct operations. Different rules apply. Remember that array initialization is legal, but aggregate array assignment is not.

```cpp
char myStr[20] = "Hello";    // OK
    ⋮
myStr = "Howdy";             // Not allowed
```

C String Input and Output

In Chapter 12, we emphasized that C++ does not provide aggregate operations on arrays. There is no aggregate assignment, aggregate comparison, or aggregate arithmetic on arrays. We also said that aggregate input/output of arrays is not possible, with one exception. C strings are that exception. Let's look first at output.

To output the contents of an array that is *not* a C string, you aren't allowed to do this:

```cpp
int alpha[100];
    ⋮
cout << alpha;    // Not allowed
```

Instead, you must write a loop and print the array elements one at a time. However, aggregate output of a null-terminated `char` array (that is, a C string) is valid. The C string can be a constant (as we've been doing since Chapter 2):

```
cout << "Results are:";
```

or it can be a variable:

```
char msg[8] = "Welcome";
   ⋮
cout << msg;
```

In both cases, the insertion operator (`<<`) outputs each character in the array until the null character is found. It is up to you to double-check that the terminating null character is present in the array. If not, the `<<` operator will march through the array and into the rest of memory, printing out bytes until—just by chance—it encounters a byte whose integer value is 0.

To input C strings, we have several options. The first is to use the extraction operator (`>>`), which behaves exactly the same as with `string` class objects. When reading input characters into a C string variable, the `>>` operator skips leading whitespace characters and then reads successive characters into the array, stopping at the first trailing whitespace character (which is not consumed, but remains as the first character waiting in the input stream). The `>>` operator also takes care of adding the null character to the end of the string. For example, assume we have the following code:

```
char firstName[31];    // Room for 30 characters plus '\0'
char lastName[31];

cin >> firstName >> lastName;
```

If the input stream initially looks like this (where ⬚ denotes a blank):

⬚⬚John⬚Smith⬚⬚⬚25

then our input statement stores 'J', 'o', 'h', 'n', and '\0' into `firstName[0]` through `firstName[4]`; stores 'S', 'm', 'i', 't', 'h', and '\0' into `lastName[0]` through `lastName[5]`; and leaves the input stream as

⬚⬚⬚25

The `>>` operator, however, has two potential drawbacks.

1. If the array isn't large enough to hold the sequence of input characters (and the '\0'), the `>>` operator will continue to store characters into memory past the end of the array.
2. The `>>` operator cannot be used to input a string that has blanks within it. (It stops reading as soon as it encounters the first whitespace character.)

To cope with these limitations, we can use a variation of the `get` function, a member of the `istream` class. We have used the `get` function to input a single character, even if it is a whitespace character:

```
cin.get(inputChar);
```

The `get` function also can be used to input C strings, in which case the function call requires two arguments. The first is the array name and the second is an `int` expression.

```
cin.get(myStr, charCount + 1);
```

The `get` function does not skip leading whitespace characters and continues until it either has read `charCount` characters or it reaches the newline character '\n', whichever comes first. It then appends the null character to the end of the string. With the statements

```
char oneLine[81];    // Room for 80 characters plus '\0'
  ⋮
cin.get(oneLine, 81);
```

the `get` function reads and stores an entire input line (to a maximum of 80 characters), embedded blanks and all. If the line has fewer than 80 characters, reading stops at '\n' but does not consume it. The newline character is now the first one waiting in the input stream. To read two consecutive lines worth of strings, it is necessary to consume the newline character:

```
char dummy;
  ⋮
cin.get(string1, 81);
cin.get(dummy);          // Eat newline before next "get"
cin.get(string2, 81);
```

The first function call reads characters up to, but not including, the '\n'. If the input of `dummy` were omitted, then the input of `string2` would read *no* characters because '\n' would immediately be the first character waiting in the stream.

Finally, the `ignore` function—introduced in Chapter 4—can be useful in conjunction with the `get` function. Recall that the statement

```
cin.ignore(200, '\n');
```

says to skip at most 200 input characters but stop if a newline was read. (The newline character *is* consumed by this function.) If a program inputs a long string from the user but only wants to retain the first four characters of the response, here is a way to do it:

```
char response[5];        // Room for 4 characters plus '\0'

cin.get(response, 5);    // Input at most 4 characters
```

```
cin.ignore(100, '\n');    // Skip remaining chars up to and
                          //   including '\n'
```

The value 100 in the last statement is arbitrary. Any "large enough" number will do.

Here is a table that summarizes the differences between the >> operator and the `get` function when reading C strings:

Statement	Skips Leading Whitespace?	Stops Reading When?
cin >> inputStr;	Yes	At the first trailing whitespace character (which is *not* consumed)
cin.get(inputStr, 21);	No	When either 20 characters are read or '\n' is encountered (which is *not* consumed)

Finally, we revisit a topic that came up in Chapter 4. Certain library functions and member functions of system-supplied classes require C strings as arguments. An example is the `ifstream` class member function named `open`. To open a file, we pass the name of the file as a C string, either a constant or a variable:

```
ifstream file1;
ifstream file2;
char     fileName[51];              // Max. 50 characters plus '\0'

file1.open("students.dat");
cin.get(fileName, 51);             // Read at most 50 characters
cin.ignore(100, '\n');            // Skip rest of input line
file2.open(fileName);
```

As discussed in Chapter 4, if our file name is contained in a `string` class object, we still can use the `open` function, *provided* we use the `string` class member function named `c_str` to convert the string to a C string:

```
ifstream inFile;
string   fileName;

cin >> fileName;
inFile.open(fileName.c_str());
```

Comparing these two code segments, you can observe a major advantage of the `string` class over C strings: A string in a `string` class object has unbounded length, whereas the length of a C string is bounded by the array size, which is fixed at compile time.

C String Library Routines

Through the header file `cstring`, the C++ standard library provides a large assortment of C string operations. In this section, we discuss three of these library functions:

strlen, which returns the length of a string; strcmp, which compares two strings using the relations less-than, equal, and greater-than; and strcpy, which copies one string to another. Here is a summary of strlen, strcmp, and strcpy:

Header File	Function	Function Value	Effect
`<cstring>`	`strlen(str)`	Integer length of `str` (excluding '\0')	Computes length of `str`
`<cstring>`	`strcmp(str1, str2)`	An integer < 0, if `str1 < str2` The integer 0, if `str1 = str2` An integer > 0, if `str1 > str2`	Compares `str1` and `str2`
`<cstring>`	`strcpy(toStr, fromStr)`	Base address of `toStr` (usually ignored)	Copies `fromStr` (including '\0') to `toStr`, overwriting what was there; `toStr` must be large enough to hold the result

The strlen function is similar to the StrLength function we wrote earlier. It returns the number of characters in a C string prior to the terminating '\0'. Here's an example of a call to the function:

```
#include <cstring>
    :
char subject[] = "Computer Science";

cout << strlen(subject);    // Prints 16
```

The strcpy routine is important because aggregate assignment with the = operator is not allowed on C strings. In the following code fragment, we show the wrong way and the right way to perform a string copy.

```
#include <cstring>
    :
char myStr[100];
    :
myStr = "Abracadabra";          // No
strcpy(myStr, "Abracadabra");   // Yes
```

In strcpy's argument list, the destination string is the one on the left, just as an assignment operation transfers data from right to left. It is the caller's responsibility to make sure that the destination array is large enough to hold the result.

The strcpy function is technically a value-returning function; it not only copies one C string to another, but also returns as a function value the base address of the destination array. The reason why the caller would want to use this function value is not at all obvious, and we don't discuss it here. Programmers nearly always ignore the function value and simply invoke strcpy as if it were a void function (as we did above). You may wish to review the Background Information box in Chapter 8 entitled "Ignoring a Function Value."

The strcmp function is used for comparing two strings. The function receives two C strings as parameters and compares them in *lexicographic* order (the order in which they would appear in a dictionary)—the same ordering used in comparing string class objects. Given the function call strcmp(str1, str2), the function returns one of the following int values: a negative integer, if str1 < str2 lexicographically; the value 0, if str1 = str2; or a positive integer, if str1 > str2. The precise values of the negative integer and the positive integer are unspecified. You simply test to see if the result is less than 0, 0, or greater than 0. Here is an example:

```
if (strcmp(str1, str2) < 0)    // If str1 is less than str2 ...
    ⋮
```

We have described only three of the string-handling routines provided by the standard library. These three are the most commonly needed, but there are many more. If you are designing or maintaining programs that use C strings extensively, you should read the documentation on strings for your C++ system.

String Class or C Strings?

When working with string data, should you use a class like string, or should you use C strings? From the standpoints of clarity, versatility, and ease of use, there is no contest. Use a string class. The standard library string class provides strings of unbounded length, aggregate assignment, aggregate comparison, concatenation with the + operator, and so forth.

However, it is still useful to be familiar with C strings. Among the thousands of software products currently in use that are written in C and C++, most (but a declining percentage) use C strings to represent string data. In your next place of employment, if you are asked to modify or upgrade such software, understanding C strings is essential. Additionally, *using* a string class is one thing; *implementing* it is another. Someone must implement the class using a concrete data representation. In your employment, that someone might be you, and the underlying data representation might very well be a C string!

Problem-Solving Case Study

Calculating Exam Statistics Revisited

PROBLEM   You are the grader in your Government class. The teacher has asked you to prepare the following statistics. (*No, this isn't a misprint!* We are going to solve the same problem in an entirely different way.)

INPUT   A file whose name is input from the keyboard containing test grades.

OUTPUT   A file whose name is input from the keyboard showing the following statistics properly labeled.

> Number of grades
> Average grade
> Lowest grade
> Highest grade
> Number of grades above the average
> Number of grades below the average

DISCUSSION   We have just designed and implemented the ADT List. Let's think of this problem in terms of a list of grades. There are the same three separate tasks to be done in this problem, but let's look at them in terms of list operations.   We need to average the values in the list, find the maximum and minimum values in the list, and go through the list counting those values above the average and those values below the average. To find the average, we sum the list of grades and divide by the number of grades. We found the minimum and maximum values in a list of numbers in the Design Studio program.   The third task involves looking at each grade, comparing it to the average, and incrementing one of two counters.

If all we had to do was find the average and the minimum and maximum grades, we could do the processing at the same time that we read the data values.   However, the task of printing the number of grades above and below the average requires that each grade be examined more than once because we don't have the average until all the values have been read.   Therefore, we must create a list of the grades so that we can access each one more than once.

We have to examine each grade twice: once to calculate the average, find the minimum value, and find the maximum value and once to compare each grade to the average.   We could do all the processing except for the number above and below the average as we initially read the grades. However, it is better style to separate the tasks into separate functions.

DATA STRUCTURES

> Simple variables
> A list of integer values

Main	Level 0

> Open files
> Input grades
> Calculate average
> Calculate highest
> Calculate lowest
> Calculate above average
> Calculate below average
> Close files

We use the same open files function we have used in the last program. However, the heading that is printed on the output needs to be changed.

Input Grades	Level 1

This function must have the file name and the list. The program needs to know the number of grades, but unlike the previous implementation, the list has a function that returns the number of items in the list.

(Inout: inData, grades)

> Read grade from inData
> WHILE inData && !grades.IsFull()
>   grades.Insert(grade);
>   Read grade from inData

Calculate Average(In: grades, numGrades)
   Out: Function value

> Set sum to 0
> Set limit to grades.Length();
> grades.Reset();
> FOR index going from 0 to limit
>   Set grade to grades.GetNextItem();
>   Set sum to sum + grade;
> Return float(sum) / float(limit);

Calculate Highest(In: grades)
Out: Function value

```
Set limit to grades.Length();
grades.Reset();
Set maxGrade to 0;
FOR index going from 0 to limit
    Set grade to grades.GetNextItem();
    IF grade > maxGrade
        Set maxGrade to grade;
Return maxGrade;
```

Calculate Lowest(In: grades)
Out: Function value

```
Set limit to grades.Length()
grades.Reset()
Set minGrade to 100
FOR index going from 0 to limit
    Set grade to grades.GetNextItem()
    IF grade < minGrade
        Set minGrade to grade;
Return minGrade;
```

Calculate Above Average(In: grades, average)
Out: Function value

```
Set roundedAverage to (int) (average+0.5)
Set limit to grades.Length()
Set number to 0
grades.Reset()
FOR index going 0 to limit
    Set grade to grades.GetNextItem()
    IF grade > roundedAverage
        Increment number
Return number
```

Calculate Below Average(In: grades, average)
Out: Function value

Set truncatedAverage to (int) (average)
Set limit to grades.Length()
Set number to 0
grades.Reset()
FOR index going 0 to limit
    Set grade to grades.GetNextItem()
    IF grade < truncatedAverage
       Increment number
Return number

Print Results(Inout: outData; In: grades, average, highest,
lowest, numberAbove, numberBelow)

Print on outdata "The number of grades is " grades.Length()
Print on outData "The average grade is " average
Print on outData "The highest grade is " highest
Print on outData "The lowest grade is " lowest
Print on outData "The number of grades above the average is "
    aboveAverage
Print on outData "The number of grades below the average is "
    belowAverage

The main module is identical to the main module in the other implementation. The changes are hidden within the functions that manipulate the structure that holds the data. The first implementation used an array of counters, one slot for each possible test score. The processing involved manipulating the array. The second implementation used a list of grades. The processing involved manipulating the values in the List ADT.

Even the Module Structure Charts are almost identical. Only the parameter list of the `InputGrades` and `PrintResults` functions need altering to remove `numGrades`.

MODULE STRUCTURE CHART

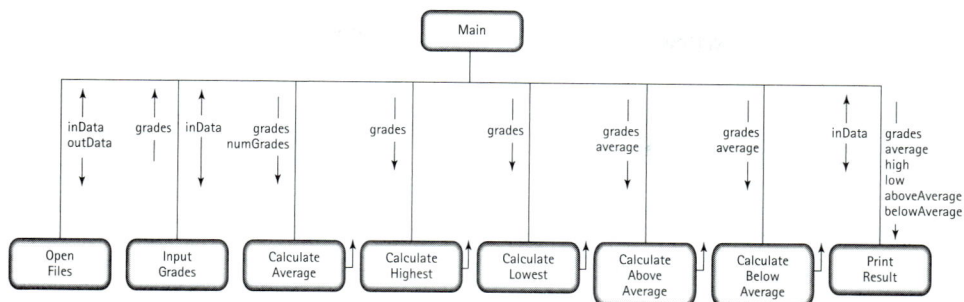

```
//*********************************************************************
// Statistics Program
// This program calculates the average, high score, low score,
// number above the average, and number below the average for
// a file of test scores.  The List ADT is used
// Assumption:  File "testScores" is not empty and does not contain
// more than MAX_GRADES values.
// To save space, we omit from each function the precondition
// comments that document the assumptions made about valid input
// parameter data. These would be included in a program intended
// for actual use.
//*********************************************************************

#include <fstream>
#include <iostream>
#include <iomanip>
#include "list.h"

using namespace std;

// Function Prototypes

void OpenFiles(ifstream& inData, ofstream& outData);
void InputGrades(List& grades, ifstream& inData);
float CalculateAverage(List grades);
int CalculateHighest(List grades);
int CalculateLowest(List grades);
int CalculateAboveAverage(List grades, float average);
int CalculateBelowAverage(List grades, float average);
void PrintResults(ofstream& outData, List grades, float average,
    int highest, int lowest, int aboveAverage, int belowAverage);
```

```cpp
int main()
{
    List grades;            // A list of grades

    float average;          // Average grade
    int highest;            // Highest grade
    int lowest;             // Lowest grade
    int aboveAverage;       // Number of grades above the average
    int belowAverage;       // Number of grades below the average

    // Declare and open files
    ifstream inData;
    ofstream outData;
    OpenFiles(inData, outData);

    // Process grades
    InputGrades(grades, inData);
    average = CalculateAverage(grades);
    highest = CalculateHighest(grades);
    lowest = CalculateLowest(grades);
    aboveAverage = CalculateAboveAverage(grades, average);
    belowAverage = CalculateBelowAverage(grades, average);
    PrintResults(outData,grades, average, highest, lowest,
        aboveAverage, belowAverage);

    inData.close();
    outData.close();
    return 0;
}


//*******************************************************************

void OpenFiles( /* inout */ ifstream& text,
                /* inout */ ofstream& outFile )

// Function OpenFiles reads in the names of the input file and
// the output file and opens them for processing
// Postcondition:
//     Files have been opened AND a label has been written on the
//     output file
if ( !inData || !outData )
{
    cout << "Files did not open successfully." << endl;
    return 1;
}
```

```cpp
{
    string inFileName;
    string outDataName;

    cout << "Enter the name of the file to be processed" << endl;
    cin >> inFileName;
    text.open(inFileName.c_str());

    cout << "Enter the name of the output file" << endl;
    cin >> outDataName;
    outFile.open(outDataName.c_str());

    //  Write label on output
    outFile << "Grade statistics using the List ADT" << endl
            << endl;
}

//********************************************************************

void InputGrades( /* inout */ List& grades,        // Grade list
                  /* inout */ ifstream& inData )  // Input file

// Grades are input from file inData and inserted into grades.
// Precondition:
//      File is not empty
// Postcondition:
//      Each grade in the file has been inserted into list of grades

{
    int grade;
    // Read grades and put them into the list
    inData >> grade;
    while (inData && !grades.IsFull())
    {
        grades.Insert(grade);
        inData >> grade;
    }
}

//********************************************************************

float CalculateAverage( /* in */ List grades )

// This function calculates the average test score
// Postcondition:
//      Return value is the average grade
```

```
    {
        int sum = 0;
        int limit = grades.Length();        // limit is the number of
                                             // grades

        int grade;

        grades.Reset();                      // Prepare for traversal

        // Add each grade to sum
        for (int index = 0; index < limit; index++)
        {
            grade = grades.GetNextItem();
            sum = sum + grade;
        }

        return float(sum) / float(limit); // Return average
    }

    //****************************************************************************

    int CalculateHighest( /* in */ List grades ) // List of grades

    // This function calculates the highest grade in the list of
    // grades
    // Postcondition:
    //     Return value is the highest grade

    {
        int limit = grades.Length();        // Number of grades
        int grade;

        grades.Reset();                      // Prepare for iteration
        int maxGrade = 0;

        // Find the maximum grade in the list
        for (int index = 0; index < limit; index++)
        {
            grade = grades.GetNextItem();
            if (grade > maxGrade)
                maxGrade = grade;
        }
        return maxGrade;
    }

    //****************************************************************************

    int CalculateLowest( /* in */ List grades ) // List of grades
```

```
// This function calculates the lowest grade in the list of
// grades
// Postcondition:
//      Return value is the lowest grade

{
    int limit = grades.Length();          // Number of grades
    int grade;

    grades.Reset();                        // Prepare for iteration
    int minGrade = 100;

    // Find the miminum grade in the list
    for (int index = 0; index < limit; index++)
    {
        grade = grades.GetNextItem();
        if (grade < minGrade)
            minGrade = grade;
    }
    return minGrade;
}


//**********************************************************************


int CalculateAboveAverage
    ( /* in */ List grades,          // List of grades
      /* inout */  float average ) // Average grade

// This function calculates the number of grades above the
// average
// Postcondition:
//      Return value is the number of grades above average

{
    int roundedAverage = (int) (average + 0.5);
    int limit = grades.Length();       // Number of grades
    int grade;
    int number = 0;

    grades.Reset();                        // Prepare for iteration

    // Calculate the number of grades above the average
    for (int index = 0; index < limit; index++)
    {
        grade = grades.GetNextItem();
        if (grade > roundedAverage)
```

```
                        number++;
        }
        return number;
}

//******************************************************************

int CalculateBelowAverage
    ( /* in */ List grades,          // List of grades
      /* inout */  float average )   // Average grade

// This function calculates the number of grades below the
// average
// Postcondition:
//     Return value is the number of grades below average

{
    int truncatedAverage = (int) (average);
    int limit = grades.Length();      // Number of grades
    int grade;
    int number = 0;

    grades.Reset();                   // Prepare for iteration

    // Calculate the number of grades below the average
    for (int index = 0; index < limit; index++)
    {
        grade = grades.GetNextItem();
        if (grade < truncatedAverage)
            number++;
    }
    return number;
}

//******************************************************************

void PrintResults( /* inout */ ofstream& outData, // Output file
                   /* in */     List grades,       // Grade list
                   /* in */     float average,     // Average
                   /* in */     int highest,       // Max grade
                   /* in */     int lowest,        // Min grade
                   /* in */     int aboveAverage,  // Number above
                   /* in */     int belowAverage ) // Number below

// Statistics are printed on file outData
// Precondition:
```

```
//      Output file has been successfully opened
// Postcondition:
//      Statistics have been written on outData, appropriately
//      labeled

{
    outData << "The number of grades is " << grades.Length()
            << endl;
    outData << fixed << setprecision(2) << "The average grade is "
            << average << endl;
    outData << "The highest grade is " << highest << endl;
    outData << "The lowest grade is " << lowest << endl;
    outData << "The number of grades above the average is "
            << aboveAverage  << endl;
    outData << "The number of grades below the average is "
            << belowAverage << endl;
}
```

TESTING   This implementation is based on a list of values. We must test for cases in which there are no grades, one grade, a few grades, and exactly the maximum number of grades. We took care of the case in which there are more grades to be stored than there are slots in the list by checking `IsFull` in function `InputGrades`. Here is a run with a few grades—the same ones we used with the last implementation. It is comforting to see that the answers are the same.

```
testScores.out - Notepad
File  Edit  Format  View  Help
Grade statistics using the List ADT

The number of grades is 18
The average grade is 71.22
The highest grade is 100
The lowest grade is 0
The number of grades above the average is 12
The number of grades below the average is 6
```

Which algorithm is more efficient? We can't answer that question because it depends on the range of possible grades and the size of the data sets. The amount of work done in the first solution is based on the range of grades. The loops go from 0 to 100 (or somewhere in between). The amount of work done in the second solution is based on the number of grades. The loops go from 0 to the number of grades. The choice of algorithm thus depends on the context in which it will be used.

Testing and Debugging

In this chapter, we have discussed, designed, and coded algorithms to construct and manipulate items in a list. In addition to the basic list operations `IsFull`, `IsEmpty`, `Length`, and an iterator pair, the algorithms included three sequential searches, a binary search, insertion into sorted and unsorted lists, deletion from sorted and unsorted lists, and a selection sort. We have already partially tested `List::Insert`, `List::Delete`, `List::Reset`, and `List::GetNextItem` in conjunction with the case study. The other searching algorithms and the functions `SortedList::Insert`, `SortedList::Delete`, and `SortedList::SelSort` need to be tested. We should test them with lists containing no components, one component, two components, MAX_LENGTH – 1 components, and MAX_LENGTH components.

When we wrote the precondition that the list was not full for operation `List::Insert`, we indicated that we could handle the problem another way—we could include an error flag in the function's parameter list. The function would call `IsFull` and set the error flag. The insertion would not take place if the error flag were set to `true`. Both options are acceptable ways of handling the problem. The important point is that we clearly state whether the calling code or the called function is to check for the error condition. However, it is the calling code that must decide what to do when an error condition occurs. In other words, if errors are handled by means of preconditions, then the user must write the code to guarantee the preconditions. If errors are handled by flags, then the user must write the code to monitor the error flags.

Testing and Debugging Hints

1. Review the Testing and Debugging Hints for Chapter 12. They apply to all one-dimensional arrays, including C strings.

2. Make sure that every C string is terminated with the null character. String constants are automatically null-terminated by the compiler. On input, the `>>` operator and the `get` function automatically add the null character. If you store characters into a C string individually or manipulate the array in any way, be sure to account for the null character.

3. Remember that C++ treats C string initialization (in a declaration) as different from C string assignment. Initialization is allowed, but assignment is not.

4. Aggregate input/output is allowed for C strings but not for other array types.

5. If you use the `>>` operator to input into a C string variable, be sure the array is large enough to hold the null character plus the longest sequence of (nonwhitespace) characters in the input stream.

6. With C string input, the `>>` operator stops at, *but does not consume,* the first trailing whitespace character. Likewise, if the `get` function stops reading early because it encounters a newline character, the newline character is not consumed.

7. When you use the `strcpy` library function, ensure that the destination array is at least as large as the array from which you are copying.

8. General-purpose functions (such as ADT operations) should be tested outside the context of a particular program, using a test driver.

9. Choose test data carefully so that you test all end conditions and some in the middle. End conditions are those that reach the limits of the structure used to store them. For example, in a list, there should be test data in which the number of components is 0, 1, and MAX_LENGTH, as well as between 1 and MAX_LENGTH.

Summary

This chapter has provided practice in working with lists stored in one-dimensional arrays. We have examined algorithms that insert, delete, search, and sort data stored in a list, and we have written functions to implement these algorithms. We can use these functions again and again in different contexts because they are members of general-purpose C++ classes (List and SortedList) that represent list ADTs.

C strings are a special case of char arrays in C++. The last significant character must be followed by a null character to mark the end of the string. C strings are less versatile than a string class. However, it pays to understand how they work because many existing programs in C and C++ use them, and string classes often use C strings as the underlying data representation.

Quick Check

1. What are the three main properties of a list? (pp. 662–669)
2. Where do we insert a new value into a list that isn't sorted? (pp. 669–673)
3. If an item isn't in the list, when does the linear search discover that it is missing? (pp. 673–678)
4. How does a sorted list ADT differ from a list ADT that includes a sort operation? (pp. 681–686)
5. With an insertion sort, what happens to the components that precede the insertion point, and the components that follow it? (pp. 684–686)
6. Where does the binary search algorithm get its name? (pp. 687–693)
7. What two members of a list class are used to represent the data in a list? (pp. 662–663)
8. What are the major steps in deleting a value from a list? (pp. 693–694)
9. What operations in a sorted list are different from the operations in an unsorted list, and how do they differ? (pp. 681–683)
10. How many For loops are there in an implementation of an selection sort? (pp. 678–681)
11. What condition ends a binary search? (pp. 687–688)

Answers

1. It is variable length, linear, and homogenous.   2. At end of the list (assuming the list isn't already full).   3. When it has examined the last element in the list.   4. The components of a sorted list are always kept in order, but the components of a regular list are only sorted after the sort operation executes, until the next insertion or deletion.   5. The components that precede the insertion point remain where they are, and the ones following the insertion point shift over one place to make room.   6. The name comes from its pattern of dividing the area of the search by two on each iteration.   7. A data array containing the specified item type in each component, and a length represented by an `int`.   8. Search for the value, delete the value, shift any succeeding values up one place.   9. There is no sort operation in the sorted list. The insert operation inserts a new value in its proper place rather than at the end of the list. The delete operation shifts the succeeding components up one place, rather than moving the last component into the vacated position. Searching in the sorted list can be done with a binary search rather than a linear search.   10. Two.   11. Either the value is found, or the first and last indexes of the search area are the same and the value has not been found.

Exam Preparation Exercises

1. Why do we say that a list is linear?
2. What do we mean when we say that a list is homogeneous?
3. If the `Length` operation associated with an *unsorted* list returns 43, and we then call the Delete operation for the list, passing it a value that matches the 21st item in the list:
   a. What is the index of the component that is deleted?
   b. What is the index of the component that takes its place?
   c. What does the `Length` operation return after the deletion?
   d. How many components in the list change their position as a result of the deletion?
4. If `ItemType` is `float`, how do we need to change the following While loop condition, as written in the sequential search, and why do we need to change it?

   ```
   while (index < length && item != data[index])
   ```

5. The following statements are supposed to swap two values in an array, but they are in the wrong order. Rearrange them into the proper order.

   ```
   data[value2] = temp;
   data[value1] = data[value2];
   temp = data[value1];
   ```

6. In a selection sort, what is accomplished by the inner loop each time it executes?
7. If the `Length` operation associated with a *sorted* list returns 43, and we then call the Delete operation for the list, passing it a value that matches the 21st item in the list:
   a. What is the index of the component that is deleted?
   b. What is the index of the component that takes its place?

   c. What does the `Length` operation return after the deletion?

   d. How many components in the list change their position as a result of the deletion?

8. On average, a sequential search of a sorted list takes the same number of iterations as searching an unsorted list. True or false?

9. We should use a binary search for large sorted lists, but a sequential search is more efficient when a list has few components. True or false?

10. What is the log (base 2) of 32?

11. Why don't we need a separate sorting operation in a sorted-list ADT?

12. A sorted list contains 16 elements, and the binary search operation is called with a value that matches the 12th value in the list. How many iterations does it take for the binary search to find this match?

13. What are the characters stored in the following C string?

```
char exam[4] = "Hop";
```

Programming Warm-Up Exercises

1. Write a C++ Boolean function named `Deleted` that has three parameters: `someItem` (of type `ItemType` as used in this chapter), `oldList`, and `newList` (both of type `List` as defined in this chapter). The function returns `true` if `someItem` is found in `oldList`, but is not present in `newList`.

2. The `List` type in this chapter allows us to store multiple copies of an item in the list. Sometimes it is useful to have a list in which any given item can appear just once. Change the implementation of the `Insert` function so that it only adds an item to the list if the item is not already there.

3. What is wrong with the following code segment, and what must be changed in type `List` to make it work correctly?

```
List inVals;
for (int count = 1; count <= 100; count++)
{
    cin >> inVal;
    inVals.Insert(inVal);
}
```

4. We would like to add a `DeleteAll` function to the `List` type that deletes all occurrences of an item from a list. Write the code that must be added to the specification file for the type to enable us to add this function.

5. Write the implementation of the `DeleteAll` function as described in Exercise 4.

6. We would like to add a `Replace` function to the `List` type that takes two parameters, `oldItem` and `newItem` of `ItemType`. The function finds `oldItem` in the list, deletes it, and inserts `newItem` in its place. The list is unchanged if `oldItem` is not present in the list. Write the code that must be added to the specification file for the type to enable us to add this function.

7. Write the implementation of the `Replace` function as described in Exercise 6.

8. The `SortedList` type keeps items in ascending order. Which function(s) would need to be changed to make the list keep the items in descending order?

9. Change the implementation of the `BinSearch` function so that it will work with a list that keeps items in descending order.

10. In Exercise 5 you wrote a `DeleteAll` function for the `List` type. Implement a `DeleteAll` function for the `SortedList` type, taking advantage of the fact that all occurrences of the item are stored in adjacent locations in the array. Note that the binary search does not necessarily return the position of the first occurrence of an item; it can return the position of any matching item. Thus, in this case, it may be more efficient to use a linear search to find the start of the matching items. Be sure that your function updates the length of the list as necessary.

11. In Exercise 7 you wrote a `Replace` function for the `List` type that deletes one value and replaces it with another. Reimplement the `Replace` function for the `SortedList` type. Note that in this case, the replacement value needs to be inserted in the proper position in the list to maintain the ordering of the items.

12. Write a code segment that fills a `SortedList` called `inData` with values that are input from a file called `unsorted`.

13. We wish to add a `FilePrint` function to the `SortedList` type. Like the `Print` operation, it outputs the contents of the list in order, but `FilePrint` takes a parameter called `outFile` of type `ofstream`, and writes the values to that file. Write the implementation of this function in the `SortedList` type.

Programming Problems

1. Write a program using the `List` class from this chapter that implements a To-Do list. The items in the list will be strings. The user should be prompted to enter a command (add an item, mark an item as done or partially done, delete an item, and print the list) and data as necessary. Simply storing items in the list is easy, but the List class doesn't directly support the recording of the status of each task. There are different ways that you might want to go about this. One would be to implement a struct or a class that represents an item and its status, and modify the `List` class to work with this struct or class as its item type. Another way would be to keep three lists: Done, Partial, and Undone. When an item is created, it enters the Undone list. When its status is changed, it moves to one of the other lists as appropriate. Choose the approach that you prefer, and implement the application using proper style, effective prompts, and sufficient documentation.

2. Many instructors like to see the distribution of scores on an exam before they assign grades. You're working for an art history professor who has asked you to develop a program that will read all of the scores from an exam and print out a bar chart that shows the distribution. The range of the scores varies from exam to exam, and there are at most 250 students in the class. Use or modify the `SortedList` class from this chapter as necessary to help you do this task. The

integer scores are entered into a file called `exams.dat` in random order. Your program's job is to read in the data, sort it, and output a bar chart with one * for each exam that has a particular score. The first bar in the chart should be the highest score, and the last bar in the chart should be the lowest score. Each line of output should start with the score value, followed by the appropriate number of stars. When there is a score value that didn't appear on any exams, just output the value and no stars, then go to the next line.

3. Enhance the program in Problem 2 as follows: The data file now contains a score and a name. Modify the `SortedList` class so that it uses a struct consisting of the score and the name as its fields. The program should input the file data into the modified list. In addition to displaying the bar chart, the program will also output the sorted list to a file called `byscore.dat`.

4. You've gathered lists of e-mail addresses from a variety of sources, and you want to send out a mass mailing to all of the addresses. However, you don't want to send out duplicate messages. All of the e-mail addresses (represented as strings) have been combined on a single file called `rawlist.dat`. You need to write a program that reads them all and discards any that already have been input. Use one of the list classes from this chapter, modifying it as necessary to work with string data, and to deal with up to 1000 items. After all of the data have been read, output the new mailing list to a file called `cleanlist.dat`.

5. You're working for the state vehicle registry, and it just has been discovered that the people who make the license plates have been mistakenly producing occasional duplicates. You have a file (`platesmade.dat`) containing a list of plate numbers, which are recorded as they are made. You need to write a program that reads this file and identifies any duplicates in the list so that notices can be sent out to recall them. The plate numbers, which consists of letters and numbers, should be stored as strings. Output the duplicates into a file called `recallplates.dat`. Use the `SortedList` class from this chapter to help you in writing this application, modifying it if necessary.

Case Study Follow-Up

1. Which of the two implementations of the statistics program (Chapter 12 or Chapter 13) do you think is more clear?
2. Revise the list solution to combine `CalculateAverage`, `CalculateHighest`, and `CalculateLowest` into one function `Calculate`.
3. Revise the list solution from Exercise 2 so that `CalculateAboveAverage` and `CalculateBelowAverage` are combined into one function `AboveBelow`.
4. Is it better to have the functions combined or left separate?

Object-Oriented Software Development

Knowledge Goals

- *To know the distinction between structured (procedural) programming and object-oriented programming.*
- *To know the characteristics of an object-oriented language.*
- *To understand the difference between static and dynamic binding of operations to objects.*

Skill Goals

To be able to:

- *Create a new C++ class from an existing class by using inheritance.*
- *Create a new C++ class from an existing class by using composition.*
- *Apply the object-oriented design methodology to solve a problem.*
- *Take an object-oriented design and code it in C++.*

In Chapter 11, we introduced the concept of data abstraction—the separation of the logical properties of a data type from the details of how it is implemented. We expanded on this concept by defining the notion of an abstract data type (ADT) and by using the C++ class mechanism to incorporate both data and operations into a single data type. In that chapter and Chapter 13, we saw how an object of a given class maintains its own private data and is manipulated by calling its public member functions.

In this chapter, we examine how classes and objects can be used to guide the entire software development process. Although the design phase precedes the implementation phase in the development of software, we reverse the order of presentation in this chapter. We begin with *object-oriented programming,* a topic that includes design but is more about implementation issues. We describe the basic principles, terminology, and programming language features associated with the object-oriented approach. After presenting these fundamental concepts, we look more closely at the design phase—*object-oriented design.*

14.1 Object-Oriented Programming

Until now, we have used functional decomposition (also called *structured design*), in which we decompose a problem into modules, where each module is a self-contained collection of steps that solves one part of the overall problem. The process of implementing a functional decomposition is often called **structured** (or **procedural**) **programming**. Some modules are translated directly into a few programming language instructions, whereas others are coded as functions with or without arguments. The end result is a program that is a collection of interacting functions (see Figure 14–1). Throughout structured design and structured programming, data is considered a passive quantity to be acted upon by control structures and functions.

> **Structured (procedural) programming** The construction of programs that are collections of interacting functions or procedures.

Structured design is satisfactory for programming in the small (a concept we discussed in Chapter 4) but often does not "scale up" well for programming in the large. In building large software systems, structured design has two important limitations. First, the technique yields an inflexible structure. If the top-level algorithm requires modification, the changes may force many lower-level algorithms to be modified as well. Second, the technique does not lend itself easily to code reuse. By *code reuse* we mean the ability to use pieces of code—either as they are or adapted slightly—in other sections of the program or in other programs. It is rare to be able to take a complicated C++ function and reuse it easily in a different context.

A methodology that often works better for creating large software systems is object-oriented design (OOD), which we introduced briefly in Chapter 4. OOD decomposes a problem into objects—self-contained entities composed of data and operations on the data. The process of implementing an object-oriented design is called **object-oriented programming (OOP)**. The end result is a program that is a collection of interacting objects (see Figure 14–2). In OOD

> **Object-oriented programming (OOP)** The use of data abstraction, inheritance, and dynamic binding to construct programs that are collections of interacting objects.

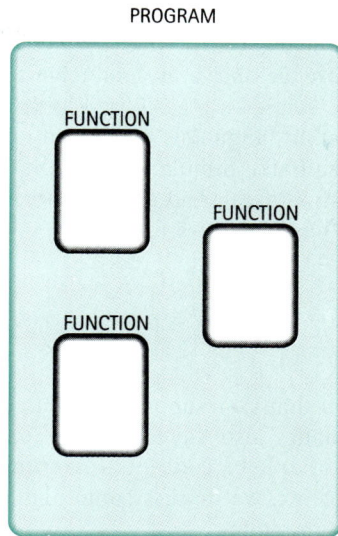

Figure 14–1   *Program Resulting from Structured (Procedural) Programming*

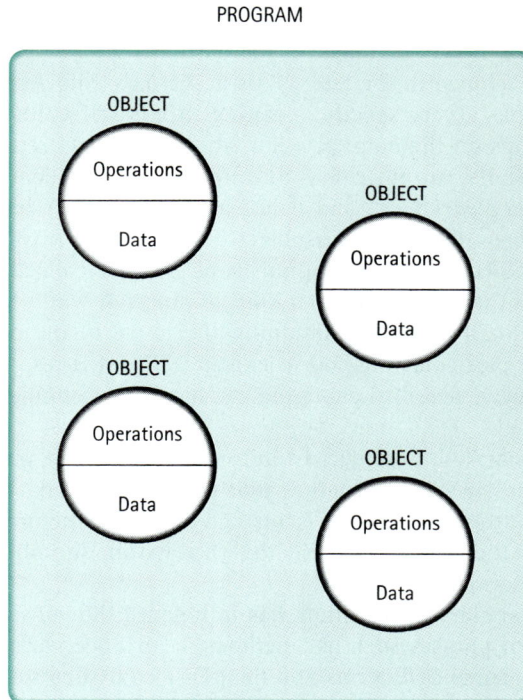

Figure 14–2   *Program Resulting from Object-Oriented Programming*

and OOP, data plays a leading role; the primary contribution of algorithms is to implement the operations on objects. In this chapter, we'll see why OOD tends to result in programs that are more flexible and conducive to code reuse than programs produced by structured design.

Several programming languages have been created specifically to support OOD and OOP: C++, Java, Smalltalk, Simula, CLOS, Objective-C, Eiffel, Actor, Object-Pascal, recent versions of Turbo Pascal, and others. These languages, called *object-oriented programming languages*, have facilities for

1. Data abstraction
2. Inheritance
3. Dynamic binding

You have already seen that C++ supports data abstraction through the class mechanism. Some non-OOP languages also have facilities for data abstraction. But only OOP languages support the other two concepts—*inheritance* and *dynamic binding.* Before we define these two concepts, we discuss some of the fundamental ideas and terminology of object-oriented programming.

14.2 Objects

The major principles of OOP originated as far back as the mid–1960s with a language called Simula. However, much of the current terminology of OOP is due to Smalltalk, a language developed in the late 1970s at Xerox's Palo Alto Research Center. In OOP, the term *object* has a very specific meaning: It is a self-contained entity encapsulating data and operations on the data. In other words, an object represents an instance of an ADT. More specifically, an object has an internal *state* (the current values of its private data, called *instance variables*), and it has a set of *methods* (public operations). Methods are the only means by which an object's state can be inspected or modified by another object. An object-oriented program consists of a collection of objects, communicating with one another by *message passing.* If object A wants object B to perform some task, object A sends a message containing the name of the object (B, in this case) and the name of the particular method to execute. Object B responds by executing this method in its own way, possibly changing its state and sending messages to other objects as well.

As you can tell, an object is quite different from a traditional data structure. A C++ struct is a passive data structure that contains only data and is acted upon by a program. In contrast, an object is an active data structure; the data and the code that manipulates the data are bound together within the object. In OOP jargon, an object knows how to manipulate itself.

The vocabulary of Smalltalk has influenced the vocabulary of OOP. The literature of OOP is full of phrases such as "methods," "instance variables," and "sending a message to." Here are some OOP terms and their C++ equivalents:

OOP	C++
Object	Class object or class instance
Instance variable	Private data member
Method	Public member function
Message passing	Function call (to a public member function)

Let's review the `Time` class that we defined in Chapter 11 to represent the ADT Time, and change it slightly to reflect object-oriented terminology and principles. There were seven operations (called responsibilities in object-oriented terminology): `Set`, `Increment`, `Write`, `Equal`, `LessThan`, and two constructors, one that takes hours, minutes, and seconds as parameters, and one that sets the time to zero.

In object-oriented terminology, there are two types of responsibilities (operations): action responsibilities and knowledge responsibilities. All of `Time`'s are actions: They do or calculate something. However, an object needs to be able to report on its own status; that is, each object should have a function that reports the internal state of each appropriate private data variable. Such functions could replace the `Write` function or supplement it. If the client code can *inspect* the internal state (not *change* it), the code can print the time in a form that is relevant to the problem using the ADT. In this case, let's add these functions rather than replace `Write`. Operations that return the state of an internal variable are knowledge responsibilities.

Let's make another change in the `Time` class. Let's add a function to prompt for and read the values from the standard input device. Here then are the revised specification and implementation files for class `Time`. We omit the documentation that hasn't changed.

```
//****************************************************************
// SPECIFICATION FILE (Time.h)
// This file gives the specification of a Time ADT with
// action responsibilities and knowledge responsibilities
//****************************************************************

class Time
{
public:
    // Action responsibilities

    void Set( /* in */ int hours,
              /* in */ int minutes,
              /* in */ int seconds );
```

```cpp
    void Increment();

    void Write() const;

    bool Equal( /* in */ Time otherTime ) const;

    bool LessThan( /* in */ Time otherTime ) const;

    Time( /* in */ int initHrs,
          /* in */ int initMins,
          /* in */ int initSecs );

    Time();

    void ReadTime();

        // Postcondition:
        //     hours, minutes, and seconds have been prompted for,
        //     read, and set

    // Knowledge responsibilities

    int Hours() const;

        // Postcondition:
        //     Return value is time

    int Minutes() const;

        // Postcondition:
        //     Return value is minutes

    int Seconds() const;

        // Postcondition:
        //     Return value is seconds


private:
    int hrs;
    int mins;
    int secs;
};
```

Here is the part of the implementation file for class `Time` that implements the changed functions.

```cpp
//******************************************************************
// IMPLEMENTATION FILE (Time.cpp)
// This file implements the Time member functions
//******************************************************************

#include "Time.h"
#include <iostream>

using namespace std;
    :

//******************************************************************

int Time::Hours() const

// Postcondition:
//     Return value is hrs

{
    return hrs;
}

//******************************************************************

int Time::Minutes() const

// Postcondition:
//     Return value is mins

{
    return mins;
}

//******************************************************************

int Time::Seconds() const

// Postcondition:
//     Return value is seconds

{
    return secs;
}
```

```
//**************************************************************

void Time::ReadTime()

// Postcondition:
//       hours, minutes, and seconds have been prompted for, read,
//       and stored into hrs, mins, and secs

{
    cout << "Enter hours (<= 23): " << endl;
    cin >> hrs;
    cout << "Enter minutes (<= 59): " << endl;
    cin >> mins;
    cout << "Enter seconds (<= 59): " << endl;
    cin >>  secs;
}

//**************************************************************
```

After this exercise we need to add three new object-oriented vocabulary items.

OOP	C++
Responsibility	An operation implemented as a function
Action responsibility	An operation that performs an action
Knowledge responsibility	An operation that returns the state of a private data variable

In C++, we define the properties and behavior of objects by using the class mechanism. Within a program, classes can be related to each other in various ways. The three most common relationships are as follows:

1. Two classes are independent of each other and have nothing in common.
2. Two classes are related by *inheritance.*
3. Two classes are related by *composition.*

The first relationship—none—is not very interesting. Let's look at the other two—inheritance and composition.

14.3 Inheritance

In the world at large, it is often possible to arrange concepts into an *inheritance hierarchy*—a hierarchy in which each concept inherits the properties of the concept immediately above it in the hierarchy. For example, we might classify different kinds of vehicles according to the inheritance hierarchy in Figure 14–3. Moving down the hierarchy, each kind of vehicle is more specialized than its *parent* (and all of its *ancestors*) and is more general than its *child* (and all of its *descendants*). A wheeled vehicle inherits properties common to all vehicles (it holds one or more people and carries them from place to place) but has an additional property that makes it more specialized (it has wheels). A car inherits properties common to all wheeled vehicles but also has additional, more specialized properties (four wheels, an engine, a body, and so forth).

The inheritance relationship can be viewed as an *is-a relationship*. Every two-door car is a car, every car is a wheeled vehicle, and every wheeled vehicle is a vehicle.

OOP languages provide a way of creating inheritance relationships among classes. In these languages, **inheritance** is the mechanism by which one class acquires the properties of another class. You can take an existing class A (called the **base class** or **superclass**) and create from it a new class B (called the **derived class** or **subclass**). The derived class B inherits all the properties of its base class A. In particular, the data and operations defined for A are now also defined for B. (Notice the is-a relationship—every B is also an A.) The idea, next, is to specialize class B, usually by adding specific properties to those already inherited from A. Let's look at an example in C++.

> **Inheritance** A mechanism by which one class acquires the properties—the data and operations—of another class.
>
> **Base class (superclass)** The class being inherited from.
>
> **Derived class (subclass)** The class that inherits.

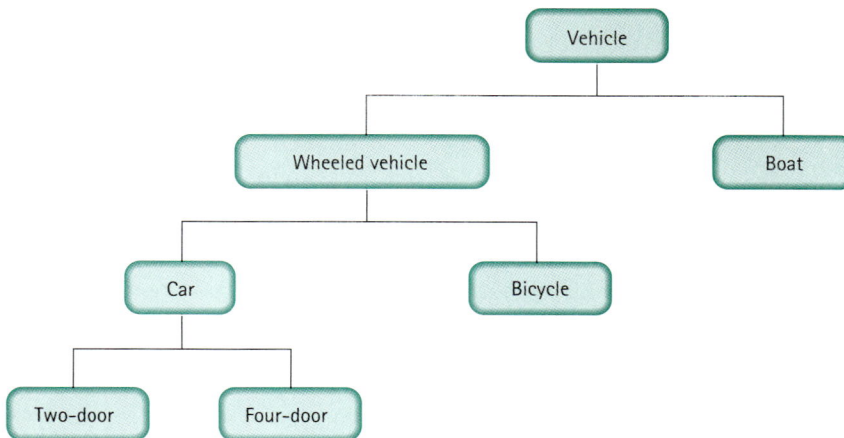

Figure 14–3 *Inheritance Hierarchy*

Deriving One Class from Another

Suppose that we want to modify the Time class in the last section by adding, as private data, a variable of an enumeration type indicating the (American) time zone—EST for Eastern Standard Time, CST for Central Standard Time, MST for Mountain Standard Time, PST for Pacific Standard Time, EDT for Eastern Daylight Time, CDT for Central Daylight Time, MDT for Mountain Daylight Time, or PDT for Pacific Daylight Time. We'll need to modify the Set function and the class constructors to accommodate a time zone value. And the Write function should print the time in the form

```
12:34:10 CST
```

The Increment function, which advances the time by one second, does not need to be changed.

To add these time zone features to the Time class, the conventional approach would be to obtain the source code found in the time.cpp implementation file, analyze in detail how the class is implemented, then modify and recompile the source code. This process has several drawbacks. If Time is an off-the-shelf class on a system, the source code for the implementation is probably unavailable. Even if it is available, modifying it may introduce bugs into a previously debugged solution. Access to the source code also violates a principal benefit of abstraction: Users of an abstraction should not need to know how it is implemented.

In C++, as in other OOP languages, there is a far quicker and safer way in which to add time zone features: Use inheritance. Let's derive a new class from the Time class and then specialize it. This new, extended time class—call it ExtTime—inherits the members of its base class, Time. Here is the declaration of ExtTime:

```
enum ZoneType {EST, CST, MST, PST, EDT, CDT, MDT, PDT};

class ExtTime : public Time
{
public:
    void Set( /* in */ int       hours,
              /* in */ int       minutes,
              /* in */ int       seconds,
              /* in */ ZoneType timeZone );
    void Write() const;
    ZoneType zone();  // Returns the time zone
    ExtTime( /* in */ int       initHrs,    // Constructor
             /* in */ int       initMins,
             /* in */ int       initSecs,
             /* in */ ZoneType initZone );
```

```
    ExtTime();                              // Default constructor,
                                            //   setting time to
private:                                    //   0:0:0 EST
    ZoneType zone;
};
```

The opening line

```
class ExtTime : public Time
```

states that ExtTime is derived from Time. The reserved word public declares Time to be a *public base class* of ExtTime. This means that all public members of Time (except constructors) are also public members of ExtTime. In other words, Time's member functions Set, Increment, and Write can also be invoked for ExtTime objects.* However, the public part of ExtTime specializes the base class by reimplementing (redefining) the inherited functions Set and Write and by providing its own constructors and a function to return the time zone.

The private part of ExtTime declares that a new private member is added: zone. The private members of ExtTime are therefore hrs, mins, secs (all inherited from Time), and zone. Figure 14–4 pictures the relationship between the ExtTime and Time classes.

This diagram shows that each ExtTime object has a Time object as a *subobject*. Every ExtTime is a Time, and more. C++ uses the terms *base class* and *derived class* instead of *superclass* and *subclass*. The terms *superclass* and *subclass* can be confusing because the prefix *sub-* usually implies something smaller than the original (for example, a subset of a mathematical set). In contrast, a subclass is often "bigger" than its superclass—that is, it has more data and/or functions.

In Figure 14–4, you see an arrow between the two ovals labeled Increment. Because Time is a public base class of ExtTime, and because Increment is not redefined by ExtTime, the Increment function available to clients of ExtTime is the same as the one inherited from Time. We use the arrow between the corresponding ovals to indicate this fact. (Notice in the diagram that Time's constructors are operations on Time, not on ExtTime. The ExtTime class must have its own constructors.)

---

*If a class declaration omits the word public and begins as

```
class DerivedClass : BaseClass
```

or if it explicitly uses the word private,

```
class DerivedClass : private BaseClass
```

then BaseClass is called a *private base class* of DerivedClass. Public members of BaseClass are *not* public members of DerivedClass. That is, clients of DerivedClass cannot invoke BaseClass operations on DerivedClass objects. We do not work with private base classes in this book.

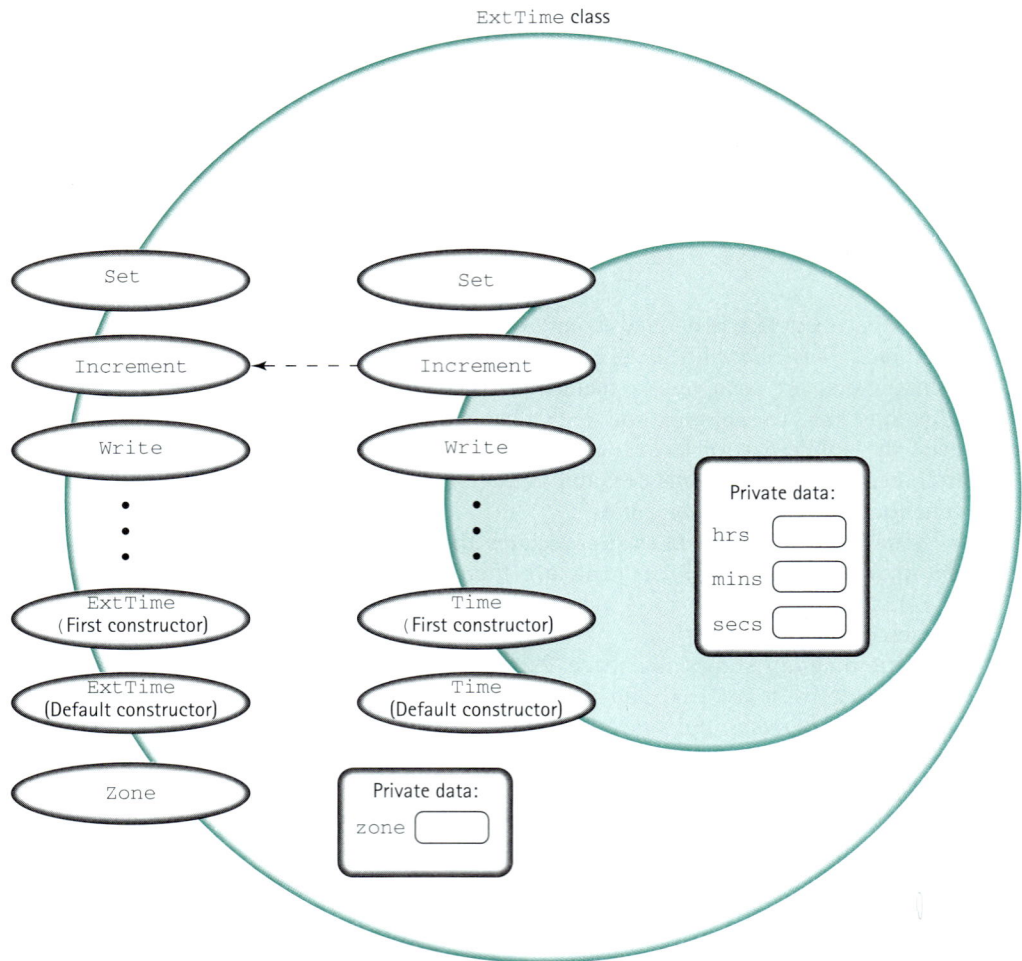

Figure 14–4   *Class Interface Diagram for* ExtTime *Class*

Software Engineering Tip

Inheritance and Accessibility

With C++, it is important to understand that inheritance does not imply accessibility. Although a derived class inherits the members of its base class, both private and public, it cannot access the private members of the base class. Figure 14–4 shows the variables `hrs`, `mins`, and `secs` to be encapsulated within the `Time` class. Neither external client code nor `ExtTime` member functions can refer to these three variables directly. If a derived class were able to access the private members of its base class, any programmer could derive a class from another and then write code to directly inspect or modify the private data, defeating the benefits of encapsulation and information hiding.

Specification of the `ExtTime` Class

Below is the fully documented specification of the `ExtTime` class. Notice that the preprocessor directive

```
#include "time.h"
```

is necessary for the compiler to verify the consistency of the derived class with its base class.

```
//**************************************************************
// SPECIFICATION FILE (exttime.h)
// This file gives the specification of an ExtTime abstract data
// type.  The Time class is a public base class of ExtTime, so
// public operations of Time are also public operations of ExtTime.
//**************************************************************
#include "time.h"

enum ZoneType {EST, CST, MST, PST, EDT, CDT, MDT, PDT};

class ExtTime : public Time
{
public:
    void Set( /* in */ int      hours,
              /* in */ int      minutes,
              /* in */ int      seconds,
              /* in */ ZoneType timeZone );
```

```
        // Precondition:
        //      0 <= hours <= 23   &&   0 <= minutes <= 59
        //   && 0 <= seconds <= 59   &&   timeZone is assigned
        // Postcondition:
        //      Time is set according to the incoming parameters

    void Write() const;
        // Postcondition:
        //      Time has been output in the form HH:MM:SS ZZZ
        //      where ZZZ is the time zone

    ZoneType Zone () const;
        // Postcondition:
        //      Return value == zone

    ExtTime( /* in */ int      initHrs,
             /* in */ int      initMins,
             /* in */ int      initSecs,
             /* in */ ZoneType initZone );
        // Precondition:
        //      0 <= initHrs <= 23   &&   0 <= initMins <= 59
        //   && 0 <= initSecs <= 59   &&   initZone is assigned
        // Postcondition:
        //      Class object is constructed
        //   && Time is set according to the incoming parameters

    ExtTime();
        // Postcondition:
        //      Class object is constructed
        //   && Time is 0:0:0 Eastern Standard Time
private:
    ZoneType zone;
};
```

With this new class, the programmer can set the time with a time zone (via a class constructor or the redefined Set function), output the time with its time zone (via the redefined Write function), and increment the time by one second (via the inherited Increment function):

```
//**********************************************************************
// TimeDemo program
// This is a very simple client of the ExtTime class
//**********************************************************************
#include <iostream>
#include "exttime.h"    // For ExtTime class
```

```
using namespace std;

int main()
{
    ExtTime time1(5, 30, 0, CDT);   // Parameterized constructor used
    ExtTime time2;                  // Default constructor used
    int      loopCount;

    cout << "time1: ";
    time1.Write();
    cout << endl << "time2: ";
    time2.Write();
    cout << endl;

    time2.Set(23, 59, 55, PST);
    cout << "New time2: ";
    time2.Write();
    cout << endl;

    cout << "Incrementing time2:" << endl;
    for (loopCount = 1; loopCount <= 10; loopCount++)
    {
        time2.Write();
        cout << ' ';
        time2.Increment();
    }
    return 0;
}
```

When executed, the TimeDemo program produces the following output.

```
time1: 05:30:00 CDT
time2: 00:00:00 EST
New time2: 23:59:55 PST
Incrementing time2:
23:59:55 PST 23:59:56 PST 23:59:57 PST 23:59:58 PST 23:59:59 PST
00:00:00 PST 00:00:01 PST 00:00:02 PST 00:00:03 PST 00:00:04 PST
```

Implementation of the `ExtTime` Class

The implementation of the `ExtTime` class needs to deal only with the new features that are different from `Time`. Specifically, we must write code to redefine the `Set` and `Write` functions and we must write the two constructors.

With derived classes, constructors are subject to special rules. At run time, the base class constructor is implicitly called first, before the body of the derived class's constructor executes. Additionally, if the base class constructor requires arguments, these arguments must be passed by the derived class's constructor. To see how these rules pertain, let's examine the implementation file `exttime.cpp` (see Figure 14–5).

Figure 14-5 *ExtTime* Implementation File

```cpp
//*****************************************************************
// IMPLEMENTATION FILE (exttime.cpp)
// This file implements the ExtTime member functions.
// The Time class is a public base class of ExtTime
//*****************************************************************
#include "exttime.h"
#include <iostream>
#include <string>

using namespace std;

// Additional private members of class:
//      ZoneType zone;


//*****************************************************************

ExtTime::ExtTime( /* in */ int      initHrs,
                  /* in */ int      initMins,
                  /* in */ int      initSecs,
                  /* in */ ZoneType initZone )

    : Time(initHrs, initMins, initSecs)

// Constructor

// Precondition:
//     0 <= initHrs <= 23   &&   0 <= initMins <= 59
//     && 0 <= initSecs <= 59   &&   initZone is assigned
// Postcondition:
//     Time is set according to initHrs, initMins, and initSecs
//         (via call to base class constructor)
//     && zone == initZone

{
    zone = initZone;
}
```

```
//*********************************************************************

ExtTime::ExtTime()

// Default constructor

// Postcondition:
//      Time is 0:0:0 (via implicit call to base class's
//      default constructor)
//   && zone == EST

{
    zone = EST;
}

//*********************************************************************

void ExtTime::Set( /* in */ int      hours,
                   /* in */ int      minutes,
                   /* in */ int      seconds,
                   /* in */ ZoneType timeZone )

// Precondition:
//      0 <= hours <= 23  &&  0 <= minutes <= 59
//   && 0 <= seconds <= 59  &&  timeZone is assigned
// Postcondition:
//      Time is set according to hours, minutes, and seconds
//   && zone == timeZone

{
    Time::Set(hours, minutes, seconds);
    zone = timeZone;
}

//*********************************************************************

    ZoneType ExtTime::Zone() const

    // Postcondition:
    //      Return value == zone

    {
        return zone;
    }
```

```
//***********************************************************************

void ExtTime::Write() const

// Postcondition:
//      Time has been output in the form HH:MM:SS ZZZ
//      where ZZZ is the time zone

{
    static string zoneString[8] =
    {
        "EST", "CST", "MST", "PST", "EDT", "CDT", "MDT", "PDT"
    };

    Time::Write();
    cout << ' ' << zoneString[zone];
}
```

In the first constructor in Figure 14–5, notice the syntax by which a constructor passes arguments to its base class constructor:

```
ExtTime::ExtTime( /* in */ int       initHrs,
                  /* in */ int       initMins,
                  /* in */ int       initSecs,
                  /* in */ ZoneType initZone )

    : Time(initHrs, initMins, initSecs)     ←    Constructor initializer

{
    zone = initZone;
}
```

After the parameter list to the `ExtTime` constructor (but before its body), you insert what is called a *constructor initializer*—a colon and then the name of the base class along with the arguments to *its* constructor. When an `ExtTime` object is created with a declaration such as

```
ExtTime time1(8, 35, 0, PST);
```

the `ExtTime` constructor receives four arguments. The first three are simply passed along to the `Time` class constructor by means of the constructor initializer. After the `Time` class constructor has executed (creating the base class subobject as shown in Figure 14–4), the body of the `ExtTime` constructor executes, setting `zone` equal to the fourth argument.

The second constructor in Figure 14–5 (the default constructor) does not need a constructor initializer; there are no arguments to pass to the base class's default constructor. When an `ExtTime` object is created with the declaration

```
ExtTime time2;
```

the `ExtTime` class's default constructor first implicitly calls `Time`'s default constructor, after which its body executes, setting `zone` to `EST`.

Next, look at the `Set` function in Figure 14–5. This function reimplements the `Set` function inherited from the base class. Consequently, there are two distinct `Set` functions, one a public member of the `Time` class, the other a public member of the `Ext-Time` class. Their full names are `Time::Set` and `ExtTime::Set`. In Figure 14–5, the `ExtTime::Set` function begins by "reaching up" into its base class and calling `Time::Set` to set the hours, minutes, and seconds. (Remember that a class derived from `Time` cannot access the private data `hrs`, `mins`, and `secs` directly; these variables are private to the `Time` class.) The function then finishes by assigning a value to `ExtTime`'s private data, the `zone` variable.

The `Write` function in Figure 14–5 uses a similar strategy. It reaches up into its base class and invokes `Time::Write` to output the hours, minutes, and seconds. Then it outputs a string corresponding to the time zone. (Recall that a value of an enumeration type cannot be output directly in C++. If we were to print the value of `zone` directly, the output would be an integer from 0 through 7—the internal representations of the `Zone-Type` values.) The `Write` function establishes an array of eight strings and selects the correct string by using `zone` to index into the array. Why is `zoneString` declared to be `static`? Remember that by default, local variables in C++ are automatic variables—that is, memory is allocated for them when the function begins execution and is deallocated when the function returns. With `zoneString` declared as `static`, the array is allocated once only, when the program begins execution, and remains allocated until the program terminates. From function call to function call, the computer does not waste time creating and destroying the array.

Now we can compile the file `exttime.cpp` into an object code file, say, `exttime.obj`. After writing a test driver and compiling it into `test.obj`, we obtain an executable file by linking three object files:

1. `test.obj`
2. `exttime.obj`
3. `time.obj`

We can then test the resulting program.

The remarkable thing about derived classes and inheritance is that modification of the base class is unnecessary. The source code for the implementation of the `Time` class may be unavailable. Yet variations of this ADT can continue to be created without that source code, in ways the creator never even considered. Through classes and inheritance, OOP languages facilitate code reuse. A class such as `Time` can be used as-is in many different contexts, or it can be adapted to a particular context by using inheritance. Inheritance allows us to create *extensible* data abstractions—a derived class typically extends the base class by including additional private data or public operations or both.

Avoiding Multiple Inclusion of Header Files

We saw that the specification file `exttime.h` begins with an `#include` directive to insert the file `time.h`:

```
#include "time.h"

enum ZoneType {EST, CST, MST, PST, EDT, CDT, MDT, PDT};

class ExtTime : public Time
{
    :
};
```

Now think about what happens if a programmer using the `ExtTime` class already has included `time.h` for other purposes, overlooking the fact that `exttime.h` also includes it:

```
#include "time.h"
#include "exttime.h"
```

The preprocessor inserts the file `time.h`, then `exttime.h`, and then `time.h` a second time (because `exttime.h` also includes `time.h`). The result is a compile-time error, because the `Time` class is defined twice.

The widely used solution to this problem is to write `time.h` this way:

```
#ifndef TIME_H
#define TIME_H
class Time
{
    :
};
#endif
```

The lines beginning with "#" are directives to the preprocessor. `TIME_H` (or any identifier you wish to use) is a preprocessor identifier, not a C++ program identifier. In effect, these directives say:

If the preprocessor identifier `TIME_H` is not already defined, then

1. define `TIME_H` as an identifier known to the preprocessor,

and

2. let the declaration of the `Time` class pass through to the compiler.

If a subsequent `#include "time.h"` is encountered, the test `#ifndef TIME_H` will fail. The `Time` class declaration will not pass through to the compiler a second time.

14.4 Composition

Earlier we said that two classes typically exhibit one of the following relationships: They are independent of each other, they are related by inheritance, or they are related by **composition**. Composition (or **containment**) is the relationship in which the internal data of one class A includes an object of another class B. Stated another way, a B object is contained within an A object.

> **Composition (containment)** A mechanism by which the internal data (the state) of one class includes an object of another class.

C++ does not have (or need) any special language notation for composition. You simply declare an object of one class to be one of the data members of another class. Let's look at an example.

Design of an Entry Class

You are developing a program to represent an appointment book. Each day object will be a sorted list of appointment objects. In preparation, you decide to build an Entry ADT with two fields, an object of a Name ADT and an object of a Time ADT. You may need to add more information for an appointment object later, but this gives you a start. Constructing this object should be easy because you already have a `Time` class and a `Name` class. For the purpose of an appointment calendar, you decide to ignore middle name or initial and the seconds in the time. You can always add the middle name later if you need it. Of course, you do need operations that return the name and time to the client program.

The operations can be `NameStr`, which returns a name composed of the first and last name, and `TimeStr`, which returns the hours and minutes with a colon between. Of course, we need constructors. How many? Well, you know that the `Name` class has two constructors, one that takes the parts of the name as parameters and one that reads the name from the standard input device (default). The same thing is true of the `Time` class. Thus, we need a default constructor for `Entry` class, which will call the default constructors for `Name` and `Time`, and a parameterized constructor, which will pass the parameters to `Name`'s and `Time`'s parameterized constructors.

```
//*******************************************************************
// SPECIFICATION FILE (Entry.h)
// This file contains the specification of the Entry ADT,
// which has two contained classes, Name and Time
//*******************************************************************

#include "Time.h"
#include "Name.h"
#include <string>

class Entry
{
public:
    string NameStr() const;
        // Returns a string made up of first name, blank, last name
        // Postcondition:
        //     Return value is first name of Name object, blank,
        //     and last name of Name object
```

```
        string TimeStr() const;
            // Returns a string made up of hour, colon, minutes
            // Postcondition:
            //     Return value is minutes from Time object, colon, and
            //     seconds of Time object
        Entry();
            // Default constructor
            // Postcondition:
            //     Entry object has been constructed

        Entry( (/* in */ string firstName,    // First name
                /* in */ string middleName,   // Middle name
                /* in */ string lastName)     // Last name
                /* in */ int  initHours,      // Hours
                /* in */ int  initMinutes,    // Minutes
                /* in */ int  initSeconds )   // Seconds
            // Parameterized constructor
            // Postcondtion:
            //     Entry object has been constructed with firstName,
            //     middleName, and lastName as arguments to Name
            //     parameterized constructor; Time object
            //     initHours, initMinutes, and initSeconds as arguments
            //     to Time parameterized constructor

    private:
        Name name;
        Time time;
    }
```

Implementing the member functions Name and Time is easy: They just involve invoking member functions of Name and Time. The specification files for each of these classes provide the interface that the functions must use. An abbreviated version of Name.h is shown below; Time.h has been shown previously in this chapter.

```
// SPECIFICATION FILE (Name.h)
...
enum RelationType{BEFORE, SAME, AFTER};
class Name
{
public:
    Name();
        // Default constructor
        // Postcondition:
        //     Name is prompted for and read from the standard input
        //     device
```

```
Name( /* in */ string firstName,
      /* in */ string middleName,
      /* in */ string lastName );
    // Parameterized constructor
    // Postcondition:
    //     first is firstName AND middle is middleName AND
    //     last is lastName
string FirstName() const;
    // Postcondition:
    //     Return value is this person's first name

string LastName() const;
    // Postcondition:
    //     Return value is this person's last name

    ...
};
```

Implementing the default class constructors involves invoking the default constructors for the `Name` object and the `Time` object. The default `Entry` constructor has nothing else to do. Thus, the body of the default constructor for `Entry` is empty. The parameterized constructor must pass the parameters to the `Name` and `Time` constructors. How is this done? We use the constructor initializer that we described in the last section. Thus, the parameterized constructor for `Entry` also has no body.

```
//*******************************************************************
// IMPLEMENTATION FILE (Entry.cpp)
// This file contains the specification of the Entry ADT,
// which has two contained classes, Name and Time
//*******************************************************************

#include "Entry.h"
#include <string>

#include <fstream>
#include <iostream>
using namespace std;
string Entry::NameStr() const

    // Returns a string made up of first name, blank, last name
    // Postcondition:
    //    Return value is first name of Name object, blank, and
    //    last name of Name object

{
    return (name.FirstName() + ' ' + name.LastName());
}
```

```cpp
string Entry::TimeStr() const

    // Returns a string made up of hour, colon, minutes
    // Postcondition:
    //     Return value is minutes from Time object, colon, and
    //     seconds of Time object

{

    return "" + time.Hours() + ":" + time.Minutes();
}

bool Entry::LessThan(Entry entry) const

    // Compares time with entry.time
    // Postcondition:
    //     Return value is true if time is less than entry.time;
    //     false otherwise

{
    return time.LessThan(entry.time);
}

bool Entry::Equal(Entry entry) const

    // Compares time with entry.time
    // Postcondition:
    //     Return value is true if self is equal to entry.time;
    //     false otherwise

{
    return time.Equal(entry.time);
}

Entry::Entry()

    // Default constructor
    // Postcondition:
    //     Entry object has been constructed
{
}

Entry::Entry( /* in */ string firstName,
              /* in */ string middleName,
              /* in */ string lastName,
```

```
                    /* in */  int   initHours,
                    /* in */  int   initMinutes,
                    /* in */  int   initSeconds )

 // Constructor initializers
  : name(firstName, middleName, lastName),
    time(initHours, initMinutes, initSeconds)

    // Parameterized constructor
    // Postcondtion:
    //     Entry object has been constructed with firstName,
    //     middleName, and lastName as arguments to Name
    //     parameterized constructor; initHours, initMinutes,
    //     and initSeconds as arguments to Time parameterized
    //     constructor

{
}
```

Testing: Here is a driver that creates two objects of class Entry and applies the appropriate functions to them.

```
//********************************************************************
// DRIVER for class Entry
// This program tests the constructors and return functions
//********************************************************************

#include <iostream>
#include "Entry.h"

using namespace std;

int main()
{
    Entry entry1("Sally", "Jane", "Smith", 12, 20, 0);
    Entry entry2("Mary", "Beth", "Jones", 10, 30, 0);

    entry1.ReadEntry();

    cout << "Entry 1: " << entry1.NameStr() << " "
         << entry1.TimeStr() << endl;
    cout << "Entry 2: " << entry2.NameStr() << " "
         << entry2.TimeStr() << endl;
    return 0;
}
```

What? Class `Entry` doesn't compile? We get the following error message:

```
Error    : illegal operand
EntryEr.cpp line 33   return "" + time.Hours() + ":" +
time.Minutes();
```

What could be wrong with this statement? We just created a string out of a string, an integer value, a colon, and another integer value. We have used concatenation to build stings since Chapter 2. Numbers are converted to strings for output. What's different about this statement? The C++ system automatically converts integers to strings *for output*, but there is no type cast from integers to strings except for output.

In order to create a string including integers, we could write it out to a file and then read it back in as a string. This would work, but it would be extremely time consuming (disk access is over a million times slower than memory access). Fortunately, the designers of the language realized that there might be times when a conversion from integers to strings would be useful. Thus they derived a class called `stringstream` from class `iostream`, which allows us to write values to a string as if we were writing them to a file. Because the data is not actually sent to a file but is kept in memory, the conversion is done quickly.

We declare an object of class `ostringstream`, and use the insertion operator (`<<`) to send the integers to the object. To get them back as a string, we use the `str` member function of class `ostringstream`. Here then is the corrected version of `TimeStr`, using an object of class `ostringstream`, followed by the output from the driver.

```cpp
#include <sstream>            // ostringstream
string Entry::TimeStr() const

// Returns a string made up of hour, colon, minutes, colon, seconds
// Postcondition:
//      Return value is minutes from Time object, colon, and
//      seconds of Time object

{
    string outStr;
    ostringstream tempOut;  // Access ostringstream

    if (time.Hours() < 10)
        tempOut << '0';
    tempOut << time.Hours() << ":";
    if (time.Minutes() < 10)
        tempOut << '0';
    tempOut << time.Minutes() << ":";
    if (time.Seconds() < 10);
        tempOut << '0';
    tempOut << time.Seconds();
```

```
        outStr = tempOut.str();
        return outStr;
}
```

Once this function is inserted, the driver produces this output.

```
EntryTest.out - Notepad                                    _ □ X
File  Edit  Format  View  Help
Entry 1: Sally Smith 12:20:00
Entry 2: Mary Jones 10:30:00
```

Constructor Initializer

We've twice seen the unusual notation—the constructor initializer—inserted between the parameter list and the body of a constructor. The first time was when we implemented the parameterized ExtTime class constructor (Figure 14–5). There, we used the constructor initializer to pass some of the incoming arguments to the base class constructor. Here, we use a constructor initializer to pass some of the arguments to member objects' (name's and time's) constructors. Whether you are using inheritance or composition, the purpose of a constructor initializer is the same: to pass arguments to another constructor. The only difference is the following: With inheritance, you specify the name of the *base class* prior to the argument list, as follows:

```
ExtTime::ExtTime( /* in */ int       initHrs,
                  /* in */ int       initMins,
                  /* in */ int       initSecs,
                  /* in */ ZoneType  initZone )

    : Time(initHrs, initMins, initSecs)
```

With composition, you specify the name of the *member object* prior to the argument list:

```
Entry::Entry( /* in */ string firstName,
              /* in */ string middleName,
              /* in */ string lastName,
              /* in */ int    initHours,
              /* in */ int    initMinutes )
// Constructor initializers
  : name(firstName, middleName, lastName),
    time(initHours, initMinutes)
```

Having discussed both inheritance and composition, we can give a complete description of the order in which constructors are executed:

Given a class X, if X is a derived class, its base class constructor is executed first. Next, constructors for member objects (if any) are executed. Finally, the body of X's constructor is executed.

When an `Entry` object is created, the constructors for its `name` member and its `time` member are first invoked. After the `name` and `time` objects are constructed, the body of `Entry`'s constructor is executed, which in this case is empty.

14.5 Dynamic Binding and Virtual Functions

Early in the chapter, we said that object-oriented programming languages provide language features that support three concepts: data abstraction, inheritance, and dynamic binding. The phrase *dynamic binding* means, more specifically, *dynamic binding of an operation to an object.* To explain this concept, let's begin with an example.

Given the `Time` and `ExtTime` classes of this chapter, the following code creates two class objects and outputs the time represented by each.

```
Time    startTime(8, 30, 0);
ExtTime endTime(10, 45, 0, CST);

startTime.Write();
cout << endl;
endTime.Write();
cout << endl;
```

This code fragment invokes two different `Write` functions, even though the functions appear to have the same name. The first function call invokes the `Write` function of the `Time` class, printing out three values: hours, minutes, and seconds. The second call invokes the `Write` function of the `ExtTime` class, printing out four values: hours, minutes, seconds, and time zone. In this code fragment, the compiler uses **static** (compile-time) **binding** of the operation (`Write`) to the appropriate object. The compiler can easily determine which `Write` function to call by checking the data type of the associated object.

> **Static binding** The compile-time determination of which function to call for a particular object.

In some situations, the compiler cannot determine the type of an object, and the binding of an operation to an object must occur at run time. One situation, which we look at now, involves passing class objects as arguments.

The basic C++ rule for passing class objects as arguments is that the argument and its corresponding parameter must be of identical type. With inheritance, though, C++ relaxes the rule. You may pass an object of a child class *C* to an object of its parent class *P*, but not the other way around—that is, you cannot pass an object of type *P* to an object of type *C*. More generally, you can pass an object of a descendant class to an object of any of its ancestor classes. This rule has a tremendous benefit—it allows us to write a single function that applies to any descendant class instead of writing a different function for each. For example, we could write a fancy Print function that takes as an argument an object of type Time or any class descended from Time:

```
void Print( /* in */ Time someTime )
{
    cout << "************************" << endl;
    cout << "** The time is ";
    someTime.Write();
    cout << endl;
    cout << "************************" << endl;
}
```

Given the code fragment

```
Time    startTime(8, 30, 0);
ExtTime endTime(10, 45, 0, CST);

Print(startTime);
Print(endTime);
```

the compiler lets us pass either a Time object or an ExtTime object to the Print function. Unfortunately, the output is not what we would like. When endTime is printed, the time zone CST is missing from the output. Let's see why.

The Slicing Problem

Our Print function uses passing by value for the parameter someTime. Passing by value sends a copy of the argument to the parameter. Whenever you pass an object of a child class to an object of its parent class using a pass by value, only the data members they have in common are copied. Remember that a child class is often "larger" than its parent—that is, it contains additional data members. For example, a Time object has three data members (hrs, mins, and secs), but an ExtTime object has four data members (hrs, mins, secs, and zone). When the larger class object is copied to the smaller parameter using a pass by value, the extra data members are discarded or "sliced off." This situation is called the *slicing problem* (see Figure 14-6).

(The slicing problem also occurs with assignment operations. In the statement

```
parentClassObject = childClassObject;
```

only the data members that the two objects have in common are copied. Additional data members contained in childClassObject are not copied.)

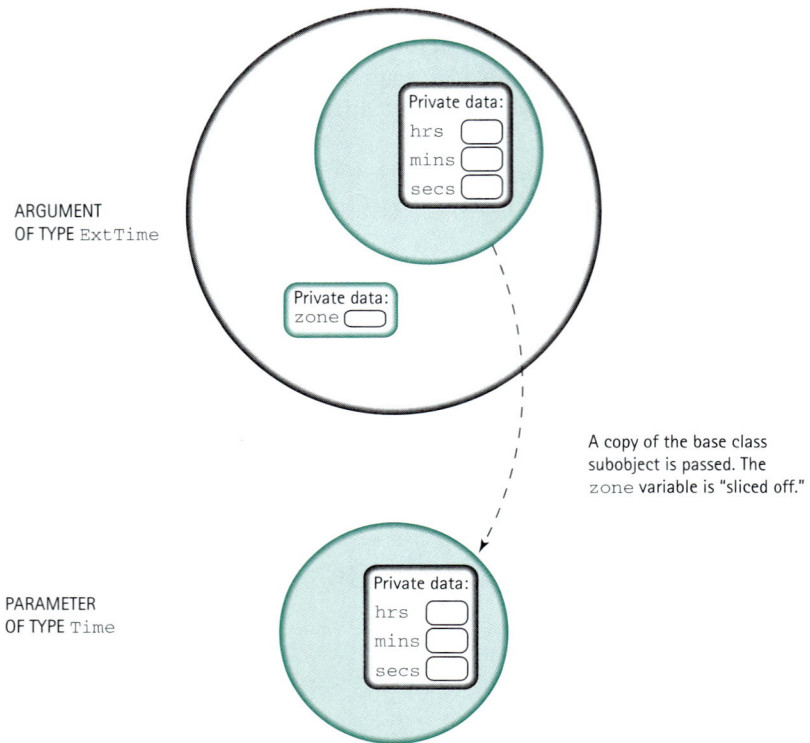

ARGUMENT
OF TYPE ExtTime

A copy of the base class
subobject is passed. The
zone variable is "sliced off."

PARAMETER
OF TYPE Time

Figure 14–6 *The Slicing Problem Resulting from Passing by Value*

With passing by reference, the slicing problem does not occur because the *address* of the caller's argument is sent to the function. Let's change the heading of our Print function so that someTime is a reference parameter:

```
void Print( /* in */ Time& someTime )
```

Now when we pass endTime as the argument, its address is sent to the function. Its time zone member is not sliced off because no copying takes place. But to our dismay, the Print function *still* prints only three of endTime's data members—hours, minutes, and seconds.

Within the Print function, the difficulty is that static binding is used in the statement

```
someTime.Write();
```

The compiler must generate machine language code for the Print function at compile time, but the type of the actual argument (Time or ExtTime) isn't known until run time.

How can the compiler know which `Write` function to use—`Time::Write` or `ExtTime::Write`? The compiler cannot know, so it uses `Time::Write` because the parameter `someTime` is of type `Time`. Therefore, the `Print` function always prints just three values—hours, minutes, and seconds—regardless of the type of the argument. Fortunately, C++ provides a very simple solution to our problem: *virtual functions.*

Virtual Functions

Suppose we make one small change to our `Time` class declaration: We begin the declaration of the `Write` function with the reserved word `virtual`.

```
class Time
{
public:
    ⋮
    virtual void Write() const;
    ⋮
private:
    ⋮
};
```

Declaring a member function to be `virtual` instructs the compiler to generate code that guarantees **dynamic** (run-time) **binding** of a function to an object. That is, the determination of which function to call is postponed until run time. (Note that to make `Write` a virtual function, the word `virtual` appears in one place only—the `Time` class declaration. It does not appear in the `Write` function definition that is located in the `time.cpp` file, nor does it appear in any descendant class—such as `ExtTime`—that redefines the `Write` function.)

> **Dynamic binding**   The run-time determination of which function to call for a particular object.

Virtual functions work in the following way. If a class object is passed *by reference* to some function, and if the body of that function contains a statement

```
param.MemberFunc( ... );
```

then

1. If `MemberFunc` is not a virtual function, the type of the *parameter* determines which function to call. (Static binding is used.)
2. If `MemberFunc` is a virtual function, the type of the *argument* determines which function to call. (Dynamic binding is used.)

With just one word—`virtual`—the difficulties we encountered with our `Print` function disappear entirely. If we declare `Write` to be a virtual function in the `Time` class, the function

```
void Print( /* in */ Time& someTime )
{
    ⋮
    someTime.Write();
    ⋮
}
```

works correctly for arguments either of type `Time` or of type `ExtTime`. The correct `Write` function (`Time::Write` or `ExtTime::Write`) is invoked because the argument carries the information necessary at run time to choose the appropriate function. Deriving a new and unanticipated class from `Time` presents no complications. If this new class redefines the `Write` function, then our `Print` function still works correctly. Dynamic binding ensures that each object knows how to print itself, and the appropriate version will be invoked. In OOP terminology, `Write` is a **polymorphic operation**—an operation that has multiple meanings depending on the type of the object that responds to it at run time.

> **Polymorphic operation** An operation that has multiple meanings depending on the type of the object to which it is bound at run time.

Here are some things to know about using virtual functions in C++:

1. To obtain dynamic binding, you must use passing by reference when passing a class object to a function. If you use passing by value, the compiler does not use the `virtual` mechanism; instead, member slicing and static binding occur.

2. In the declaration of a virtual function, the word `virtual` appears only in the base class, not in any derived class.

3. If a base class declares a virtual function, it *must* implement that function, even if the body is empty.

4. A derived class is not required to provide its own reimplementation of a virtual function. In this case, the base class's version is used by default.

5. A derived class cannot redefine the function return type of a virtual function.

14.6 Object-Oriented Design

We have looked at language features that let us implement an object-oriented design. Now let's turn to the phase that precedes implementation—OOD itself.

A computer program usually models some real-life activity or concept. A banking program models the real-life activities associated with a bank. A spreadsheet program models a real spreadsheet, a large paper form used by accountants and financial planners. A robotics program models human perception and human motion.

Nearly always, the aspect of the world that we are modeling (the *application domain* or *problem domain*) consists of objects—checking accounts, bank tellers, spreadsheet rows, spreadsheet columns, robot arms, robot legs. The computer program that solves the real-life problem also includes objects (the *solution domain*)—counters, lists, menus, windows, and so forth. OOD is based on the philosophy that programs are easier to write and understand if the major objects in a program correspond closely to the objects in the problem domain.

There are many ways in which to perform object-oriented design. Different authors advocate different techniques. Our purpose is not to choose one particular technique or to present a summary of all the techniques. Rather, our purpose is to describe a three-step process that captures the essence of OOD:

1. Identify the objects and operations.
2. Determine the relationships among objects.
3. Design the driver.

In this section, we do not show a complete example of an object-oriented design of a problem solution—we save that for the Problem-Solving Case Study at the end of the chapter. Instead, we describe the important issues involved in each of the three steps.

Step 1: Identify the Objects and Operations

Recall that structured design (functional decomposition) begins with identification of the major actions the program is to perform. In contrast, OOD begins by identifying the major objects and the associated operations on those objects. In both design methods, it is often difficult to see where to start.

To identify solution-domain objects, a good way to start is to look at the problem domain. More specifically, go to the problem definition and look for important nouns and verbs. The nouns (and noun phrases) may suggest objects; the verbs (and verb phrases) may suggest operations. For example, the problem definition for a banking program might include the following sentences:

... The program must handle a customer's savings account. The customer is allowed to deposit funds into the account and withdraw funds from the account, and the bank must pay interest on a quarterly basis. ...

In these sentences, the key nouns are

Savings account
Customer

and the key verb phrases are

Deposit funds
Withdraw funds
Pay interest

Although we are working with a very small portion of the entire problem definition, the list of nouns suggests two potential objects: savingsAccount and customer. The operations on a savingsAccount object are suggested by the list of verb phrases— namely, Deposit, Withdraw, and PayInterest. What are the operations on a customer object? We would need more information from the rest of the problem definition in order to answer this question. In fact, customer may not turn out to be a useful object at all. The nouns-and-verbs technique is only a starting point—it points us to *potential* objects and operations.

Determining which nouns and verbs are significant is one of the most difficult aspects of OOD. There are no cookbook formulas for doing so, and there probably never will be. Not all nouns become objects, and not all verbs become operations. The nouns-and-verbs technique is imperfect, but it does give us a first approximation to a solution.

The solution domain includes not only objects drawn from the problem domain but also *implementation-level* objects. These are objects that do not model the problem domain but are used in building the program itself. In systems with graphical user interfaces—Microsoft Windows or the Macintosh operating system, for example—a program may need several kinds of implementation-level objects: window objects, menu objects, objects that respond to mouse clicks, and so on. Objects such as these are often available in class libraries so that we don't need to design and implement them from scratch each time we need them in different programs.

Step 2: Determine the Relationships Among Objects

After selecting potential objects and operations, the next step is to examine the relationships among the objects. In particular, we want to see whether certain objects might be related either by inheritance or by composition. Inheritance and composition relationships not only pave the way for code reuse—as we emphasized in our discussion of OOP—but also simplify the design and allow us to model the problem domain more accurately. For example, the banking problem may require several kinds of savings accounts—one for general customers, another for preferred customers, and another for children under the age of 12. If these are all variations on a basic savings account, the is-a relationship (and, therefore, inheritance) is probably appropriate. Starting with a `SavingsAccount` class that provides operations common to any savings account, we could design each of the other accounts as a child class of `SavingsAccount`, concentrating our efforts only on the properties that make each one different from the parent class.

On the other hand, composition was the only choice for class `Entry`. An `Entry` object contains a `Time` object and a `Name` object.

Step 3: Design the Driver

The final step is to design the driver—the top-level algorithm. In OOD, the driver is the glue that puts the objects (along with their operations) together. When implementing the design in C++, the driver becomes the `main` function.

Notice that structured design *begins* with the design of the top-level algorithm, whereas OOD *ends* with the top-level algorithm. In OOD, most of the control flow has already been designed in steps 1 and 2; the algorithms are located within the operations on objects. As a result, the driver often has very little to do but process user commands or input some data and then delegate tasks to various objects.

> ## Software Engineering Tip
>
> *The Iterative Nature of Object-Oriented Design*
>
> Software developers, researchers, and authors have proposed many different strategies for performing OOD. Common to nearly all of these strategies are three fundamental steps:
>
> 1. Identify the objects and operations.
> 2. Determine the relationships among objects.
> 3. Design the driver.
>
> Experience with large software projects has shown that these three steps are not necessarily sequential—step 1, step 2, step 3, then we are done. In practice, step 1 occurs first, but only as a first approximation. During steps 2 and 3, new objects or operations may be discovered, leading us back to step 1 again. It is realistic to think of steps 1 through 3 not as a sequence but as a loop.
>
> Furthermore, each step is an iterative process within itself. Step 1 may entail working and reworking our view of the objects and operations. Similarly, steps 2 and 3 often involve experimentation and revision. In any step, we may conclude that a potential object is not useful after all. Or we might decide to add or eliminate operations on a particular object.
>
> There is always more than one way to solve a problem. Iterating and reiterating through the design phase leads to insights that produce a better solution.

14.7 Implementing the Design

In OOD, when we first identify an object, it is an *abstract object.* We do not immediately choose an exact data representation for that object. Similarly, the operations on objects begin as *abstract operations,* because there is no initial attempt to provide algorithms for these operations.

Eventually, we have to implement the objects and operations. For each abstract object, we must

- Choose a suitable data representation.
- Create algorithms for the abstract operations.

To select a data representation for an object, the C++ programmer has three options:

1. Use a built-in data type.
2. Use an existing ADT.
3. Create a new ADT.

For a given object, a good rule of thumb is to consider these three options in the order listed. A built-in type is the most straightforward to use and understand, and operations on these types are already defined by the language. If a built-in type is not adequate to represent an object, you should survey available ADTs in a class library (either the system's or your own) to see if any are a good match for the abstract object. If no suitable ADT exists, you must design and implement a new ADT to represent the object.

Fortunately, even if you must resort to option 3, the mechanisms of inheritance and composition allow you to combine options 2 and 3. When we needed an `ExtTime` class earlier in the chapter, we used inheritance to build on an existing `Time` class. And when we created an `Entry` class, we used composition to include a `Time` object and `Name` object in the private data.

In addition to choosing a data representation for the abstract object, we must implement the abstract operations. With OOD, the algorithms that implement the abstract operations are often short and straightforward. We have seen numerous examples in this chapter and in Chapters 11 and 13 in which the code for ADT operations is only a few lines long. But this is not always the case. If an operation is extremely complex, it may be best to treat the operation as a new problem and use functional decomposition on the control flow. In this situation, it is appropriate to apply both functional decomposition and object-oriented methodologies together. Experienced programmers are familiar with both methodologies and use them either independently or in combination with each other. However, the software development community is becoming increasingly convinced that although functional decomposition is important for designing low-level algorithms and operations on ADTs, the future in developing huge software systems lies in OOD and OOP.

Problem–Solving Case Study

Creating an Appointment Calendar

PROBLEM   Create an appointment calendar with the following operations:

Given a date, insert a time and name pair.
Given a date, return the day's time and name pairs in order of time.
Given a date and a time, return true if the time is free, false otherwise.

DISCUSSION   What are the objects in this description? A date, a time, a name, and a collection of time/name pairs for each date. All of the operations begin "Given a date" and involve doing something with name/time pairs. Let's simplify this problem by implementing a list of name/time pairs first. The next step would be to combine the list of name/time pairs with a date to create a day's list of appointments.

We already have a `Name` class, a `Time` class, and an `Entry` class made up of `Name` and `Time` objects. Collection is another name for a list. We have a `List` class. It looks like this problem is simply putting building blocks together, where the building blocks are classes. We can use each of these classes directly except for the `List` class.

The `List` class is a list of `ItemType` objects in which `ItemType` is set by a Typedef statement. In the case study in the last chapter, we used the `List` class to hold a list of integers. Here we have a list of `Entry` objects, which should be ordered by time. That's OK; we have a `SortedList` class we can use. No, it isn't OK. The `SortedList` operations `Insert` and `BinSearch` involve comparing two items using the relational operators. Our `Time` class has comparison operators `Equal` and `LessThan`; the relational operators are not defined on `Time` objects. This means that we must add two functions to class `Entry`: `LessThan` and `Equal`.

While we are enhancing class `Entry`, let's add a `ReadEntry` function to the class. An `Entry` object should have an action responsibility to read values into itself.

Here are the prototypes for the new functions:

```
bool LessThan( Entry entry ) const;

    // Compares time with entry.time
    // Postcondition:
    //     Return value is true if time is less than entry.time;
    //     false otherwise

bool Equal( Entry entry ) const;

    // Compares time with entry.time
    // Postcondition:
    //     Return value is true if time is equal to entry.time;
    //     false otherwise

void ReadEntry();

    // Postcondition:
    //     Values have been read from the keyboard and stored
    //     into name and time
```

LessThan(In: entry)

> Return time.LessThan(entry.time)

Equal(In: entry)

> Return time.Equal(entry.time)

ReadEntry()

> time.ReadName()
> name.ReadTime()

SORTEDLIST Is our current `SortedList` class useless? No; we must rewrite two of the functions using the appropriate comparisons `LessThan` and `Equal` from the `Entry` class, thus specializing the list, but we can use the operations that do not require a comparison as is. There are several advanced features of C++ that allow us to solve this problem by creating a general list. We look at one of them in Chapter 17.

The operations that need to be rewritten are `Insert` and `BinSearch`. What about `Delete`? Our problem doesn't indicate that we need to delete an appointment, but we should anticipate such an operation in the future. However, as `Delete` uses `BinSearch`, it doesn't have to be changed. Note that "item" is of class `Entry`, and our comparisons are on time, so `LessThan` and `Equal` in class `Entry` just call `LessThan` and `Equal` in class `Time`.

Insert(In: item)

```
Set index to length – 1
WHILE index ≥ 0 AND item.LessThan(data[index])
    Set data[index + 1] to data[index]
    Decrement index
Set data[index + 1] to item
Increment length
```

BinSearch(In: item; InOut: found, position)

```
Set found to false
Set first to 0
Set last to length-1
WHILE last >= first AND NOT found
    Set middle to (first + last)/2
    IF item.LessThan(data[middle])
        Set last to middle-1
    ELSE IF data[middle].LessThan(item)
        Set first to middle + 1
    ELSE
        Set found to true
IF found
    Set position to middle
```

DRIVER The calls to the `SortedList` functions to implement the tasks go into the driver at the moment. When we incorporate what we have done here into the bigger task, the driver will become part of the class that manipulates a day's events.

Main

> Get time/name pairs
> Return time/name pairs
> Time free?
> Delete
> Return time/name pairs

Get Pairs

We need a loop to input time/name pairs. Since this is a driver and not a real program, we can arbitrarily set up a loop: Let's input 5 pairs.

> FOR count going from 1 to 5
>   ReadEntry()
>   Insert entry into list

Return Pairs

This operation gives access to the list items. We have no idea what the final program will do with the data, but we can let the driver print out the pairs.

> Set limit to list.length()
> Reset list
> FOR count going from 1 to limit
>   Set entry to list.GetNextItem()
>   Print entry

Time Free(In: item)
    Out: Function value

> Return NOT list.IsPresent(item)

Delete(In: entry)

> list.Delete(entry)

PUTTING IT ALL TOGETHER   Most of the work for this program was done elsewhere. We just had to put the pieces together. The Name class and the Time class had already been tested and were not altered. We have added three new functions to class Entry, and changed two functions in class `SortedList`. We need to retest the current version of class `Entry` before we try running the driver. Here is the implementation file for the expanded class `Entry`, the driver to test it, and the output from the driver.

```cpp
//****************************************************************
// IMPLEMENTATION FILE (Entry.cpp)
// This file contains the specification of the Entry ADT,
// which has two contained classes, Name and Time
//****************************************************************

#include "Entry.h"
#include <string>
#include <fstream>
#include <iostream>
#include <sstream>              // ostringstream

using namespace std;

string Entry::NameStr() const

// Returns a string made up of first name, blank, last name
// Postcondition:
//      Return value is first name of Name object, blank, and
//      last name of Name object

{
    return (name.FirstName() + ' ' + name.LastName());
}

string Entry::TimeStr() const

// Returns a string made up of hour, colon, minutes, colon, seconds
// Postcondition:
//      Return value is minutes from Time object, colon, and
//      seconds of Time object

{
    string outStr;
    ostringstream tempOut;  // Access ostringstream class
    if (time.Hours() < 10)
        tempOut << '0';
    tempOut << time.Hours() << ":";
    if (time.Minutes() < 10)
        tempOut << '0';
```

```
        tempOut << time.Minutes() << ":";
        if (time.Seconds() < 10)
            tempOut << '0';
        tempOut << time.Seconds();
        outStr = tempOut.str();
        return outStr;
}

void Entry::ReadEntry()

// Postcondition:
//      Values have been read from the keyboard into name and time.

{
    name.ReadName();
    time.ReadTime();
}

bool Entry::LessThan(Entry entry) const

// Compares time with entry.time
// Postcondition:
//      Return value is true if time is less than entry.time;
//      false otherwise

{
    return time.LessThan(entry.time);
}

bool Entry::Equal(Entry entry) const

// Compares time with entry.time
// Postcondition:
//      Return value is true if self is equal to entry.time;
//      false otherwise

{
    return time.Equal(entry.time);
}

Entry::Entry()

// Default constructor
```

```cpp
// Postcondition:
//      Entry object has been constructed
{
}

Entry::Entry( /* in */ string firstName,
              /* in */ string middleName,
              /* in */ string lastName,
              /* in */ int   initHours,
              /* in */ int   initMinutes,
              /* in */ int   initSeconds )

    // Constructor initializers
    : name(firstName, middleName, lastName),
      time(initHours, initMinutes, initSeconds)

// Parameterized constructor
// Postcondition:
//      Entry object has been constructed with firstName,
//      middleName, and lastName as arguments to Name
//      parameterized constructor; initHours, initMinutes,
//      and initSeconds as arguments to Time parameterized
//      constructor

{
}

//*****************************************************************
// DRIVER for expanded class Entry (File ExpEntryDr.cpp)
// This program tests the constructors and return functions
//*****************************************************************

#include <iostream>
#include "Entry.h"
using namespace std;

int main()
{
    Entry entry1;
    Entry entry2("Mary", "Beth", "Jones", 10, 30, 0);

    entry1.ReadEntry();

    // Testing consructors and ReadEntry
    cout << "Entry 1: " << entry1.NameStr() << " "
         << entry1.TimeStr() << endl;
```

```
    cout << "Entry 2: " << entry2.NameStr() << " "
         << entry2.TimeStr() << endl;

    // Testing LessThan
    if (entry1.LessThan(entry2))
        cout << "Entry 1 is less than Entry 2" << endl;
    else
        cout << "Entry 1 is not less than Entry 2" << endl;
    if (entry2.LessThan(entry1))
        cout << "Entry 2 is less than Entry 1" << endl;
    else
        cout << "Entry 2 is not less than Entry 1" << endl;

    // Testing Equal
    if (entry1.Equal(entry2))
        cout << "Entry 1 equals Entry 2" << endl;
    else
        cout << "Entry 1 does not equal Entry 2" << endl;

    entry1 = entry2;
    cout << "entry1 set to entry2" << endl;
    if (entry1.Equal(entry2))
        cout << "Entry 1 equals Entry 2" << endl;
    else
        cout << "Entry 1 does not equal Entry 2" << endl;

    return 0;
}
```

```
C:\PPSC++\2-22-04\Ch14\EntryTest.exe                          _ □ ×
Enter first name: Susy
Enter middle name: Sunshine
Enter last name: Smith
Enter hours (<= 23):
9
Enter minutes (<= 59):
30
Enter seconds (<= 59):
0
Entry 1: Susy Smith 09:30:00
Entry 2: Mary Jones 10:30:00
Entry 1 is less than Entry 2
Entry 2 is not less than Entry 1
Entry 1 does not equal Entry 2
entry1 set to entry2
Entry 1 equals Entry 2
```

Now that the expanded class Entry has been tested, we can continue with the rest of the problem. Here are the implementations of the changed functions in class `SortedList`.

```
//*****************************************************************

void SortedList::Insert( /* in */ ItemType& item )

// Inserts item into the SortedList

// Precondition:
//      length < MAX_LENGTH
//   && data[0..length-1] are in ascending order
// Postcondition:
//      item is in the SortedList
//   && length == length@entry + 1
//   && data[0..length-1] are in ascending order

{
    int index;      // Index and loop control variable
    index = length - 1;
    while (index >= 0 && item.LessThan(data[index]))
    {
        data[index+1] = data[index];
        index--;
    }
    data[index+1] = item;            // Insert item
    length++;
}

//*****************************************************************

void SortedList::BinSearch(
        /* in */  ItemType item,           // Item to be found
        /* out */ bool&     found,          // True if item is found
        /* out */ int&      position ) const // Location if found

// Searches list for item, returning the index of item if item was
// found.

// Precondition:
//      length <= INT_MAX / 2
//   && data[0..length-1] are in ascending order
// Postcondition:
//      IF item is in the list
//          found == true  &&  data[position] contains item
```

```
//      ELSE
//          found == false  &&  position is undefined

{
    int first = 0;              // Lower bound on list
    int last = length - 1;      // Upper bound on list
    int middle;                 // Middle index

    found = false;
    while (last >= first && !found)
    {
        middle = (first + last) / 2;
        if (item.LessThan(data[middle]))
            // Assert: item is not in data[middle..last]
            last = middle - 1;
        else if (data[middle].LessThan(item))
            // Assert: item is not in data[first..middle]
            first = middle + 1;
        else
            // Assert: item == data[middle]
            found = true;
    }
    if (found)
        position = middle;
}
```

TESTING   In order to test the list of class `Entry` items, we must create a another driver. The driver that incorporates calls to class `SortedList` is shown below. Entries are read in, inserted into the list, accessed one at a time and printed, compared to another entry, and deleted. The output screen from this driver is shown below the code.

```
//**************************************************************
// DRIVER for List of Entry class objects
// Four entries are read from the keyboard and inserted into the
// list of entries.  The entries are accessed one at a time and
// printed.  A time that is in the list is checked; a time that is
// not in the list is checked.  An item is deleted and the list is
// printed to show that the item is gone.
//**************************************************************

#include <iostream>
#include "SortedList.h"
using namespace std;
```

```cpp
int main()
{
    int limit;              // Number of items in the list
    Entry nameTime;
    SortedList list;
    for (int count = 1; count <= 3; count++) // Enter data
    {
        nameTime.ReadEntry();
        list.Insert(nameTime);
    }

    // Prepare and iterate through the list, printing items
    limit = list.Length();
    list.Reset();                           // Prepare for iteration
    for (int count = 0; count < limit; count++)
    {
        nameTime = list.GetNextItem();
        cout << "Name: " << nameTime.NameStr() << " Time: "
            << nameTime.TimeStr() << endl;
    }

    // Item is in the list
    if (list.IsPresent(nameTime))
        cout << nameTime.TimeStr() << " is not free." << endl;
    else
        cout << nameTime.TimeStr() << " is free. " << endl;

    // Item is not in the list
    Entry entry2("Nell", "Boylan", "Dale", 0, 0, 0);
    if (list.IsPresent(entry2))
        cout << entry2.TimeStr() << " is not free." << endl;
    else
        cout << entry2.TimeStr() << " is free. " << endl;

    // Delete and iterate through the list, printing items
    list.Delete(nameTime);
    list.Reset();                           // Prepare for iteration
    limit = list.Length();
    for (int count = 0; count < limit; count++)
    {
        nameTime = list.GetNextItem();
        cout << "Name: " << nameTime.NameStr() << " Time: "
            << nameTime.TimeStr() << endl;
    }
    return 0;
}
```

```
C:\PPSC++\EntryListTest.exe                                    _ □ ×
Enter first name: Sarah
Enter middle name: Jane
Enter last name: Jones
Enter hours (<= 23):
10
Enter minutes (<= 59):
30
Enter seconds (<= 59):
00
Enter first name: Susan
Enter middle name: Margaret
Enter last name: Smith
Enter hours (<= 23):
9
Enter minutes (<= 59):
30
Enter seconds (<= 59):
00
Enter first name: Judy
Enter middle name: Dale
Enter last name: David
Enter hours (<= 23):
3
Enter minutes (<= 59):
00
Enter seconds (<= 59):
0
Name: Judy David Time: 03:00:00
Name: Susan Smith Time: 09:30:00
Name: Sarah Jones Time: 10:30:00
10:30:00 is not free.
00:00:00 is free.
Name: Judy David Time: 03:00:00
Name: Susan Smith Time: 09:30:00
```

PROBLEM   As we keyed in the data for the driver, we realize that we have a problem. Class `Time` represents hours, minutes, and seconds; that is, it represents *active* time. To create or set or read a time, the user must enter hours, minutes, and seconds. There is an operation to increment time by one second. For our appointment calendar, we don't care about seconds or incrementing time by a second. Appointment times are different; they are *static* times. We are only interested in hours and minutes. How do we solve this problem? We could define a derived class and redefine the operations to work only with hours and minutes. However, this isn't the natural use for inheritance. A static time isn't a dynamic time *and more*. Let's just define a class `AptTime`, in which we remove the increment operation and change the other operations to just work with hours and minutes. Do we have to make corresponding changes in class `Entry`? Yes; we need to remove seconds from the constructor and the time string and change the Include statement. We leave the coding and testing of class `AptTime` to the Case Study Follow-Up Exercises.

Here is the screen shot from the same input, using `AptTime` rather than `Time`. The only difference is that the user is not prompted to enter seconds.

```
C:\PPSC++\EntryListTest.exe                                    _ □ ×
Enter first name: Sarah
Enter middle name: Jane
Enter last name: Jones
Enter hours (<= 23):
10
Enter minutes (<= 59):
30
Enter first name: Susan
Enter middle name: Margaret
Enter last name: Smith
Enter hours (<= 23):
9
Enter minutes (<= 59):
30
Enter first name: Judy
Enter middle name: Dale
Enter last name: David
Enter hours (<= 23):
3
Enter minutes (<= 59):
00
Name: Judy David Time: 03:00:00
Name: Susan Smith Time: 09:30:00
Name: Sarah Jones Time: 10:30:00
10:30:00 is not free.
00:00:00 is free.
Name: Judy David Time: 03:00:00
Name: Susan Smith Time: 09:30:00
```

Testing and Debugging

Testing and debugging an object-oriented program is largely a process of testing and debugging the C++ classes on which the program is built. The top-level driver also needs testing, but this testing is usually uncomplicated—OOD tends to result in a simple driver.

To review how to test a C++ class, you should refer back to the Testing and Debugging section of Chapter 11. There we walked through the process of testing each member function of a class. We made the observation that you could write a separate test driver for each member function or you could write just one test driver that tests all of the member functions. The latter approach is recommended only for classes that have a few simple member functions.

When an object-oriented program uses inheritance and composition, the order in which you test the classes is, in a sense, predetermined. If class X is derived from class Y or contains an object of class Y, you cannot test X until you have designed and implemented Y. Thus, it makes sense to test and debug the lower-level class (class Y) before testing class X. This chapter's Problem-Solving Case Study demonstrated this sequence of testing. We tested the lowest level class—the `Time` class—first. Next, we tested the `TimeCard` class, which contains a `Time` object. Finally, we tested the `TimeCardList` class, which contains an array of `TimeCard` objects. The general principle is that if class X is built on class Y (through inheritance or composition), the testing of X is simplified if Y is already tested and is known to behave correctly.

Testing and Debugging Hints

1. Review the Testing and Debugging Hints for Chapter 11. They apply to the design and testing of C++ classes, which are at the heart of OOP.

2. When using inheritance, don't forget to include the word `public` when declaring the derived class:

```
class DerivedClass : public BaseClass
{
    ⋮
};
```

The word `public` makes `BaseClass` a public base class of `DerivedClass`. That is, clients of `DerivedClass` can apply any public `BaseClass` operation (except constructors) to a `DerivedClass` object.

3. The header file containing the declaration of a derived class must `#include` the header file containing the declaration of the base class.

4. Although a derived class inherits the private and public members of its base class, it cannot directly access the inherited private members.

5. If a base class has a constructor, it is invoked before the body of the derived class's constructor is executed. If the base class constructor requires arguments, you must pass these `arguments` using a constructor initializer:

```
DerivedClass::DerivedClass( ... )
    : BaseClass(arg1, arg2)
{
    ⋮
}
```

If you do not include a constructor initializer, the base class's default constructor is invoked.

6. If a class has a member that is an object of another class and this member object's constructor requires arguments, you must pass these arguments using a constructor initializer:

```
SomeClass::SomeClass( ... )
    : memberObject(arg1, arg2)
{
    ⋮
}
```

If there is no constructor initializer, the member object's default constructor is invoked.

7. To obtain dynamic binding of an operation to an object when passing class objects as arguments, you must

- Pass the object by reference, not by value.
- Declare the operation to be `virtual` in the base class declaration.

8. If a base class declares a virtual function, it *must* implement that function even if the body is empty.

9. A derived class cannot redefine the function return type of a virtual function.

Summary

Object-oriented design (OOD) decomposes a problem into objects—self-contained entities in which data and operations are bound together. In OOD, data is treated as an active, rather than passive, quantity. Each object is responsible for one part of the solution, and the objects communicate by invoking each other's operations.

OOD begins by identifying potential objects and their operations. Examining objects in the problem domain is a good way to begin the process. The next step is to determine the relationships among the objects using inheritance (to express is-a relationships) and composition (to express has-a relationships). Finally, a driver algorithm is designed to coordinate the overall flow of control.

Object-oriented programming (OOP) is the process of implementing an object-oriented design by using language mechanisms for data abstraction, inheritance, and dynamic binding. Inheritance allows any programmer to take an existing class (the base class) and create a new class (the derived class) that inherits the data and operations of the base class. The derived class then specializes the base class by adding new private data, adding new operations, or reimplementing inherited operations—all without analyzing and modifying the implementation of the base class in any way. Dynamic binding of operations to objects allows objects of many different derived types to respond to a single function name, each in its own way. Together, inheritance and dynamic binding have been shown to reduce dramatically the time and effort required to customize existing ADTs. The result is truly reusable software components whose applications and lifetimes extend beyond those conceived of by the original creator.

Quick Check

1. How do structured programs differ from object-oriented programs in terms of the components that interact with each other to solve a problem? (pp. 724–726)
2. What are the three main facilities that are provided by an object-oriented language that enable object-oriented programming? (pp. 724–726)
3. Is a virtual function bound statically or dynamically? (pp. 750–754)
4. If you have a class called `Phone` and you want to extend it to support a country code, calling the new class `InternationalPhone`, how would you write the class heading for the new subclass? (pp. 731–734)

5. Suppose that in Quick Check 4, you wanted to create `InternationalPhone` as a separate class that contains an instance of `Phone`, rather than making it a subclass of phone. Describe how you would go about doing this. (pp. 742–749)
6. What are the three major steps in designing an object-oriented solution to a problem? (pp. 754–755)
7. Given a design for an object that lists the data that it contains and provides algorithms for the operations that it performs, what C++ construct would you use to represent the object, its data, and its operations? (pp. 726–727)

Answers

1. In a structured program, functions interact with one another and with the data in the program. In an object-oriented program, objects (which bind operations and data together) are the components that interact. 2. Data abstraction, inheritance, and dynamic binding. 3. Dynamically. 4. `class InternationalPhone : public Phone` 5. By placing a member field within `InternationalPhone` that is of class `Phone`. 6. Identify the objects and operations, determine the relationships among the objects, design the driver. 7. The object would be represented by a class. Its data would be represented by member fields of the class. The object's operations would be represented by member functions of the class.

Exam Preparation Exercises

1. Match the following terms with the definitions given below.
   a. Structured program
   b. Object-oriented program
   c. Inheritance
   d. Superclass
   e. Subclass
   f. Composition
   g. Static binding
   h. Dynamic binding
   i. Polymorphic
      i. Determining, at run time, from which class to call a function.
      ii. A class from which properties are acquired.
      iii. A collection of classes designed using abstraction, inheritance, and polymorphism.
      iv. An operation that has different meanings depending on its binding to an object.
      v. Including an object of one class within another class.
      vi. A class that acquires properties from another class.
      vii. Determining, at compile time, from which class to call a function.
      viii. A collection of functions, designed using functional decomposition.
      ix. Acquiring the properties of another class.
2. Structured programming is better suited to developing small programs while object-oriented programming is better for writing large programs. True or false?
3. Inheritance allows us to reuse functions from a base class, and add new functions. But we cannot replace functions in the base class with new implementations. True or false?

4. To solve the slicing problem we use a combination of pass-by-reference and virtual functions? True or false?

5. If we want a function to be virtual, where do we write the keyword? In the base class declaration file, in the base class definition file, in the derived class declaration file, or in the derived class definition file?

6. What C++ language mechanism implements composition?

7. Suppose you have a subclass that contains several data members that are not defined in its superclass. What happens to those data members if you assign an object of the subclass to a variable of the superclass?

8. A client is supplied with the following declaration for a base class and a derived class.

```
class BaseClass
{
public:
    void PrintFields() const;
    ⋮
};


class DerivedClass : BaseClass
{
public:
    void NewFunction();
    DerivedClass( /* in */ int StartValue);
    ⋮
};
```

So, the client writes the following code to call the constructor for an object of type DerivedClass, and then prints the fields in the newly created object.

```
DerivedClass anObject(10);
anObject.PrintFields();
```

But the compiler reports an error for the second statement. What's wrong? How would you fix this problem?

9. Consider the following base and derived class declarations.

```
class BaseClass
{
public:
    void BaseAlpha();
private:
    void BaseBeta();
    float baseField;
};


class DerivedClass : public BaseClass
{
```

```
public:
    void DerivedAlpha();
    void DerivedBeta();
private:
    int derivedField;
};
```

For each class, do the following:
a. List all private data members.
b. List all private data members that the class's member functions can reference directly.
c. List all functions that the class's member functions can invoke.
d. List all member functions that a client of the class may invoke.

10. A class called `DerivedClass` is a subclass of a class called `BaseClass`. `DerivedClass` also has a member field that is an object of class `ComposedClass`.
   a. Which class's constructor is called first when an object of class `DerivedClass` is created?
   b. Which class's constructor is called last when an object of class `DerivedClass` is created?

11. Why does slicing occur with pass-by-value but not with pass-by-reference when a derived class object is being passed to a parameter of its base class?

12. What's wrong with the following class declarations?

```
class BaseClass
{
public:
    virtual void BaseAlpha();
private:
    float baseField;
};

class DerivedClass : public BaseClass
{
public:
    virtual void BaseAlpha();
private:
    int derivedField;
};
```

13. Explain the difference between an *is-a* relationship and a *has-a* relationship.

14. When we code a derived class in separate files, which of the following do we do?
   a. Include the base class specification and implementation file in both the derived class specification file and its implementation files.
   b. Include the base class specification file in the derived class specification file, and include the base class implementation file in the derived class implementation file.

c. Include the base class specification file in the derived class specification file.
d. Include the base class implementation file in the derived class implementation file.

Programming Warm-Up Exercises

1. Given the following declaration for a test score class, write a derived class declaration called `IDScore` that adds an integer student ID number as a private member, and that supplies a constructor that has parameters corresponding to the three member fields, and an observer that returns the ID number.

```
class TestScore
{
public:
    TestScore(/* in */ string name,
              /* in */ int score);
    string GetName() const;
    int GetScore() const;
private:
    string studentName;
    int studentScore;
};
```

2. Write the implementation file for the `TestScore` class in Exercise 1. The constructor just assigns its parameters to the private data members, and the observers simply return the corresponding member.

3. Write the implementation file for the `IDScore` class in Exercise 1. The constructor just assigns its parameters to the private data members, and the observer simply returns the corresponding member.

4. Write the specification file for a class called `Exam` that uses composition to create an array of 100 objects of class `IDScore` as defined in Exercise 1. The class can use the default constructor, and will have a function that assigns an `IDScore` object to a location in the array, given the object and the location as parameters. The class should also have an observer that returns the `IDScore` object at the position specified by its parameter.

5. Write the implementation file for class `Exam` as defined in Exercise 4.

6. The following class represents a telephone number in the United States.

```
// SPECIFICATION FILE (phone.h)

enum PhoneType (HOME, OFFICE, CELL, FAX, PAGE);

class Phone
{
public:
    Phone( /* in */ int newAreaCode,
           /* in */ int newNumber,
```

```
            /* in   */ PhoneType newType);
    void Write () const;
private:
    int areaCode;
    int number;
    PhoneType type;
}
```

Using inheritance, we want to derive an international phone number class, InternPhone, from the Phone class. For this exercise, we assume that the only change necessary is to add a country code (an integer) that identifies the country or region. The public operations of InternPhone are Write, which reimplements the Write function from the base class, and a class constructor that takes four parameters corresponding to the four member fields in the class. Write the class declaration for the InternPhone class.

7. Implement the InternPhone class constructor as described in Exercise 6.

8. Implement the Write function of the InternPhone class as described in Exercise 6.

9. Write a global function WritePhone that takes a single parameter and uses dynamic binding to print either a U.S. phone number (Phone class) or an international phone number (InternPhone class). Make the necessary change(s) in the declaration of the Phone class from Exercise 6 so that WritePhone executes correctly.

10. Given the following declaration for a class that represents a computer in a company's inventory, write a derived class declaration (for a class called InstallRecord) that adds a string field representing the location of the computer, and a field of class SimpleDate that holds the installation date. The new class should provide observers for each of the new fields. It should also reimplement the Write function.

```
class Computer
{
public:
    Computer(
        /* in */ string newName,
        /* in */ string newBrand,
        /* in */ string newModel,
        /* in */ int    newSpeed,
        /* in */ string newSerial,
        /* in */ int    newNumber);
    string GetName() const;
    string GetBrand() const;
    string GetModel() const;
    int GetSpeed() const;
    string GetSerial() const;
    int GetNumber() const;
    void Write() const;
```

```
private:
    string name;
    string brand;
    string model;
    int speed;
    string serialNumber;
    int inventoryNumber;
};
```

11. Implement the constructor for the `Computer` class declared in Exercise 10.
12. Implement the constructor for the `InstallRecord` class declared in Exercise 10.
13. Implement the `Write` function for the `Computer` class declared in Exercise 10. It should output each member field on a separate line.
14. Implement the Write function for the `InstallRecord` class declared in Exercise 10. It should output each member field on a separate line. Assume that the `SimpleDate` class provides a `void` function called `Write()` that outputs the date in a standard format.
15. Expand class `ExtTime` by redefining function `ReadTime`.

Programming Problems

1. Use object-oriented programming to develop a game application that simulates a roulette table. The roulette table has 36 numbers (1 to 36) that are arranged in three columns of 12 rows. The first row has the numbers 1 through 3, the second row contains 4 through 6, and so on. There is also a number 0 that is outside of the table of numbers. The numbers in the table are colored red and black (0 is green). The red numbers are 1, 3, 5, 7, 9, 12, 14, 16, 18, 19, 21, 23, 25, 27, 30, 32, 34, 36. The other half of the numbers are black. In a simplified set of rules, players can bet on an individual number (including 0), the red numbers, the black numbers, the even numbers, the odd numbers, the numbers 1 to 18, the numbers 19 to 36, and any of the columns or rows in the table.

   The user should be allowed to enter one of the bets, and the application uses the `rand` function from `<cstdlib>` as the basis for computing the number that would be rolled on the wheel. It then compares this number to the bet, and reports whether it won or lost. The process repeats until the user enters a quit command.

2. Use object-oriented programming to develop an extension to the application of Problem 1. The new application also should allow the user to enter an initial amount of money into an account. In addition to placing a bet, the user specifies an amount to go with the bet. The amount is deducted from the account. Any winnings are added to the account. The current winnings or losses (difference from the original amount) should be displayed in addition to the value of the account. Winnings are computed as follows:

Single number bets pay 36 times the amount placed
Row bets pay 12 times
Column bets pay 3 times
Odd/Even, Red/Black, High/Low half bets pay 2 times the amount

The user should not be allowed to bet more than is in the account.

3. Use object-oriented programming to develop a game application that plays the children's game of rock, paper, scissors. The user enters a letter, indicating their choice. When a choice is entered, the `rand` function from `<cstdlib>` is used to pick a value in the range of 1 through 3, with 1 corresponding to rock, 2 corresponding to paper, and 3 corresponding to scissors. The computer's choice is compared to the user's choice according to the rules: rock breaks scissors, scissors cut paper, paper covers rock. Choices that match are ties. Output a count of the wins by the user and the computer, and of the ties. The application ends when the user enters an invalid choice.

4. Use object-oriented programming to develop an extension to the application of Problem 3. The new application should accept either the original single letter, or the full words (rock, paper, scissors). The capitalization of the words should not matter. The extended application also should end only when the user enters "q" or "quit" as a choice and should prompt the user for one of the valid choices if an invalid value is entered.

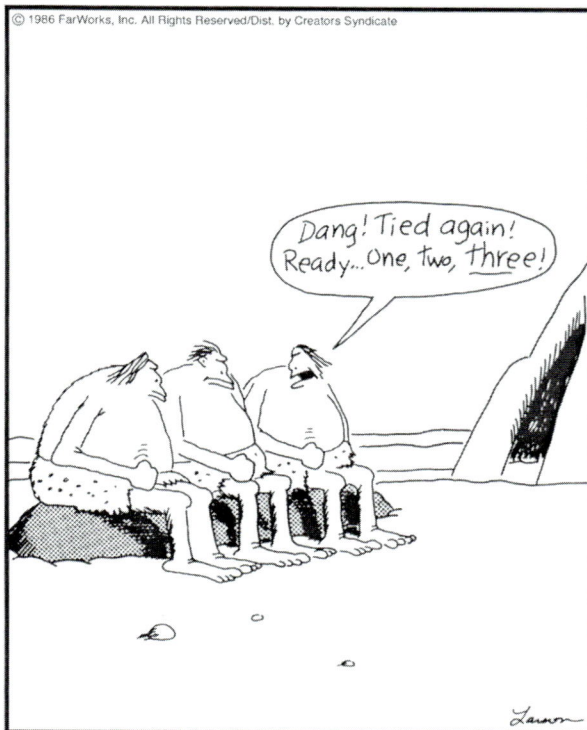

THE FAR SIDE®   By GARY LARSON

Before paper and scissors

5. Use the `Computer` and `InstallRecord` classes declared in Programming Warm-Up Exercises 10 to 14, together with the `SortedList` class developed in Chapter 13 as the basis for an object-oriented program that keeps track of a company's computer inventory. The company has at most 500 computers. Operations that should be supported are:

Add a new computer to the list.
Delete a computer from the list.
Change the location of a computer.
Print a list of all computers in inventory-number order.
Print a list of all computers in a given location.
Print a list of all computers of a particular brand.
Print a list of all computers installed before a given date.

The application should keep the list sorted by inventory number. It should read an initial list from a file called `original.dat`. At the end of processing, it should write the current data in the list onto a file called `update.dat` in a format that could be read back in by the program as an initial list. You will also need to develop the `SimpleDate` class to the degree necessary to support the application.

Case Study Follow-Up

1. Implement and test class `AptTime`.
2. It is not appropriate for `AptTime` (a static time) to inherit from `Time` (an active time). Would it be appropriate for an active time to inherit from a static time? Explain.
3. As you look at the output from the driver, you see that the times look strange. 03:00 certainly is technically less than 09:30, but surely the appointment time is 03:00 in the afternoon and should come after 09:30. The time is specified as a 24-hour clock. We could tell the user to enter the times on a 24-hour basis or we could change class `AptTime` to have an additional field that contains PM or AM or we could derive a class from AptTime that has a PM or AM field. Think about this solution and outline what would have to be changed to implement time on a 12-hour clock.
4. Implement your solution to Problem 3.
5. Write a driver and test the new class developed in Problem 4.
6. Substitute the new class from Problem 4 into the driver for the Case Study and rerun that test.

Pointers, Dynamic Data, and Reference Types

Knowledge Goals

- *To understand how pointers can be used to improve program efficiency.*
- *To understand the difference between deep and shallow copy operations.*
- *To understand how C++ defines the term initialization.*
- *To know and understand the four member functions that should be present in any class that manipulates dynamic data.*

Skill Goals

To be able to:

- *Declare variables of pointer types.*
- *Take the addresses of variables and access the variables through pointers.*
- *Write an expression that selects a member of a class, struct, or union that is pointed to by a pointer.*
- *Create and access dynamic data.*
- *Destroy dynamic data.*
- *Declare and initialize variables of reference types.*
- *Access variables that are referenced by reference types.*

Goals

In the preceding chapters, we have looked at the simple types and structured types available in C++. There are only two built-in data types left to cover: **pointer types** and reference types (see Figure 15–1). These types are simple data types, yet in Figure 15–1 we list them separately from the other simple types because their purpose is so special. We refer to pointer types and reference types as *address types*. A variable of one of these types does not contain a data value; it contains the *memory address* of another variable or structure. Address types have two main purposes: They can make a program more efficient—either in terms of speed or in terms of memory usage—and they can be used to build complex data structures. In this chapter, we demonstrate how they make a program more efficient. Chapter 16 explains how to build complex structures using address types.

> **Pointer type**   A simple data type consisting of an unbounded set of values, each of which addresses or otherwise indicates the location of a variable of a given type. Among the operations defined on pointer variables are assignment and testing for equality.

15.1 Pointers

In many ways, we've saved the best till last. Pointer types are the most interesting data types of all. Pointers are what their name implies: variables that tell where to find something else; that is, pointers contain the addresses or locations of other variables.

Let's begin this discussion by looking at how pointer variables are declared in C++.

Pointer Variables

Surprisingly, the word *pointer* isn't used in declaring pointer variables; the symbol * is used instead. The declaration

```
int* intPtr;
```

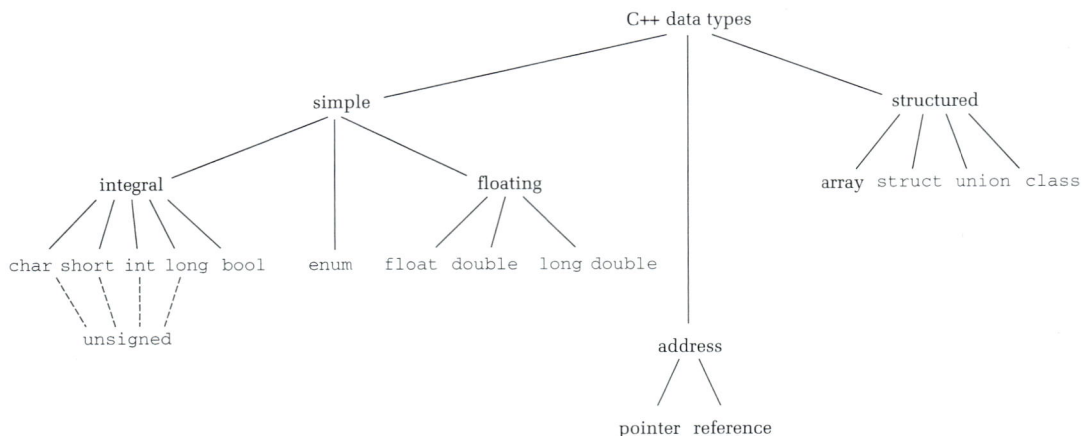

Figure 15–1   *C++ Data Types*

states that `intPtr` is a variable that can point to (that is, contain the address of) an `int` variable. Here is the syntax template for declaring pointer variables:

PointerVariableDeclaration

```
 ┌ DataType* Variable ;
 ┤
 └ DataType *Variable , *Variable . . . ;
```

The syntax template shows two forms, one for declaring a single variable and the other for declaring several variables. In the first form, the compiler does not care where the asterisk is placed. Both of the following declarations are equivalent:

```
int* intPtr;
int *intPtr;
```

Although C++ programmers use both styles, we prefer the first. Attaching the asterisk to the data type name instead of the variable name readily suggests that `intPtr` is of type "pointer to `int`."

According to the syntax template, if you declare several variables in one statement you must precede each variable name with an asterisk. Otherwise, only the first variable is taken to be a pointer variable. The compiler interprets the statement

```
int* p, q;
```

as if it were written

```
int* p;
int  q;
```

To avoid unintended errors when declaring pointer variables, it is safest to declare each variable in a separate statement.

Given the declarations

```
int  beta;
int* intPtr;
```

we can make `intPtr` point to `beta` by using the unary `&` operator, which is called the *address-of* operator. At run time, the assignment statement

```
intPtr = &beta;
```

MEMORY

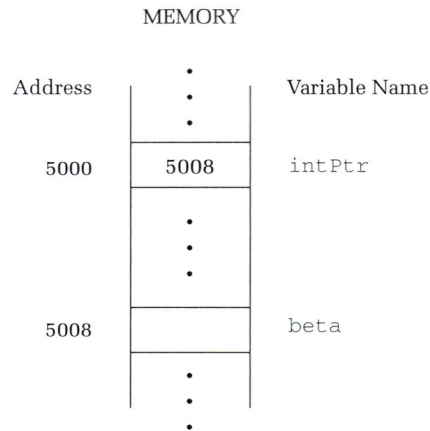

Figure 15–2   *Machine-Level View of a Pointer Variable*

takes the memory address of `beta` and stores it into `intPtr`. Alternatively, we could initialize `intPtr` in its declaration as follows:

```
int   beta;
int*  intPtr = &beta;
```

Suppose that `intPtr` and `beta` happen to be located at memory addresses 5000 and 5008, respectively. Then storing the address of `beta` into `intPtr` results in the relationship pictured in Figure 15–2.

Because actual numeric addresses are generally unknown to the C++ programmer, it is more common to display the relationship between a pointer and a pointed-to variable by using rectangles and arrows as in Figure 15–3.

To access a variable that a pointer points to, we use the unary `*` operator—the *dereference* or *indirection* operator. The expression

```
*intPtr
```

denotes the variable pointed to by `intPtr`. In our example, `intPtr` currently points to `beta`, so the statement

```
*intPtr = 28;
```

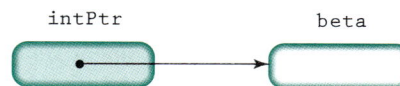

Figure 15–3   *Abstract Diagram of a Pointer Variable*

dereferences `intPtr` and stores the value 28 into `beta`. This statement represents **indirect addressing** of `beta`; the machine first accesses `intPtr`, then uses its contents to locate `beta`. In contrast, the statement

> **Indirect addressing** Accessing a variable in two steps by first using a pointer that gives the location of the variable.
>
> **Direct addressing** Accessing a variable in one step by using the variable name.

```
beta = 28;
```

represents **direct addressing** of `beta`. Direct addressing is like opening a post office box (P.O. Box 15, for instance) and finding a package, whereas indirect addressing is like opening P.O. Box 15 and finding a note that says your package is sitting in P.O. Box 23.

Continuing with our example, if we execute the statements

```
*intPtr = 28;
cout << intPtr << endl;
cout << *intPtr << endl;
```

then the output is

```
5008
28
```

The first output statement prints the contents of `intPtr` (5008); the second prints the contents of the variable pointed to by `intPtr` (28).

Let's look at a more involved example of declaring pointers, taking addresses, and dereferencing pointers. The following program fragment declares several types and variables. In this code, the `TimeType` class is the C++ class we developed in Chapter 11, with member functions `Set`, `Increment`, `Write`, `Equal`, and `LessThan`.

```
#include "timetype.h"    // For TimeType class
   ⋮
enum ColorType {RED, GREEN, BLUE};
struct PatientRec
{
    int idNum;
    int height;
    int weight;
};

int         alpha;
ColorType   color;
PatientRec  patient;
TimeType    startTime(8, 30, 0);

int*        intPtr = &alpha;
```

```
ColorType*   colorPtr = &color;
PatientRec*  patientPtr = &patient;
TimeType*    timePtr = &startTime;
```

The variables `intPtr`, `colorPtr`, `patientPtr`, and `timePtr` are all pointer variables. `intPtr` points to (contains the address of) a variable of type `int`, `colorPtr` points to a variable of type `Color`, `patientPtr` points to a struct variable of type `PatientRec`, and `timePtr` points to a class object of type `TimeType`.

The expression `*intPtr` denotes the variable pointed to by `intPtr`. The pointed-to variable can contain any `int` value. The expression `*colorPtr` denotes a variable of type `ColorType`. It can contain RED, GREEN, or BLUE. The expression `*patientPtr` denotes a struct variable of type `PatientRec`. Furthermore, the expressions `(*patientPtr).idNum`, `(*patientPtr).height`, and `(*patientPtr).weight` denote the `idNum`, `height`, and `weight` members of `*patientPtr`. Notice how the accessing expression is built.

`patientPtr`	A pointer variable of type "pointer to `PatientRec`."
`*patientPtr`	A struct variable of type `PatientRec`.
`(*patientPtr).weight`	The `weight` member of a struct variable of type `PatientRec`.

The expression `(*patientPtr).weight` is a mixture of pointer dereferencing and struct member selection. The parentheses are necessary because the dot operator has higher precedence than the dereference operator (see Appendix B for C++ operator precedence). Without the parentheses, the expression `*patientPtr.weight` would be interpreted wrongly as `*(patientPtr.weight)`.

When a pointer points to a struct (or a class or a union) variable, enclosing the pointer dereference within parentheses can become tedious. In addition to the dot operator, C++ provides another member selection operator: `->`. This *arrow operator* consists of two consecutive symbols: a hyphen and a greater-than symbol. By definition,

   PointerExpression -> MemberName

is equivalent to

   (*PointerExpression).MemberName

Therefore, we can write `(*patientPtr).weight` as `patientPtr->weight`.

The general guideline for choosing between the two member selection operators (dot and arrow) is the following:

> Use the dot operator if the first operand denotes a struct, class, or union variable; use the arrow operator if the first operand denotes a *pointer* to a struct, class, or union variable.

If we want to increment and print the `TimeType` class object pointed to by `timePtr`, we could use either the statements

```
(*timePtr).Increment();
(*timePtr).Write();
```

or the statements

```
timePtr->Increment();
timePtr->Write();
```

And if we had declared an array of pointers

```
PatientRec* patPtrArray[20];
```

and initialized the array elements, then we could access the `idNum` member of the fourth patient as follows:

```
patPtrArray[3]->idNum
```

Pointed-to variables can be used in the same way as any other variable. The following statements are all valid:

```
*intPtr = 250;
*colorPtr = RED;
patientPtr->idNum = 3245;
patientPtr->height = 64;
patientPtr->weight = 114;
patPtrArray[3]->idNum = 6356;
patPtrArray[3]->height = 73;
patPtrArray[3]->weight = 185;
```

Figure 15–4 shows the results of these assignments.

At this point, you may be wondering why we should use pointers at all. Instead of making `intPtr` point to `alpha` and storing 250 into `*intPtr`, why not just store 250 directly into `alpha`? The truth is that there is no good reason to program this way; on the contrary, the examples we have shown would make a program more roundabout and confusing. The major use of pointers in C++ is to manipulate *dynamic variables*—variables that come into existence at execution time only as they are needed. Later in the chapter, we show how to use pointers to create dynamic variables. In the meantime, let's continue with some of the basic aspects of pointers themselves.

Pointer Expressions

You learned in the early chapters that an arithmetic expression is made up of variables, constants, operator symbols, and parentheses. Similarly, pointer expressions are composed of pointer variables, pointer constants, certain allowable operators, and parentheses. We have already discussed pointer variables—variables that hold addresses of other variables. Let's look now at pointer constants.

In C++, there is only one literal pointer constant: the value 0. The pointer constant 0, called the *null pointer,* points to absolutely nothing. The statement

```
intPtr = 0;
```

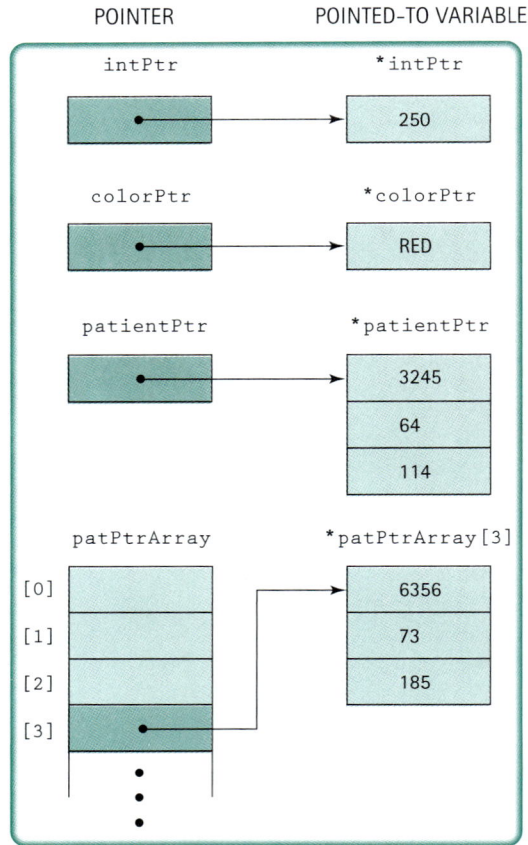

Figure 15–4 *Results of Assignment Statements*

stores the null pointer into `intPtr`. This statement does *not* cause `intPtr` to point to memory location zero; the null pointer is guaranteed to be distinct from any actual memory address. Because the null pointer does not point to anything, we diagram the null pointer as follows, instead of using an arrow to point somewhere:

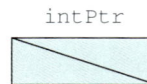

Instead of using the constant 0, many programmers prefer to use the named constant `NULL` that is supplied by the standard header file `cstddef`:

```
#include <cstddef>
    ⋮
intPtr = NULL;
```

As with any named constant, the identifier NULL makes a program more self-document-ing. Its use also reduces the chance of confusing the null pointer with the integer con-stant 0.

It is an error to dereference the null pointer, as it does not point to anything. The null pointer is used only as a special value that a program can test for:

```
if (intPtr == NULL)
    DoSomething();
```

We'll see examples of using the null pointer later in this chapter and in Chapter 16.

Although 0 is the only literal constant of pointer type, there is another pointer expression that is considered to be a constant pointer expression: an array name with-out any index brackets. The value of this expression is the base address (the address of the first element) of the array. Given the declarations

```
int   arr[100];
int* ptr;
```

the assignment statement

```
ptr = arr;
```

has exactly the same effect as

```
ptr = &arr[0];
```

Both of these statements store the base address of arr into ptr.

Although we did not explain it at the time, you have already used the fact that an array name without brackets is a pointer expression. Consider the following code, which calls a ZeroOut function to zero out an array whose size is given as the second argument:

```
int main()
{
    float velocity[30];
      ⋮
    ZeroOut(velocity, 30);
      ⋮
}
```

In the function call, the first argument—an array name without index brackets—is a pointer expression. The value of this expression is the base address of the velocity array. This base address is passed to the function. We can write the ZeroOut function in one of two ways. The first approach—one that you have seen many times—declares the first parameter to be an array of unspecified size.

```
void ZeroOut( /* out */ float arr[],
              /* in */  int   size )
{
    int i;

    for (i = 0; i < size; i++)
        arr[i] = 0.0;
}
```

Alternatively, we can declare the parameter to be of type `float*`, because the parameter simply holds the address of a `float` variable (the address of the first array element).

```
void ZeroOut( /* out */ float* arr,
              /* in */  int   size )
{
    ⋮   // Function body is unchanged
}
```

Whether we declare the parameter as `float arr[]` or as `float* arr`, the result is exactly the same to the C++ compiler: Within the `ZeroOut` function, `arr` is a simple variable that points to the beginning of the caller's actual array (see Figure 15–5).

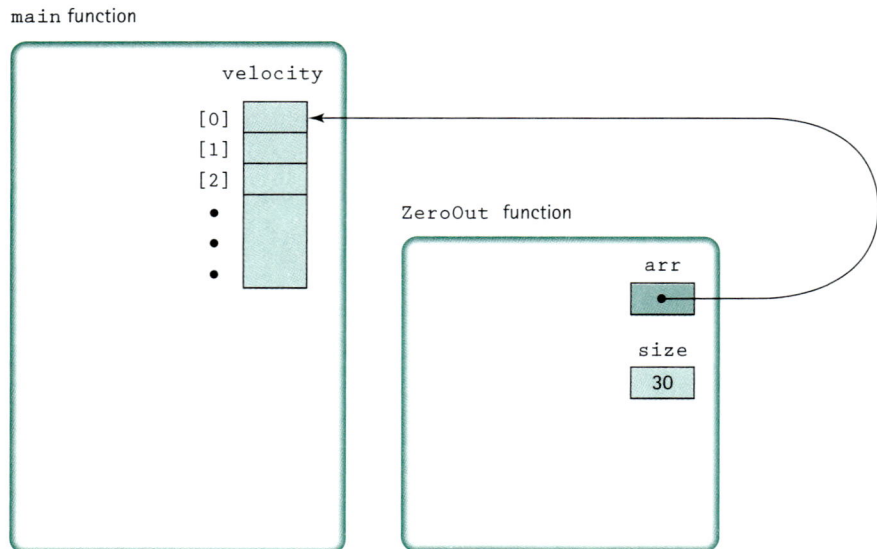

Figure 15–5   *A Parameter Pointing to the Caller's Argument*

Even though `arr` is a pointer variable within the `ZeroOut` function, we are still allowed to attach an index expression to the name `arr`:

```
arr[i] = 0.0;
```

Indexing a pointer variable is made possible by the following rule in C++:

> Indexing is valid for *any* pointer expression, not only an array name. (However, indexing a pointer makes sense only if the pointer points to an array.)

We have now seen four C++ operators that are valid for pointers: =, *, ->, and [].
The following table lists the most common operations that may be applied to pointers.

Operator	Meaning	Example	Remarks
=	Assignment	`ptr = &someVar;` `ptr1 = ptr2;` `ptr = 0;`	Except for the null pointer, both operands must be of the same data type.
*	Dereference	`*ptr`	
==, !=, <, <=, > and >=	Relational operators	`ptr1 == ptr2`	The two operands must be of the same data type.
!	Logical NOT	`!ptr`	The result is `true` if the operand is 0 (the null pointer), else the result is `false`.
[]	Index (or subscript)	`ptr[4]`	The indexed pointer should point to an array.
->	Member selection	`ptr->height`	Selects a member of the class, struct, or union variable that is pointed to.

Notice that the logical NOT operator can be used to test for the null pointer:

```
if ( !ptr )
    DoSomething();
```

Some people find this notation confusing because `ptr` is a pointer expression, not a Boolean expression. We prefer to phrase the test this way for clarity:

```
if (ptr == NULL)
    DoSomething();
```

When looking at the table, it is important to keep in mind that the operations listed are operations on pointers, *not* on the pointed-to variables. For example, if `intPtr1` and `intPtr2` are variables of type `int*`, the test

```
if (intPtr1 == intPtr2)
```

compares the pointers, not what they point to. In other words, we are comparing memory addresses, not ints. To compare the integers that intPtr1 and intPtr2 point to, we would need to write

```
if (*intPtr1 == *intPtr2)
```

In addition to the operators we have listed in the table, the following C++ operators may be applied to pointers: ++, --, +, -, +=, and -=. These operators perform arithmetic on pointers that point to arrays. For example, the expression ptr++ causes ptr to point to the next element of the array, regardless of the size in bytes of each array element. And the expression ptr + 5 accesses the array element that is five elements beyond the one currently pointed to by ptr. We'll say no more about these operators or about pointer arithmetic; the topic of pointer arithmetic is off the main track of what we want to emphasize in this chapter. Instead, we proceed now to explore one of the most important uses of pointers: the creation of dynamic data.

15.2 Dynamic Data

In Chapter 8, we described two categories of program data in C++: static data and automatic data. Any global variable is static, as is any local variable explicitly declared as static. The lifetime of a static variable is the lifetime of the entire program. In contrast, an automatic variable—a local variable not declared as static—is allocated (created) when control reaches its declaration and deallocated (destroyed) when control exits the block in which the variable is declared.

> **Dynamic data** Variables created during execution of a program by means of special operations. In C++, these operations are new and delete.

With the aid of pointers, C++ provides a third category of program data: **dynamic data**. Dynamic variables are not declared with ordinary variable declarations; they are explicitly allocated and deallocated at execution time by means of two special operators, new and delete. When a program requires an additional variable, it uses new to allocate the variable. When the program no longer needs the variable, it uses delete to deallocate it. The lifetime of a dynamic variable is therefore the time between the execution of new and the execution of delete. The advantage of being able to create new variables at execution time is that we don't have to create any more of them than we need.

The new operation has two forms, one for allocating a single variable and one for allocating an array. Here is the syntax template:

AllocationExpression

```
{ new DataType

  new DataType [ IntExpression ]
```

The first form is used for creating a single variable of type DataType. The second form creates an array whose elements are of type DataType; the desired number of array elements is given by IntExpression. Here is an example that demonstrates both forms of the `new` operation:

```
int*  intPtr;
char* nameStr;
```

`intPtr = new int;`	Creates a variable of type `int` and stores its address into `intPtr`.
`nameStr = new char[6];`	Creates a six-element `char` array and stores the base address of the array into `nameStr`.

Normally, the `new` operator does two things: It creates an uninitialized variable (or an array) of the designated type, and it returns a pointer to this variable (or the base address of an array). However, if the computer system has run out of space available for dynamic data, the program terminates with an error message.*

Variables created by `new` are said to be on the **free store** (or **heap**), a region of memory set aside for dynamic variables. The `new` operator obtains a chunk of memory from the free store, and, as we will see, the `delete` operator returns it to the free store.

> **Free store (heap)** A pool of memory locations reserved for allocation and deallocation of dynamic data.

A dynamic variable is unnamed and cannot be directly addressed. It must be indirectly addressed through the pointer returned by the `new` operator. Below is an example of creating dynamic data and then accessing the data through pointers. The code begins by initializing the pointer variables in their declarations.

```
#include <cstring>    // For strcpy()
    ⋮
int*  intPtr = new int;
char* nameStr = new char[6];

*intPtr = 357;
strcpy(nameStr, "Ben");
```

---

*Technically, if the `new` operator finds that no more memory is available, it generates what is called a `bad_alloc` exception–a topic we cover in Chapter 17. Unless we write additional program code to deal explicitly with this `bad_alloc` exception, the program simply terminates with a message such as "ABNORMAL PROGRAM TERMINATION."

In pre-standard C++, an entirely different approach was used. If `new` found no more memory available, it returned the null pointer rather than a pointer to a newly allocated object. The code invoking `new` could then test the returned pointer to see whether the allocation succeeded.

Recall from Chapter 13 that the `strcpy` library function requires two arguments, each being the base address of a `char` array. For the first argument, we are passing the base address of the dynamic array on the free store. For the second argument, the compiler passes the base address of the anonymous array where the C string "Ben" (including the terminating null character) is located. Figures 15-6a and 15-6b picture the effect of executing this code segment.

Dynamic data can be destroyed at any time during the execution of a program when it is no longer needed. The built-in operator `delete` is used to destroy a dynamic variable. The `delete` operation has two forms, one for deleting a single variable, the other for deleting an array:

DeallocationExpression

{
delete Pointer

delete [ ] Pointer
}

a. `int*   intPtr = new int;`
   `char* nameStr = new char[6];`

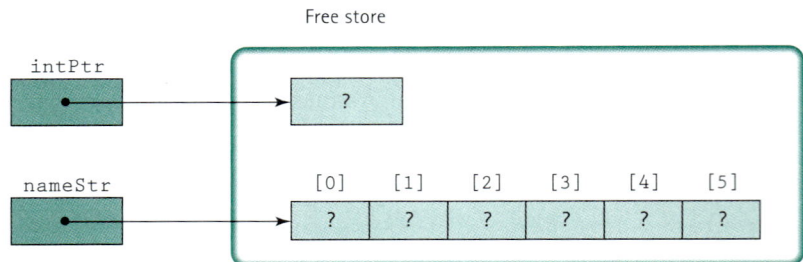

Free store

intPtr

?

nameStr

[0]	[1]	[2]	[3]	[4]	[5]
?	?	?	?	?	?

b. `*intPtr = 357;`
   `strcpy(nameStr, "Ben");`

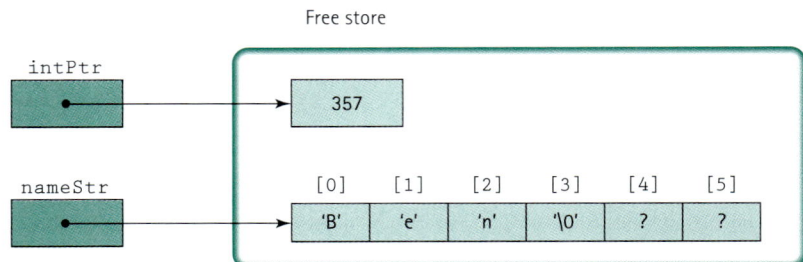

Free store

intPtr

357

nameStr

[0]	[1]	[2]	[3]	[4]	[5]
'B'	'e'	'n'	'\0'	?	?

Figure 15-6 *Allocating Dynamic Data on the Free Store*

Using the previous example, we can deallocate the dynamic data pointed to by `intPtr` and `nameStr` with the following statements.

`delete intPtr;`	Returns the variable pointed to by `intPtr` to the free store to be used again. The value of `intPtr` is then undefined.
`delete [] nameStr;`	Returns the array pointed to by `nameStr` to the free store to be used again. The value of `nameStr` is then undefined.*

After execution of these statements, the values of `intPtr` and `nameStr` are undefined; they may or may not still point to the deallocated data. Before using these pointers again, you must assign new values to them (that is, store new memory addresses into them).

Until you gain experience with the `new` and `delete` operators, it is important to pronounce the statement

```
delete intPtr;
```

accurately. Instead of saying "Delete `intPtr`," it is better to say "Delete the variable *pointed to* by `intPtr`." The `delete` operation does not delete the pointer; it deletes the pointed-to variable.

When using the `delete` operator, you should keep two rules in mind.

1. Applying `delete` to the null pointer does no harm; the operation simply has no effect.

2. Excepting rule 1, the `delete` operator must only be applied to a pointer value that was obtained previously from the `new` operator.

The second rule is important to remember. If you apply `delete` to an arbitrary memory address that is not in the free store, the result is undefined and could prove to be very unpleasant.

Finally, remember that a major reason for using dynamic data is to economize on memory space. The `new` operator lets you create variables only as they are needed. When you are finished using a dynamic variable, you should `delete` it. It is counterproductive to keep dynamic variables when they are no longer needed—a situation known as a **memory leak**. If this is done too often, you may run out of memory.

> **Memory leak**   The loss of available memory space that occurs when dynamic data is allocated but never deallocated.

_____

*The syntax for deallocating an array, `delete [] nameStr`, may not be accepted by some prestandard compilers. Early versions of the C++ language required the array size to be included within the brackets: `delete [6] nameStr`. If your compiler complains about the empty brackets, include the array size.

Let's look at another example of using dynamic data.

```
int* ptr1 = new int;     // Create a dynamic variable
int* ptr2 = new int;     // Create a dynamic variable

*ptr2 = 44;              // Assign a value to a dynamic variable
*ptr1 = *ptr2;           // Copy one dynamic variable to another
ptr1 = ptr2;             // Copy one pointer to another
delete ptr2;             // Destroy a dynamic variable
```

Here is a more detailed description of the effect of each statement:

`int* ptr1 = new int;`	Creates a pair of dynamic variables of type `int` and stores their locations into `ptr1` and `ptr2`.
`int* ptr2 = new int;`	The values of the dynamic variables are undefined even though the pointer variables now have values (see Figure 15–7a).
`*ptr2 = 44;`	Stores the value 44 into the dynamic variable pointed to by `ptr2` (see Figure 15–7b).
`*ptr1 = *ptr2;`	Copies the contents of the dynamic variable `*ptr2` to the dynamic variable `*ptr1` (see Figure 15–7c).
`ptr1 = ptr2;`	Copies the contents of the pointer variable `ptr2` to the pointer variable `ptr1` (see Figure 15–7d).
`delete ptr2;`	Returns the dynamic variable `*ptr2` back to the free store to be used again. The value of `ptr2` is undefined (see Figure 15–7e).

In Figure 15–7d, notice that the variable pointed to by `ptr1` before the assignment statement is still there. It cannot be accessed, however, because no pointer is pointing to it. This isolated variable is called an **inaccessible object**. Leaving inaccessible objects on the free store should be considered a logic error and is a cause of memory leaks.

> **Inaccessible object** A dynamic variable on the free store without any pointer pointing to it.
>
> **Dangling pointer** A pointer that points to a variable that has been deallocated.

Notice also that in Figure 15–7e `ptr1` is now pointing to a variable that, in principle, no longer exists. We call `ptr1` a **dangling pointer**. If the program later dereferences `ptr1`, the result is unpredictable. The pointed-to value might still be the original one (44), or it might be a different value stored there as a result of reusing that space on the free store.

Both situations shown in Figure 15–7e—an inaccessible object and a dangling pointer—can be avoided by deallocating `*ptr1` before assigning `ptr2` to `ptr1`, and by setting `ptr1` to NULL after deallocating `*ptr2`. (See the code on page 798.)

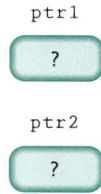

INITIAL CONDITIONS

a. `int* ptr1 = new int;`
   `int* ptr2 = new int;`

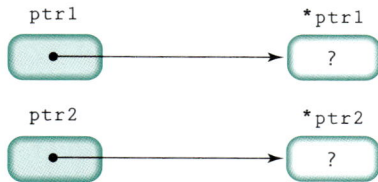

d. `ptr1 = ptr2;`

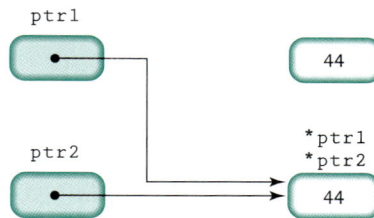

b. `*ptr2 = 44;`

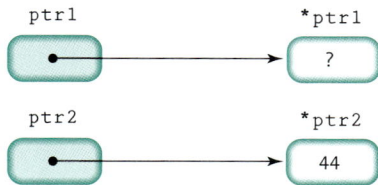

e. `delete ptr2;`

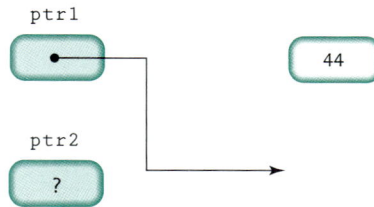

c. `*ptr1 = *ptr2;`

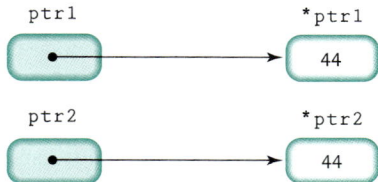

Figure 15-7 *Results from Sample Code Segment*

```
#include <cstddef>      // For NULL
    ⋮
int* ptr1 = new int;
int* ptr2 = new int;

*ptr2 = 44;
*ptr1 = *ptr2;
delete ptr1;            // Avoid an inaccessible object
ptr1 = ptr2;
delete ptr2;
ptr1 = NULL;            // Avoid a dangling pointer
```

Figure 15–8 shows the results of executing this revised code segment.

15.3 Reference Types

According to Figure 15–1, there is only one built-in type remaining: the **reference type**. Like pointer variables, reference variables contain the addresses of other variables. The statement

```
int& intRef;
```

declares that `intRef` is a variable that can contain the address of an `int` variable. Here is the syntax template for declaring reference variables:

Reference type   A simple data type consisting of an unbounded set of values, each of which is the address of a variable of a given type. The only operation defined on a reference variable is initialization, after which every appearance of the variable is implicitly dereferenced.

ReferenceVariableDeclaration

$\Big\{$ DataType& Variable ;

   DataType &Variable , &Variable ... ;

Although reference variables and pointer variables both contain addresses of data objects, there are two fundamental differences. First, the dereferencing and address-of operators (* and &) are not used with reference variables. After a reference variable has been declared, the compiler *invisibly* dereferences every single appearance of that reference variable. This difference is illustrated on page 800.

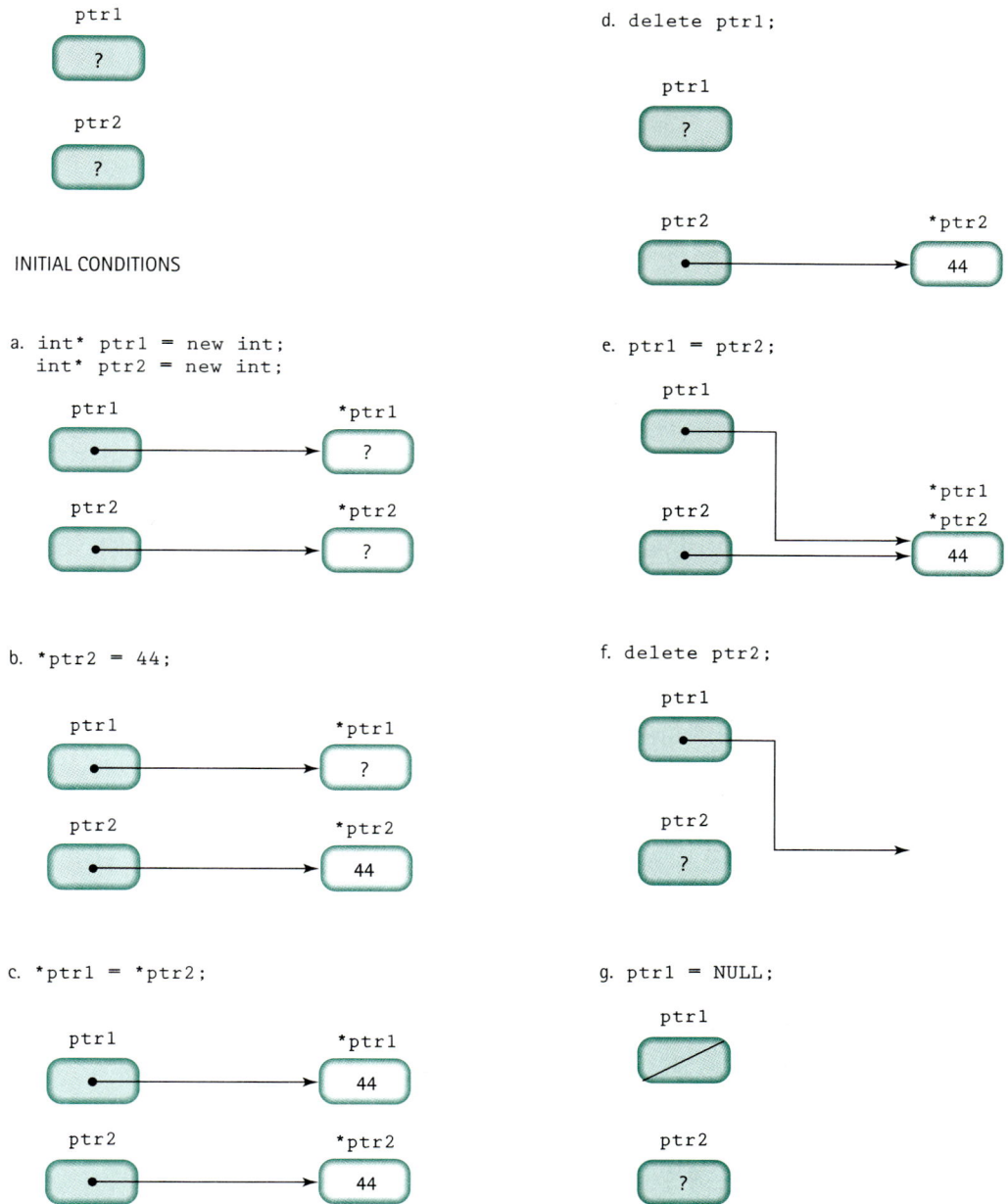

INITIAL CONDITIONS

a. `int* ptr1 = new int;`
   `int* ptr2 = new int;`

b. `*ptr2 = 44;`

c. `*ptr1 = *ptr2;`

d. `delete ptr1;`

e. `ptr1 = ptr2;`

f. `delete ptr2;`

g. `ptr1 = NULL;`

Figure 15–8   *Results from Sample Code Segment After It Was Modified*

Using a Reference Variable	Using a Pointer Variable
| ```
int   gamma = 26;
int& intRef = gamma;
// Assert: intRef points
//            to gamma
``` | ```
int   gamma = 26;
int* intPtr = &gamma;
// Assert: intPtr points
//            to gamma
``` |
| ```
intRef = 35;
// Assert: gamma == 35
``` | ```
*intPtr = 35;
// Assert: gamma == 35
``` |
| ```
intRef = intRef + 3;
// Assert: gamma == 38
``` | ```
*intPtr = *intPtr + 3;
// Assert: gamma == 38
``` |

Some programmers like to think of a reference variable as an *alias* for another variable. In the preceding code, we can think of intRef as an alias for gamma. After intRef is initialized in its declaration, everything we do to intRef is actually happening to gamma.

The second difference between reference and pointer variables is that the compiler treats a reference variable as if it were a *constant* pointer. It cannot be reassigned after being initialized. In fact, absolutely no operations apply directly to a reference variable except initialization. (In this context, C++ defines initialization to mean (a) explicit initialization in a declaration, (b) implicit initialization by passing an argument to a parameter, or (c) implicit initialization by returning a function value.) For example, the statement

```
intRef++;
```

does not increment intRef; it increments the variable to which intRef points. Why? Because the compiler implicitly dereferences each appearance of the name intRef.

The principal advantage of reference variables, then, is notational convenience. Unlike pointer variables, reference variables do not require the programmer to continually prefix the variable with an asterisk in order to access the pointed-to variable.

A common use of reference variables is to pass nonarray arguments by reference instead of by value (as we have been doing ever since Chapter 7). Suppose the programmer wants to exchange the contents of two float variables with the function call

```
Swap(alpha, beta);
```

Because C++ normally passes simple variables by value, the following code fails:

```
void Swap( float x, float y )
// Caution: This routine does not work
{
    float temp = x;

    x = y;
    y = temp;
}
```

By default, C++ passes the two arguments by value. That is, *copies* of alpha's and beta's values are sent to the function. The local contents of x and y are exchanged within the function, but the caller's arguments alpha and beta remain unchanged. To correct this situation, we have two options. The first is to send the addresses of alpha and beta explicitly by using the address-of operator (&):

```
Swap(&alpha, &beta);
```

The function must then declare the parameters to be pointer variables:

```
void Swap( float* px, float* py )
{
    float temp = *px;

    *px = *py;
    *py = temp;
}
```

This approach is necessary in the C language, which has pointer variables but not reference variables.

The other option is to use reference variables to eliminate the need for explicit dereferencing:

```
void Swap( float& x, float& y )
{
    float temp = x;

    x = y;
    y = temp;
}
```

In this case, the function call does not require the address-of operator (&) for the arguments:

```
Swap(alpha, beta);
```

The compiler implicitly generates code to pass the addresses, not the contents, of alpha and beta. This method of passing nonarray arguments by reference is the one that we have been using all along and continue to use throughout the book.

By now, you have probably noticed that the ampersand (&) has several meanings in the C++ language. To avoid errors, it pays to keep these meanings distinct from each other. Following is a table that summarizes the different uses of the ampersand. Note that a *prefix* operator is one that precedes its operand(s), an *infix* operator lies between its operands, and a *postfix* operator comes after its operand(s).

Position	Usage	Meaning
Prefix	&Variable	Address-of operation
Infix	Expression & Expression	Bitwise AND operation (mentioned, but not explored, in Chapter 10)
Infix	Expression && Expression	Logical AND operation
Postfix	DataType&	Data type (specifically, a reference type)
		Exception: To declare two variables of reference type, the & must be attached to each variable name: int &var1, &var2;

15.4 Classes and Dynamic Data

When programmers use C++ classes, it is often useful for class objects to create dynamic data on the free store. Let's consider a class Message, which is made up of a Time object and a message.

To keep the example simple, we supply only a bare minimum of public member functions. We begin with the class declaration for a Message class, abbreviated by leaving out the function preconditions and postconditions.

```
class Message
{
public:
    void Print() const;                        // Output operation
    Message( /* in */ Time        time,    // Constructor
             /* in */ const char* msgStr );
private:
    Time time;
    char* msg;
};
```

In the class constructor's parameter list, we could just as well have declared msgStr as

```
const char[] msgStr
```

instead of

```
const char* msgStr
```

Remember that both of these declarations are equivalent as far as the C++ compiler is concerned. They both mean that the parameter being received is the base address of a C string.

As you can see in the private part of the class declaration, the private variable `msg` is a pointer, not a `char` array. If we declared `msg` to be an array of fixed size, say, 30, the array might be either too large or too small to hold the `msgStr` string that the client passes through the constructor's argument list. Instead, the class constructor will dynamically allocate a `char` array of just the right size on the free store and make `msg` point to this array. Here is the implementation of the class constructor as it would appear in the implementation file:

```
#include <cstring>    // For strcpy() and strlen()
   :
 Message::Message( /* in */ Time          newTime,    // Constructor
                   /* in */ const char* msgStr );
{
    time = newTime
    msg = new char[strlen(msgStr) + 1];
    // Assert:
    //     Storage for dynamic C string is now on free store
    //     and its base address is in msg
    strcpy(msg, msgStr);
    // Assert:
    //     Incoming string has been copied to free store
}
```

The constructor begins by copying the first incoming parameter into the appropriate private variable. Next, we use the `new` operator to allocate a `char` array on the free store. (We add 1 to the length of the incoming string to leave room for the terminating `'\0'` character.) Finally, we use `strcpy` to copy all the characters from the `msgStr` array to the new dynamic array. If the client code declares two class objects with the statements,

```
Message msg1(10, 30, 0, "Call Bobby");
Message msg2(10, 35, 30, "Call Sue");
   :
```

then the two class objects point to dynamic char arrays as shown in Figure 15–9.

Figure 15–9 illustrates an important concept: a `Message` class object does not encapsulate an array—it only encapsulates *access* to the array. The array itself is located externally (on the free store), not within the protective abstraction barrier of the class object. This arrangement does not violate the principle of information hiding, however. The only access to the array is through the pointer variable `msg`, which is a private class member and is therefore inaccessible to clients.

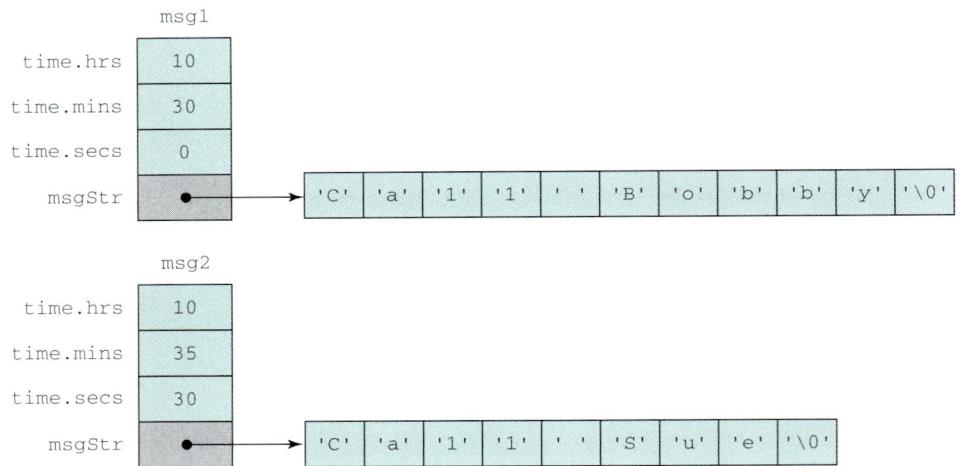

Figure 15–9   *Class Objects Pointing to Dynamically Allocated C Strings*

Notice that the `Message` class allocates dynamic data, but we have made no provision for deallocating the dynamic data. To deal adequately with class objects that point to dynamic data, we need more than just a class constructor. We need an entire group of class member functions: a class constructor, a *class destructor*, a *deep copy operation*, and a *class copy-constructor*. One by one, we will explain each of these new functions. But first, here is the overall picture of what our new class declaration looks like:

```
class Message
{
public:
    void Print() const;                             // Output operation

    void CopyFrom( /* in */ Message otherMsg );
    // Deep copy operation
    Message( /* in */ Time newTime;
             /* in */ const char* msgStr );
    Message( const Message& otherMsg );     // Copy-constructor
    ~Message();                             // Destructor
private:
    Time   time;
    char* msg;
};
```

This class declaration includes function prototypes for all four of the member functions we said we are going to need: constructor, destructor, deep copy operation, and copy-constructor. Before proceeding, let's define more precisely the semantics of each member function by furnishing the function preconditions and postconditions.

```cpp
//*********************************************************************
// SPECIFICATION FILE (Message.h)
// This file gives the specification of a Message abstract data
// type representing a time and a message
//*********************************************************************

#include "Time.h"

class Message
{
public:
    void Print() const;
        // Postcondition:
        //      Message and time have been output in the form
        //         hours, minutes, seconds, and message

    void CopyFrom( /* in */ Message otherMsg );
        // Postcondition:
        //      This message is a copy of otherMsg, including
        //      the message string

    Message( /* in */ Time newTime,
             /* in */ const char* msgStr  );
        // Constructor
        // Postcondition:
        //      New class object is constructed with time set to
        //      newTime and msg set to msgStr

    Message( const Message& otherMsg );
        // Copy-constructor
        // Postcondition:
        //      New class object is constructed with time and
        //      message string the same as otherMsg's
        // Note:
        //      This constructor is implicitly invoked whenever a
        //      Message object is passed by value, is returned as a
        //      function value, or is initialized by another
        //      Message object in a declaration

    ~Message();
        // Destructor
        // Postcondition:
```

```
                //      Message string is destroyed
private:
    Time time;
    char* msg;
};
```

Here is a client program that demonstrates calls to member functions of the Mes-sage class.

```
//************************************************************
// MessageDemo program
// This is a very simple client of the Message class
//************************************************************
#include <iostream>
#include <string>            // For string class
#include "Message.h"         // For Message class

using namespace std;

int main()
{
    Time time;          // Time object
    string msg;         // Input message

    // Construct object msg1, and print it
    time.ReadTime();
    cout << "Enter message " << endl;
    cin >> msg;
    Message msg1(time, msg.c_str());
    cout << "Message 1: ";
    msg1.Print();
    cout << endl;

    // Construct object msg2, then make it a copy of msg2
    time.Set(5, 30, 0);
    Message msg2(time, "Old");

    cout << "Old Message 2: ";
    msg2.Print();
    cout << endl;

    msg2.CopyFrom(msg1);
    cout << "New Message 2: ";
    msg2.Print();       // Should be same as msg1
```

```
    cout << endl;

    return 0;
}
```

Class Destructors

The `Message` class provides a destructor function named `~Message`. A class destructor, identified by a tilde (~) preceding the name of the class, can be thought of as the opposite of a constructor. Just as a constructor is implicitly invoked when control reaches the declaration of a class object, a destructor is implicitly invoked when the class object is destroyed. A class object is destroyed when it "goes out of scope." (An automatic object goes out of scope when control leaves the block in which it is declared. A static object goes out of scope when program execution terminates.) The following block— which might be a function body, for example—includes remarks at the locations where the constructor and destructor are invoked:

```
{
    Time time;

    time.ReadTime();
    Message myMsg(time, "Remember meeting");   ← Constructor is invoked here
      :
}   ← Destructor is invoked here because myMsg goes out of scope
```

In the implementation file `Message.cpp`, the implementation of the class destructor is very simple:

```
Message::~Message()

// Destructor

// Postcondition:
//      Array pointed to by msg is no longer on the free store
{
    delete [] msg;
}
```

You cannot pass arguments to a destructor and, as with a class constructor, you must not declare the data type of the function.

With the `Message` class, four data items are enclosed within the abstraction barrier— the hours, minutes, and seconds of time and the pointer to the message, but the array is not (see Figure 15–9). Without the destructor function `~Message`, destruction of a class object would deallocate the *pointer* to the dynamic array, but would not deallocate the array itself. The result would be a memory leak; the dynamic array would remain allocated but no longer accessible.

Shallow Versus Deep Copying

Next, let's look at the `CopyFrom` function of the `Message` class. This function is designed to copy one class object to another, *including the dynamic message array*. With the built-in assignment operator (`=`), assignment of one class object to another copies only the class members; it does *not* copy any data pointed to by the class members. For example, given the `msg1` and `msg2` objects of Figure 15–9, the effect of the assignment statement

```
msg1 = msg2;
```

is shown in Figure 15–10. The result is called a **shallow copy** operation. The pointer is copied, but the pointed-to data is not.

Shallow copying is perfectly fine if none of the class members are pointers. But if one or more members are pointers, then shallow copying may be erroneous. In Figure 15–10, the dynamic array originally pointed to by the `msg1` object has been left inaccessible.

What we want is a **deep copy** operation—one that duplicates not only the class members, but also the pointed-to data. The `CopyFrom` function of the `Message` class performs a deep copy.

> **Shallow copy**   An operation that copies one class object to another without copying any pointed-to data.
>
> **Deep copy**   An operation that not only copies one class object to another, but also makes copies of any pointed-to data.

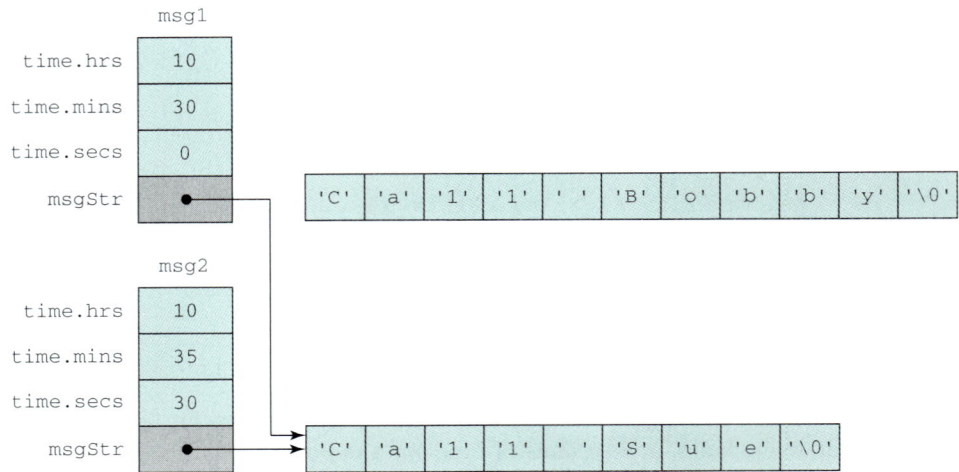

Figure 15–10   *A Shallow Copy Caused by the Assignment msg1 = msg2*

Here is the function implementation:

```
void Message::CopyFrom( /* in */ Message otherMsg )

// Postcondition:
//     time == otherMsg.time
//  && msg points to a duplicate of otherMsg's message string
//     on the free store

{
    time = otherMsg.time;
    delete [] msg;                          // Deallocate original
    msg = new char[strlen(otherMsg.msg) + 1];
    // Allocate new array
    strcpy(msg, otherMsg.msg);              // Copy the chars
}
```

First, the function copies the `Time` object from the `otherMsg` object into the current object. Next, the function deallocates the current object's dynamic array from the free store, allocates a new dynamic array, and copies all elements of `otherMsg`'s array into the new array. The result is therefore a deep copy—two identical class objects pointing to two identical (but *separate*) dynamic arrays. Given our `msg1` and `msg2` objects of Figure 15–9, the statement,

```
msg1.CopyFrom(msg2);
```

yields the result shown in Figure 15–11. Compare this figure with the shallow copy pictured in Figure 15–10.

Class Copy-Constructors

As we have just discussed, the built-in assignment operator (=) leads to a shallow copy when class objects point to dynamic data. The issue of deep versus shallow copying also can appear in another context: initialization of one class object by another. C++ defines initialization to mean the following:

1. Initialization in a variable declaration

   ```
   Message msg1 = msg2;
   ```

2. Passing a copy of an argument to a parameter (that is, passing by value)

3. Returning an object as the value of a function

   ```
   return someObject;
   ```

By default, C++ performs such initializations using shallow copy semantics. In other words, the newly created class object is initialized via a member-by-member copy of the

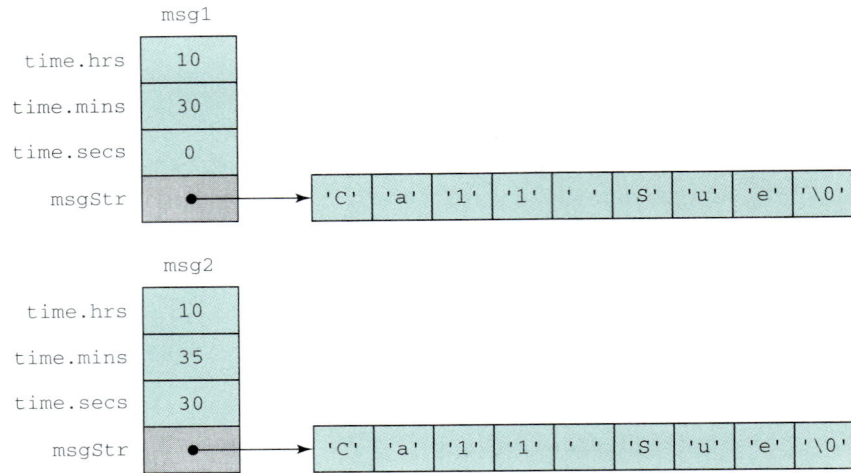

Figure 15-11   *A Deep Copy*

old object without regard for any data to which the class members may point. For our `Message` class, the result would again be two class objects pointing to the same dynamic data.

To handle this situation, C++ has a special kind of constructor known as a *copy-constructor*. In a class declaration, its prototype has the following form:

```
class SomeClass
{
public:
    :
    SomeClass( const SomeClass& someObject );   // Copy-constructor
    :
};
```

Notice that the function prototype does not use any special words to suggest that this is a copy-constructor. You simply have to recognize the pattern of symbols: the class name followed by a parameter list, which contains a single parameter of type

```
const SomeClass&
```

For example, our Message class declaration shows the prototype of the copy-constructor to be

```
Message( const Message& otherMsg );
```

If a copy-constructor is present, the default method of initialization (member-by-member copying) is inhibited. Instead, the copy-constructor is implicitly invoked whenever one class object is initialized by another. The following implementation of the copy-constructor for the `Message` class shows the steps that are involved:

```
Message::Message( const Message& otherMsg )

// Copy-constructor

// Postcondition:
//      time = otherMsg.time
//   && msg points to a duplicate of otherMsg's message string
//      on the free store

{
    time = otherMsg.time;
    msg = new char[strlen(otherMsg.msg) + 1];
    strcpy(msg, otherMsg.msg);
}
```

The body of the copy-constructor function differs from the body of the `CopyFrom` function in only one line of code. The `CopyFrom` function executes

```
delete [] msg;
```

before allocating a new array. The difference between these two functions is that `Copy-From` is copying to an *existing* class object (which is already pointing to a dynamic array that must be deallocated), whereas the copy-constructor is creating a new class object that doesn't already exist.

Notice the use of the reserved word `const` in the parameter list of the copy-constructor. The word `const` ensures that the function cannot alter `otherMsg`, even though `otherMsg` is passed by reference.

As with any nonarray variable in C++, a class object can be passed to a function either by value or by reference. Because C++ defines initialization to include passing by value, copy-constructors are vitally important when class objects point to dynamic data. Assume that we did not include a copy-constructor for the `Message` class, and assume that the following call to the `DoSomething` function uses a pass by value:

```
int main()
{
    Time time;
    time.Set(10, 30, 0);
    Message quizMsg(time, "Geography quiz");
       :
```

```
DoSomething(quizMsg);
    :
```

Without a copy-constructor, `quizMsg` would be copied to the `DoSomething` function's parameter using a shallow copy. A copy of `quizMsg`'s dynamic array would *not* be created for use within `DoSomething`. Both `quizMsg` and the parameter within `DoSomething` would point to the same dynamic array (see Figure 15–12). If the `DoSomething` function were to modify the dynamic array (thinking it is working on a *copy* of the original), then after the function returns, `quizMsg` would point to a corrupted dynamic array.

In summary, the default operations of assignment and initialization may be dangerous when class objects point to dynamic data on the free store. Member-by-member assignment and initialization cause only pointers to be copied, not the pointed-to data. If a class allocates and deallocates data on the free store, it almost certainly needs the following suite of member functions to ensure deep copying of dynamic data:

```
class SomeClass
{
public:
        :
```

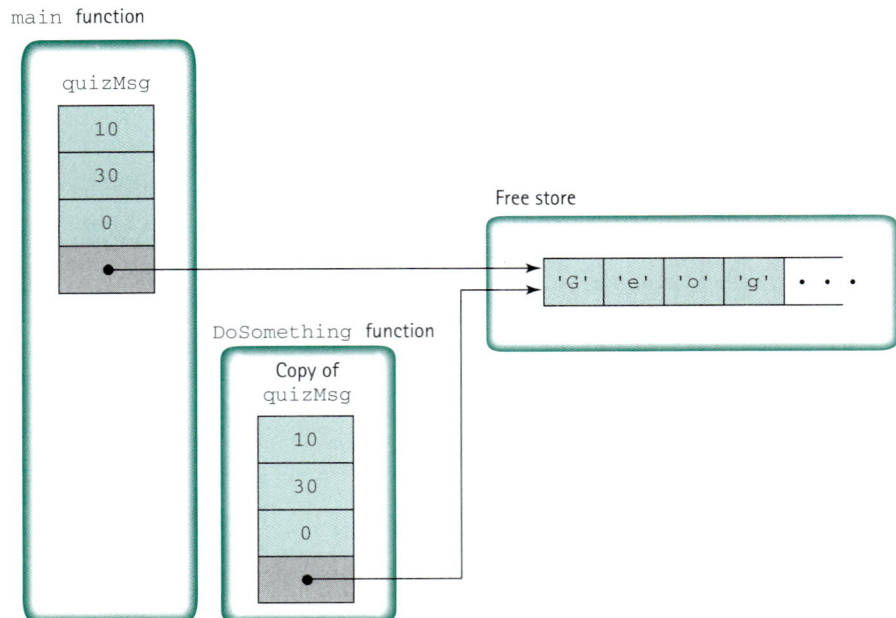

Figure 15–12   *Shallow Copy Caused by a Pass by Value without a Copy-Constructor*

```
      void CopyFrom( SomeClass anotherObject );
          // A deep copy operation

      SomeClass( ... );
          // Constructor, to create data on the free store

      SomeClass( const SomeClass& anotherObject );
          // Copy-constructor, for deep copying in initializations

      ~SomeClass();
          // Destructor, to clean up the free store
  private:
      ⋮
  };
```

At the beginning of this chapter, we said that pointers are used for two reasons: to make a program more efficient—either in speed or in memory usage—and to create complex data structures (called *linked structures*). We give examples of the use of pointers to make a program more efficient in the case study in this chapter. Linked structures are covered in Chapter 16.

Problem–Solving Case Study

Creating an Appointment Calendar Continued

PROBLEM   In the last chapter we created one part of a future appointment calendar. It contained a list of name/time pairs ordered by time. The next step is to extend the appointment calendar to represent a complete day, which would contain a date and a list of entries. Expanding the appointment calendar to a list of days can come later.

DISCUSSION   We should have guessed that we would eventually need a Date abstract data type. A date is an object like name and time that occurs frequently in problems. So creating a Date class is the first order of business.

Creating a Date Class   What sort of operations will we need in our ADT Date? Of course, we need a default constructor and a parameterized constructor that takes month, day, year as parameters. We probably should have a transformer operation to reset the date. We should have observer operations that let us observe the values for month, day, and year. We should also have an operation that let's us compare two dates. The informal specification of the ADT is given on the next page.

TYPE
>   Date

DOMAIN
>   Each Date value is a single date after the year 1582 A.D. in the form of month, day, and year.

OPERATIONS
>   Construct a new Date instance.
>   Set the date.
>   Inspect the date's month.
>   Inspect the date's day.
>   Inspect the date's year.
>   Compare two dates for "before," "equal," or "after."

SPECIFICATION OF THE ADT   The domain of our ADT is the set of all dates after the year 1582 A.D. in the form of a month, a day, and a year. We restrict the year to be after 1582 A.D. in order to simplify the ADT operations (10 days were skipped in 1582 in switching from the Julian to the Gregorian calendar).

To represent the Date ADT as program code, we use a C++ class named `Date`. The ADT operations become public member functions of the class. Let's now specify the operations more carefully.

Construct a new Date instance   For this operation, we use a C++ default constructor that initializes the date to January 1 of the year 1583. The client code can reset the date at any time using the "Set the date" operation.

Set the date   The client must supply three arguments for this operation: month, day, and year. Although we haven't yet determined a concrete data representation for a date, we must decide what data types the client should use for these arguments. We choose integers, where the month must be in the range 1 through 12, the day must be in the range 1 through the maximum number of days in the month, and the year must be greater than 1582. Notice that these range restrictions will become the precondition for invoking this operation.

Inspect the date's month, inspect the date's day, and inspect the date's year   All three of these operations are observer operations. They give the client access, indirectly, to the private data. In the Date class, we represent these operations as value-returning member functions with the following prototypes:

```
int Month();
int Day();
int Year();
```

Why do we need these observer operations? Why not simply let the data representation of the month, day, and year be public instead of private so that the client can access the values directly? We have seen this question before and the answer is the same: The client should be allowed to inspect *but not modify* these values. If the data were public, a client could manipulate the data incorrectly (such as incrementing January 31 to January 32), thereby compromising the correct behavior of the ADT.

Compare two dates This operation compares two dates and determines whether the first one comes before the second one, they are the same, or the first one comes after the second one. To indicate the result of the comparison, we define an enumeration type with three values:

```
enum RelationType {BEFORE, SAME, AFTER};
```

Then we can code the comparison operation as a class member function that returns a value of type RelationType. Here is the function prototype:

```
RelationType ComparedTo( /* in */ Date otherDate ) const;
```

Because this is a class member function, the date being compared to otherDate is the class object for which the member function is invoked. For example, the following client code tests to see whether date1 comes before date2.

```
Date date1;
Date date2;
  ⋮
if (date1.ComparedTo(date2) == BEFORE)
    DoSomething();
```

We are now almost ready to write the C++ specification file for our Date class. The simplest representation for a date is three int values—one each for the month, day, and year. Here, then, is the specification file containing the Date class declaration (along with the declaration of the RelationType enumeration type).

```
//**************************************************************
// SPECIFICATION FILE (Date.h)
// This file gives the specification of a Date abstract data
// type and provides an enumeration type for comparing dates.
// To save space, we omit from each function the precondition
// comments that document the assumptions made about valid input
// parameter data. These would be included in a program intended
// for actual use.
//**************************************************************

enum RelationType {BEFORE, SAME, AFTER};

class Date
{
public:
```

```cpp
void Set( /* in */ int newMonth,
          /* in */ int newDay,
          /* in */ int newYear  );
    // Precondition:
    //     1 <= newMonth <= 12
    //  && 1 <= newDay <= maximum no. of days in month newMonth
    //  && newYear > 1582
    // Postcondition:
    //     Date is set according to the incoming parameters

int Month() const;
    // Postcondition:
    //     Return value is this date's month

int Day() const;
    // Postcondition:
    //     Return value is this date's day

int Year() const;
    // Postcondition:
    //     Return value is this date's year

RelationType ComparedTo( /* in */ Date otherDate ) const;
    // Postcondition:
    //     Return value is
    //         BEFORE, if this date is before otherDate
    //         SAME, if this date equals otherDate
    //         AFTER, if this date is after otherDate

Date();
    // Postcondition:
    //     New Date object is constructed with a
    //     month, day, and year of 1, 1, and 1583

Date( /* in */ int newMonth,
      /* in */ int newDay,
      /* in */ int newYear  );
    // Precondition:
    //     1 <= newMonth <= 12
    //  && 1 <= newDay <= maximum no. of days in month newMonth
    //  && newYear > 1582
    // Postcondition:
    //     Date is set according to the incoming parameters
```

```
private:
    int month;
    int day;
    int year;
};
```

IMPLEMENTATION OF THE ADT   We have already chosen a concrete data representation for a date, shown in the specification file as the int variables month, day, and year. Now we must implement each class member function, placing the function definitions into a C++ implementation file named Date.cpp. As we implement the member functions, we also discuss testing strategies that can help to convince us that the implementations are correct.

The class constructor, Set, Month, Day, and Year functions   The implementations of these functions are so straightforward that no discussion is needed.

Date ( )

> Set month to 1
> Set day to 1
> Set year to 1583

Date(In: newMonth, newDay, newYear)

> Set month to newMonth
> Set day to newDay
> Set year to newYear

Set (In: newMonth, newDay, newYear)

> Set month to newMonth
> Set day to newDay
> Set year to newYear

Month ( )
  Out: Function value

> Return month

Day ( )

   Out: Function value

> Return day

Year ( )

   Out: Function value

> Return year

TESTING   The `Month`, `Day`, and `Year` observer functions can be used to verify that the class constructor and `Set` functions work correctly. The code

```
Date someDate;
Date otherDate(12, 24, 2004);

cout << someDate.Month() << ' ' << someDate.Day() << ' '
     << someDate.Year() << endl;
cout << otherDate.Month() << ' ' << otherDate.Day() << ' '
     << otherDate.Year() << endl;
```

should print out 1 1 1583 and 12 24 2004. To test the `Set` function, it is sufficient to set a `Date` object to a few different values (obeying the precondition for the `Set` function), then print out the month, day, and year as above.

The ComparedTo function   If we were to compare two dates in our heads, we would look first at the years. If the years were different, we would immediately know which date came first. If the years were the same, we would look at the months. If the months were the same, we would have to look at the days. As so often happens, we can use this algorithm directly in our function.

ComparedTo (In: otherDate)

   Out: Function value

> IF year < otherDate.year
>   Return BEFORE
> IF year > otherDate.year
>   Return AFTER
>
> //Years are equal. Compare months
> IF month < otherDate.month
>   Return BEFORE
> IF month > otherDate.month
>   Return AFTER

```
//Years and months are equal. Compare days
IF day < otherDate.day
    Return BEFORE
IF day > otherDate.day
    Return AFTER

//Years, months, and days are equal
Return SAME
```

TESTING   In testing this function, we should ensure that each path is taken at least once. Case Study Follow-Up Exercise 1 asks you to design test data for this function and to write a driver that does the testing.

```cpp
//******************************************************************
// IMPLEMENTATION FILE (Date.cpp)
// This file implements the Date member functions
//******************************************************************

#include "Date.h"
#include <iostream>

using namespace std;

// Private members of class:
//      int month;
//      int day;
//      int year;

int DaysInMonth( int, int );  // Prototype for auxiliary function


//******************************************************************

Date::Date()

// Constructor

// Postcondition:
//      month is 1  &&  day is 1  &&  year is 1583

{
    month = 1;
    day   = 1;
    year  = 1583;
}
```

```cpp
//*******************************************************************

void Date::Set( /* in */ int newMonth,
                /* in */ int newDay,
                /* in */ int newYear  )

// Precondition:
//      1 <= newMonth <= 12
//   && 1 <= newDay <= maximum no. of days in month newMonth
//   && newYear > 1582
// Postcondition:
//      month is newMonth  AND  day is newDay  AND  year is newYear

{
    month = newMonth;
    day   = newDay;
    year  = newYear;
}


//*******************************************************************

int Date::Month() const

// Postcondition:
//      Return value is month

{
    return month;
}

//*******************************************************************

int Date::Day() const

// Postcondition:
//      Return value is day

{
    return day;
}

//*******************************************************************

int Date::Year() const
```

```
// Postcondition:
//      Return value is year

{
    return year;
}


RelationType Date::ComparedTo( /* in */ Date otherDate ) const

// Postcondition:
//      Return value is BEFORE, if this date is
//                              before otherDate
//                 is SAME, if this date equals otherDate
//                 is AFTER, if this date is
//                              after otherDate

{
    if (year < otherDate.year)        // Compare years
        return BEFORE;
    if (year > otherDate.year)
        return AFTER;

    if (month < otherDate.month)      // Years are equal. Compare
        return BEFORE;                //    months
    if (month > otherDate.month)
        return AFTER;

    if (day < otherDate.day)          // Years and months are equal.
        return BEFORE;                //    Compare days
    if (day > otherDate.day)
        return AFTER;

    return SAME;                      // Years, months, and days
                                      //    are equal
}
```

Changes in class SortedList Our SortedList class had the maximum number of items set by a constant. Now that we know how to create a structure at run time using new, let's rewrite the class so that there is a default constructor that sets the number of cells to a fixed size, say 20, and a parameterized constructor that takes the size of the array as a parameter. Here are the changes in the private part of the class.

```
class SortedList
{
...
```

```
        SortedList( /* in */ int numElements );

    // Postcondition:
    //      data has been created
    //      size has been set to numElements
    //      length has been set to 0

private:
    int         length;
    int         currentPos;
    int         size;
    ItemType* data;
    void        BinSearch( ItemType, bool&, int& ) const;
};
```

Notice that `data` is now a pointer variable, not an array name. It points to the first element of a dynamically allocated array. Remember in C++, however, you can attach an index expression to any pointer—not only an array name—as long as the pointer points to an array. Thus, `data` can be indexed exactly as it was when it was defined as an array of type `ItemType`.

Because the `IsFull` function needs to know how large the array is, we need to store the parameter value or the default value. We call that variable `size` (see Figure 15–13). The changed functions in class `SortedList` are shown on the next page.

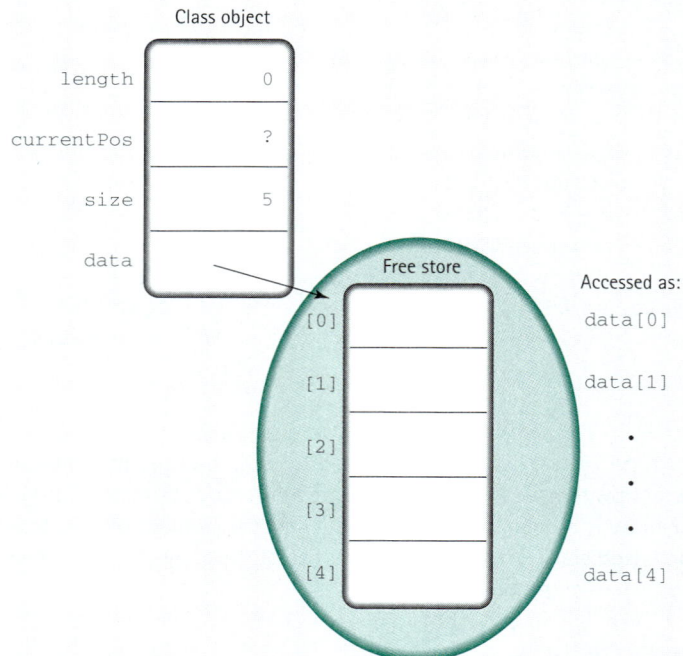

Figure 15–13   *An Empty List in Dynamically Allocated Space*

```
//*********************************************************************

SortedList::SortedList()

// Constructor

// Postcondition:
//      length is set to zero
//      size is set to 20
//      data is created with 20 slots

{
    length = 0;
    size = 20;
    data = new ItemType[size];
}

//*********************************************************************

SortedList::SortedList( /* in */ int numElements )

// Constructor

// Postcondition:
//      data has been created with numElements slots
//      size has been set to numElements
//      length has been set to 0

{
    length = 0;
    size = numElements;
    data = new ItemType[numElements];
}

//*********************************************************************

bool SortedList::IsFull() const

// Reports whether SortedList is full

// Postcondition:
//      Return value is true, if length equals size;
//      is false, otherwise
```

```
{
    return (length == size);
}
```

//***

List of Date Entry pairs   Now we have all the pieces: objects of class `Entry`, objects of class `Date`, and a `SortedList` object to which we can pass the number of places in the array at run time. We need to combine them into a Day ADT. What operations do we need? Given a date, we need to apply each of the operations that were applied in the driver in the case study in Chapter 14: Insert an entry, delete an entry, determine if a time is free, and iterate through the list of entries. Because we know that the next stage in the processing includes a list of class `Day` objects ordered by date, we should include a comparison operation, which compares two objects by date.

The internal representation of the `Day` class contains a `Date` object and a `SortedList` of `Entry` objects, which are made up of `AptTime` objects and `Name` objects. This is getting rather complicated. Let's look at the structure before we start writing specifications. The tail of the arrow is a variable and the head is its type. The types of the variables with no arrows coming from them are built-in types `int` or `string`.

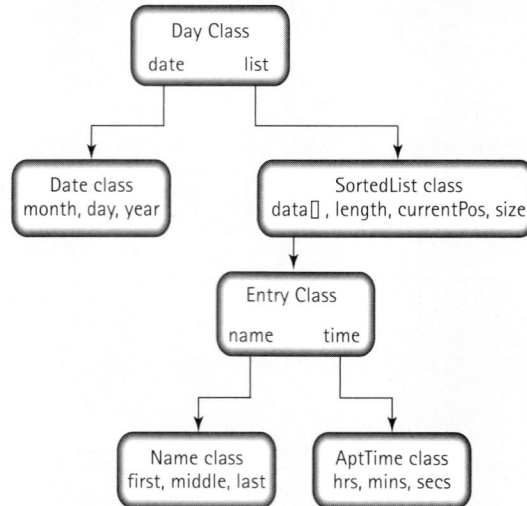

When so many classes are grouped together via containment, there is always the possibility that there will be some duplication. In this case, both class `Date` and class `Name` define the enumerated type `RelationType`. This duplication will keep class `Day` from compiling. We can solve this problem by moving the definition of `RelationType` into a header file surrounded by the compiler directives discussed in Chapter 14. Both class `Name` and class `Date` can include this file. The compiler directives prohibit duplication. In fact, it would be a good idea to protect each of our general classes, such as `Name`, `AptTime`, and `Date`, with these directives.

```
//****************************************************************
// SPECIFICATION FILE for RelationType (relType.h)
// There is no implementation file
//****************************************************************
#ifndef ENUM
#define ENUM
enum RelationType{BEFORE, SAME, AFTER};
#endif
```

Here then is the specification file for class Day. You will note that there are three constructors: one default constructor, one that takes a date and the number of array items, and one that takes a date, an entry, and the number of array items.

```
//****************************************************************
// SPECIFICATION FILE (Day.h)
// This file contains the specification of the Day ADT,
// which has two contained classes, Date and a SortedList
// of objects of class Entry
// To save space, we omit from each function the precondition
// comments that document the assumptions made about valid input
// parameter data. These would be included in a program intended
// for actual use.
//****************************************************************
#include "SortedList.h"
#include "Date.h"
#include "relType.h"

class Day
{
public:
    //  Constructors

    Day();

        // Postcondition:
        //     date and list have been initialized to 20 slots

    Day( /* in */ Date newDate,
         /* in */ int numAppts );

        // Postcondition:
        //     date is set to newDate
        //     list is created with numAppts slots
```

```
Day( /* in */ Date newDate,
     /* in */ Entry newEntry,
     /* in */ int numAppts );

    // Postcondition:
    //     date is set to newDate
    //     newEntry is inserted in list

// Other member functions

void InsertEntry( /* in */ Entry newEntry );

    // Precondition:
    //     time field in newEntry is free
    // Postcondition:
    //     newEntry is inserted in list

void Delete( /* inout */ Entry entry);

    // Precondition:
    //     entry is in the list
    // Postcondition:
    //     entry is no longer in the list

Date DateIs() const;

    // Postcondition:
    //     Return value is this day's date

RelationType ComparedTo( /* in */ Day otherDay ) const;

    // Postcondition:
    //     Return value is BEFORE, if this day's date is
    //                                    before otherDay's date
    //                   is SAME, if this day's date
    //                                    equals otherDay's date
    //                   is AFTER, if this day's date is
    //                                    after otherDay's date

int NumberOfEntries();

    // Postcondition:
    //     Return value is the length of the list of entries

void ResetEntries();
```

```
    // Postcondition:
    //      Iteration is initialized

Entry GetNextItem();

    // Precondition:
    //      Iteration has been initialized by call to
    //      ResetEntries;
    //      No transformers have been invoked since last call
    // Postcondition:
    //      Returns item at the current position in the list
    //      on entry;
    //      If last item has been returned, the next call will
    //      return the first item.

bool TimeFree(AptTime time);

    // Postcondition:
    //      Return value is true if an entry with time is not
    //      in list; false otherwise

private:
    Date        date;
    SortedList  list;
};
```

All of these operations, except for the observer that returns the `Date` member, involve list manipulations. In fact they just call the parallel list functions. The only one that is slightly different is `TimeFree`, which takes an `AptTime` object, rather than an `Entry` object. An `Entry` object must be constructed to pass to the `SortedList IsPresent` function. Here then is the implementation file. Notice that we used a constructor initializer to pass array size to the `SortedList` constructor.

```
//*****************************************************************
// IMPLEMENTATION FILE (Day.cpp)
// This file contains the implementation of the Day ADT,
// which has two contained classes, Date and SortedList
//*****************************************************************
#include "Day.h"

void Day::InsertEntry( /* in */ Entry newEntry )

// Precondition:
```

```
//      time field in newEntry is free
// Postcondition:
//      newEntry is inserted in list

{
    list.Insert(newEntry);
}


Day::Day() : list(24)

//      date and list have been initialized to 24 slots

{
}


Day::Day( /* in */ Date newDate,
          /* in */ int numAppts ) : list(numAppts)

// Postcondition:
//      date is set to newDate
//      list is created with numAppts slots

{
    date = newDate;
}


Day::Day( /* in */ Date newDate,
          /* in */ Entry newEntry,
          /* in */ int numAppts )  : list(numAppts)

// Postcondition:
//      date is set to newDate; newEntry is inserted in list

{
    list.Insert(newEntry);
    date = newDate;
}


void Day::Delete( /* inout */ Entry entry)

// Precondition:
//      entry is in the list
// Postcondition:
//      entry is no longer in the list
```

```
{
    list.Delete(entry);
}

Date Day::DateIs() const
// Postcondition:
//      Return value is this day's date

{
    return date;
}

RelationType Day::ComparedTo( /* in */ Day otherDay ) const

// Postcondition:
//      Return value is BEFORE, if this day's date is
//                              before otherDay's date
//                  is SAME, if this day's date
//                              equals otherDay's date
//                  is AFTER, if this day's date is
//                              after otherDay's date

{
    return date.ComparedTo(otherDay.date);
}

int Day::NumberOfEntries()

// Postcondition:
//      Return value is the length of the list of entries

{
    return list.Length();
}

void Day::ResetEntries()

// Postcondition:
//      Iteration is initialized

{
    list.Reset();
}
```

```cpp
Entry Day::GetNextItem()

// Precondition:
//      Iteration has been initialized by call to ResetEntries;
//      No transformers have been invoked since last call
// Postcondition:
//      Returns item at the current position in the list
//      on entry;
//      If last item has been returned, the next call will
//      return the first item

{
    return list.GetNextItem();
}


bool Day::TimeFree(AptTime time)

// Postcondition:
//      Return value is true if an entry with time is not
//      in list; false otherwise

{
    Entry entry(" ", " ", " ", time.Hours(),
                time.Minutes());
    return !(list.IsPresent(entry));
}
```

Day class Driver   The driver for the Day class must test each of the functions.   Because none of the functions contain loops or branches, the test plan can be quite simple. Here is a driver that calls all of the Day member functions. Examine this driver very carefully. The complex structure of this problem means that you have to be very careful when you build your accessing expressions.

```cpp
//******************************************************************
// DRIVER for Day class (DayDriver.cpp)
// Three entries are read from the keyboard and inserted into the
// list of entries.  The entries are accessed one at a time and
// printed.  A time that is in the list  is checked; a time that is
// not in the list is checked.  An item is deleted and the list is
// printed to show that the item is gone.
//******************************************************************

#include <iostream>
#include "Day.h"
using namespace std;
```

```cpp
int main()
{

    Entry nameTime;

    AptTime time(10, 30);
    Date date;
    date.Set(12, 3, 2004);      // Set date to 12 3 2004
    Day day(date, 5);           // Set day to date with 5 appointments

    SortedList list;
    for (int count = 1; count <= 3; count++)
    {
        nameTime.ReadEntry();
        day.InsertEntry(nameTime);
    }
    // Prepare and iterate through the list, printing items
    int limit = day.NumberOfEntries();
    day.ResetEntries();                     // Prepare for iteration

    cout << "Entries for " << day.DateIs().Month() << " "
         << day.DateIs().Day()
         << ", " << day.DateIs().Year()  << endl;
    for (int count = 0; count < limit; count++)
    {
        nameTime = day.GetNextItem();
        cout << "Name: " << nameTime.NameStr() << " Time: "
             << nameTime.TimeStr() << endl;
    }

    // Item is in the list
    if (day.TimeFree(time))
        cout << time.Hours() << ":" << time.Minutes()
             << " is free." << endl;
    else
        cout << time.Hours() << ":" << time.Minutes()
             << " is not free. " << endl;
    // Item is not in the list
    time.Set(0, 0);
    if (day.TimeFree(time))
        cout << time.Hours() << ":" << time.Minutes()
             << " is free." << endl;
    else
        cout << time.Hours() << ":" << time.Minutes()
             << " is not free. " << endl;
```

```
        // Delete and iterate through the list, printing items
        day.Delete(nameTime);
        day.ResetEntries();              // Prepare for iteration
        limit = day.NumberOfEntries();

        for (int count = 0; count < limit; count++)
        {
            nameTime = day.GetNextItem();
            cout << "Name: " << nameTime.NameStr() << " Time: "
                << nameTime.TimeStr() << endl;
        }
        return 0;
}
```

The driver was run with the same data as in Chapter 14. Here is the screen shot.

```
C:\PPSC++\DayDriver.exe                                    - □ ×
Enter first name: Sarah
Enter middle name: Jane
Enter last name: Jones
Enter hours (<= 23):
10
Enter minutes (<= 59):
30
Enter first name: Susan
Enter middle name: Margaret
Enter last name: Smith
Enter hours (<= 23):
9
Enter minutes (<= 59):
30
Enter first name: Judy
Enter middle name: Dale
Enter last name: David
Enter hours (<= 23):
3
Enter minutes (<= 59):
0
Entries for 12 3, 2004
Name: Judy David Time: 03:00
Name: Susan Smith Time: 09:30
Name: Sarah Jones Time: 10:30
10:30 is not free.
0:0 is free.
Name: Judy David Time: 03:00
Name: Susan Smith Time: 09:30
```

How is this output different from the last? We have a date printed as a heading to the output. At least that is what you see. The underlying list structure has been changed so that the array containing the list elements is generated at run time using the new operator, and the user is requested to input the maximum number of appointments for a particular date.

Testing and Debugging

Programs that use pointers are more difficult to write and debug than programs without pointers. Indirect addressing never seems quite as "normal" as direct addressing when you want to get at the contents of a variable.

The most common errors associated with the use of pointer variables are as follows:

1. Confusing the pointer variable with the variable it points to
2. Trying to dereference the null pointer or an uninitialized pointer
3. Inaccessible objects
4. Dangling pointers

Let's look at each of these in turn.

If `ptr` is a pointer variable, care must be taken not to confuse the expressions `ptr` and `*ptr`. The expression

```
ptr
```

accesses the variable `ptr` (which contains a memory address). The expression

```
*ptr
```

accesses the variable that `ptr` points to.

`ptr1 = ptr2`	Copies the contents of `ptr2` into `ptr1`.
`*ptr1 = *ptr2`	Copies the contents of the variable pointed to by `ptr2` into the variable pointed to by `ptr1`.
`*ptr1 = ptr2`	Illegal—one is a pointer and one is a variable being pointed to.
`ptr1 = *ptr2`	Illegal—one is a pointer and one is a variable being pointed to.

The second common error is to dereference the null pointer or an uninitialized pointer. On some systems, an attempt to dereference the null pointer produces a run-time error message such as "NULL POINTER DEREFERENCE," followed immediately by termination of the program. When this event occurs, you have at least some notion of what went wrong with the program. The situation is worse, though, if your program dereferences an uninitialized pointer. In the code fragment

```
int   num;
int*  intPtr;

num = *intPtr;
```

the variable `intPtr` has not been assigned any value before we dereference it. Initially, it contains some meaningless value such as 315988, but the computer does not know that it is meaningless. The machine simply accesses memory location 315988 and copies whatever it finds there into `num`. There is no way to test whether a pointer variable contains an undefined value. The only advice we can give is to check the code carefully to make sure that every pointer variable is assigned a value before being dereferenced.

The third error—leaving inaccessible objects on the free store—usually results from either a shallow copy operation or incorrect use of the `new` operator. In Figure 15-11, we showed how the built-in assignment operator causes a shallow copy; the dynamic data object originally pointed to by one pointer variable remains allocated but inaccessible. Misuse of the `new` operator also can leave dynamic data inaccessible. Execution of the code fragment

```
float* floatPtr;

floatPtr = new float;
*floatPtr = 38.5;
floatPtr = new float;
```

creates an inaccessible object: the dynamic variable containing 38.5. The problem is that we assigned a new value to `floatPtr` in the last statement without first deallocating the variable it pointed to. To guard against this kind of error, examine every use of the `new` operator in your code. If the associated variable currently points to data, `delete` the pointed-to data before executing the `new` operation.

Finally, dangling pointers are a source of errors and can be difficult to detect. One cause of dangling pointers is deallocating a dynamic data object that is pointed to by more than one pointer. Figures 15–7d and 15–7e pictured this situation. A second cause of dangling pointers is returning a pointer to an automatic variable from a function. The following function, which returns a function value of type `int*`, is erroneous.

```
int* Func()
{
    int n;
      ⋮
    return &n;
}
```

Remember that automatic variables are implicitly created at block entry and implicitly destroyed at block exit. The above function returns a pointer to the local variable `n`, but `n` disappears as soon as control exits the function. The caller of the function therefore receives a dangling pointer. Dangling pointers are hazardous for the same reason that uninitialized pointers are hazardous: When your program dereferences incorrect pointer values, it will access memory locations whose contents are unknown.

Testing and Debugging Hints

1. To declare two pointer variables in the same statement, you must use

   ```
   int *p, *q;
   ```

   You cannot use

   ```
   int* p, q;
   ```

Similarly, you must use

```
int &m, &n;
```

to declare two reference variables in the same statement.

2. Do not confuse a pointer with the variable it points to.

3. Before dereferencing a pointer variable, be sure it has been assigned a meaningful value other than NULL.

4. Pointer variables must be of the same data type to be compared or assigned to one another.

5. In an expression, an array name without any index brackets is a pointer expression; its value is the base address of the array. The array name is considered a *constant* expression, so it cannot be assigned to. The following code shows correct and incorrect assignments.

```
int   arrA[5] = {10, 20, 30, 40, 50};
int   arrB[5] = {60, 70, 80, 90, 100};
int* ptr;

ptr = arrB;      // OK--you can assign to a variable
arrA = arrB;     // Wrong--you cannot assign to a constant
```

6. If `ptr` points to a struct, union, or class variable that has an `int` member named `age`, the expression

```
*ptr.age
```

is incorrect. You must either enclose the dereference operation in parentheses:

```
(*ptr).age
```

or use the arrow operator:

```
ptr->age
```

7. The `delete` operator must be applied to a pointer whose value was previously returned by `new`. Also, the `delete` operation leaves the value of the pointer variable undefined; do not use the variable again until you have assigned it a new value.

8. A function must not return a pointer to automatic local data, or else a dangling pointer will result.

9. If `ptrA` and `ptrB` point to the same dynamic data object, the statement

```
delete ptrA;
```

makes `ptrB` a dangling pointer. You should now assign `ptrB` the value NULL rather than leave it dangling.

10. Deallocate dynamic data when it is no longer needed. Memory leaks can cause you to run out of memory space.

11. Inaccessible objects—another cause of memory leaks—are caused by

   a. shallow copying of pointers that point to dynamic data. When designing C++ classes whose objects point to dynamic data, be sure to provide a deep copy operation and a copy-constructor.

   b. using the `new` operation when the associated variable already points to dynamic data. Before executing `new`, use `delete` to deallocate the data that is currently pointed to.

Summary

Pointer types and reference types are simple data types for storing memory addresses. Variables of these types do not contain data; rather, they contain the addresses of other variables or data structures. Pointer variables require explicit dereferencing using the `*` operator. Reference variables are dereferenced implicitly and are commonly used to pass nonarray arguments by reference.

A powerful use of pointers is to create dynamic variables. The pointer is created at compile time, but the data to which the pointer points is created at run time. The built-in operator `new` creates a variable on the free store (heap) and returns a pointer to that variable. A dynamic variable is not given a name, but rather is accessed through a pointer variable.

The use of dynamic data saves memory space because a variable is created only when it is needed at run time. When a dynamic variable is no longer needed, it can be deallocated (using `delete`) and the memory space can be used again. The use of dynamic data can also save machine time when large structures are being sorted. The pointers to the large structures, rather than the large structures themselves, can be rearranged.

When C++ class objects point to data on the free store, it is important to distinguish between shallow and deep copy operations. A shallow copy of one class object to another copies only the pointers and results in two class objects pointing to the same dynamic variable. A deep copy results in two distinct copies of the pointed-to data. Therefore, classes that manipulate dynamic data usually require a complete collection of support routines: one or more constructors, a destructor (for cleaning up the free store), a deep copy operation, and a copy-constructor (for deep copying during initialization of one class object by another).

Quick Check

1. Why is it more efficient to create a list of structs using pointers rather than directly? (pp. 792–795)
2. If you want to copy all of the pointed-to data in a struct, should you use deep or shallow copying? (pp. 808–813)
3. Two of the ways that C++ defines initialization are initialization in a variable declaration and passing an argument by value. What is the third way that C++ defines initialization? (pp. 809–813)

4. Every class that manipulates dynamic data should have a constructor, a destructor, and what other two types of member functions? (pp. 804–807)
5. In declaring a pointer variable called `compass` that points to an `int`, there are two ways that you can write the declaration in C++. What are they? (pp. 782–783)
6. If you want `compass` to point to the variable `north`, how would you write the assignment that accomplishes this? (pp. 783–784)
7. If `installRecord` points to a `struct` with a member called `location`, what are the two ways that C++ allows you to write an indirect access to this member? (pp. 785–787)
8. What is the keyword that we use in writing a C++ allocation expression? (pp. 792–793)
9. What is the keyword that we use in writing a C++ deallocation expression? (pp. 794–795)
10. In declaring a reference variable called `dictionary` that refers to a `string`, there are two ways that you can write the declaration in C++. What are they? (pp. 798–802)
11. If `dictionary` refers to a variable called `firstWord`, how would you use the reference variable to assign the value "aardvark" to `firstWord`? (pp. 798–802)

Answers
1. Because pointers allow us to dynamically create the list to be only as long as necessary.
2. Deep copying. 3. Returning an object as the value of a function. 4. A deep copy, and a copy-constructor. 5. `int* compass; int *compass;` 6. `compass = &north;` 7. `(*install-Record).location` or `installRecord -> location` 8. `new` 9. `delete` 10. `string& dictionary; string &dictionary;` 11. `dictionary = "aardvark";`

Exam Preparation Exercises

1. Match the following terms with the definitions given below.
   a. Pointer type
   b. Indirect addressing
   c. Direct addressing
   d. Reference type
   e. Shallow copy
   f. Deep copy
      i. Accessing a variable using its name.
      ii. Assigning the value of one object to another object, including the duplication of any pointed-to data.
      iii. Accessing a variable using an address stored in a pointer.
      iv. A simple type that can only be initialized with the address of a variable.
      v. A simple type that can be assigned the address of a variable.
      vi. Assigning the value of one object to another without duplicating any pointed-to data.

2. Match the following terms with the definitions given below.
   a. Heap
   b. Memory leak
   c. Inaccessible object
   d. Dangling pointer
   e. Destructor
   f. Dynamic data
      i. The loss of available space that occurs when dynamic data is not deallocated properly.
     ii. The area of memory used for allocation and deallocation of dynamic data.
    iii. An object that has been allocated but has no pointer pointing to it.
    iv. Variables created with the new operation.
     v. A pointer that points to a deallocated object.
    vi. A member function invoked when an object goes out of scope.

3. Assigning the NULL to a pointer causes it to point to nothing. True or false?

4. An index expression (like those used with arrays) can be attached to any pointer variable, even if it doesn't point to an array. True or false?

5. A reference variable can be reassigned a new address value at any time. True or false?

6. When an object goes out of scope, its pointer variables are automatically deleted, but their pointed-to values are not automatically deleted. True or false?

7. Does delete return the pointer to the heap or the pointed-to data?

8. What happens to the pointer(s) and pointed-to data in an object if it goes out of scope without applying delete to the corresponding pointer(s)?

9. What is wrong with the following code segment?

```
int* needle;
needle = new int;
*needle 100;
cout << *needle;
needle = new int;
*needle = 32;
cout << * needle;
```

10. What is wrong with the following code segment?

```
int* birdDog;
int* germanShortHair;
birdDog = new int;
germanShortHair = birdDog;
*birdDog = 42;
cout << *birdDog;
delete birdDog;
cout << *germanShortHair;
```

11. What does the following code do?

```
int number;
int& atlas = number;
number = 212;
atlas++;
```

  a. Increments the contents of atlas.
  b. Increments the contents of number.
  c. Increments the contents of both atlas and number.
  d. Adds two to number.
  e. Produces a dangling pointer.

12. What does the following code do?

```
int number;
int* weathervane;
weathervane = &number;
number = 180;
(*weathervane)++;
```

  a. Increments the contents of weathervane.
  b. Increments the contents of number.
  c. Increments the contents of both weathervane and number.
  d. Adds two to number.
  e. Produces a dangling pointer.

13. What does the following code do?

```
int number;
int* finger;
finger = &number;
number = 2;
*finger++;
```

  a. Increments the contents of finger.
  b. Increments the contents of number.
  c. Increments the contents of both finger and number.
  d. Adds two to number.
  e. Produces a dangling pointer.

14. The copy constructor for class faxLog should have one parameter. What should the type of this parameter be?

15. Why is it a problem if you perform a shallow copy of one object to another object and then delete the first object and all of its pointed-to dynamic data?

16. What kind of member function does the following heading declare?

```
~phoneTree();
```

17. Applying delete to the null pointer produces an error message. True or false?

18. In the following expression, `index` is a pointer to an array and `book` is a member of a `struct` of type `libraryRecord`.

    ```
    index[12] -> book[5]
    ```

    What is the type of the components that are contained in the array that `index` points to?

Programming Warm-Up Exercises

1. Declare a pointer variable `intPointer` and initialize it to point to an `int` variable named `someInt`. Write two assignment statements, the first of which stores the value 451 directly into `someInt` and the second of which indirectly stores 451 into the variable pointed to by `intPointer`.

2. Declare a pointer variable `charArrPointer` and initialize it to point to the first element of a 4-element `char` array named `initials`. Write assignment statements to indirectly store `'A'`, `'E'`, and `'W'` into the first three elements of the array pointed to by `charArrPointer`.

3. Declare a pointer variable `structPointer` and initialize it to point to a `struct` variable called `newPhone`, of type `Phone`, that has three `int` fields called `country`, `area`, and `number`. Also write the declaration of the `Phone` type. Then write assignment statements to indirectly store the values 1, 888, and 5551212 into these fields.

4. Declare a reference variable `structReference` and initialize it to point to a `struct` variable called `newPhone`, of type `Phone`, that has three `int` fields called `country`, `area`, and `number`. Also write the declaration of the `Phone` type. Then write assignment statements to indirectly store the values 1, 888, and 5551212 into these fields.

5. Write a Boolean value-returning function called `ShallowCompare` that takes two variables of type `structPointer`, as defined in Exercise 3, and returns true if they point to the same struct, and false otherwise.

6. Write a Boolean value-returning function called `DeepCompare` that takes two variables of type `structPointer`, as defined in Exercise 3, and returns true if the structs that they point to have identical values in their corresponding fields.

7. Write a for loop that scans through a dynamically allocated `int` array, pointed to by a variable called `data`, keeping track of the greatest value in a static `int` variable `max`. The array contains 100 values. At the end of the loop, the array should be deleted.

8. Wrap the loop written in Exercise 7 in an `int`-returning function called `Greatest` that takes the array and its size as parameters and returns the value in `max` after the array is deleted. Be sure to change the loop to work with the given array size rather than the constant 100.

9. Write an `int`-returning function that prompts the user for the number of values to be entered, then creates an `int` array of that size, and reads that many values into it. The function then passes this array to the `Greatest` function defined in

Exercise 8, and returns the result from that function as its own result. Call the function `GetGreatestInput`.

10. A class called `Circuit` has two private dynamic array data members called `source` and `sink`. Write a destructor for the class that ensures that the dynamic data are destroyed.

11. Write a code segment that checks whether the pointer `oldValue` actually points to a valid memory location. If it does, then its contents are assigned to `newValue`. If not, then `newValue` is assigned a new `int` variable from the heap.

12. Write a code segment that checks whether the pointers `oldValue` and `newValue` point to different locations. If they do, then delete the value pointed to by `oldValue`, otherwise do nothing.

Programming Problems

1. You are working for your state's motor vehicle registry, and it has been discovered that some people in the driver's license database have multiple records. The license records are stored in alphabetical order on a set of files, one per letter in the alphabet. The first file is `licensesa.dat`, and the last is `licensesz.dat`. The files differ in size, with the first line of each being an integer that specifies the number of records in the file. For this problem, we'll just focus on getting the program to work for the `licensesa.dat` file. Some of the duplicate records are due to slight differences in spelling of names, so each file needs to be sorted into order by license number (an 8-digit integer) to find the duplicates. Each record consists of a license number, a name, and an address, all on a single line. For the purposes of this problem, the name and address can be stored in a single string because they are not processed separately. The license number and the corresponding string should be kept together in a struct.

   Change the `SortedList` class from Chapter 13 so that the list array is dynamically created to be the necessary length for the data on the particular file. Each component of the list will be a license `struct` type. Also add to the `SortedList` class a function that returns values from the list in successive order (called `GetNext`), and a companion function (called `Restart`) that resets the other function to begin again at the first component of the list.

   Once the data have been read from a file into the `SortedList`, use the new functions to scan through the list, comparing each license number with the one before it to see if they are the same. Keep a count of the number of duplicate records discovered. Then output this count to an output file called `duplicensesa.dat`. Restart the scanning of the list from the beginning and this time, as each duplicate record is found, it should be written on the output file. Remember to delete the dynamic array and close the file at the end of the program.

2. Extend the program from Problem 1 in two ways. The first extension is to make it automatically process all 26 data files. The second extension is to have the duplicate records be output in alphabetical order so that the output file has the same organization as the input file. To do this, after the first pass through the list, you need to create a second `SortedList` that is the proper length to hold

all of the duplicate records, and this list must sort on the string field of the license `struct`. Once all of the duplicate records have been copied to this list, you can delete the first list, and then output the second list to the file.

3. You're working for a company that wants to take client contact information as it is entered by a salesperson from a stack of business cards that he or she has collected, and output the information to a file (`contacts.dat`) in alphabetical order. Assume that there are never more than 100 cards to enter. The program should prompt the salesperson for each of the following values for each card:

Last name
First name
Middle name or initial
Title
Company name
Street address
City
State
Zip code
Phone number
Fax number
Email address

After the data are entered for each card, the user should be asked if there is another card to enter. This data should be sorted by last name, using a version of the `SortedList` class from Chapter 13 that will hold up to 100 `struct` values, each with a member corresponding to an item in the list above. Because the `struct` is so large, however, it will be more efficient if each element of the list array is a pointer to one of the `struct` values, and the class merely rearranges the pointers within the array in order to do the sorting. You should dynamically create a new `struct` for each component of the list array to point to as the cards are input. Thus, the program won't allocate `struct` memory for any more cards than are entered. The `Print` function of the class will need to be modified to output the list to the `contacts.dat` file instead of `cout`. Each member of the `struct` should be written on a separate line. The function should also write the number of cards that are in the list as the first line of the file.

4. You are working for a company that has a collection of files, each of which contains information from up to 100 business cards. The files are created by another program (see Problem 3 for a description of what this program outputs). There are no more than 100 of these files. The company would like to merge the files into a single file, sorted alphabetically by last name. The user should be prompted to enter the names of the files, until a file name of "done" is entered. For each file name that is entered, dynamically create a `struct` (of type `fileRecord`) whose members are an `int length`, and an `ifstream` object. Assign a pointer to the `struct` to the next available component of an array. Each component of the array is a `fileRecord*`. Open the `ifstream` in the most recently-created `struct`, using the name provided by the user, and then read the first

line of the file into the `length` member of the `struct`. Once all of the file names have been entered, and the files are open, go through all of the `structs` pointed to by the array, adding up the number of cards in all of the files, as given by their `length` members.

Modify the `SortedList` from Chapter 13 to use a dynamic array that contains a specified number of components. Each component of the list should be a pointer to a `struct` type as described in Problem 3. These pointers are the only values that will be rearranged by the sorting process. Use the count of cards among all of the files as the size of the array in the `SortedList`. Then go through the array of `fileRecord` values, reading all of the data from each file into the `SortedList`. Once all of the data are input, write the sorted data back out to a file called `mergedcontacts.dat`. The `Print` function of the `SortedList` class will need to be modified to output the list to the `mergedcontacts.dat` file instead of `cout`. Each member of the `struct` should be written on a separate line. The function should also write the number of cards that are in the combined list as the first line of the file.

5. Modify the program in Problem 4 so that after the data have been input, it scans through the list and deletes all duplicate records before writing out the list. A record is a duplicate if the last name, first name, middle name or initial, and company name are the same as in another record. Be sure that you properly delete any dynamically allocated data that are removed from the list.

Case Study Follow-Up

1. Write and implement a test plan for class `Date`.
2. We did not include a copy constructor nor a destructor in the revised `SortedList` class. Should we have? Explain.
3. The classes in this case study have been built up over several chapters. Does this demonstrate top-down design or object-oriented design? Explain.
4. Outline the next step in constructing an appointment calendar. How might a list of days ordered by date be implemented?

Linked Structures

Knowledge Goals

■ *To understand the concept of a linked data structure.*

Skill Goals

To be able to:

■ *Declare the data types and variables needed for a dynamic linked list.*

■ *Print the contents of a linked list.*

■ *Insert new items into a linked list.*

■ *Delete items from a linked list.*

Goals

In the last chapter, we saw that C++ has a mechanism for creating dynamic variables. These dynamic variables, which can be of any simple or structured type, can be created or destroyed at any time during execution of the program using the operators `new` and `delete`. A dynamic variable is referenced not by a name but through a pointer that contains its location (address). Every dynamic variable has an associated pointer by which it can be accessed. We used dynamic variables to save space and machine time. In this chapter, we see how to use them to build data structures that can grow and shrink as the program executes.

16.1 Sequential Versus Linked Structures

As we have pointed out in previous chapters, many problems in computing involve lists of items. A list is an abstract data type (ADT) with certain allowable operations: searching the list, sorting it, printing it, and so forth. The structure we have used as the concrete data representation of a list is the array, a sequential structure. By *sequential structure* we mean that successive components of the array are located next to each other in memory.

If the list we are implementing is a sorted list—one whose components must be kept in ascending or descending order—certain operations are efficiently carried out using an array representation. For example, searching a sorted list for a particular value is done quickly by using a binary search. However, inserting and deleting items from a sorted list are inefficient with an array representation. To insert a new item into its proper place in the list, we must shift array elements down to make room for the new item (see Figure 16–1). Similarly, deleting an item from the list requires that we shift up all the array elements following the one to be deleted.

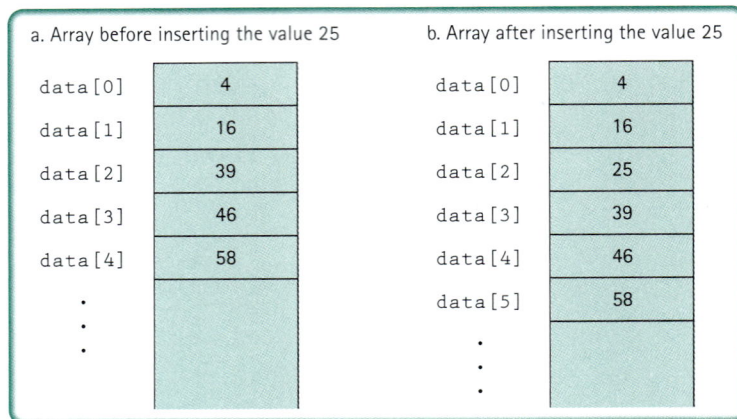

a. Array before inserting the value 25		b. Array after inserting the value 25	
data[0]	4	data[0]	4
data[1]	16	data[1]	16
data[2]	39	data[2]	25
data[3]	46	data[3]	39
data[4]	58	data[4]	46
.		data[5]	58
.		.	
.		.	
		.	

Figure 16–1   *Inserting into a Sequential Representation of a Sorted List*

When insertions and deletions are frequent, there is a better data representation for a list: the **linked list**. A linked list is a collection of items, called *nodes*, that can be scattered about in memory, not necessarily in consecutive memory locations. Each node, typically represented as a struct, consists of two members:

> **Linked list**   A list in which the order of the components is determined by an explicit link member in each node, rather than by the sequential order of the components in memory.

1. A component or item member, which contains one of the data values in the list
2. A link member, which gives the location of the next node in the list

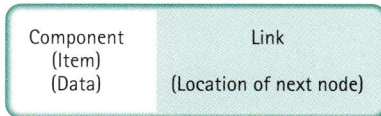

Figure 16-2 shows an abstract diagram of a linked list. An arrow is used in the link member of each node to indicate the location of the next node. The slash (/) in the link member of the last node signifies the end of the list. The separate variable `head` is not a node in the linked list; its purpose is to give the location of the first node.

Accessing the items in a linked list is a little like playing the children's game of treasure hunt—each child is given a clue to the hiding place of the next clue, and the chain of clues eventually leads to the treasure.

As you look at Figure 16-2, you should observe two things. First, we have deliberately arranged the nodes in random positions. We have done this to emphasize the fact that the items in a linked list are not necessarily in adjacent memory locations (as they are in the array representation of Figure 16-1). Second, you may already be thinking of pointers when you see the arrows in the figure because we drew pointer variables this way in Chapter 15. But so far, we have carefully avoided using the word *pointer*; we said only that the link member of a node gives the location of the next node. As we will see, there are two ways in which to implement a linked list. One way is to store it in an array of structs, a technique that does not use pointers at all. The second way is to use dynamic data and pointers. Let's begin with the first of these two techniques.

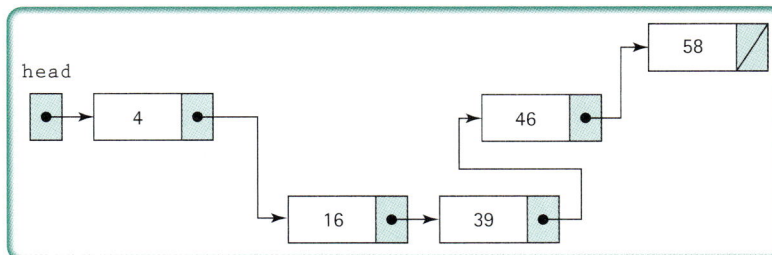

Figure 16-2   *A Linked List*

16.2 Array Representation of a Linked List

A linked list can be represented as an array of structs. For a linked list of `int` components, we use the following declarations:

```
struct NodeType
{
    int component;
    int link;
};


NodeType node[1000];    // Max. 1000 nodes
int      head;
```

The nodes all reside in an array named `node`. Each node has two members: `component` (in this example, an `int` data value) and `link`, which contains the *array index* of the next node in the list. The last node in the list will have a `link` member of −1. Because −1 is not a valid array index in C++, it is suitable as a special "end-of-list" value. The variable `head` contains the array index of the first node in the list. Figure 16–3 illustrates an array representation of the linked list of Figure 16–2.

Compare Figures 16–1 and 16–3. Figure 16–1 shows a list represented directly as an array. Figure 16–3 shows a list represented as a linked list, which, in turn, is represented as an array (of structs). We said that when insertions and deletions occur frequently, it is better to use a linked list to represent a list than it is to use an array directly. Let's see why.

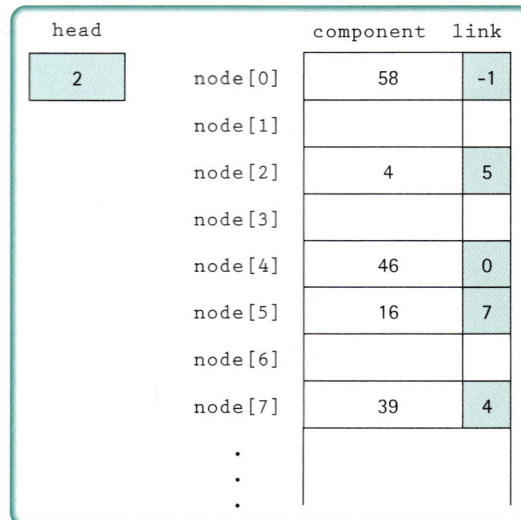

Figure 16–3   *Array Representation of a Linked List*

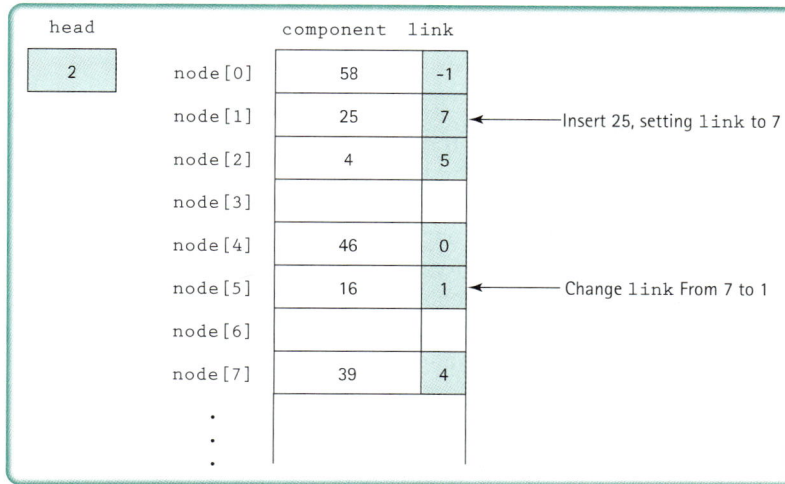

Figure 16–4   *Array Representation of Linked List After 25 Was Inserted*

Figure 16-1 showed the effect of inserting 25 into the list; we had to shift array elements 2, 3, 4,... down to insert the value 25 into element 2. If the list is long, we might have to move hundreds or thousands of numbers. In contrast, inserting the value 25 into the linked list of Figure 16-3 requires *no* movement of existing data. We simply find an unused slot in the array, store 25 into the component member, and adjust the link member of the node containing 16 (see Figure 16-4).

Before we introduce the second technique for implementing a linked list—the use of dynamic data and pointers—let's step back and look at the big picture. We are interested in the list as an ADT. Because it is an ADT, we must implement it using some existing data representation. One data representation is the built-in array, a sequential structure. Another data representation is the linked list, a linked structure. But a linked list is, itself, an ADT and requires a concrete data representation—an array of structs, for example. To help visualize all these relationships, we use an *implementation hierarchy diagram*, such as the one shown in Figure 16-5. In this diagram, each data type is implemented by using the data type(s) directly below it in the hierarchy.

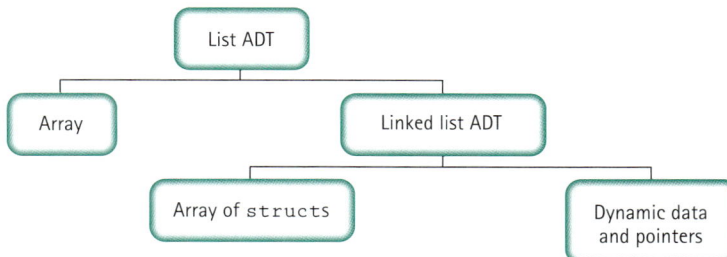

Figure 16–5   *Implementation Hierarchy for a List ADT*

16.3 Dynamic Data Representation of a Linked List

Representing a list either as an array or as a linked list stored in an array of structs has a disadvantage: The size of the array is fixed and cannot change while the program is executing. Yet when we are working with lists, we often have no idea how many components we will have. The usual approach in this situation is to declare an array large enough to hold the maximum amount of data we can logically expect. Because we usually have less data than the maximum, memory space is wasted on the unused array elements.

There is an alternative technique in which the list components are dynamic variables that are created only as they are needed. We represent the list as a linked list whose nodes are dynamically allocated on the free store, and the link member of each node contains the memory address of the next dynamic node. In this data representation, called a **dynamic linked list**, the arrows in the diagram of Figure 16–2 really do represent pointers (and the slash in the last node is the null pointer). We access the list with a pointer variable that holds the address of the first node in the list. This pointer variable, named head in Figure 16–2, is called the **external pointer** or **head pointer**. Every node after the first node is accessed by using the link member in the node before it.

> **Dynamic linked list**   A linked list composed of dynamically allocated nodes that are linked together by pointers.
>
> **External (head) pointer**   A pointer variable that points to the first node in a dynamic linked list.
>
> **Dynamic data structure**   A data structure that can expand and contract during execution.

Such a list can expand or contract as the program executes. To insert a new item into the list, we allocate more space on the free store. To delete an item, we deallocate the memory assigned to it. We don't have to know in advance how long the list will be. The only limitation is the amount of available memory space. Data structures built using this technique are called **dynamic data structures**.

To create a dynamic linked list, we begin by allocating the first node and saving the pointer to it in the external pointer. We then allocate a second node and store the pointer to it into the link member of the first node. We continue this process—allocating a new node and storing the pointer to it into the link member of the previous node—until we have finished adding nodes to the list.

Let's look at how we can use C++ pointer variables to create a dynamic linked list of float values. We begin with the declarations

```
typedef float ComponentType;

struct NodeType
{
    ComponentType  component;
    NodeType*      link;
};
typedef NodeType* NodePtr;
```

```
NodePtr head;               // External pointer to list
NodePtr currPtr;            // Pointer to current node
NodePtr newNodePtr;         // Pointer to newest node
```

The order of these declarations is important. The Typedef for `NodePtr` refers to the identifier `NodeType`, so the declaration of `NodeType` must come first. (Remember that C++ requires every identifier to be declared before it is used.) Within the declaration of `NodeType`, we would like to declare `link` to be of type `NodePtr`, but we can't because the identifier `NodePtr` hasn't been declared yet. However, C++ allows *forward* (or *incomplete*) *declarations* of structs, classes, and unions:

```
typedef float ComponentType;

struct  NodeType;           // Forward (incomplete) declaration
typedef NodeType* NodePtr;

struct NodeType             // Complete declaration
{
    ComponentType component;
    NodePtr       link;
};
```

The advantage of using a forward declaration is that we can declare the type of `link` to be `NodePtr` just as we declare `head`, `currPtr`, and `newNodePtr` to be of type `NodePtr`.

Given the declarations above, the following code fragment creates a dynamic linked list with the values 12.8, 45.2, and 70.1 as the components in the list.

```
#include <cstddef>    // For NULL
   ⋮
head = new NodeType;
head->component = 12.8;
newNodePtr = new NodeType;
newNodePtr->component = 45.2;
head->link = newNodePtr;
currPtr = newNodePtr;
newNodePtr = new NodeType;
newNodePtr->component = 70.1;
currPtr->link = newNodePtr;
newNodePtr->link = NULL;
currPtr = newNodePtr;
```

Let's go through each of these statements, describing in words what is happening and showing the linked list as it appears after the execution of the statement.

`head = new NodeType;`

A dynamic variable of type `NodeType` is created. The pointer to this new node is stored into `head`. Variable `head` is the external pointer to the list we are building.

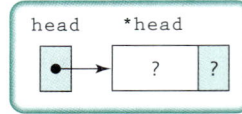

`head->component = 12.8;`

The value 12.8 is stored into the `component` member of the first node.

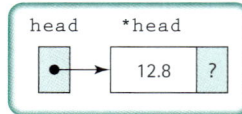

`newNodePtr = new NodeType;`

A dynamic variable of type `NodeType` is created. The pointer to this new node is stored into `newNodePtr`.

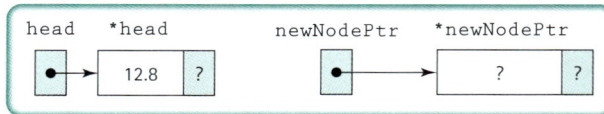

`newNodePtr->component = 45.2;`

The value 45.2 is stored into the `component` member of the new node.

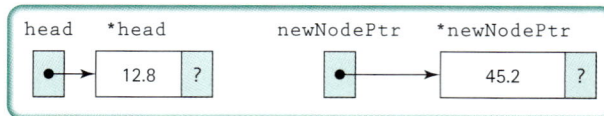

`head->link = newNodePtr;`

The pointer to the new node containing 45.2 in its `component` member is copied into the `link` member of `*head`. Variable `newNodePtr` still points to this new node. The node can be accessed either as `*newNodePtr` or as `*(head->link)`.

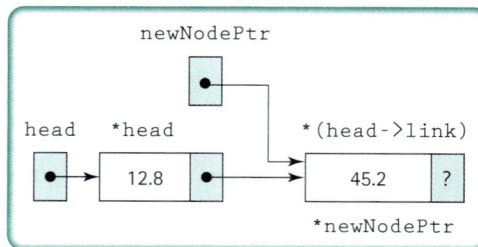

`currPtr = newNodePtr;`

The pointer to the new node is copied into `currPtr`. Now `currPtr`, `newNodePtr`, and `head->link` all point to the node containing 45.2 as its component.

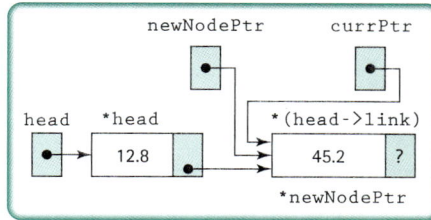

`newNodePtr = new NodeType;`

A dynamic variable of type `NodeType` is created. The pointer to this new node is stored into `newNodePtr`.

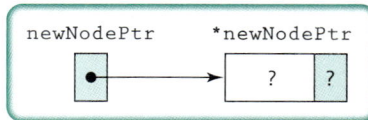

`newNodePtr->component = 70.1;`

The value 70.1 is stored into the `component` member of the new node.

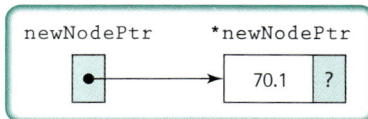

`currPtr->link = newNodePtr;`

The pointer to the new node containing 70.1 in the `component` member is copied into the `link` member of the node that contains 45.2.

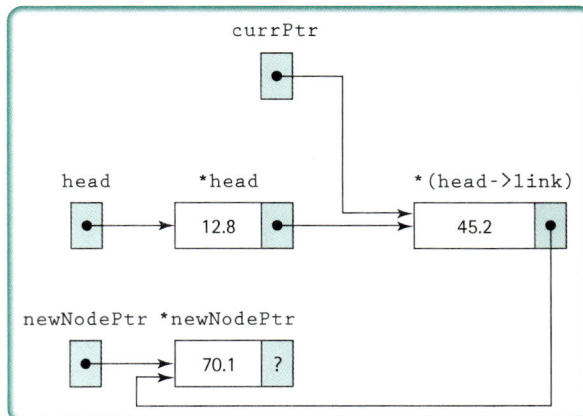

`newNodePtr->link = NULL;`

The special pointer constant `NULL` is stored into the `link` member of the last node in the list. When used in the `link` member of a node, `NULL` means the end of the list. `NULL` is shown in the diagram as a / in the `link` member.

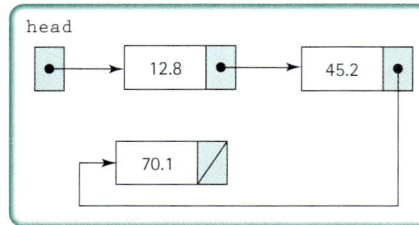

`currPtr = newNodePtr;`

`currPtr` is updated.

We would like to generalize this algorithm so that we can use a loop to create a dynamic linked list of any length. In the algorithm, we used three pointers:

1. `head`, which was used in creating the first node in the list and became the external pointer to the list.

2. `newNodePtr`, which was used in creating a new node when it was needed.

3. `currPtr`, which was updated to always point to the last node in the linked list.

When building any dynamic linked list by adding each new node to the end of the list, we always need three pointers to perform these functions. The algorithm that we used is generalized below to build a linked list of `int` numbers read from the standard input device. It is assumed that the user types in at least one number.

```
Set head = new NodeType
Read head->component
Set currPtr = head

Read inputVal
WHILE NOT EOF
    Set newNodePtr = new NodeType
    Set newNodePtr->component = inputVal
    Set currPtr->link = newNodePtr
    Set currPtr = newNodePtr
    Read inputVal
Set currPtr->link = NULL
```

The following code segment implements this algorithm. For variety, we define the component type to be `int` rather than `float`.

```
typedef int ComponentType;

struct  NodeType;                  // Forward declaration
typedef NodeType* NodePtr;

struct NodeType
{
    ComponentType component;
    NodePtr       link;
};

NodePtr        head;              // External pointer to list
NodePtr        newNodePtr;        // Pointer to newest node
NodePtr        currPtr;           // Pointer to last node
ComponentType inputVal;

head = new NodeType;
cin >> head->component;
currPtr = head;

cin >> inputVal;
while (cin)
{
    newNodePtr = new NodeType;         // Create new node
    newNodePtr->component = inputVal;  // Set its component value
    currPtr->link = newNodePtr;        // Link node into list
    currPtr = newNodePtr;              // Set currPtr to last node
    cin >> inputVal;
}
currPtr->link = NULL;                  // Mark end of list
```

Let's do a code walk-through and see just how this algorithm works.

`head = new NodeType;`	A variable of type `NodeType` is created. The pointer is stored into `head`. Variable `head` will remain unchanged as the pointer to the first node (that is, `head` is the external pointer to the list).
`cin >> head->component;`	The first number is read into the `component` member of the first node in the list.
`currPtr = head;`	`currPtr` now points to the last node (the only node) in the list.

`cin >> inputVal;`	The next number (if there is one) is read into variable `inputVal`.
`while (cin)` `{`	An event-controlled loop is used to read input values until end-of-file occurs.
`newNodePtr = new NodeType;`	Another variable of type `NodeType` is created, with `newNodePtr` pointing to it.
`newNodePtr->component = inputVal;`	The current input value is stored into the `component` member of the newly created node.
`currPtr->link = newNodePtr;`	The pointer to the new node is stored into the `link` member of the last node in the list.
`currPtr = newNodePtr;`	`currPtr` is again pointing to the last node in the list.
`cin >> inputVal;`	The next input value (if there is one) is read in.
`}`	The loop body repeats again.
`currPtr->link = NULL;`	The `link` member of the last node is assigned the special end-of-list value `NULL`.

Following is the linked list that results when the program is run with the numbers 32, 78, 99, and 21 as data. The final values are shown for the auxiliary variables.

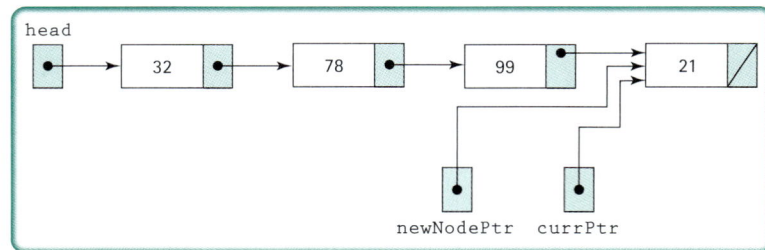

Algorithms on Dynamic Linked Lists

Now that we have looked at two examples of creating a dynamic linked list, let's look at algorithms that process nodes in a linked list. We need to be able to insert a node into a list, delete a node from a list, print the data values in a list, and so forth. For each of these operations, we make use of the fact that NULL is in the link member of the last node. NULL can be assigned to any pointer variable. It means that the pointer points to nothing. Its importance lies in the fact that we can compare the link member of each node to NULL to see when we have reached the end of the list.

As we develop these algorithms, we do so in the following context. We want to write a C++ class for a list (not linked list) ADT. As emphasized in Figure 16–5, a list ADT can be implemented in several ways. We choose a dynamic linked list as the data representation for a list, and we create the `HybridList` class whose specification is shown in Figure 16–6. We call it a "HybridList" because it has two insert operations and two delete operations.

Figure 16–6   *Specification of the `HybridList` Class*

```
//***********************************************************************
// SPECIFICATION FILE (hybrid.h)
// This file gives the specification of a hybrid list abstract data
// type with two insert operations and two delete operations. The
// list components are maintained in ascending order of value
//***********************************************************************

typedef int ComponentType;    // Type of each component
                              //    (a simple type or the string type)

struct NodeType;              // Forward declaration
                              //    (Complete declaration is
                              //    hidden in implementation file)
class HybridList
{
public:
    bool IsEmpty() const;
        // Postcondition:
        //      Function value == true, if list is empty
        //                     == false, otherwise

    void Print() const;
        // Postcondition:
        //      All components (if any) in list have been output

    void InsertAsFirst( /* in */ ComponentType item );
        // Precondition:
        //      item < first component in list
        // Postcondition:
        //      item is first component in list
        //   && List components are in ascending order

    void Insert( /* in */ ComponentType item );
        // Postcondition:
        //      item is in list
        //   && List components are in ascending order
```

```
        void RemoveFirst( /* out */ ComponentType& item );
            // Precondition:
            //     NOT IsEmpty()
            // Postcondition:
            //     item == first component in list at entry
            //  && item is no longer in list
            //  && List components are in ascending order

        void Delete( /* in */ ComponentType item );
            // Precondition:
            //     item is somewhere in list
            // Postcondition:
            //     First occurrence of item is no longer in list
            //  && List components are in ascending order

        HybridList();
            // Constructor
            // Postcondition:
            //     Empty list is created

        HybridList( const SortedList2& otherList );
            // Copy-constructor
            // Postcondition:
            //     List is created as a duplicate of otherList

        ~HybridList();
            // Destructor
            // Postcondition:
            //     List is destroyed
    private:
        NodeType* head;
    };
```

In the class declaration, notice that the preconditions and postconditions of the member functions mention nothing about linked lists. The abstraction is a list, not a linked list. The user of the class is interested only in manipulating lists of items and does not care how we implement a list. If we change to a different implementation—an array, for example—the public interface remains valid.

The private data of the HybridList class consists of a single item: a pointer variable head. This variable is the external pointer to a dynamic linked list. As with any C++ class, different class objects have their own copies of the private data. For example, suppose the client code declares and manipulates two class objects as in the following program.

```
//*************************************************************************
// ListDemo program
// This is a very simple client of the HybridList class
//*************************************************************************
#include <iostream>
#include "hybrid.h"    // For HybridList class

using namespace std;

int main()
{
    HybridList    list1;    // First list, initially empty
    HybridList    list2;    // Second list, initially empty
    ComponentType item;     // One list item

    list1.Insert(-35);
    list1.Insert(100);
    list1.Insert(12);
    cout << "First list:" << endl;
    list1.Print();                        // Prints -35, 12, and 100
                                          //    in that order

    while ( !list1.IsEmpty() )
    {
        list1.RemoveFirst(item);
        if (item > 0)
            list2.Insert(item);
    }
    cout << endl;
    cout << "First list:" << endl;
    list1.Print();                        // No output (list is empty)
    cout << "Second list:" << endl;
    list2.Print();                        // Prints 12 and 100
                                          //    in that order

    return 0;
}
```

Then in the ListDemo program, each of the two objects `list1` and `list2` has its own private `head` variable and maintains its own dynamic linked list on the free store.

In Figure 16–6, the specification file `hybridList.h` declares a type `NodeType`, but only as a forward declaration. The only reason we need to declare the identifier `NodeType` in the specification file is so that the data type of the private variable `head` can be specified. In the spirit of information hiding, we place the complete declaration of `NodeType` into the implementation file `hybridList.cpp`. The complete declaration

is an implementation detail that the user does not need to know about. Here's how
hybridList.cpp starts out:

```
//**********************************************************************
// IMPLEMENTATION FILE (hybrid.cpp)
// This file implements the HybridList class member functions
// List representation: a linked list of dynamic nodes
//**********************************************************************
#include "hybridList.h"
#include <iostream>
#include <cstddef>      // For NULL

using namespace std;

typedef NodeType* NodePtr;
struct NodeType
{
    ComponentType component;
    NodePtr       link;
};

// Private members of class:
//      NodePtr head;                    External pointer to linked list
    ⋮
```

To illustrate some commonly used algorithms on dynamic linked lists, let's look at
the implementations of the HybridList member functions. Creating an empty linked
list is the easiest of the algorithms, so we begin there.

Creating an Empty Linked List   To create a linked list with no nodes, all that is
necessary is to assign the external pointer the value NULL. For the HybridList class,
the appropriate place to do this is in the class constructor:

```
HybridList::HybridList()

// Constructor

// Postcondition:
//      head == NULL

{
    head = NULL;
}
```

As we discussed in Chapter 13, the implementation assertions (the preconditions and postconditions appearing in the implementation file) are often stated differently from the abstract assertions (those located in the specification file). Abstract assertions are written in terms that are meaningful to the user of the ADT; implementation details should not be mentioned. In contrast, implementation assertions can be made more precise by referring directly to variables and algorithms in the implementation code. In the case of the `HybridList` class constructor, the abstract postcondition is simply that an empty list (not a linked list) has been created. On the other hand, the implementation postcondition

```
// Postcondition:
//      head == NULL
```

is phrased in terms of our private data (`head`) and our particular list implementation (a dynamic linked list).

Testing for an Empty Linked List   The `HybridList` member function `IsEmpty` returns `true` if the list is empty and `false` if the list is not empty. Using a dynamic linked list representation, we return `true` if `head` contains the value `NULL`, and `false` otherwise:

```
bool HybridList::IsEmpty() const

// Postcondition:
//      Return value == true, if head == NULL
//                   == false, otherwise

{
    return (head == NULL);
}
```

Printing a Linked List   To print the components of a linked list, we need to access the nodes one at a time. This requirement implies an event-controlled loop, where the event that stops the loop is reaching the end of the list. The loop control variable is a pointer that is initialized to the external pointer and is advanced from node to node by setting it equal to the link member of the current node. When the loop control pointer equals `NULL`, the last node has been accessed.

Print ( )

Set currPtr = head
WHILE currPtr doesn't equal NULL
    Print component member of *currPtr
    Set currPtr = link member of *currPtr

Note that this algorithm works correctly even if the list is empty (head equals NULL).

```
void HybridList::Print() const

// Postcondition:
//      Component members of all nodes (if any) in linked list
//      have been output

{
    NodePtr currPtr = head;      // Loop control pointer

    while (currPtr != NULL)
    {
        cout << currPtr->component << endl;
        currPtr = currPtr->link;
    }
}
```

Let's do a code walk-through using the following list.

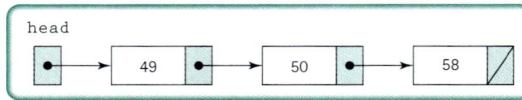

currPtr = head;   currPtr and head both point to the first
                                         node in the list.

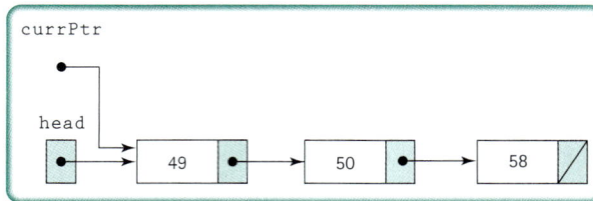

while (currPtr != NULL)   The loop body is entered because currPtr
                                         is not NULL.

cout << currPtr->component << endl;   The number 49 is printed.

currPtr = currPtr->link;   currPtr now points to the second node in
                                         the list.

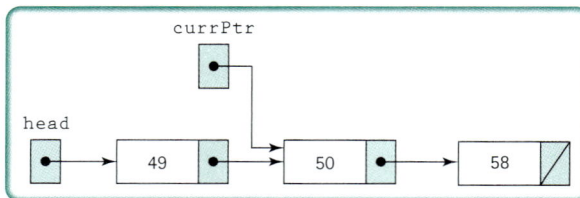

`while (currPtr != NULL)`	The loop body repeats because `currPtr` is not NULL.
`cout << currPtr->component << endl;`	The number 50 is printed.
`currPtr = currPtr->link;`	`currPtr` now points to the third node in the list.

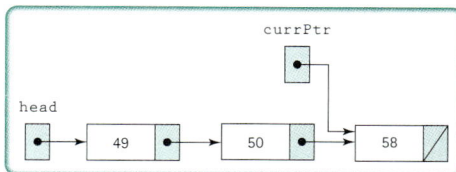

`while (currPtr != NULL)`	The loop body repeats because `currPtr` is not NULL.
`cout << currPtr->component << endl;`	The number 58 is printed.
`currPtr = currPtr->link;`	`currPtr` is now NULL.

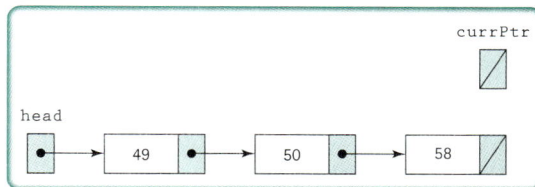

`while (currPtr != NULL)`	The loop body is not repeated because `currPtr` is NULL.

Inserting into a Linked List   A function for inserting a component into a linked list must have an argument: the item to be inserted. The phrase *inserting into a linked list* could mean either inserting the component at the top of the list (as the first node) or inserting the component into its proper place according to some ordering (alphabetic or numeric). Let's examine these two situations separately.

Inserting a component at the top of a list is easy because we don't have to search the list to find where the item belongs.

InsertAsFirst (In: item)

> Set newNodePtr = new NodeType
> Set component member of *newNodePtr = item
> Set link member of *newNodePtr = head
> Set head = newNodePtr

This algorithm is coded in the following function.

```
void HybridList::InsertAsFirst( /* in */ ComponentType item )

// Precondition:
//     Component members of list nodes are in ascending order
//     && item < component member of first list node
// Postcondition:
//     New node containing item is at top of linked list
//     && component members of list nodes are in ascending order

{
    NodePtr newNodePtr = new NodeType;    // Temporary pointer

    newNodePtr->component = item;
    newNodePtr->link = head;
    head = newNodePtr;
}
```

The function precondition states that `item` must be smaller than the value in the first node. This precondition is not a requirement of linked lists in general. However, the `HybridList` abstraction we are implementing is a sorted list. The precondition/postcondition contract states that *if* the client sends a value smaller than the first one in the list, then the function guarantees to preserve the ascending order. If the client violates the precondition, the contract is broken.

The following code walk-through shows the steps in inserting a component with the value 20 as the first node in the linked list that was printed in the last section.

`newNodePtr = new NodeType;`   A new node is created.

`newNodePtr->component = item;`   The number 20 is stored into the `component` member of the new node.

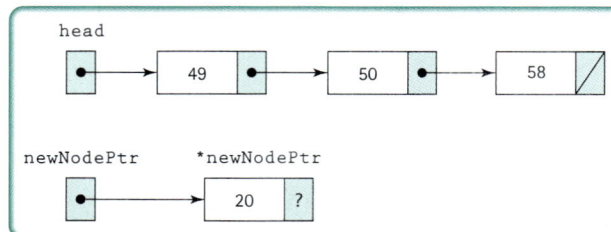

`newNodePtr->link = head;`   The `link` member of `*newNodePtr` now points to the first node in the list.

(see diagram next page)

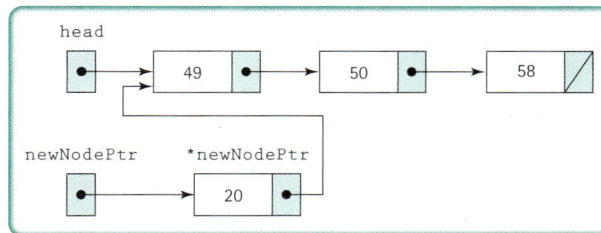

`head = newNodePtr;`

The external pointer to the list now points to the node containing the new component.

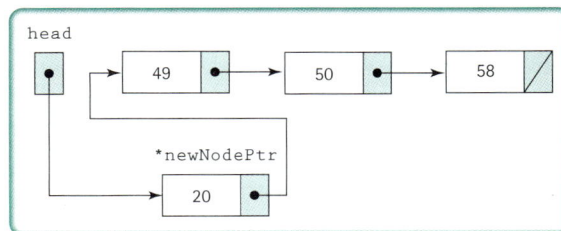

To insert a component into its proper place in a sorted list, we have to loop through the nodes until we find where the component belongs. Because the `HybridList` class keeps components in ascending order, we can recognize where a component belongs by finding the node that contains a value greater than the one being inserted. Our new node should be inserted directly before the node with that value; therefore, we must keep track of the node before the current one in order to insert our new node. We use a pointer `prevPtr` to point to this previous node. This method leads to the following algorithm:

Insert (In: item)

```
Set newNodePtr = new NodeType
Set component member of *newNodePtr = item
Set prevPtr = NULL
Set currPtr = head
WHILE item > component member of *currPtr
      Set prevPtr = currPtr
      Set currPtr = link member of *currPtr
Insert *newNodePtr between *prevPtr and *currPtr
```

This algorithm is basically sound, but there are problems with it in special cases. If the new component is larger than all other components in the list, the event that stops the loop (finding a node whose component is larger than the one being inserted) does not occur. When the end of the list is reached, the While condition tries to dereference currPtr, which now contains NULL. On some systems, the program will crash. We can take care of this case by using the following expression to control the While loop:

currPtr isn't NULL AND item > component member of *currPtr

This expression keeps us from dereferencing the null pointer because C++ uses short-circuit evaluation of logical expressions. If the first part evaluates to false—that is, if currPtr equals NULL—the second part of the expression, which dereferences currPtr, is not evaluated.

There is one more point to consider in our algorithm: the special case in which the list is empty or the new value is less than the first component in the list. The variable prevPtr remains NULL in this case, and *newNodePtr must be inserted at the top instead of between *prevPtr and *currPtr.

The following function implements our algorithm with these changes incorporated.

```cpp
void HybridList::Insert( /* in */ ComponentType item )

// Precondition:
//      Component members of list nodes are in ascending order
// Postcondition:
//      New node containing item is in its proper place
//         in linked list
//    && component members of list nodes are in ascending order

{
    NodePtr currPtr;        // Moving pointer
    NodePtr prevPtr;        // Pointer to node before *currPtr
    NodePtr newNodePtr;     // Pointer to new node

    // Set up node to be inserted

    newNodePtr = new NodeType;
    newNodePtr->component = item;

    // Find previous insertion point

    prevPtr = NULL;
    currPtr = head;
    while (currPtr != NULL && item > currPtr->component)
```

```
    {
        prevPtr = currPtr;
        currPtr = currPtr->link;
    }

    // Insert new node

    newNodePtr->link = currPtr;
    if (prevPtr == NULL)
        head = newNodePtr;
    else
        prevPtr->link = newNodePtr;
}
```

Let's go through this code for each of the three cases: inserting at the top (`item` is 20), inserting in the middle (`item` is 60), and inserting at the end (`item` is 100). Each insertion begins with the list below.

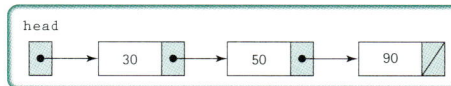

Insert(20)

```
newNodePtr = new NodeType;
newNodePtr->component = item;
prevPtr = NULL;
currPtr = head;
```

These four statements initialize the variables used in the searching process. The variables and their contents are shown below.

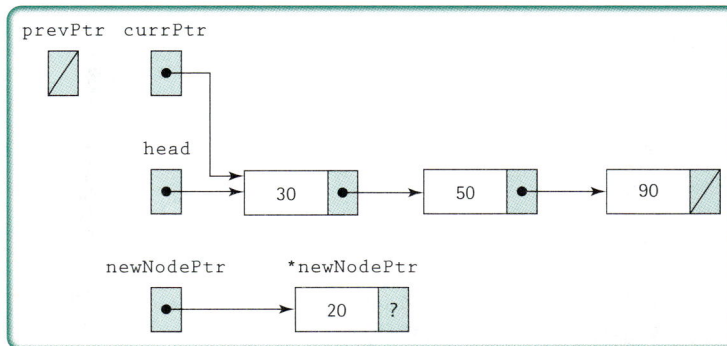

```
while (currPtr != NULL &&
    item > currPtr->component)
```

Because 20 is less than 30, the expression is `false` and the loop body is not entered.

```
newNodePtr->link = currPtr;
```
link member of *newNodePtr now points to *currPtr.

```
if (prevPtr == NULL)
    head = newNodePtr;
```
Because prevPtr is NULL, the then-clause is executed and 20 is inserted at the top of the list.

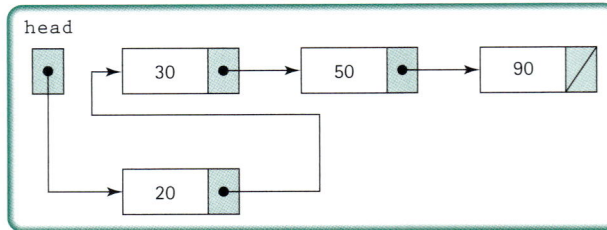

Insert(60)

```
newNodePtr = new NodeType;
newNodePtr->component = item;
prevPtr = NULL;
currPtr = head;
```
These four statements initialize the variables used in the searching process. The variables and their contents are shown below.

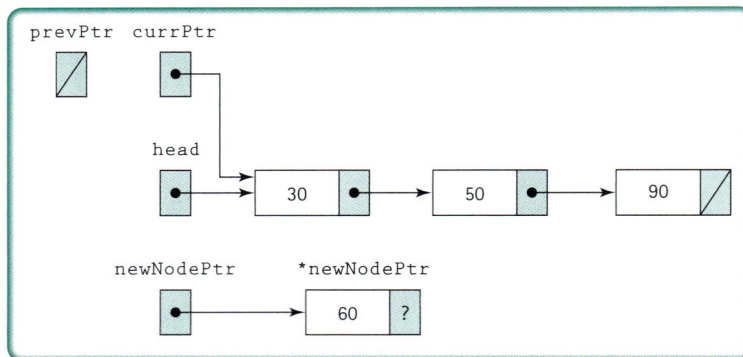

```
while (currPtr != NULL &&
    item > currPtr->component)

prevPtr = currPtr;
currPtr = currPtr->link;
```
Because 60 is greater than 30, this expression is true and the loop body is entered.

Pointer variables are advanced.

(see diagram next page)

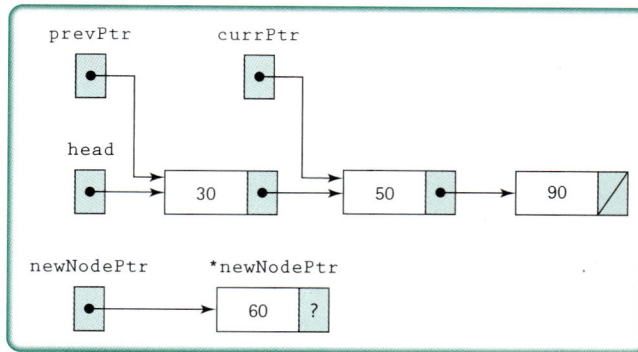

```
while (currPtr != NULL &&
    item > currPtr->component)
prevPtr = currPtr;
currPtr = currPtr->link;
```

Because 60 is greater than 50, this expression is **true** and the loop body is repeated. Pointer variables are advanced.

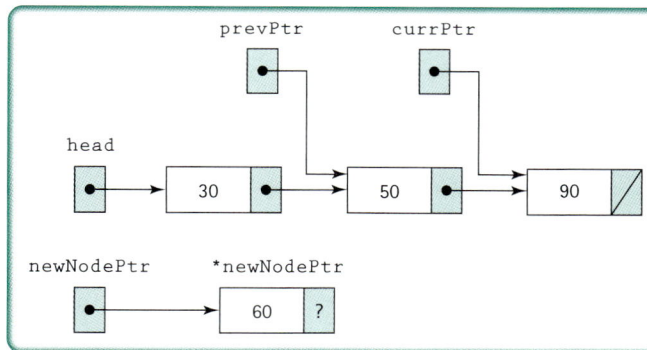

```
while (currPtr != NULL &&
    item > currPtr->component)
```

Because 60 is not greater than 90, the expression is **false** and the loop body is not repeated.

```
newNodePtr->link = currPtr;
```

link member of *newNodePtr now points to *currPtr.

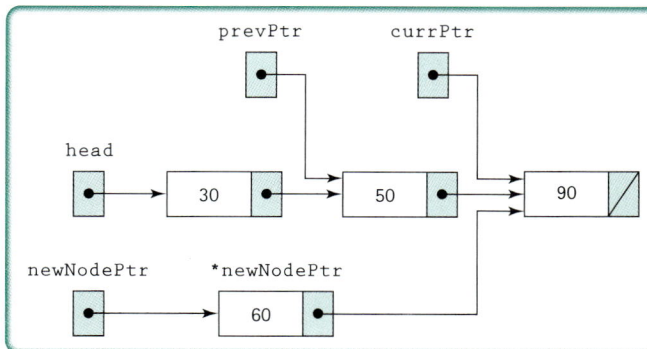

```
if (prevPtr == NULL)
prevPtr->link = newNodePtr;
```

Because `prevPtr` does not equal `NULL`, the else-clause is executed. The completed list is shown with the auxiliary variables removed.

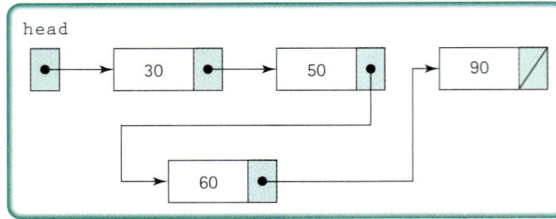

Insert(100)

We do not repeat the first part of the search, but pick up the walk-through where `prevPtr` is pointing to the node whose component is 50, and `currPtr` is pointing to the node whose component is 90.

```
while (currPtr != NULL &&
    item > currPtr->component)

prevPtr = currPtr;
currPtr = currPtr->link;
```

Because 100 is greater than 90, this expression is `true` and the loop body is repeated.

The pointer variables are advanced.

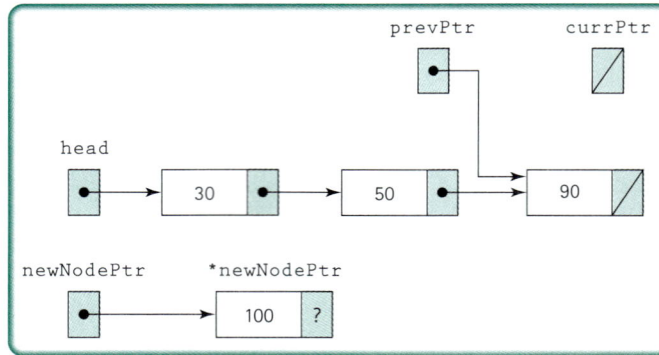

```
while (currPtr != NULL &&
    item > currPtr->component)
```

Because `currPtr` equals `NULL`, the expression is `false` and the loop body is not repeated.

```
newNodePtr->link = currPtr;
```

`NULL` is copied into `link` member of `*newNodePtr`.

```
if (prevPtr == NULL)
    prevPtr->link = newNodePtr;
```

Because `prevPtr` does not equal `NULL`, the else-clause is executed. Node `*newNodePtr` is inserted after `*prevPtr`. The list is shown with auxiliary variables removed.

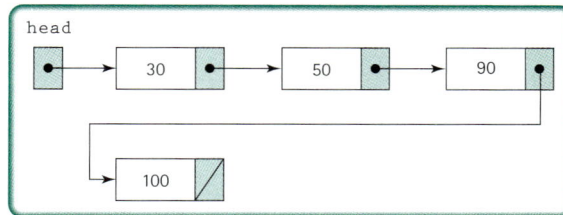

Deleting from a Linked List To delete an existing node from a linked list, we have to loop through the nodes until we find the node we want to delete. We look at the mirror image of our insertions: deleting the top node and deleting a node whose component is equal to an incoming parameter.

To delete the first node, we just change the external pointer to point to the second node (or to contain `NULL` if we are deleting the only node in a one-node list). The value in the node being deleted can be returned as an outgoing parameter. Notice the precondition for the following function: The client must not call the function if the list is empty.

```
void HybridList::RemoveFirst( /* out */ ComponentType& item )

// Precondition:
//     Linked list is not empty (head != NULL)
//  && component members of list nodes are in ascending order
// Postcondition:
//     item == component member of first list node at entry
//  && Node containing item is no longer in linked list
//  && component members of list nodes are in ascending order

{
    NodePtr tempPtr = head;    // Temporary pointer

    item = head->component;
    head = head->link;
    delete tempPtr;
}
```

We don't show a complete code walk-through because the code is so straightforward. Instead, we show the state of the data structure in two stages: after the first two statements and at the end. We use one of our previous lists. Following is the data structure after the execution of the first two statements in the function.

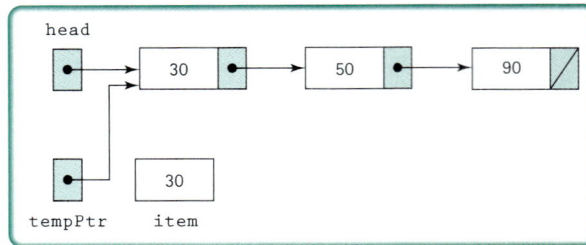

After the execution of the function, the structure is as follows:

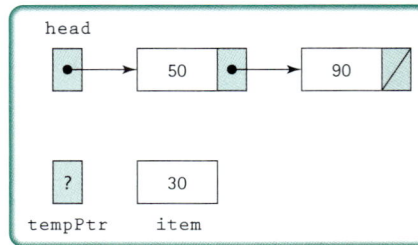

The function for deleting a node whose component contains a certain value is similar to the `Insert` function. The difference is that we are looking for a match, not a `component` member greater than our `item`. Because the function precondition states that the component we are looking for is definitely in the list, our loop control is simple. We don't have to worry about dereferencing the null pointer.

As in the `Insert` function, we need the node before the one that is to be deleted so we can change its `link` member. In the following function, we demonstrate another technique for keeping track of the previous node. Instead of comparing `item` with the `component` member of `*currPtr`, we compare it with the `component` member of the node pointed to by `currPtr->link`; that is, we compare `item` with `currPtr->link->component`. When `currPtr->link->component` is equal to `item`, `*currPtr` is the previous node.

```
void HybridList::Delete( /* in */ ComponentType item )

// Precondition:
//      item == component member of some list node
//   && component members of list nodes are in ascending order
// Postcondition:
//      Node containing first occurrence of item is no longer in
//         linked list
//   && component members of list nodes are in ascending order
```

```
{
    NodePtr delPtr;        // Pointer to node to be deleted
    NodePtr currPtr;       // Loop control pointer

    // Check if item is in first node

    if (item == head->component)
    {
        // Delete first node

        delPtr = head;
        head = head->link;
    }
    else
    {
        // Search for node in rest of list

        currPtr = head;
        while (currPtr->link->component != item)
            currPtr = currPtr->link;

        // Delete *(currPtr->link)

        delPtr = currPtr->link;
        currPtr->link = currPtr->link->link;
    }
    delete delPtr;
}
```

Let's delete the node whose component is 90. The structure is shown below, with the nodes labeled as they are when the While statement is reached.

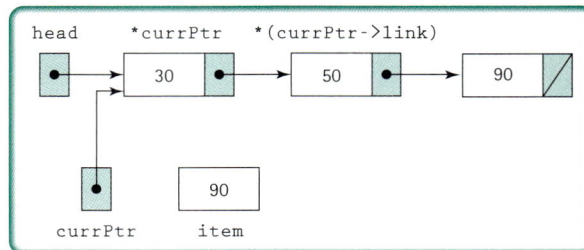

```
while (currPtr->link->component != item)       Because 50 is not equal to 90, the
                                               loop body is entered.
```

```
currPtr = currPtr->link;
```
Pointer is advanced.

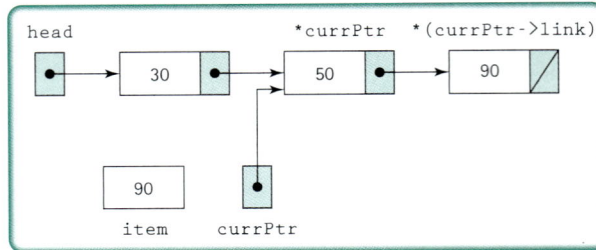

```
while (currPtr->link->component != item)
```
Because 90 is equal to 90, the loop is exited.

```
delPtr = currPtr->link;
currPtr->link = currPtr->link->link;
```
The `link` member of the node whose component is 90 is copied into the `link` member of the node whose component is 50. The `link` member equals NULL in this case.

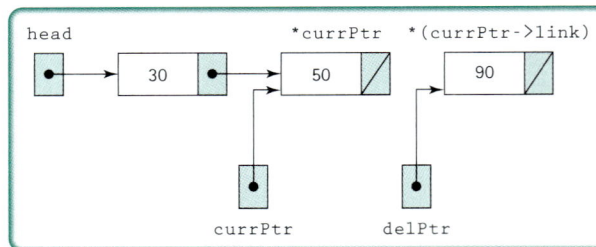

```
delete delPtr;
```
Memory allocated to `*delPtr` (the node that was deleted) is returned to the free store. The value of `delPtr` is undefined.

Note that NULL was stored into `currPtr->link` only because the node whose component is 90 was the last one in the list. If there had been more nodes beyond this one, a pointer to the next node would have been stored into `currPtr->link`.

Pointer Expressions

As you can see from the `HybridList::Delete` function, pointer expressions can be quite complex. Let's look at some examples.

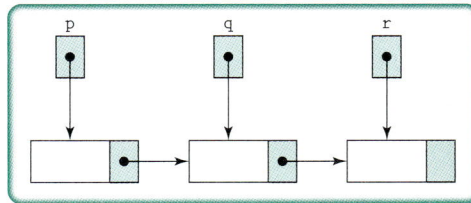

p, q, and r point to nodes in a dynamic linked list. The nodes themselves are *p, *q, and *r. Use the preceding diagram to convince yourself that the following are true.

```
p->link == q
*(p->link) is the same node as *q
p->link->link == r
*(p->link->link) is the same node as *r
q->link == r
*(q->link) is the same node as *r
```

And remember the semantics of assignment statements for pointers.

p = q;   Assigns the contents of pointer q to pointer p.
*p = *q;   Assigns the contents of the variable pointed to by q to the variable pointed to by p.

Classes and Dynamic Linked Lists

In Chapter 15, we said that classes whose objects manipulate dynamic data on the free store should provide not only a class constructor but also a destructor, a deep copy operation, and a copy-constructor. The HybridList class includes all of these except (to keep the example simpler) a deep copy operation. Let's look at the class destructor.

The purpose of the destructor is to deallocate the dynamic linked list when a HybridList class object is destroyed. Without a destructor, the linked list would be left behind on the free store, still allocated but inaccessible. The code for the destructor is easy to write. Using the existing member functions IsEmpty and DeleteTop, we simply march through the list and delete each node:

```
HybridList::~HybridList()

// Destructor

// Postcondition:
//      All linked list nodes have been deallocated from free store
```

```
{
    ComponentType temp;     // Temporary variable

    while ( !IsEmpty() )
        RemoveFirst(temp);
}
```

The copy-constructor is harder to write. Before we look at it, we must stress the importance of providing a copy-constructor whenever we also provide a destructor. Pretend that `HybridList` doesn't have a copy-constructor, and suppose that a client passes a class object to a function using a pass by value. (Remember that passing an argument by value sends a *copy* of the value of the argument to the function.) Within the function, the parameter is initialized to be a copy of the caller's class object, including the caller's value of the private variable `head`. At this point, both the argument and the parameter are pointing to the same dynamic linked list. When the client function returns, the class destructor is invoked for the parameter, destroying the only copy of the linked list. Upon return from the function, the caller's linked list has disappeared!

By providing a copy-constructor, we ensure deep copying of an argument to a parameter whenever a pass by value occurs. The implementation of the copy-constructor, shown below, employs a commonly used algorithm for creating a new linked list as a copy of another.

```
HybridList::HybridList( const SortedList2& otherList )

// Copy-constructor

// Postcondition:
//     IF otherList.head == NULL  (i.e., the other list is empty)
//        head == NULL
//     ELSE
//        head points to a new linked list that is a copy of
//        the linked list pointed to by otherList.head

{
    NodePtr fromPtr;    // Pointer into list being copied from
    NodePtr toPtr;      // Pointer into new list being built

    if (otherList.head == NULL)
    {
        head = NULL;
        return;
    }
```

```
    // Copy first node

    fromPtr = otherList.head;
    head = new NodeType;
    head->component = fromPtr->component;

    // Copy remaining nodes

    toPtr = head;
    fromPtr = fromPtr->link;
    while (fromPtr != NULL)
    {
        toPtr->link = new NodeType;
        toPtr = toPtr->link;
        toPtr->component = fromPtr->component;
        fromPtr = fromPtr->link;
    }
    toPtr->link = NULL;
}
```

16.4 Choice of Data Representation

We have looked in detail at two ways of representing lists of components: one in which the components are physically next to each other (a direct array representation, as in Figure 16–1), and one in which the components are only logically next to each other (a linked list). Furthermore, a linked list is an abstraction that can be implemented either by using an array of structs or by using dynamically allocated structs and pointers (a dynamic linked list).

Let's compare the array representation with the dynamic linked list representation. (Throughout this discussion, we use *array* to mean a direct array representation, not an array of structs forming a linked list.) We look at common operations on lists and examine the advantages and disadvantages of each representation for each operation.

Common Operations

1. Read the components into an initially empty list.
2. Access all the components in the list in sequence.
3. Insert or delete the first component in a list.
4. Insert or delete the last component in a list.
5. Insert or delete the *n*th component in a list.
6. Access the *n*th component in a list.
7. Sort the components in a list.
8. Search the list for a specific component.

Reading components into a list is faster with an array representation than with a dynamic linked list because the `new` operation doesn't have to be executed for each component. Accessing the components in sequence takes approximately the same time with both structures.

Inserting or deleting the first component is much faster using a linked representation. Remember that with an array, all the other list items have to be shifted down (for an insertion) or up (for a deletion). Conversely, inserting or deleting the last component is much more efficient with an array; there is direct access to the last component, and no shifting is required. In a linked representation, the entire list must be searched to find the last component.

On average, the time spent inserting or deleting the nth component is about equal for the two types of lists. A linked representation would be better for small values of n, and an array representation would be better for values of n near the end of the list.

Accessing the nth element is *much* faster in an array representation. We can access it directly by using $n - 1$ as the index into the array. In a linked representation, we have to access the first $n - 1$ components sequentially to reach the nth one.

For many sorting algorithms, including the selection sort, the two representations are approximately equal in efficiency. However, there are some sophisticated, very fast sorting algorithms that rely on direct access to array elements by using array indexes. These algorithms are not suitable for a linked representation, which requires sequential access to the components.

In general, searching a sorted list for a specific component is much faster in an array representation because a binary search can be used. When the components in the list to be searched are not in sorted order, the two representations are about the same.

When you are trying to decide whether to use an array representation or a linked representation, determine which of these common operations are likely to be applied most frequently. Use your analysis to determine which structure would be better in the context of your particular problem.

An additional point to consider when deciding whether to use an array or a dynamic linked list: How accurately can you predict the maximum number of components in the list? Does the number of components in the list fluctuate widely? If you know the maximum and it remains fairly constant, an array representation is fine in terms of memory usage. Otherwise, it is better to choose a dynamic linked representation in order to use memory more efficiently.

There is one final point that should be considered when deciding between an array-based or a linked implementation. An array-based structure can be written to a file and read back in later. A linked structure is valid only for the run of the program in which it is formed. Because the links are memory addresses, and memory may be allocated differently each time a program is executed, we cannot directly write a linked list to a file to be used later. Of course, the *components* can be written to a file, but the program would have to recreate the list each time it executes.

Problem-Solving Case Study

The Appointment Calendar Completed

PROBLEM Complete the Appointment Calendar by creating a list of objects of class Day.

DISCUSSION We are finally there! We have all the pieces; we just need to complete the list of Day objects. Before we look at the structure, let's determine the operations that we need. We are defining the final level now, so we need those operations that one does with an appointment calendar.

> Create the calendar
> Insert a day
> Insert an appointment, given a date
> Delete an appointment, given a date and a time
> Test to see if a time is free, given a date
> Print a day's appointments, given a date

DATA STRUCTURES We certainly know by now how to create a list of objects. In each stage of building this appointment calendar, we have changed and enhanced the list structure as we have learned new techniques. Let's leave class Day as it is for now, and just look at the structure for the list of days. We could create an array-based list like we have used for the list of objects of class Entry. We could make a linked list of days sorted by date. We also have another, not quite so obvious, choice.

There are always 12 months in a year, but the number of days with appointments varies by number of days in a month, the number of weekends, and the number of holidays. An efficient structure would be a 12-item array of months in which each cell contains a pointer to a list of days ordered by day. That is, the month would be an index into the place in the array for that month's appointments. The list of appointments would be a linked list of Day objects ordered by day of the month. See Figure 16–7. The linked structure pointed to from calendar[0] is repeated for each month for which you have an appointment.

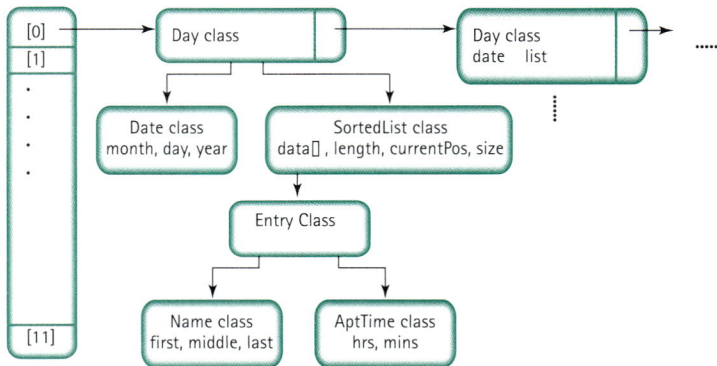

Figure 16–7

What other information do we need in our final program in addition to array `calendar`? It would be nice to have the name of the month, not just the month number on the output list. We can declare an array of strings for the names of the months and access it by the month number minus one, the same value that indexes the list of appointments for the month. Since only the print operation needs this information, we can make this structure local to that operation.

This is a very complex structure! Let's first create a list of days. Once we have this structure coded and tested, we can design the main program that declares an array of 12 of these lists.

Linked List of Days   Can we use the operations in the Hybrid list ADT in this chapter? Let's see. We need to insert a day into the list and find a day in order to implement all those operations that say "given a date." There are two insert operations in the Hybrid list, one of which inserts an object into its proper place. However, no separate search operation is defined and none of the other operations are useful to us here. Let's just cannibalize the code and define an insert and a search for our list of days. (Remember: Never reinvent the wheel.)

Here is the specification file for class `DayList`, incorporating all of the operations that we defined in our discussion.

```
//*****************************************************************
// SPECIFICATION FILE (DayList.h)
// This file gives the specification of the DayList class, which
// is a list of objects of class Day.  Two functions operate on
// class DayList itself: InsertDay and FindDay.  The other
// functions operate on the components in the list.
// To save space, we omit from each function the precondition
// comments that document the assumptions made about valid input
// parameter data. These would be included in a program intended
// for actual use.
//*****************************************************************

#include <iostream>
#include <fstream>
#include "Date.h"

using namespace std;

struct NodeType;

class DayList
{
public:
    void InsertDay(Date date);

        // Precondition:
        //      Component members of list of days are in ascending
        //      day order
```

```
    // Postcondition:
    //      New node containing date is in its proper place
    //      in list of days
    //   && component members of day list are in ascending day
    //      order

void InsertApt(Date date);

    // Precondition:
    //      Component members of list of days are in ascending
    //      day order
    //   && list of entries for day are in time order
    // Postcondition:
    //      A user-entered entry is inserted into the entry
    //      list for the given day
    //   && entry list is in ascending time order

bool IsFree(Date date);

    // Precondition:
    //      Component members of list of days are in ascending
    //      day order
    //   && list of entries for day are in time order
    // Postcondition:
    //      Return value is true if user-entered time is free on
    //      given day; false otherwise

void PrintDay(ofstream& outFile, Date date);

    // Precondition:
    //      Component members of list of days are in ascending
    //      day order
    // Postcondition:
    //      Entry list for day has been written on outFile

void DeleteApt(Date date);

    // Precondition:
    //      Component members of list of days are in ascending
    //      day order
    //   && list of entries for date are in time order
    // Postcondition:
    //      Day has been deleted from the list of days
```

```
      DayList();

          // Postcondition:
          //      Empty list is created

  private:
      NodeType* dayList;

      NodeType* FindDay(Date date);

          // Precondition:
          //      Component members of list of days are in ascending
          //      day order
          // Postcondition:
          //      Return value is a pointer to the day for the given
          //      date or NULL if day not found.
  };
```

Read the documentation carefully. Notice that the preconditions state the order of the list elements that they are manipulating. Although the original operations are in terms of a date, our structure guarantees that the list of days contains only those dates in the same month.

Create a `DayList` The only data item in class `DayList` is a pointer; we must set it to NULL to represent the empty list. We did not include a destructor or a copy constructor for this problem. The list of days is not passed as a parameter, is not the return value of a function, and is declared at the top level. It goes out of scope when the program is completed.

Inserting a `Day` object into the List We can use the algorithm for this operation that was already given on page 863.

Finding a `Day` object with a given `Day` We must set a moving pointer to the beginning of the list and keep moving the pointer through the list until the date is found or the end of the list is reached.

FindDay(In: date)
  Out: Function value

Set currPtr to dayList
WHILE currPtr != NULL AND currPtr->component.DateIs() != date
    Increment currPtr
Return currPtr

We must make this function return a pointer to the node we want and not the node itself. Why? If we send back the node itself, there will be an error if the day with the given date is not found.

InsertApt   We can use the `FindDay` operation to find the day with the given date, prompt the user for the name and time, and insert the entry into the date.

InsertApt(In: date)

```
Set day to FindDay(date)
IF day is NULL
    Write "Day has not been initialized"
ELSE
    entry.ReadEntry()
    day->component.InsertEntry(entry)
```

DeleteApt   This operation is identical to the InsertApt operation except that you apply `Delete` rather than `InsertEntry`.

IsFree   This operation just applies the `TimeFree` function to the returned component.

Print the Appointments for a Day   We use `FindDay` to find the day to print. If NULL is returned, an error message should be printed; otherwise, we iterate through the list printing each component.

PrintDay(Inout: outFile; In: date)

```
Set day to FindDay(date)
IF day is NULL
    Write on outFile "Day has not been initialized"
ELSE
    Write heading on outFile
    Set limit to Number of Entries
    ResetEntries
    WHILE limit is not 0
        Set entry to next item
        Write on outFile name and time
        Decrement limit
```

Here is the implementation file for class `DayList`.

```cpp
//***********************************************************************
// IMPLEMENTATION FILE (DayList.cpp)
// This file implements the DayList class, which is a
// linked list of objects of class Day.
//***********************************************************************
#include "DayList.h"
#include <iostream>
#include "Day.h"
#include <cstddef>                    // For NULL
using namespace std;

typedef NodeType* NodePtr;

struct NodeType
{
    Day component;
    NodePtr link;
};

DayList::DayList()

// Constructor

// Postcondition:
//     dayList is NULL

{
    dayList = NULL;
}

NodePtr DayList::FindDay(Date date)

// Precondition:
//     component members of list are in ascending date order
// Postcondition:
//     Return value is a pointer to the day for the given date or
//     NULL if day not found.

{
    NodePtr currPtr = dayList;
```

```
    while (currPtr != NULL &&
            currPtr->component.DateIs().ComparedTo(date) != SAME)
        currPtr = currPtr->link;
    return currPtr;
}


void DayList::InsertApt(Date date)

// Precondition:
//     component members of day list nodes are in ascending date
//   && list of entries for date is in time order
// Postcondition:
//     New node containing entry is inserted in entry list
//   && component members of list are in ascending time order

{
    Entry entry;
    NodePtr day;

    day = FindDay(date);
    if (day == NULL)
        cout << "Day has not been initialized" << endl;
    else
    { // Insert entry into list of entries for date
        entry.ReadEntry();
        day->component.InsertEntry(entry);
    }
}


void DayList::InsertDay(Date date)

// Precondition:
//     component members of list of days are in ascending date
//     order
// Postcondition:
//     New node containing item is in its proper place
//     in list of days
//   && component members of day list are in ascending date order

{
    int numberOfApts;
    cout << "How many appointments can be made on this date?"
        << endl;
    cin >> numberOfApts;
```

```
                    Day day(date, numberOfApts);

                    NodePtr currPtr;        // Moving pointer
                    NodePtr prevPtr;        // Pointer to node before *currPtr
                    NodePtr newNodePtr;     // Pointer to new node

                    // Set up node to be inserted

                    newNodePtr = new NodeType;
                    newNodePtr->component = day;

                    // Find insertion point
                    prevPtr = NULL;
                    currPtr = dayList;
                    while (currPtr != NULL &&
                        date.ComparedTo(currPtr->component.DateIs()) == AFTER)
                    {
                        prevPtr = currPtr;
                        currPtr = currPtr->link;
                    }

                    // Insert new node

                    newNodePtr->link = currPtr;
                    if (prevPtr == NULL)
                        dayList = newNodePtr;
                    else
                        prevPtr->link = newNodePtr;
                }

                void DayList::DeleteApt(Date date)

                // Precondition:
                //     Component members of day list are in ascending date
                //     && list of entries for date are in time order
                // Postcondition:
                //     Time read from the keyboard is removed from the entry list
                //     for date if present; otherwise an error message is written

                {
                    AptTime time;
                    time.ReadTime();
                    Entry entry(" ", " ", " ", time.Hours(), time.Minutes());
```

```
    NodePtr  day;

    day = FindDay(date);

    if (day == NULL)
        cout << "Day has not been initialized" << endl;
    else
        day->component.Delete(entry);
}

bool DayList::IsFree(Date date)

// Precondition:
//     Component members of day list are in ascending date order
//  && list of entries for date are in time order
// Postcondition:
//     Return value is true if user-entered time is free on
//     given day; false otherwise

{

    AptTime time;
    time.ReadTime();

    NodePtr day;

    day = FindDay(date);

    if (day == NULL)
    {
        cout << "Day has not been initialized " << endl;
        return true;
    }
    else
        return day->component.TimeFree(time);
}

void DayList::PrintDay(ofstream& outFile, Date date)

// Precondition:
//     Component members of day list are in ascending date order
// Postcondition:
//     Entry list for date has been written on outFile if present;
//     otherwise error message has been written
```

```
{
    static string  months[12] = {"January", "February", "March",
        "April", "May", "June", "July", "August", "September",
        "October", "November", "December"};

    int limit;
    Entry entry;
    NodePtr day;

    day = FindDay(date);

    if (day == NULL)
        outFile << "Day has not been initialized " << endl;
    else
    {
        outFile << "Appointments for " << months[date.Month() -1]
                << " " << date.Day()
                << ", " << date.Year() << endl;

        limit = day->component.NumberOfEntries();
        day->component.ResetEntries();
        while (limit != 0)
        {
            entry = day->component.GetNextItem();
            outFile << entry.NameStr() << " at "
                    << entry.TimeStr() << endl;
            limit--;
        }
        outFile << endl;
    }
}
```

TESTING   A driver should be constructed that tests each of the operations in the class. We do not show it here, but an appropriate driver is available from the publisher's website.

Main Program   Finally, we can write the main program for our appointment calendar! The data structure is declared as follows.

```
DayList calendar[12];
```

The main program is just a driver that prompts the user to enter a command. The command, a string, is converted into an enumerated type that can be used on a Switch statement. The various cases in the Switch statement get a date if needed and call the appropriate DayList operations. All of this processing is enclosed within a loop.

Main

```
Set notQuit to true

WHILE notQuit
    Print menu
    Get the operation
    SWITCH (Convert(operation))
        case INSERT_DAY
            GetDate(date)
            calendar[date.Month()-1].InsertDay(date)
        case INSERT_APT
            GetDate(date)
            calendar[date.Month()-1].InsertApt(date)
        case DELETE_APT
            GetDate(date)
            calendar[date.Month()-1].DeleteApt(date)
        case IS_FREE
            GetDate(date)
            IF calendar[date.Month()-1].IsFree(date)
                Write "Time is free"
            ELSE
                Write "Time is not free"
        case PRINT_DAY
            GetDate(date)
            calendar[date.Month()-1].PrintDay(outFile, date)
        case QUIT
            Set notQuit to false
        case ERROR
            Write "Input string was not valid.  Read menu and try again."
```

Which of the operations here need expanding? Print menu must be expanded to give instructions to the user about what to enter. Get the operation can be a simple string read. Convert(operation) must be coded as a function that takes a string and returns the appropriate enumerated type. GetDate(date) must prompt for and read the date.

PrintMenu

Write "Menu Options"
Write "InsertDay sets up a new day"
Write "InsertApt inserts a new entry"
Write "DeleteApt deletes an entry"
Write "IsFree checks to see if a time is free"
Write "PrintDay prints all the appointments for a day"
Write "Quit ends the processing"
Write "Type in the appropriate string"

Convert(In: operation)
Out: Function value

IF operation equals "InsertDay"
    Return INSERT_DAY
ELSE IF operation equals "InsertApt"
    Return INSERT_APT
ELSE IF operation equals "DeleteApt"
    Return DELETE_APT
ELSE IF operation equals "IsFree"
    Return IS_FREE
ELSE IF operation equals "PrintDay"
    Return PRINT_DAY
ELSE IF operation equals "Quit"
    Return QUIT
ELSE
    Return ERROR

GetDate(Out: date)

Write "Enter month, day, year in that order"
Get month, day, year
date.Set(month, day, year)

At last we are ready to code our appointment calendar.

```cpp
//****************************************************************
// APPOINTMENT CALENDAR PROGRAM
// This file implements an appointment calendar.
//****************************************************************

#include "DayList.h"
#include <fstream>
#include <string>
#include <iostream>
#include <cstddef>       // For NULL
using namespace std;

enum Operations{INSERT_DAY, INSERT_APT, DELETE_APT, IS_FREE,
                PRINT_DAY, QUIT, ERROR};

// Function prototypes
Operations Convert(string operation);
void GetDate(Date& date);
void PrintMenu();

int main()
{
    DayList calendar[12];
    bool notQuit = true;
    Date date;

    string operation;
    ofstream outData;
    ofstream outList;
    outData.open("Appointments");

    while (notQuit)
    {
        PrintMenu();
        cin >> operation;
        switch (Convert(operation))
```

```
                    {
                        case INSERT_DAY:
                            GetDate(date);
                            calendar[date.Month()-1].InsertDay(date);
                            break;
                        case INSERT_APT:
                            GetDate(date);
                            calendar[date.Month()-1].InsertApt(date);
                            break;
                        case DELETE_APT:
                            GetDate(date);
                            calendar[date.Month()-1].DeleteApt(date);
                            break;
                        case IS_FREE:
                            GetDate(date);
                            if (calendar[date.Month()-1].IsFree(date))
                                cout << "Time is free" << endl;
                            else
                                cout << "Time is not free" << endl;
                            break;
                        case PRINT_DAY:
                            GetDate(date);
                            calendar[date.Month()-1].PrintDay(outData, date);
                            break;
                        case QUIT:
                            notQuit = false;
                            break;
                        case ERROR:
                            cout << "Input string was not valid."
                                 << endl
                                 << "Read menu and try again."
                                 << endl;
                    }
                }
                outData.close();
                outList.close();
                return 0;

            }

        void GetDate(Date& date)
        {
            int month;
            int day;
            int year;
```

```
        cout << "Enter month, day, and year in that order" << endl;
        cin >> month >> day >> year;
        date.Set(month, day, year);
}


void PrintMenu()
{
        cout << "Menu Options" << endl;
        cout << "        InsertDay sets up a new day " << endl;
        cout << "        InsertApt inserts a new entry" << endl;
        cout << "        DeleteApt deletes an entry " << endl;
        cout << "        IsFree checks to see if a time is free"
             << endl;
        cout << "        PrintDay prints all of the appointments "
             << " for a day" << endl;
        cout << "        Quit ends the processing" << endl;
        cout << "Type in the appropriate string " << endl << endl;
}


Operations Convert(string operation)
{
        if (operation == "InsertDay")
            return INSERT_DAY  ;
        else if (operation == "InsertApt")
            return INSERT_APT;
        else if (operation == "DeleteApt")
            return DELETE_APT;
        else if (operation == "IsFree")
            return IS_FREE;
        else if (operation == "PrintDay")
            return PRINT_DAY;
        else if (operation == "Quit")
            return QUIT;
        else return ERROR;
}
```

TESTING   A minimum test plan would require that each operation be tested at least once and several at least twice.

Reason for test case	Input values	Expected output	Observed output
Insert day		None expected	
one month	InsertDay 1 3 2004 5		
another month	InsertDay 4 5 2004 6		
InsertApt		None expected	
one month	InsertApt 1 3 2004 Sarah Jane Jones 10:30		
same month	InsertApt 1 3 2004 Susan Margaret Smith 9:30		
another month	InsertApt 4 5 2004 Judy Dale David 3:00		
PrintDay			
month with one	PrintDay 4 5 2004	Judy Dale David 3:00	
month with more	PrintDay 1 3 2004	Susan Margaret Smith 9:30 Sarah Jane Jones 10:30	
day not there	PrintDay 2 3 2004	Day has not been initialized	
DeleteApt			
appointment there	DeleteApt 1 3 2004 9:30 PrintDay 1 3 2004	Sarah Jane Jones 10:30	
apt. not there	DeleteApt 1 3 2004 12:30 PrintDay 1 3 2004	Sarah Jane Jones 10:30	
day not there	DeleteApt 3 3 2004 12:30	Day has not been initialized	
IsFree			
time is free	IsFree 1 3 2004 4:30	Time is free	
time is not free	IsFree 1 3 2004 10:30	Time is not free	
day not there	IsFree 1 6 2004 1:30	Day has not been initialized	
Error in input	DeletApt	Input string was not valid. Read menu and try again.	
Quit	Quit		

Because the output is five pages long, we only show excerpts, with the menu removed.

```
Menu Options
      InsertDay sets up a new day
      InsertApt inserts a new entry
      DeleteApt deletes an entry
      IsFree checks to see if a time is free
      PrintDay prints all of the appointments  for a day
      Quit ends the processing
Type in the appropriate string
```

```
InsertDay
Enter month, day, and year in that order
1 3 2004
How many appointments can be made on this date?
5


...
InsertDay
Enter month, day, and year in that order
4 5 2004
How many appointments can be made on this date?
6


...

InsertApt
Enter month, day, and year in that order
1 3 2004
Enter first name: Sarah
Enter middle name: Jane
Enter last name: Jones
Enter hours (<= 23):
10
Enter minutes (<= 59):
30


...

InsertApt
Enter month, day, and year in that order
1 3 2004
Enter first name: Susan
Enter middle name: Margaret
Enter last name: Smith
Enter hours (<= 23):
9
Enter minutes (<= 59):
30


...


InsertApt
Enter month, day, and year in that order
4 5 2004
```

```
Enter first name: Judy
Enter middle name: Dale
Enter last name: David
Enter hours (<= 23):
3
Enter minutes (<= 59):
0


...


PrintDay
Enter month, day, and year in that order
4 5 2004


...


PrintDay
Enter month, day, and year in that order
1 3 2004


...


PrintDay
Enter month, day, and year in that order
2 3 2004
Day has not been initialized


...


DeleteApt
Enter month, day, and year in that order
1 3 2004
Enter hours (<= 23):
9
Enter minutes (<= 59):
30


...


PrintDay
Enter month, day, and year in that order
1 3 2004


...
```

```
DeleteApt
Enter month, day, and year in that order
1 3 2004
Enter hours (<= 23):
12
Enter minutes (<= 59):
30

...

PrintDay
Enter month, day, and year in that order
1 3 2004

...

DeleteApt
Enter month, day, and year in that order
3 3 2004
Enter hours (<= 23):
12
Enter minutes (<= 59):
30
Day has not been initialized

...

IsFree
Enter month, day, and year in that order
1 3 2004
Enter hours (<= 23):
4
Enter minutes (<= 59):
30
Time is free

...

IsFree
Enter month, day, and year in that order
1 3 2004
Enter hours (<= 23):
10
```

```
Enter minutes (<= 59):
30
Time is not free


. . .

IsFree
Enter month, day, and year in that order
1 6 2004
Enter hours (<= 23):
1
Enter minutes (<= 59):
30
Day has not been initialized
Time is free


. . .

DeletApt
Input string was not valid.
Read menu and try again.


. . .

Quit
```

Here are the contents of file Appointments.

```
Appointments for April 5, 2004
Judy David at 03:00

Appointments for January 3, 2004
Susan Smith at 09:30
Sarah Jones at 10:30

Appointments for January 3, 2004
Sarah Jones at 10:30

Appointments for January 3, 2004
Sarah Jones at 10:30
```

Testing and Debugging

Testing and debugging a linked structure is complicated by the fact that each item in the structure contains not only a data portion but also a link to the next item. Algorithms must correctly account for both the data and the link.

When linked lists are implemented with dynamic data and pointers, the errors discussed in Chapter 15 can crop up: memory leaks, dangling pointers, and attempts to dereference a null pointer or an uninitialized pointer. Below are suggestions to help you locate such errors or avoid them in the first place.

Testing and Debugging Hints

1. Review the Testing and Debugging Hints for Chapter 15. They apply to the pointers and dynamic data that are used in dynamic linked lists.

2. Be sure that the link member in the last node of a dynamic linked list has been set to NULL.

3. When visiting the components in a dynamic linked list, be sure that you test for the end of the list in such a way that you don't try to dereference the null pointer. On many systems, dereferencing the null pointer causes a run-time error.

4. Be sure to initialize the external pointer to each dynamic data structure.

5. Do not use

   ```
   currPtr++;
   ```

   to make currPtr point to the next node in a dynamic linked list. The list nodes are not necessarily in consecutive memory locations on the free store.

6. Keep close track of pointers. Changing pointer values prematurely may cause problems when you try to get back to the pointed-to variable.

7. If a C++ class that points to dynamic data has a class destructor but not a copy-constructor, do not pass a class object to a function using pass by value. A shallow copy occurs, and both the parameter and the argument point to the same dynamic data. When the function returns, the parameter's destructor is executed, destroying the argument's dynamic data.

Summary

Dynamic data structures grow and contract during run time. They are made up of nodes that contain two kinds of members: the component, and one or more pointers to nodes of the same type. The pointer to the first node is saved in a variable called the external pointer to the structure.

A linked list is a data structure in which the components are logically next to each other rather than physically next to each other as they are in an array. A linked list can be represented either as an array of structs or as a collection of dynamic nodes, linked

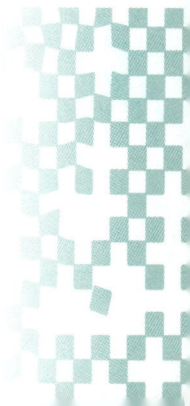

together by pointers. The end of a dynamic linked list is indicated by the special pointer constant NULL. Common operations on linked lists include inserting a node, deleting a node, and traversing the list (visiting each node from first to last).

In this chapter, we used linked lists to implement lists. But linked lists are also used to implement many data structures other than lists. The study of data structures forms a major topic in computer science. Entire books and courses are developed to cover the subject. A solid understanding of the fundamentals of linked lists is a prerequisite to creating more complex structures.

Quick Check

1. Describe a situation in which we can't just use a dynamically allocated array to implement a list instead of using a dynamic linked list. (pp. 877–878)
2. What member do we need in addition to the data members of a struct to use the struct as a node in a linked list? (pp. 846–847)
3. What are the general steps that a program must go through to print the components of a linked list? (pp. 861–863)
4. What are the general steps necessary to insert a new node into a linked list following a specific node? (pp. 865–871)
5. What are the general steps necessary to delete a node from a linked list following a specific node? (pp. 871–874)

Answers

1. When we don't know in advance how much data will be stored in the list.   2. A pointer to the next node in the list.   3. Set the current position pointer to the head of the list, then iteratively print the node and advance the current position to the next node by setting it equal to the node pointer within the current node.   4. Allocate a new node. Assign the value from the node pointer of the current node to the node pointer of the new node. Assign the node pointer of the current node to equal the address of the new node. Assign any data members to the new node as appropriate.   5. Assign the value of the node pointer of the current node to a temporary pointer. Assign the value of the node pointer from the node pointed to by the node pointer field of the current node to the node pointer field of the current node. (Assign the address of the node following the one to be deleted to the node pointer of the current node.) Delete the data associated with the temporary pointer.

Exam Preparation Exercises

1. Define the following terms:

   Node
   Component member
   Link member
   Current pointer

2. We only need a head pointer for a dynamic linked list. With an array-based linked list, we can find the head automatically. True or false?

3. Using a forward declaration of the node pointer type allows us to avoid using an anonymous type to declare the link field within the `struct` representing the node. True or false?

4. What value does each of the following expressions access? The variable names have the same meanings as we have used them elsewhere in this chapter.
   a. `currPtr->link`
   b. `currPtr->component`
   c. `currPtr->link->component`
   d. `currPtr->link->link`
   e. `currPtr->link->link->component`
   f. `head->link->link->link->component`

5. a. In an array implementation of a linked list, does the link field store the address of the next node or the index of the next node?
   b. In a dynamic data implementation of a linked list, does the link field store the address of the next node or the index of the next node?

6. a. What special state of a list does the condition `head == NULL` test for?
   b. What special condition does the expression `currPtr == NULL` test for?

7. What are the algorithmic steps for inserting a new node into a sorted linked list?

8. What are the algorithmic steps for deleting the successor of the current node, assuming that the current node is not the last node in the list?

9. For each of the following operations, decide which is faster: a direct array representation of a list, or a linked representation.
   a. Inserting near the head of the list.
   b. Deleting the last element of the list.
   c. Accessing the *n*th element
   d. Searching for an item in a sorted list

10. Explain the difference between a direct array implementation of a list and an array implementation of a linked list.

11. Why does the following code segment produce a compiler error? What is missing from the declarations?

```
typedef NodeType* NodePtr;
struct NodeType
{
    ComponentType component;
    NodePtr link;
};
```

12. For each of the following, decide whether a direct array implementation or a dynamic linked list representation would be the best choice. Assume that memory capacity is limited, and good speed is desirable.
    a. A list of CD titles in a personal library, with not more than 500 albums. CDs are rarely deleted, added occasionally, and the most frequent operation on the list is to search for a specific title.
    b. A list of shipping orders to be processed. The orders are inserted as they come in, and they are deleted as they are shipped. The list can be quite large just

before the December holidays, and may be nearly empty in January. The list is occasionally searched for a specific item, to check its status.

c. An itinerary of customer visits for a sales person. Visits may be added anywhere within the itinerary, and are deleted from the head after they have been done. The itinerary can be of any length.

Programming Warm-Up Exercises

1. Given the array implementation of a linked list shown below, write expressions that do the following, assuming that `currPtr` is somewhere in the middle of the list:

   a. Access the component member of the first list element.
   b. Advance `currPtr` to point to the next element.
   c. Access the component member of the next element (the one that follows the current element).
   d. Access the component member of the element that follows the next element.

   ```
   struct NodeType
   {
       int component;
       int link;
   };
   NodeType node[100];
   int head;
   int currPtr;
   ```

2. Given the dynamic linked implementation of a linked list shown below, write expressions that do the following, assuming that `currPtr` is somewhere in the middle of the list:

   a. Access the component member of the first list element.
   b. Advance `currPtr` to point to the next element.
   c. Access the component member of the next element (the one that follows the current element).
   d. Access the component member of the element that follows the next element.

   ```
   typedef int ComponentType;

   struct NodeType;
   typedef NodeType* NodePtr;

   struct NodeType
   {
       ComponentType component;
       NodePtr link;
   }
   ```

```
NodePtr head;
NodePtr currPtr;
NodePtr newNodePtr;
```

3. Given the declarations in Exercise 2, write a code segment that creates a new node, assigns the value 100 to the component member, links `head` to the new node, and sets `currPtr` to also point to the node.

4. Given the declarations in Exercise 2, and that the first node has been inserted into the list, as in Exercise 3, write a code segment that creates a new node with the component value equal to 212, and inserts it at the end of the list, updating any pointers as necessary.

5. Given the declarations in Exercise 2, assume that the list has a large collection of members, and that `currPtr` is somewhere in the middle of the list. Write a code segment to insert a new node with the component value of 32 following the node pointed to by `currPtr`, and update `currPtr` to point to the new node.

6. Given the declarations in Exercise 2, assume that the list has a large collection of members, and that `currPtr` is somewhere in the middle of the list. Write a code segment to remove the node following the node pointed to by `currPtr` and reinsert it at the head of the list.

7. Given the declarations in Exercise 2, assume that the list has a large collection of members, and that `currPtr` is anywhere in the list. Write a code segment that declares a new pointer, `auxPtr`, and that scans from `currPtr` to the end of the list, and then deletes the last element of the list.

8. Rewrite the code segment in Exercise 7 to work without any assumption about the number of elements in the list. That is, assuming the list could be empty, or have one or more elements.

9. Given the declarations in Exercise 2, write a void function that sorts the elements of the list in ascending order. The sort algorithm will scan the list, keeping a pointer to the lowest value seen thus far. When the end of the list is reached, the lowest value will be removed from that point and be inserted at the end of a new list. After all of the elements have been moved from the original list to the sorted list, change `head` and `currPtr` to point to the first element of the new list. That way, when the function returns, the client code will simply see the list as having been sorted.

10. Given the declarations in Exercise 2, write a code segment that declares the variables for managing a second list and then copies the elements of the list to the new list in reverse order.

Programming Problems

1. This problem has you rewrite the program from Problem 1 of Chapter 15 using a dynamic linked list. Because the list can vary in size, we no longer need to know the length of the data file in advance. Here is the problem, restated in this new context.

You are working for your state's motor vehicle registry, and it has been discovered that some people in the driver's license database have multiple records. The license records are stored in alphabetical order on a set of files, one per letter in the alphabet. The first file is `licensesa.dat`, and the last is `licensesz.dat`. For this problem, we'll just focus on getting the program to work for the `licensesa.dat` file. Some of the duplicate records are due to slight differences in spelling of names, so each file needs to be sorted into order by license number (an 8-digit integer) to find the duplicates. Each record consists of a license number, a name, and an address, all on a single line. For the purposes of this problem, the name and address can be stored in a single string because they are not processed separately. The license number and the corresponding string should be kept together in a `struct`.

Use the `HybridList` class from this Chapter so that the list array is dynamically created to be the necessary length for the data on the particular file. Each component of the list will be a license `struct` type. Also, add to the `HybridList` class a function that returns values from the list in successive order (called `GetNext`), and a companion function (called `Restart`) that resets the other function to begin again at the first component of the list.

Once the data have been read from a file into the `HybridList`, use the new functions to scan through the list, comparing each license number with the one before it to see if they are the same. As each duplicate record is found, it should be written to an output file called `duplicensesa.dat`. Keep a count of the number of duplicate records discovered and write it to `cout`. Remember to close the file at the end of the program.

2. Extend the program from Problem 1 in two ways. The first extension is to make it automatically process all 26 data files. The second extension is to have the duplicate records be output in alphabetical order so that the output file has the same organization as the input file. To do this, after the first pass through the list, you need to create a second `HybridList` that is the proper length to hold all of the duplicate records, and this list must sort on the string member of the license `struct`. Once all of the duplicate records have been copied to this list, you can delete the first list, and then output the second list to the file.

3. This problem has you rewrite the program from Problem 3 of Chapter 15 using a dynamic linked list. Because the list can vary in size, we no longer need to limit the maximum number of business cards. There is also no reason to output the number of entries to the output file. Here is the problem, restated in this new context.

You're working for a company that wants to take client contact information as it is entered by a salesperson from a stack of business cards that he or she has collected, and output the information to a file (`contacts.dat`) in alphabetical order. The program should prompt the salesperson for each of the following values for each card:

Last name
First name
Middle name or initial
Title
Company name
Street address
City
State
Zip code
Phone number
Fax number
Email address

After the data are entered for each card, the user should be asked if there is another card to enter. These data should be sorted by last name, using a version of the HybridList class from this Chapter that will hold struct values, each with a member corresponding to an item in the list above. The Print function of the class will need to be modified to output the list to the contacts.dat file instead of cout. Each member of the struct should be written on a separate line.

4. This problem has you rewrite the program from Problem 4 of Chapter 15 using a dynamic linked list. Because the list is not fixed in size, we no longer need to determine the total number of records on the files in advance of allocating the storage space. Here is the problem, restated in this new context.

You are working for a company that has a collection of files, each of which contains information from business cards. The files are created by another program (see Problem 3 for a description of what this program outputs). The company would like to merge the files into a single file, sorted alphabetically by last name. The user should be prompted to enter the names of the files, until a file name of "done" is entered.

Modify the HybridList from this Chapter so that each node of the list contains a struct type as described in Problem 3. As each filename is input by the user, open the file, and read the data, creating and inserting nodes into the sorted list. Once all of the data are input, write the sorted data back out to a file called mergedcontacts.dat. The Print function of the HybridList class will need to be modified to output the list to the mergedcontacts.dat file instead of cout. Each member of the struct should be written on a separate line.

5. Modify the program in Problem 4 so that after the data have been input, it scans through the list and deletes all duplicate records before writing out the list. A record is a duplicate if the last name, first name, middle name or initial, and company name are the same as in another record. Be sure that you properly delete any dynamically allocated data that are removed from the list.

Case Study Follow-Up

1. Could we have implemented the list of days using a list class that we have already implemented? Explain your answer. (Think very carefully about this question; it is not as simple as it appears.)

2. The user is asked how many appointments may be made on a day when the day is initialized, yet this value is never taken advantage of. Add a test to the InsertApt function that writes an error message on the screen if the user tries to insert more than the allowed number of appointments.

3. Prompting for and inputting the first name, middle name, and last name became quite tedious. Derive a class that inherits from Name that has a ReadName operation that prompts the user to enter the first name and last name with a blank in between.

4. Prompting for and inputting hours and minutes also became quite tedious. Alter class AptTime so that function ReadTime prompts the user to input the hours and minutes with a blank in between.

5. Rerun the appointment program using the sample data used in the case study with the class derived from Name and the altered AptTime class. Was the input much easier?

6. We have compared dates rather than days even though we know that the months are the same. Would it be more efficient to access the day fields of the date and component and compare them using the equality operator? Explain.

Templates and Exceptions

Knowledge Goals

- *To understand the concept of a template.*
- *To understand the concept of an exception.*

Skill Goals

To be able to:

- *Write a C++ function template.*
- *Write code that instantiates a function template.*
- *Write a user-defined specialization of a function template.*
- *Write a C++ class template.*
- *Write code that instantiates a class template.*
- *Write function definitions for members of a template class.*
- *Define an exception class and write code that throws an exception.*
- *Write an exception handler.*

This chapter introduces two C++ language features that can have a powerful impact on how we design and implement software: *templates* and *exceptions*. Templates and exceptions are basically unrelated concepts, and a separate chapter could be devoted to each one. However, this book is intended as an introduction to computer science and software design, and we present both topics in a single chapter, exploring each in less detail than a textbook for a more advanced course might.

A template, as the name suggests, is a pattern from which we can create multiple instances of something. In earlier chapters, we have used the phrase "multiple instances" when talking about data types. We have said that a data type is a pattern from which we create multiple instances (variables or class objects) of that type. The C++ template mechanism carries the concept of "instance" to a higher level. Instead of the instances being variables or class objects, the instances are entire functions or C++ class types. In this chapter, you learn how to define a *function template* from which the compiler creates multiple versions of a function. Similarly, you'll see how to define a *class template* from which the compiler creates multiple versions of a class type.

Exceptions are unusual events, often errors, that may occur while a program is executing. The C++ exception-handling mechanism allows one part of a program to inform another part of the program that an exception has occurred in case the problem can't be handled locally. As you'll discover, the topic of exception handling employs some colorful terminology. The part of the program that detects an error is said to *throw* an exception, hoping that another part of the program (an exception handler) will *catch* the exception.

If you are jumping to this chapter from another part of the book, here are the prerequisite topics. Section 17.1 (Template Functions) assumes you have already read through Chapter 10 of the book, Section 17.2 (Template Classes) assumes you have read through Chapter 13, and Section 17.3 (Exceptions) assumes you have read through Chapter 11.

17.1 Template Functions

Sometimes as we are designing or testing software, we find a need for a single algorithm that might be applied to objects of different data types at different times. We want to be able to describe the algorithm without having to specify the data types of the items being manipulated. Such an algorithm is often referred to as a **generic algorithm**. C++ supports generic algorithms by providing two mechanisms: *function overloading* and *template functions*.

> **Generic algorithm** An algorithm in which the actions or steps are defined but the data types of the items being manipulated are not.

Function Overloading

> **Function overloading** The use of the same name for different C++ functions, distinguished from each other by their parameter lists.

Function overloading is the use of the same name for different functions, as long as their parameter types are sufficiently different for the compiler to tell them apart.

Let's look at an example. We are debugging a program and want to trace its execution by printing the values of certain variables as the program executes. The variables we want to trace are of the following six data types: char, short, int, long, float, and double. We could create six functions with different names in order to output values of different types:

```cpp
void PrintInt( int n )
{
    cout << "***Debug" << endl;
    cout << "Value is " << n << endl;
}
void PrintChar( char ch )
{
    cout << "***Debug" << endl;
    cout << "Value is " << ch << endl;
}
void PrintFloat( float x )
{
    ⋮
}
void PrintDouble( double d )
{
    ⋮
}
    ⋮
```

At places in the program where we want to output the traced values, we would insert calls to the various functions as follows:

```cpp
    ⋮
sum = alpha + beta + gamma;
PrintInt(sum);
    ⋮
PrintChar(initial);
    ⋮
PrintFloat(angle);
```

Instead of having to invent different names for all these similar functions, we can use function overloading by giving them all the same name, Print:

```cpp
void Print( int n )
{
    cout << "***Debug" << endl;
    cout << "Value is " << n << endl;
}
void Print( char ch )
```

```
{
    cout << "***Debug" << endl;
    cout << "Value is " << ch << endl;
}
void Print( float x )
{
 ⋮
}
 ⋮
```

The code that calls these functions now looks like this:

```
Print(someInt);
Print(someChar);
Print(someFloat);
```

We can think of `Print` as a generic algorithm in the sense that the algorithm itself—printing the string `"***Debug"` and then the value of a variable—is independent of the data type of the variable being printed. As we program, we only have to use one name for this algorithm (`Print`), even though there really are six distinct functions.

How does function overloading work? When our program is compiled, the compiler encounters six different functions named `Print` but gives them six different names internally. We don't know what those internal names are, but for the sake of this discussion, let's assume the names are `Print_int`, `Print_char`, and so on. When the compiler encounters the function call

```
Print(someVar);
```

it must determine which of our six functions to invoke. To do so, the compiler compares the type of the actual argument with the types of the formal parameters of the six functions. Above, if `someVar` is of type `int`, then the compiler generates code to call the `Print` function that has an `int` parameter (the one with internal name `Print_int`). If `someVar` is of type `float`, the compiler generates code to call the `Print` function that has a `float` parameter (the one with internal name `Print_float`), and so forth.

As you can see, function overloading benefits the programmer by eliminating the need to come up with many different names for functions that perform identical tasks (identical except for operating on variables of different data types). Overloading also reduces the chance of unexpected results caused by using the wrong function name—for example, calling `PrintInt` when passing a `float` variable as an argument.

Despite the benefits of function overloading in our `Print` function example, we still had to supply six distinct function definitions. This entails a tedious amount of typing or using copy-and-paste in an editor, and the resulting source code file is cluttered with a group of nearly identical function definitions. We now look at a much cleaner way of implementing generic algorithms in C++: template functions.

Defining a Function Template

In C++, a function template allows you to write a function definition with "blanks" left in the definition to be filled in by the calling code. Most often, the "blanks" to be filled in are the names of data types. Here is a function template for our Print function:

> **Function template**   A C++ language construct that allows the compiler to generate multiple versions of a function by allowing parameterized data types.

```
template<class SomeType>
void Print( SomeType val )
{
    cout << "***Debug" << endl;
    cout << "Value is " << val << endl;
}
```

This function template begins with template<class SomeType>, and SomeType is known as the *template parameter*. You can use any identifier for the template parameter; we use SomeType in this example.

Here is the syntax for a function template:

FunctionTemplate

```
template < TemplateParamList >
FunctionDefinition
```

where FunctionDefinition is an ordinary function definition. The full syntax description of TemplateParamList in C++ is quite complicated, and we simplify it for our purposes as follows. TemplateParamList is a sequence of one or more parameter declarations separated by commas, where each is defined as follows:

TemplateParamDeclaration

```
{ class
  typename }    Identifier
```

Notice in the syntax template for FunctionTemplate that the angle brackets are required but the parameter list is optional. We discuss later why you would want to omit the parameter list.

Instantiating a Function Template

Given that we have written our `Print` function template, we can make function calls as follows:

```
Print<int>(sum);
Print<char>(initial);
Print<float>(angle);
```

In this code, the data type name enclosed in angle brackets is called the *template argument*. At compile time, the compiler generates (*instantiates*) three different functions and gives its own internal name to each of the functions. The three new functions are called *template functions* or *generated functions* (as opposed to the *function template* from which they were created). Also, a version of a template for a particular template argument is called a *specialization*.

When the compiler instantiates a template, it literally substitutes the template argument for the template parameter throughout the function template, just as you would do a search-and-replace operation in a word processor or text editor. For example, the first time the compiler encounters `Print<float>` in the calling code, it generates a new function by substituting `float` for every occurrence of `SomeType` in the function template:

```
                                    ──── float

void Print( (SomeType) val )
{
    cout << "***Debug" << endl;
    cout << "Value is " << val << endl;
}
```

There are two things to note about template parameters. First, the function template uses the reserved word `class` in its parameter list: `template<class SomeType>`. However, the word `class` in this context is simply required syntax and does not mean that the caller's template argument must be the name of a C++ class. (In fact, you can use the reserved word `typename` instead of `class` if you wish.) The template argument can be the name of any data type, built-in or user-defined. In our example of calling code, we used `int`, `char`, and `float` as template arguments. Second, observe that these template arguments are data type names, not variable names. This seems strange at first, because when we pass arguments to functions, we always pass variable names or expressions, not data type names. Furthermore, note that passing an argument to a template has an effect at *compile time* (the compiler generates a new function definition from the template), whereas passing an argument to a function has an effect at *run time*.

Here is the syntax template for a call to a template function:

TemplateFunctionCall

```
FunctionName  <  TemplateArgList  >  ( FunctionArgList )
```

As you can see, the template argument list in angle brackets is optional. In fact, programmers generally omit it. In that case, the compiler is said to *deduce* the template argument(s) by examining the *function argument* list. For example, our earlier example of calling code using explicit template arguments would more likely be written as follows:

```
Print(sum);        // Implicit: Print<int>(sum)
Print(initial);    // Implicit: Print<char>(initial)
Print(angle);      // Implicit: Print<float>(angle)
```

In this code, when the compiler encounters `Print(sum)`, it looks at the data type of the function argument `sum` (which is `int`) and deduces that the template argument must be `int`. Therefore, the function call is to the `Print<int>` specialization of the template.

Enhancing the `Print` Template

With our current version of `Print`, if the variable `sum` contains the value 38 and the variable `angle` contains the value 64.5, the function calls

```
Print(sum);
Print(angle);
```

produce the following output:

```
***Debug
Value is 38
***Debug
Value is 64.5
```

This output is not as helpful as it could be; it doesn't indicate the name of the variable whose value is being output. Let's rewrite the `Print` template so that it outputs both the name of a variable and its current value:

```
template<class SomeType>
void Print( string    vName,    // Name of the variable
            SomeType val   )    // Value of the variable
{
    cout << "***Debug" << endl;
    cout << "Value of " << vName << " = " << val << endl;
}
```

Here, we are telling the compiler that the first function parameter is always of a specific type (type `string`), whereas the second is of a parameterized type. Therefore, when the template is instantiated in the calling code, the compiler should look at the second function argument in order to deduce the template argument. In other words, in the calling code

```
Print("sum", sum);
Print("angle", angle);
```

the first function call implicitly calls the `Print<int>` specialization because the argument `sum` is of type `int`, and the second one calls the `Print<float>` specialization. The output from these two function calls is

```
***Debug
Value of sum = 38
***Debug
Value of angle = 64.5
```

User-Defined Specializations

We began this chapter by supposing that we needed to output—for debugging purposes—the values of variables of six data types: `char`, `short`, `int`, `long`, `float`, and `double`. We have looked at three ways to accomplish the task. The first was to write six different function definitions with different function names. The second was to write six different function definitions, all with the same function name (function overloading). The third was to write only one function definition (a function template) and let the compiler do the work of generating the individual functions from the template. The last method—using template functions—is the most compact and convenient for the programmer. Furthermore, template functions support the concept of generic algorithms because they let us focus more on the algorithms and less on the specifics of the data types they manipulate.

We think of our `Print` template function as a generic function because it can output a value of any data type. However, the "any data type" part isn't quite true. The body of the `Print` function uses the `<<` operator to output a value to the stream `cout`. Unfortunately, the `<<` operator is only defined for built-in types and certain library classes such as `string`. If our program has defined an enumeration type (Chapter 10) and a variable of that type as follows:

```
enum StatusType {OK, OUT_OF_STOCK, BACK_ORDERED};
StatusType currentStatus;
```

then our `Print` template function cannot be passed an argument of type `StatusType`. (Recall that a variable of an enumeration type cannot be output directly by the `<<` operator.) To force the `Print` function to accommodate an argument of type `StatusType`, we use the following code:

```
template<>
void Print( string     vName,    // Name of the variable
            StatusType val    )   // Value of the variable
{
    cout << "***Debug" << endl;
    cout << "Value of " << vName << " = ";
    switch (val)
    {
        case OK            : cout << "OK";
                             break;
        case OUT_OF_STOCK : cout << "OUT_OF_STOCK";
                             break;
        case BACK_ORDERED : cout << "BACK_ORDERED";
                             break;
        default           : cout << "Invalid value";
    }
    cout << endl;
}
```

The prefix `template<>` says that this is an alternative definition of the `Print` template that takes no template parameter and should be used whenever the second argument in a call to `Print` is of type `StatusType`. Such a template is called a *user-defined special-ization*, or just *user specialization*. Given our two template definitions for `Print`—the general one and the one specialized for `StatusType` variables—the compiler treats the following calling code as shown in the comments:

```
Print("sum", sum);                          // Call the Print<int>
                                            //   specialization
Print("currentStatus", currentStatus);      // Call the user-defined
                                            //   specialization
```

Organization of Program Code

Given both of our `Print` function templates, where do we place them physically in a program? There are three possibilities, described here in increasing order of desirability (in our opinion). The first is to place the template definitions near the beginning of the program file, prior to the `main` function.

```
// myprog1.cpp
#include <iostream>
#include <string>
using namespace std;

enum StatusType {OK, OUT_OF_STOCK, BACK_ORDERED};
```

```cpp
template<class SomeType>
void Print( string    vName,
            SomeType val    )
{
  ⋮
}
template<>
void Print( string     vName,
            StatusType val    )
{
  ⋮
}

int main()
{
    int intVar;
    StatusType status;
      ⋮
    Print("intVar", intVar);
    Print("status", status);
      ⋮
}
```

This organization would not be used by programmers who prefer to place the `main` function first, followed by other functions. Thus, the second approach is to place function prototypes (forward declarations) of the templates first, then the `main` function, and finally the template definitions.

```cpp
// myprog2.cpp
#include <iostream>
#include <string>
using namespace std;

enum StatusType {OK, OUT_OF_STOCK, BACK_ORDERED};

template<class SomeType>                    // Prototypes first
void Print( string vName, SomeType val );

template<>
void Print( string vName, StatusType val );

int main()                                  // Then main()
{
    int intVar;
```

```
    StatusType status;
       ⋮
    Print("intVar", intVar);
    Print("status", status);
       ⋮
}
template<class SomeType>                    // Then template
void Print( string    vName,                //   definitions
            SomeType val    )
{
  ⋮
}
template<>
void Print( string     vName,
            StatusType val    )
{
  ⋮
}
```

The third and, in our opinion, best approach is to tuck the template definitions away in a header (.h) file and then simply use #include to insert that file into our program. If we place the #include directive before the main function, we don't need template prototypes because the compiler will have seen the template definitions before it encounters the calls to the template functions. Here is the header file:

```
// templs.h -- Header file containing template definitions
#include <iostream>
#include <string>
using namespace std;

template<class SomeType>
void Print( string    vName,
            SomeType val    )
{
  ⋮
}
template<>
void Print( string     vName,
            StatusType val    )
{
  ⋮
}
```

Given this header file, our main program file can simply #include it as follows.

```cpp
// myprog3.cpp -- Main program file
#include <iostream>
#include <string>
using namespace std;

enum StatusType {OK, OUT_OF_STOCK, BACK_ORDERED};

#include "templs.h"     // Insert template definitions AFTER
                        //    StatusType is defined
int main()
{
    int intVar;
    StatusType status;
      ⋮
    Print("intVar", intVar);
    Print("status", status);
      ⋮
}
```

Two important benefits of using this header file approach are (1) the main program file is less cluttered with code, and (2) we can simply #include the file templs.h in any of our other program files when we need debugging output.

17.2 Template Classes

In Chapter 13, we defined a List abstract data type (ADT) that represented a list of unsorted components, each of type ItemType. We coded this ADT as a C++ class named List, and the header file List.h was written as follows (abbreviated here by omitting the function preconditions and postconditions):

```cpp
const int MAX_LENGTH = 50;       // Maximum possible number of
                                 //    components needed
typedef int ItemType;            // Type of each component
                                 //    (a simple type or string class)
class List
{
public:
    bool IsEmpty() const;
    bool IsFull() const;
    int  Length() const;
    void Insert( /* in */ ItemType item );
    void Delete( /* in */ ItemType item );
    bool IsPresent( /* in */ ItemType item ) const;
    void Reset();
    ItemType GetNextItem();
```

```
    void SelSort();
    List();                      // Constructor
private:
    int     length;
    int     currentPos;
    ItemType data[MAX_LENGTH];
};
```

The `typedef` statement lets us choose a particular type for `ItemType`, as long as it is a simple type or the `string` class. (The reason for the restriction is that the `List` member functions use relational operators to compare list items and use the `<<` operator to output list items. `ItemType` cannot be an array type, for example, because relational operations and the `<<` operation cannot be applied to an entire array as an aggregate.)

The `List` class is similar to a **generic data type** in the sense that the list items can be of (almost) any data type. If we change `Item-Type` by changing the `typedef` statement, we can recompile the class without changing any of the algorithms in the member functions.

However, the `List` class as written has two serious limitations. First, once the class is compiled using, say, `int` as `ItemType`, a client program's `List` objects can only be

> **Generic data type** A type for which the operations are defined but the data types of the items being manipulated are not.
>
> **Class template** A C++ language construct that allows the compiler to generate multiple versions of a class by allowing parameterized data types.

lists of `ints`. There is no way for the client to maintain lists of `ints`, lists of `floats`, and lists of `chars`, all within the same program. Second, a client program cannot specify or change `ItemType`; a human must go into the file `list.h` with an editor and change it manually.

To make a class such as `List` a truly generic type, we would like a language construct that allows `ItemType` to be a parameter to the class declaration. Fortunately, C++ provides such a construct: the **class template.**

Here is an example of a class template (the name `GList` stands for generic list):

```
template<class ItemType>
class GList
{
public:
    bool IsEmpty() const;
    bool IsFull() const;
    int  Length() const;
    void Insert( /* in */ ItemType item );
    void Delete( /* in */ ItemType item );
    bool IsPresent( /* in */ ItemType item ) const;
    void SelSort();
    void Reset();
    ItemType GetNextItem();
    GList();                     // Constructor
```

```
private:
    int       length;
    int       currentPos;
    ItemType data[MAX_LENGTH];
};
```

As you can see, this template looks just like the class declaration for the `List` type except that it is preceded by `template<class ItemType>`. Here, `ItemType` (or whatever identifier you wish to use throughout the template) is the template parameter. As with function templates, you can use either the word `class` or the word `typename` to declare a template parameter.

Instantiating a Class Template

Given the `GList` class template, the client program can use code like the following to create several lists whose components are of different data types:

```
// Client code

GList<int> list1;
GList<float> list2;
GList<string> list3;


list1.Insert(356);
list2.Insert(84.375);
list3.Insert("Muffler bolt");
```

In the declarations of `list1`, `list2`, and `list3`, the data type name enclosed in angle brackets is the *template argument.* Class template arguments *must* be explicit; they cannot be implicit as with template functions. (Recall that a function template argument usually is omitted, and the compiler deduces the argument by looking at the function's argument list.)

When the compiler encounters the declarations of `list1`, `list2`, and `list3` above, it generates (instantiates) three distinct class types and gives its own internal name to each of the three types. You might imagine that the declarations are transformed internally into something like this:

```
GList_int list1;
GList_float list2;
GList_string list3;
```

In C++ terminology, the three new class types are called *template classes* or *generated classes* (as opposed to the *class template* from which they were created). As with function templates, a version of a template for a particular template argument is called a *specialization.*

When the compiler instantiates a template, it literally substitutes the template argument for the template parameter throughout the class template. For example, the first time the compiler encounters GList<int> in the client code, it generates a new class by substituting int for every occurrence of ItemType in the class template:

```
class GList_int
{
public:
         ⋮
    void  Insert(  /*  in  */  ItemType  item  );
    void  Delete(  /*  in  */  ItemType  item  );
    bool  IsPresent(  /*  in  */  ItemType  item  )  const;
         ⋮
private:
    int         length;
    ItemType  data [MAX_LENGTH];
};
```

A useful perspective on class templates is this: Whereas an ordinary class declaration is a pattern for stamping out individual variables or objects, a class template is a pattern for stamping out individual data types.

Now that we've seen how to write the definition of a class template, what do we do about the definitions of the class member functions? We need to write them as *function templates* so that the compiler can associate each one with the proper template class. For example, we code the Insert function as the following function template:

```
template<class ItemType>
void GList<ItemType>::Insert(  /*  in  */  ItemType  item  )
{
    data [length]  =  item;
    length++;
}
```

Within the function template, every occurrence of GList as a class name must have <ItemType> appended to it. If the client has declared a type GList<float>, the compiler generates a function definition similar to the following:

```
void GList<float>::Insert(  /*  in  */  float  item  )
{
    data [length]  =  item;
    length++;
}
```

Organization of Program Code

When working with template classes, we must change the ground rules regarding which file(s) we put the source code into. Previously, we placed the class declaration into a header file `list.h` and the member function definitions into an implementation file `list.cpp`. As a result, `list.cpp` could be compiled into object code independently of any client code. This strategy won't work with templates. The compiler cannot instantiate a function template unless it knows the argument to the template, and this argument is located in the client code. Different compilers have different mechanisms to solve this problem.

A general solution that works with any compiler is to compile client code and the class member functions at the same time. With our `GList` template, one technique is to dispense with an implementation file `glist.cpp`, and place the class template and the member function definitions all into the same file, `glist.h`. Another technique is to retain two distinct files, `glist.h` and `glist.cpp`, as before but place the directive `#include "glist.cpp"` at the end of the file `glist.h`. Either way, when the client code specifies `#include "glist.h"`, the compiler has all the source code—both the client code and the member function definitions—available to it at once.

In the following code for the `GList` template, we use the second technique—namely, keeping two separate files and having the `.h` file use `#include` at the end to insert the contents of the `.cpp` file. Here is the header file, with the preconditions and postconditions omitted to save space:

```
//******************************************************************
// SPECIFICATION FILE (glist.h)
// This file gives the specification of a generic list ADT.
// The list components are not assumed to be in order by value
//******************************************************************

const int MAX_LENGTH = 50;         // Maximum possible number of
                                   //    components needed

// Below, ItemType must be a simple type or string class

template<class ItemType>
class GList
{
public:
    bool IsEmpty() const;
    bool IsFull() const;
    int  Length() const;
    void Insert( /* in */ ItemType item );
    void Delete( /* in */ ItemType item );
    bool IsPresent( /* in */ ItemType item ) const;
    void SelSort();
    void Reset();
    ItemType GetNextItem();
    GList();                            // Constructor
```

```
private:
    int       length;
    int       currentPos;
    ItemType  data[MAX_LENGTH];
};

#include "glist.cpp"    // Inserts member function definitions
```

Next is the implementation file, glist.cpp. Much of the internal documentation has been omitted to save space. The fully documented version can be found on the program disk for this book or at the publisher's Web site. In the following, pay close attention to the required syntax of the member function definitions.

```
//**********************************************************************
// IMPLEMENTATION FILE (glist.cpp)
// This file implements the GList class member functions
// List representation: a one-dimensional array and a length
//                      variable
//**********************************************************************

// Warning: This file is #included by glist.h, so
// DO NOT use #include "glist.h" in this file, and
// DO NOT compile this file separately from the client code file

#include <iostream>

using namespace std;

template<class ItemType>
GList<ItemType>::GList()    // Constructor
{
    length = 0;
}

template<class ItemType>
bool GList<ItemType>::IsEmpty() const
{
    return (length == 0);
}

template<class ItemType>
bool GList<ItemType>::IsFull() const
{
    return (length == MAX_LENGTH);
}

template<class ItemType>
int GList<ItemType>::Length() const
{
```

```cpp
    return length;
}

template<class ItemType>
void GList<ItemType>::Insert( /* in */ ItemType item )
{
    data[length] = item;
    length++;
}

template<class ItemType>
void GList<ItemType>::Delete( /* in */ ItemType item )
{
    int index = 0;

    while (index < length && item != data[index])
        index++;
    if (index < length)
    {                                          // Remove item
        data[index] = data[length-1];
        length--;
    }
}

template<class ItemType>
bool GList<ItemType>::IsPresent( /* in */ ItemType item ) const
{
    int index = 0;

    while (index < length && item != data[index])
        index++;
    return (index < length);
}

template<class ItemType>
void GList<ItemType>::Reset()
{
    currentPos = 0;
}

template<class ItemType>
ItemType GList<ItemType>::GetNextItem()
{
    ItemType item;
    item = data[currentPos];
    if (currentPos == length - 1)
        currentPos = 0;
    else
```

```
            currentPos++;
        return item;
}

template<class ItemType>
void GList<ItemType>::SelSort()
{
    ItemType temp;
    int       passCount;
    int       searchIndx;
    int       minIndx;

    for (passCount = 0; passCount < length - 1; passCount++)
    {
        minIndx = passCount;
        for (searchIndx = passCount + 1; searchIndx < length;
             searchIndx++)
            if (data[searchIndx] < data[minIndx])
                minIndx = searchIndx;

        temp = data[minIndx];
        data[minIndx] = data[passCount];
        data[passCount] = temp;
    }
}
```

A Caution

If you develop your programs using an IDE (integrated development environment) in which the editor, compiler, and linker are bundled into one application, you must be careful when using templates. With an IDE, you typically are asked to define a "project"—a list of the individual files that constitute a program. With Chapter 13's List class comprising two files (list.h and list.cpp) and your client code located in a file myprog.cpp, you would specify myprog.cpp and list.cpp in your project. The idea is that these two files are compiled *separately* and then their object code files are linked (by the linker) to form an executable file.

With templates, the situation may change. Given the files glist.h and glist.cpp just shown, we do *not* want to compile myprog.cpp and glist.cpp separately. As stated before, we cannot compile glist.cpp all by itself because the template arguments are located in a different file (myprog.cpp). Therefore, if we specify both myprog.cpp and glist.cpp in a project, we'll get compiler and/or linker error messages. The solution in this case is to specify *only* myprog.cpp in the project. (Because myprog.cpp says to include glist.h, and glist.h in turn says to include glist.cpp, we want the compiler to receive only one large chunk of source code to compile.)

We now turn our attention away from templates to another useful language feature provided by C++: *exceptions*.

17.3 Exceptions

Suppose we're writing a program in which we frequently need to divide two integers and obtain the quotient. In every case, we need to check for division by 0, so we write a function named `Quotient` that returns the quotient of any two integers unless the denominator is 0:

```cpp
int Quotient( /* in */ int numer,       // The numerator
              /* in */ int denom )      // The denominator
{
    if (denom != 0)
        return numer / denom;
    else
        // What to do??
}
```

We are faced with a problem: What should this function do if the denominator is 0? This is not an easy question to answer. Here are some possibilities, none of which is entirely satisfactory:

1. Don't perform the division, and silently return to the calling code.
2. Print an error message and return an arbitrary integer value.
3. Return a special value such as −9999 to the caller as a signal that something went wrong.
4. Rewrite the function with a third parameter, a Boolean flag indicating success or failure.
5. Print an error message and halt the program.

Choice 1 is clearly irresponsible. Choice 2 might help the human running the program by displaying an error message but will not notify the calling code that anything was wrong. Choice 3 might be all right in some circumstances but in general is not a good solution. If the numerator and denominator are allowed to be any integers, then −9999 is a perfectly valid quotient and cannot be distinguished from a special signal value. Choice 4 is a reasonable approach and is used quite often by programmers. The disadvantage in our case is that we must change our value-returning function (which returns just one value) into a void function so that *two* values can be returned through the parameter list as reference parameters: the quotient and the Boolean flag. Choice 5 is almost never satisfactory. The calling code, not the called function, should be allowed to decide what to do in case of an error. Perhaps the caller would like to take steps to recover from the error and keep executing rather than terminate the program.

One way out of our dilemma is to eliminate the dilemma! Use a function precondition as follows:

```
int Quotient( /* in */ int numer,     // The numerator
              /* in */ int denom )     // The denominator

// Precondition:
//      denom != 0
// Postcondition:
//      Return value == numer / denom

{
    return numer / denom;
}
```

Here, the caller must ensure that the precondition is true before calling the function, and the function therefore does not have to do any error detection. With this approach, the caller is responsible for both error detection and error handling. Throughout this book, we have used this strategy of using preconditions to eliminate error detection from called functions. However, there are situations in which errors can be detected only *after* an action has been attempted, not before. For example, a function ReadInt that is supposed to read an integer value from the keyboard may find that the user has erroneously typed some letters of the alphabet (in which case the input variable is not changed, and the cin stream goes into the fail state). In this case, we cannot state a precondition for ReadInt that "The next input value is a valid integer" because there is no way for the caller of ReadInt to predict what the human at the keyboard will type. To deal with errors of this kind (and for programmers who prefer not to use the precondition approach), the C++ language provides what is called an *exception-handling* mechanism.

In the world of software, an **exception** is an unusual event, often an error, that requires special processing. A section of program code that provides that special processing is called an **exception handler**. When a section of code announces that an exception has occurred, it is said to **throw** (or **raise**) an exception, hoping that another section of code (the exception handler) will **catch** the exception and process it. If no exception handler exists for that particular exception, the entire program terminates with an error message. Let's look now at the mechanisms C++ provides for throwing and catching exceptions.

> **Exception**   An unusual, often unpredictable event, detectable by software or hardware, that requires special processing; also, in C++, a variable or class object that represents an exceptional event.
>
> **Exception handler**   A section of program code that is executed when a particular exception occurs.
>
> **Throw**   To signal the fact that an exception has occurred; also called *raise*.
>
> **Catch**   To process a thrown exception. (The catching is performed by an exception handler.)

The throw **Statement**

In C++, the word *exception* not only has the general meaning of an unusual event but also has a more specific meaning: a variable or class object that represents such an event. To throw (raise) an exception, the programmer uses a `throw` statement, whose syntax is as follows:

ThrowStatement

```
throw  Expression ;
```

In the `throw` statement, Expression can be a value or a variable of any data type, built-in or user-defined. Let's look at three examples of `throw` statements. Here is Example 1:

```
throw 5;
```

In this example, we are throwing an exception of type `int` with the expectation that one or more exception handlers wants to catch an exception of type `int` (we see how this is done in the next section). In Example 2 below, we throw an exception of type `string`, the standard library class:

```
string str = "Invalid customer age";
throw str;
```

Finally, Example 3 throws an exception of a class type that we define ourselves:

```
class SalaryError
{};                    // Member list is empty
    ⋮
SalaryError sal;
throw sal;
```

In Example 3, observe how we first declare a class object named `sal` and then throw that object. More commonly, C++ programmers do the following:

```
class SalaryError
{};                    // Member list is empty
    ⋮
throw SalaryError();
```

In this code, the `throw` statement creates an anonymous (unnamed) object of type `SalaryError` by explicitly calling its default constructor (signified by the empty argument list) and then passes this anonymous object to an exception handler. It would be a syntax error to leave off the parentheses:

```
throw SalaryError;    // Invalid
```

because the syntax template for the `throw` statement shows that we need an expression, not the name of a data type.

Finally, notice in the syntax template that Expression is optional. We discuss later what happens if the `throw` expression is absent.

The `try-catch` Statement

If one part of a program throws an exception, how does another part of the program catch the exception and process it? The answer is by using a `try-catch` statement, which has the following form:

TryCatchStatement

```
try
   Block
catch ( FormalParameter )
   Block
catch ( FormalParameter )
   Block
      ⋮
```

The syntax of FormalParameter is as follows:

FormalParameter

```
{ DataType  VariableName
{ . . .
```

(In the latter syntax template, the three dots are literally three periods that are typed into the program.)

As the first syntax template shows, the `try-catch` statement consists of a *try-clause* followed by one or more *catch-clauses*. The try-clause consists of the reserved word `try` and a block (a { } pair enclosing any number of statements). Each catch-clause consists of the reserved word `catch`, a single parameter declaration enclosed in parentheses, and a block. Each catch-clause is, in fact, an exception handler.

When a statement or group of statements in a program might result in an exception, we enclose them in a try-clause. For each type of exception that can be produced by the statements, we write a catch-clause (exception handler). Here is an example of a `try-catch` statement involving the three types of exceptions (`int`, `string`, and `SalaryError`) discussed previously with the `throw` statement:

```
try
{
    ⋮          // Statements that process personnel data and may throw
               // exceptions of type int, string, and SalaryError
}
```

```
catch ( int )
{
    :          // Statements to handle an int exception
}
catch ( string s )
{
    cout << s << endl;  // Prints "Invalid customer age"
    :          // More statements to handle an age error
}
catch ( SalaryError )
{
    :          // Statements to handle a salary error
}
```

The `try-catch` statement is meant to sound like the coach telling the gymnast, "Go ahead and try this somersault, and I'll catch you if you fall." We are telling the computer to try executing some operations that might fail, and then we're providing code to catch the potential exceptions.

Execution of `try-catch`   Execution of the preceding `try-catch` statement works as follows. If none of the statements in the try-clause throws an exception, then control transfers to the statement following the entire `try-catch` statement. That is, we try some statements, and if everything goes according to plan, we just continue with the succeeding statements. However, if an exception is thrown by a statement in the try-clause, control immediately transfers to the appropriate exception handler (catch-clause). It is important to understand that control jumps directly from whatever statement caused the exception to the exception handler. If there are statements in the try-clause following the one that caused the exception, they are skipped. When control reaches the exception handler, statements to deal with the exception are executed, and if these statements do not cause any new exceptions and do not transfer control elsewhere (as with a `return` statement), then control passes to the next statement following the entire `try-catch` structure.

Formal Parameters in Exception Handlers   When an exception is thrown, how does the computer know which of several exception handlers is appropriate? It looks at the data type of the formal parameter declared in each handler and selects the first one whose data type matches that of the thrown exception. A formal parameter consisting solely of an ellipsis (three dots or periods), as shown earlier in the syntax template for FormalParameter, is a "wild card"—it matches any exception type. Because the computer searches the exception handlers for a matching parameter in sequential or "north-to-south" order, a final exception handler with an ellipsis parameter serves as a "catch-all" handler for any exception whose type hasn't been listed:

```
try
{
    ⋮          // Statements that may throw an exception
}
catch ( Type1 )
{
    ⋮          // Handle a Type1 exception
}
catch ( Type2 )
{
    ⋮          // Handle a Type2 exception
}
catch ( ... )                     // Catch-all handler
{
    cout << "Panic! Unexpected exception." << endl;
    ⋮          // Statements to deal with this situation
}
```

Note that the "north-to-south" search for a matching parameter type requires us to place the catch-all handler last. If we placed it first, it would trap *every* exception, and the remaining handlers would be ignored.

Another issue regarding formal parameters in exception handlers is this: Should the parameter declaration include a name for the parameter or not? (If you go back and look at the syntax template for FormalParameter, you'll see that the parameter's data type is required but its name is optional.) The answer is that the parameter's name is needed only if statements in the body of the exception handler use that variable. In our earlier example of catching int, string, and SalaryError exceptions, the parameter lists for the first and third exception handlers contain data type names only, whereas the parameter list for the second handler specifies string s. The reason is that the body of that handler uses the statement

```
cout << s << endl;   // Prints "Invalid customer age"
```

to print the message contained in s.

Finally, we address a very important issue in the programming of exceptions: the data types of the exceptions themselves. In our int, string, and SalaryError example, we used all three exception types simply to demonstrate the possibilities for the programmer and to show how exception handlers are written in order to catch exceptions of these types. In practice, exceptions of built-in types (int, float, and so on) and even of class string are of limited usefulness. If a try-clause throws several exceptions of type int with different integer values, then an exception handler receiving an int value becomes complicated. It must include logic that tests the integer to determine exactly what kind of error occurred. Furthermore, statements such as

```
throw 23;
```

are much less readable and self-documenting than statements like

```
throw SalaryError();
```

Consequently, it is a better idea to use only user-defined classes (and structs) as exception types, defining one type for each kind of exception and using descriptive identifiers:

```
class SalaryError     // Exception class
{};
class BadRange        // Exception class
{};
  ⋮
if ( condition )
    throw SalaryError();
  ⋮
if ( condition )
    throw BadRange();
```

Nonlocal Exception Handlers

In our discussion so far, we have assumed that a throw statement is physically located within the try-catch statement that is intended to catch the exception. In that case, if the exception is thrown, control transfers to the catch-clause with the corresponding data type.

However, it is more common in C++ programs for the throw to occur inside a function that is *called* from within a try-clause, as shown with functions Func3 and Func4 in Figure 17–1. At run time, the computer first looks for a catch within Func4. When it fails to find one, it causes Func4 to return immediately and pass the exception back to its caller, Func3. The computer then looks around the point where Func4 was called, finds an appropriate catch-clause, and executes the catch. As you can see, the exception was thrown in Func4, but the exception handler is nonlocal (it's in the calling function, Func3).

Suppose in Figure 17–1 that there were no matching catch-clause in Func3. Then Func3 would return immediately and pass the exception back to *its* caller, perhaps Func2. This process is like the child's game of "Hot Potato." Each function that doesn't know how to deal with the problem passes the potato (the exception) back to the previous function. This sequence of returns continues back through the chain of function calls until either a matching exception handler is found or control reaches main. If main fails to catch the exception (a situation known as an *uncaught exception*), the system terminates the program and displays a relatively unhelpful message like "ABNORMAL PROGRAM TERMINATION." Figures 17–2a and 17–2b illustrate this process.

```
void Func3()
{
    :
    try
    {
        :
        Func4();
        :
    }
    catch ( ErrType )
    {
        :
    }
    :
}
```

Function
call

Normal
return

Return from
throw exception

```
void Func4()
{
    :

    if (error)
        throw ErrType();
    :
}
```

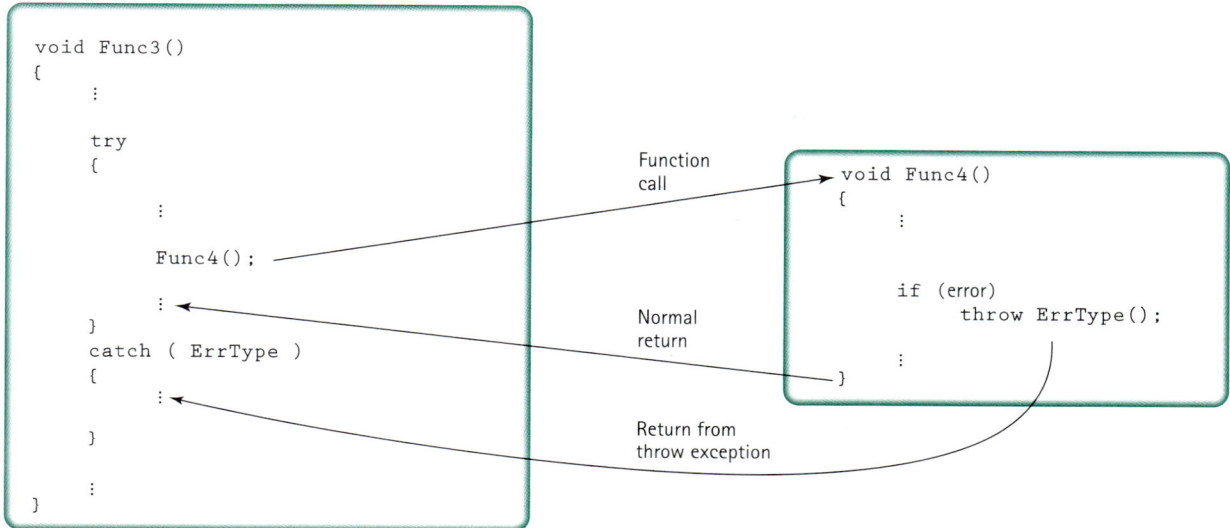

Figure 17–1 *Throwing an Exception to be Caught by the Calling Code*

Note that even if a `throw` statement *is* physically present in the try-clause of a `try-catch` but there is no matching exception handler in that `try-catch` statement, the result is the same as we have just described—namely, the enclosing function returns immediately and passes the exception back up the calling chain.

You may wonder why we said that it's most common for C++ programs to use non-local exception handlers. The reason lies at the very heart of exception handling, no matter what programming language is used. The fundamental purpose of exceptions is to allow one part of a program to report an error to another part of the program if the error cannot be handled locally. When one function calls another function, the two generally exhibit a master-slave relationship. The master (the calling function) tells the slave (the called function) to do something for it. If the slave encounters an exceptional situation, it may not have enough information about the "outside world" to know how to recover from the error. Thus, the slave gives up and simply reports the error to the master by throwing an exception. If the master knows how to recover from the error, it catches the exception with an exception handler; otherwise, it passes the exception back to *its* master, and so on. Often, the exception must be passed all the way back to `main` before a decision can be made to either terminate the program or recover from the error and continue executing.

(a) Function Func1 has a handler for ErrType

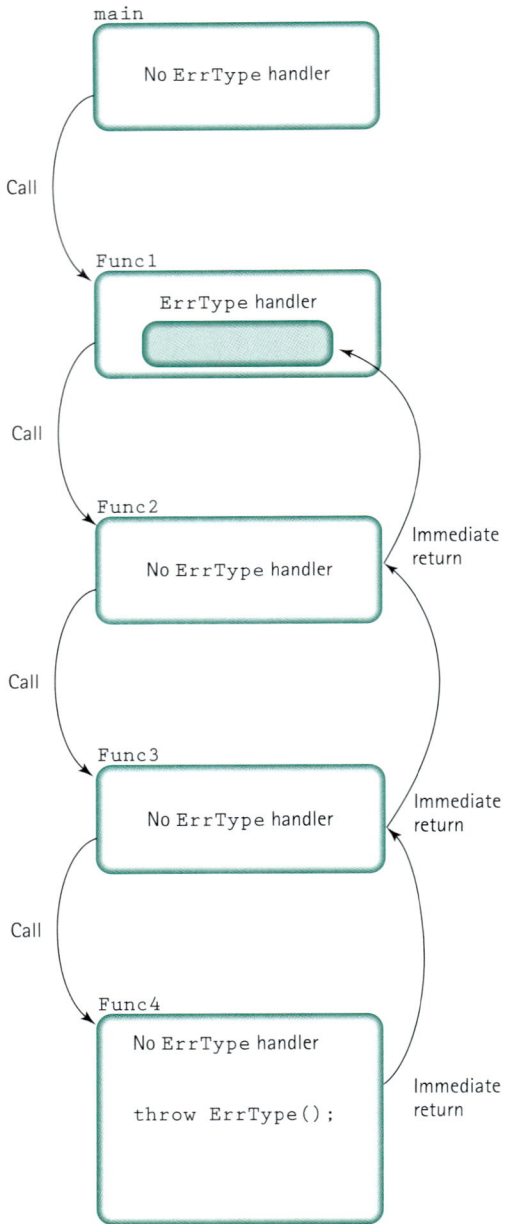

(b) No function has a handler for ErrType

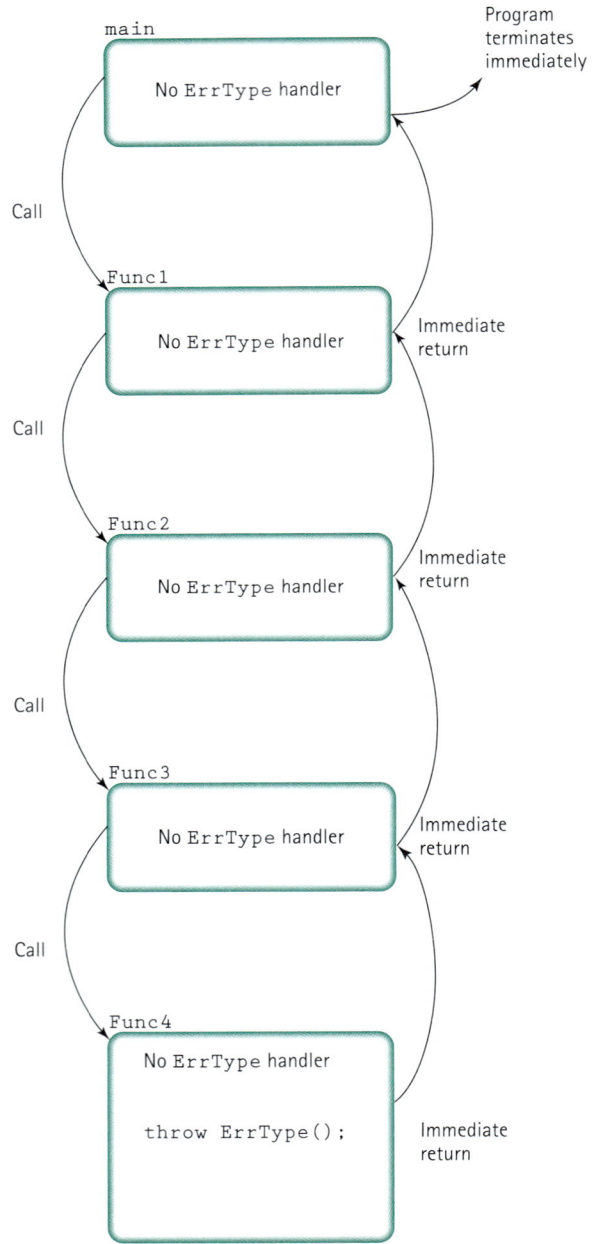

Figure 17-2 *Passing an Exception Up the Chain of Function Calls*

Re-Throwing an Exception

We have been using `throw` statements of the following form:

```
throw SalaryError();
```

The syntax template for the `throw` statement, presented earlier in the chapter, shows that we use the word `throw`, followed *optionally* by an expression. Therefore, the `throw` expression may be omitted, as in the statement

```
throw;
```

This statement is used within an exception handler that has caught an exception and performed some actions, and then wishes to pass the exception along to its caller (*re-throw* the exception) for further processing. Here is an example:

```
void WriteToFile( parameters )
{
    ⋮   // Open a file for output
    try
    {
        while ( condition )
        {
            DoSomething( arguments );   // May throw a BadData
                                        // exception
        ⋮   // Write to output file
        }
    }
    catch ( BadData )
    {
        ⋮         // Write message to output file and close it
        throw;   // Re-throw the exception
    }
    ⋮   // Continue processing
        //   and close the output file
}
```

Re-throwing an exception is C++'s way of allowing *partial exception handling.* In the code above, the catch-clause handles the `BadData` exception partially (by writing an error message to the file and closing it) and then returns, re-throwing the exception up the chain of function calls until it is caught.

What would happen in the code above if we deleted the `throw` statement? What would happen if we changed `throw` to `return`? An Exam Preparation exercise at the end of this chapter asks you to consider these questions.

Standard Exceptions

Not all exceptions are defined by us as C++ programmers. Several exception classes are predefined in the C++ standard library and are thrown either by C++ operations or by code that is supplied in standard library routines.

Exceptions Thrown by the Language   Certain C++ operations throw exceptions if errors occur during their execution. These operations are `new`, `dynamic_cast`, `typeid`, and something called an exception specification. The last three are not covered in this book, so we discuss only the `new` operator here. If you have not read about dynamic allocation of data in Chapter 15, you may want to skip this discussion.

In Chapter 15, we said that the `new` operator obtains a chunk of memory from the free store (heap) and returns a pointer to (the address of) the beginning of that chunk. For example, the code

```
int* intPtr;
intPtr = new int[1000];
```

creates a 1000-element `int` array on the free store and assigns the base address of the array to `intPtr`. We also said that if the system has run out of space on the free store, execution of `new` causes the program to terminate with an error message. Now that we know about exceptions, we can describe more completely what happens. If `new` finds that the free store is exhausted, it throws an exception of type `bad_alloc`, a C++ class that is predefined in the standard library. If this exception is not caught by any exception handler, then, as with any uncaught exception, the program halts with a generic message such as "ABNORMAL PROGRAM TERMINATION." On the other hand, our program can catch the exception and take some corrective action (or at least display a more specific error message). For example, we might write code such as the following in our `main` function:

```
float* arr;
try
{
    arr = new float[50000];
}
catch ( bad_alloc )
{
    cout << "*** Out of memory. Can't allocate array." << endl;
    return 1;    // Terminate the program
}
: // Continue. Allocation succeeded
```

Observe the `return` statement in the exception handler. This statement will terminate the program only if it is in the `main` function. If we want the above code to be located in some other function, we must change the `return` statement into something else. We could re-throw the `bad_alloc` exception to a higher-level function or throw a new exception (naming it, say, `OutOfMem`) for a higher-level function to catch.

Note: At the time of this writing, not all C++ compilers fully implement the ISO/ANSI C++ language standard with regard to the `new` operator. Some compilers still use the old (prestandard) definition of `new` in which a failed memory allocation returns the null pointer (0) instead of throwing an exception. If you are using such a compiler, you would rewrite the preceding code as follows:

```
float* arr;

arr = new float[50000];
if (arr == 0)
{
    cout << "*** Out of memory. Can't allocate array." << endl;
    return 1;    // Terminate the program
}
⋮ // Continue. Allocation succeeded
```

Exceptions Thrown by Standard Library Routines   The C++ standard library is really two libraries: facilities inherited from the C language (called the C library) and facilities designed specifically for C++. In general, header files beginning with the letter c— cmath, cstddef, and cctype, for example—are part of the C library, and all other header files are specific to C++. (One header file named complex does not fit this pattern. It begins with c but is C++-specific.) Library routines in the C library do not throw exceptions because exceptions are not part of the C language. Instead, they employ a global integer variable named errno that is set to a nonzero value if an error occurs in a library routine. The exact value assigned to errno depends on the particular library routine being executed, and the programmer can look it up in the documentation for the C library. However, we often are interested only in whether an error occurred (errno is nonzero) or did not occur. Here is a way to simulate throwing exceptions from C library routines, even though the C library doesn't do so. Begin by setting errno to 0. Call the library routine, and then check errno. If errno is still 0, no error occurred. If it is nonzero, throw your own exception. In the following code, *C_lib_routine* would be replaced by the name of an actual C library routine such as sqrt or abs:

```
class CLibErr     // Our own exception class
{};
  ⋮
void SomeFunc( parameters )
{
    ⋮
    errno = 0;
    C_lib_routine( arguments );
    if (errno != 0)
        throw CLibErr();
    ⋮
}
```

The other portion of the C++ standard library—the portion with facilities that are specific to C++—defines several exception classes, and various library routines throw objects of those classes when errors occur. The exception classes are `bad_alloc`, `out_of_range`, `length_error`, `domain_error`, and others. Other than `bad_alloc`, discussed in the previous section, the only exception types that relate to material covered in this book are `out_of_range` and `length_error`. These exceptions can be thrown when working with objects of class `string`, available through the header file named `string`. Let's look at these exceptions now.

Near the end of Chapter 3, we examined a `string` class member function named `substr`. We said that if `str` is a `string` object, the expression `str.substr(pos, len)` returns a new `string` object that is the substring of `str` starting at position `pos` and of length `len`. We said that if `pos` is too large, the program terminates with an error message. In more detail, what happens is that if `pos` is too large, an `out_of_range` exception is thrown. If this exception is not caught, then, as with any uncaught exception, it's true that the program terminates with a vague error message. But we can catch the exception if we wish and then handle it in some way.

Another exception that can be thrown by the `string` class is `length_error`, and it can happen as follows. Recall that the integer positions of individual characters within a `string` object are represented by an unsigned integer type `string::size_type`. The range of values in this type is 0 through `string::npos−1`, where `string::npos` is a constant whose value on many machines is about 4 billion. In the (unlikely) event that your program tries to construct a string whose length is greater than `string::npos`, a `length_error` exception is thrown. One way this could happen would be for your program to repeatedly concatenate large strings (using expressions like `str1 + str2`) in an unconstrained manner. Thus, to guard against range errors and length errors when working with `string` objects, we might write code like the following:

```
void SomeFunc( parameters )
{
    string s1, s2;
    try
    {
        ⋮
        s2 = s1.substr(pos, len);   // May throw out_of_range()
        s1 = s1 + s1 + s2;          // May throw length_error()
        ⋮
    }
    catch ( out_of_range )
    {
        cout << "Exception: out_of_range in SomeFunc" << endl;
        throw;     // Re-throw exception to a caller
    }
    catch ( length_error )
    {
        cout << "Exception: length_error in SomeFunc" << endl;
```

```
        throw;     // Re-throw exception to a caller
    }
    ⋮   // Continue if no errors
}
```

Although we've looked at only two exception classes as used by the string class, there are several other standard exception classes that are used by other standard library facilities. As you work more with the C++ standard library in the future, you will learn of these exception types.

Back to the Division-by-Zero Problem

We began the topic of exceptions by proposing a Quotient function that returns the quotient of two integers unless the divisor is 0. We said that if the divisor is 0, it's not clear how the function should deal with the error. We said that one solution was to make the problem go away by means of a precondition (that the caller must not send an argument of 0 as the divisor). We now present another solution that puts together what we've learned about exceptions. We define our own exception class DivByZero, and the function throws an exception of this type if it discovers a 0 divisor. The idea is that the Quotient function cannot know whether the program should be terminated or not, so it throws an exception and lets a higher-level function decide what to do. The following is a rather simple program that prompts the user for a pair of integers and outputs their quotient, doing so repeatedly until the user types the end-of-file keystrokes. In this program, it's the decision of main *not* to terminate the program if it catches an exception. Rather, an error message is displayed to the user, and the loop continues.

```cpp
// quotient.cpp -- Quotient program

#include <iostream>
#include <string>

using namespace std;

int Quotient( int, int );

class DivByZero     // Exception class
{};

int main()
{
    int numer;     // Numerator
    int denom;     // Denominator

    cout << "Enter numerator and denominator: ";
    cin >> numer >> denom;
    while (cin)
```

```
    {
        try
        {
            cout << "Their quotient: "
                 << Quotient(numer, denom) << endl;
        }
        catch ( DivByZero )
        {
            cout << "*** Denominator can't be 0" << endl;
        }
        cout << "Enter numerator and denominator: ";
        cin >> numer >> denom;
    }
    return 0;
}

int Quotient( /* in */ int numer,      // The numerator
              /* in */ int denom )     // The denominator
{
    if (denom == 0)
        throw DivByZero();
    return numer / denom;
}
```

Problem–Solving Case Study

Re-Implement SortedList Specification and
Enhance Appointment Calendar

PROBLEM   There are two parts to this case study. First, in order to prove that changing the underlying implementation of a class does not affect the client code using the class, take the specification file of the SortedList class we used in the case study in Chapter 14, change the data representation and implement the specification using a linked list. Test the implementation by running the same driver with the new implementation.

After the SortedList class has been tested, go back to the appointment calendar and make any changes to the specification that you think would make the ADT more robust. Implement and test the changes.

Linked Implementation of SortedList

DISCUSSION   The first thing to do is look at the specifications again and make notes of what changes are required. We make the comments within the text of the specification.

```
//*********************************************************************
// SPECIFICATION FILE (SortedList.h)
// This file gives the specification of a SortedList abstract data
// type. The SortedList items are assumed to be in order by
// value
//*********************************************************************

#include "Entry.h"

const int MAX_LENGTH =100;        // Maximum possible number of
                                  //    items needed
```

In an array-based list, the maximum number of cells must be known when the array is created: either at compile time or when the array is created using `new` during run time. In a linked-list the number of items does not need to be known; however, for certain applications a maximum number might be useful.

```
typedef Entry ItemType;           // Type of each item
                                  //    (a simple type or string class)
```

Now that we know how to use templates and make the type a parameter to the class, let's do so here. The only change that will be required in the program is to include the type as a parameter when the structure is declared. The constraint that the type be simple was so that the relational operators would be defined. That is an implementation issue that we will take up later.

```
class SortedList
{
public:
    bool IsEmpty() const;
    // Postcondition:
    //      Return value is true, if SortedList is empty;
    //      false, otherwise

    bool IsFull() const;
    // Postcondition:
    //      Return value is true, if SortedList is full;
    //      false, otherwise
```

If we don't have a maximum number of items in the list, we really don't need an `IsFull` operation. If we want to make all of the operations available for consistency's sake, we could just have `IsFull` return `false`. If we decide that we should give the user the option of setting a maximum, then `IsFull` would check against this value. For now, we just return `false`.

```
int Length() const;
    // Postcondition:
    //      Return value is length of SortedList

void Insert( /* in */ ItemType& item );
    // Inserts item into the SortedList
    // Precondition:
    //      length < MAX_LENGTH
    //   && data[0..length-1] are in ascending order
    // Postcondition:
    //      item is in the SortedList
    //   && length == length@entry + 1
    //   && data[0..length-1] are in ascending order
```

Of course, the documentation for the array-based list will no longer apply.

```
void Delete( /* in */ ItemType item );
    // Precondition:
    //      NOT IsEmpty()
    // Postcondition:
    //      IF item is in SortedList at entry
    //           First occurrence of item is no longer in
    //           SortedList
    //        && Length() == Length()@entry - 1
    //      ELSE
    //           SortedList is unchanged
```

The Delete is a "delete if there." The algorithm given for the Delete function in the linked version given in Chapter 17 is a "delete, it is there."

```
bool IsPresent( /* in */ ItemType item ) const;
    // Precondition:
    //      item is assigned
    // Postcondition:
    //      Return value == true, if item is in SortedList
    //                   == false, otherwise

void Reset();
    // Postcondition:
    //      Iteration is initialized

ItemType GetNextItem();
    // Precondition:
    //      No transformers have been invoked since last call
```

```
        // Postcondition:
        //     Returns item at the current position in the SortedList

    SortedList();
        // Constructor
        // Postcondition:
        //     Empty SortedList is created
private:
    int      length;
    int      currentPos;
    ItemType data[MAX_LENGTH];
    void     BinSearch( ItemType, bool&, int& ) const;
};
```

In an array-based list, the length variable must be there to distinguish the list from the array in which the items are stored. In a linked list, we have two choices. We can keep a length variable, which we increment and decrement with each insert and delete. Alternatively, we can count the number of items each time the Length function is called. Which is better? It depends on how many times the Length function is called. If there are lots of inserts and deletes and the Length function is called only a few times, then counting is best. Let's use a length variable here.

We still need some way of keeping track of the current position in the list during a traversal. However, this variable will contain a pointer rather than an index. Rather than an array variable to hold the items, we have a pointer to the head of the linked list. Clearly, the binary search algorithm is not needed. In fact, it can't be used. You cannot apply a binary search to a linked list.

Because the implementation is linked, we should include a copy constructor and a destructor. Here is the specification file for SortedList2.

```
//**************************************************************
// SPECIFICATION FILE (SortedList2.h)
// This file gives the specification of a sorted list abstract data
// type. The list items are maintained in ascending order of
// value
// Assumption: ItemType must implement LessThan and Equal.
//**************************************************************

#include "Entry.h"

template<class ItemType>
struct NodeType;                   // Forward declaration

template<class ItemType>
class SortedList2
{
public:
```

```
                        // Assumption: ItemType must implement LessThan and Equal.
        bool IsEmpty() const;
            // Postcondition:
            //      Return value is true, if list is empty;
            //      false, otherwise

        bool IsFull() const;
            // Postcondition:
            //      Return value is true, if list is full;
            //      false, otherwise

        void Insert( /* in */ ItemType item );
            // Precondition:
            //      item is assigned
            // Postcondition:
            //      item is in list
            //   && List components are in ascending order

        void Delete( /* in */ ItemType item );
            // Precondition:
            //      item is somewhere in list
            // Postcondition:
            //      First occurrence of item is no longer in list
            //   && List components are in ascending order

        void Reset();
            // Postcondition:
            //      Iteration is initialized

        ItemType GetNextItem();
            // Precondition:
            //      No transformers have been invoked since last call
            // Postcondition:
            //      Returns component at the current position
            //      in the SortedList

        int Length() const;
            // Postcondition:
            //      Return value is length of list

        bool IsPresent(ItemType item) const;

        // Searches the list for item, reporting whether it was found
        // Postcondition:
```

```
//       Return value is true, if item is the list;
//       false, otherwise

SortedList2();
    // Constructor
    // Postcondition:
    //     Empty list is created

SortedList2( const SortedList2& otherList );
    // Copy-constructor
    // Postcondition:
    //     List is created as a duplicate of otherList

~SortedList2();
    // Destructor
    // Postcondition:
    //     List is destroyed
private:
    NodeType<ItemType>* head;
    NodeType<ItemType>* currentPos;
    int length;
};

#include "SortedList2.cpp"
```

In Chapter 17, all of the algorithms were given except for Reset and GetNextItem. What is analogous to setting index to zero in the array-based version? Setting the pointer to NULL. What is analogous to incrementing an index in an array-based version? Setting the pointer to the next link.

Reset

Set currentPos to NULL

GetNextItem
Out: Function value

IF currentPos is NULL
    curentPos is head
Set item to currentPos->item
Set currentPos to currentPost->link

Does the change in precondition change the Delete algorithm? Yes it does. The technique used to find the component to delete depends on the item being in the list. If this function is applied and the item is not in the list, a NULL pointer results. We must have a trailing pointer to use in the delete as we did in the insert. We also need to change the relational operator to `Equal`, because the list of entries is ordered by time. We must be sure to add the assumption that `ItemType` implements `LessThan` and `Equal` to the specification file header documentation.

Delete(In: item)

```
Set currentPtr to head
Set prevPtr to NULL
WHILE currentPtr != NULL AND !(currentPtr->item.Equal(item))
    Set prevPtr to currentPtr
    Set currentPtr to currentPtr->link
IF currentPtr != NULL
    Set prevPtr->link to currentPtr->link
    Decrement length
```

The algorithm given for Insert also used a relational operator. We must go into the insert algorithm, replace the relational operator < with `LessThan`, and recode the algorithm. This is so straightforward (dare we say algorithmic?) that we skip to the code.

```cpp
//*************************************************************************
// IMPLEMENTATION FILE (SortedList2.cpp)
// This file implements the SortedList2 class member functions
// List representation: a linked list of templated dynamic nodes
//*************************************************************************
#include <iostream>
#include <cstddef>      // For NULL

using namespace std;

template<class ItemType>
struct NodeType
{
    ItemType item;
    NodeType<ItemType>* link;
};

// Private members of class:
//      NodeType* head; External pointer to linked list


//*************************************************************************

template<class ItemType>
SortedList2<ItemType>::SortedList2()
```

```cpp
// Constructor

// Postcondition:
//     head == NULL

{
    head = NULL;
    length = 0;
}

//********************************************************************

template<class ItemType>
SortedList2<ItemType>::SortedList2
    ( const SortedList2<ItemType>& otherList )

// Copy-constructor

// Postcondition:
//     IF otherList.head == NULL  (i.e., the other list is empty)
//         head == NULL
//     ELSE
//         head points to a new linked list that is a copy of
//         the linked list pointed to by otherList.head

{
    NodeType<ItemType>* fromPtr;  // Pointer original list
    NodeType<ItemType>* toPtr;    // Pointer into new list being
                                  //    built

    if (otherList.head == NULL)
    {
        head = NULL;
        return;
    }

    // Copy first node

    fromPtr = otherList.head;
    head = new NodeType<ItemType>;
    head->item = fromPtr->item;

    // Copy remaining nodes

    toPtr = head;
    fromPtr = fromPtr->link;
```

```
        while (fromPtr != NULL)
        {
            toPtr->link = new NodeType<NodeType>;
            toPtr = toPtr->link;
            toPtr->item = fromPtr->item;
            fromPtr = fromPtr->link;
        }
        toPtr->link = NULL;
        length = otherList.length;
        currentPos = otherList.currentPos;
}

//******************************************************************

template<class ItemType>
SortedList2<ItemType>::~SortedList2()

// Destructor

// Postcondition:
//      All linked list nodes have been deallocated from free store

{
    NodeType<ItemType>* temp;      // Temporary variable

    while ( !IsEmpty() )
    {
        temp = head;
        head = head->link;
        delete temp;
    }
}
//******************************************************************

template<class ItemType>
bool SortedList2<ItemType>::IsEmpty() const

// Postcondition:
//      Return value is true, if head == NULL; false, otherwise

{
    return (head == NULL);
}

//******************************************************************
```

```cpp
template<class ItemType>
bool SortedList2<ItemType>::IsFull() const

// Postcondition:
//      Return value is false

{
    return false;
}


//**********************************************************************


template<class ItemType>
void SortedList2<ItemType>::Insert( /* in */ ItemType item )

// Precondition:
//      item members of list nodes are in ascending order
//   && item is assigned
// Postcondition:
//      New node containing item is in its proper place
//          in linked list
//   && item members of list nodes are in ascending order

{
    NodeType<ItemType>* currentPtr;     // Moving pointer
    NodeType<ItemType>* prevPtr;        // Pointer to previous node
    NodeType<ItemType>* newNodePtr;     // Pointer to new node

    // Set up node to be inserted

    newNodePtr = new NodeType<ItemType>;
    newNodePtr->item = item;

    // Find previous insertion point
    prevPtr = NULL;
    currentPtr = head;
    while (currentPtr != NULL && currentPtr->item.LessThan(item))
    {
        prevPtr = currentPtr;
        currentPtr = currentPtr->link;
    }

    // Insert new node

    newNodePtr->link = currentPtr;
    if (prevPtr == NULL)
```

```
                head = newNodePtr;
        else
            prevPtr->link = newNodePtr;
        length++;
}

//*********************************************************************

template<class ItemType>
void SortedList2<ItemType>::Delete( /* in */ ItemType item )

// Precondition:
//      item == item member of some list node
//   && item members of list nodes are in ascending order
// Postcondition:
//      Node containing first occurrence of item is no longer in
//         linked list
//   && item members of list nodes are in ascending order

{
    NodeType<ItemType>* currentPtr;
    NodeType<ItemType>* prevPtr;

    currentPtr = head;
    prevPtr = NULL;

    while (currentPtr != NULL && !(currentPtr->item.Equal(item)))
    {
        prevPtr = currentPtr;
        currentPtr = currentPtr->link;
    }

    if (currentPtr != NULL)
    {
        prevPtr->link = currentPtr->link;
        length--;
    }

}

//*********************************************************************

template<class ItemType>
void SortedList2<ItemType>::Reset()

// Postcondition:
//      Iteration is initialized
```

```cpp
{
    currentPos = NULL;
}

template<class ItemType>
ItemType SortedList2<ItemType>::GetNextItem()

//******************************************************************
// Precondition:
//     No transformers have been invoked since last call
// Postcondition:
//     Returns item at the current position in the SortedList and
//     resets current to next position or first position if
//     last item is returned

{
    ItemType item;
    if (currentPos == NULL)
        currentPos = head;
    item = currentPos->item;
    currentPos = currentPos->link;
    return item;
}

//******************************************************************
template<class ItemType>
int SortedList2<ItemType>::Length() const

// Postcondition:
//     Return value is length

{
    return length;
}

//******************************************************************
template<class ItemType>
bool SortedList2<ItemType>::IsPresent(ItemType item) const

// Searches the list for item, reporting whether it was found
// Postcondition:
//     Return value is true, if item is the list;
//     false, otherwise

{
    NodeType<ItemType>* currentPtr;        // Moving pointer

    // Search for item
```

```
            currentPtr = head;
            while (currentPtr != NULL && currentPtr->item.LessThan(item))
                currentPtr = currentPtr->link;


            if (currentPtr == NULL)
                return false;
            return currentPtr->item.Equal(item);
        }
```

Go back and look at the driver for class Entry in Chapter 14. We changed two statements.

```
#include "SortedList2.h"
SortedList2<Entry> list;
```

Here is the input/output screen. This exercise demonstrates the value of using classes to encapsulate the implementation of a structure.

```
C:\PPSC++\LinkedEntry.exe                                              _ □ ×
Enter first name: Sarah
Enter middle name: Jane
Enter last name: Jones
Enter hours (<= 23):
10
Enter minutes (<= 59):
30
Enter seconds (<= 59):
00
Enter first name: Susan
Enter middle name: Margaret
Enter last name: Smith
Enter hours (<= 23):
9
Enter minutes (<= 59):
30
Enter seconds (<= 59):
00
Enter first name: Judy
Enter middle name: Dale
Enter last name: David
Enter hours (<= 23):
3
Enter minutes (<= 59):
00
Enter seconds (<= 59):
00
Name: Judy David Time: 03:00:00
Name: Susan Smith Time: 09:30:00
Name: Sarah Jones Time: 10:30:00
10:30:00 is not free.
00:00:00 is free.
Name: Judy David Time: 03:00:00
Name: Susan Smith Time: 09:30:00
```

Enhancing the Appointment Calendar

DISCUSSION Let's think of ways that we could make our appointment calendar more robust by adding exceptions. For example, the lists that we have been using allow duplicates. When we are talking about appointment times, this doesn't make sense. There is a precondition on function `InsertEntry` in class `Day` that states that the time is free. It would be safer to remove that precondition and throw an exception if the time is not free. Couldn't we just leave the precondition in and check anyway? No. A precondition is a contract that is not checked unless the consequences are life-threatening.

There are several occasions in which we write messages on the screen when a day has not been defined. We should make each of these cases an exception. The recognition of an illegal input string also should be an exception. What about a duplicate day? Yes, this also should be an exception. And finally, we should test to be sure that there is room to insert an entry before doing so in class `Day`. Here then are our exception classes.

```
class DuplicateTime
{};

class UndefinedDay
{};

class DuplicateDay
{};

class UndefinedString
{};

class EntryListIsFull
{};
```

Where should these errors be thrown?   A duplicate time and a full list should be detected in the `InsertEntry` function of `Day` class. An undefined or duplicate day should be detected in the appropriate functions in the `DayList` class. The undefined string is detected in the main program. A full list should be detected in class `Day`.

Where should these errors be caught?   The error message should be written on the screen for the user to see. As all of the functions have access to `cout`, the exceptions could be caught in the functions where they are detected. However, as we discussed in the chapter, it is better for an exception detected in a low-level operation in a complex structure to just report that the error has occurred and leave the handling to a higher authority. In this case, we catch the exceptions in the main program, where the appropriate message is written on the screen.

DayList: Add the checks for duplicate and undefined days in class DayList.
Day:
  Check for full list in InsertEntry and throw EntryListIsFull exception if it is.
  Check for duplicate time in the InsertFunction and throw a DuplicateTime exception if it is.
Appointments (main):
  Change the main program to throw an exception if a string cannot be decoded.
  Enclose the entire main loop in a try-catch statement.
  Insert the catch-clauses.

Let's look at each of these in order. We need to catch both undefined days and duplicate days in class DayList and throw the appropriate exceptions. These cases come up in all but the constructors. Each of these functions use helper function FindDay. If the day is found in InsertDay, a DuplicateDay exception has occurred. If a day is *not* found in InsertApt, DeleteApt, IsFree, and PrintDay, an UndefinedDay exception is thrown. We don't bother to show the code here, but it is on the Web.

The checks for a full list and duplicate time are very straightforward.

```
void Day::InsertEntry( /* in */ Entry newEntry )

// Postcondition:
//     If list is full, EntryListIsfull exception is thrown; if
//     time is already filled, DuplicateTime exception is thrown;
//     else newEntry is inserted in list

{
    if (list.IsFull())
        throw EntryListIsFull();
    else
        if (list.IsPresent(newEntry))
            throw DuplicateTime();
        else
          list.Insert(newEntry);
}
```

Throwing an exception when an input string is not a command can be accomplished by throwing an exception in the Switch statement when enumerated type ERROR is returned. Placing the loop within a Try-Catch statement needs no explanation. What about the Catch clauses? We just place the original output string within the Catch clauses for the cases we have checked previously and insert appropriate strings for the new ones. Here then is the revised Appointment Calendar program. Go over the code of this program very carefully. It contains several new syntactic constructs.

```
//****************************************************************
// APPOINTMENT CALENDAR PROGRAM
// This file implements an appointment calendar.  Exceptions are
// thrown if duplicate days or times are defined, if an entry list
```

```
// is full when trying to insert an entry, and an operation code
// cannot be decoded
//********************************************************************

#include "DayList.h"
#include <fstream>
#include <string>
#include <iostream>
#include <cstddef>        // For NULL
using namespace std;

enum Operations{INSERT_DAY, INSERT_APT, DELETE_APT, IS_FREE,
                PRINT_DAY, QUIT, ERROR};

// Function prototypes
Operations Convert(string operation);
void GetDate(Date& date);
void PrintMenu();

int main()
{
    DayList calendar[12];
    bool notQuit = true;
    Date date;

    string operation;
    ofstream outData;
    ofstream outList;
    outData.open("Appointments");

    while (notQuit)
    {
        try
        {
            PrintMenu();
            cin >> operation;
            switch (Convert(operation))
            {
                case    INSERT_DAY    :
                    GetDate(date);
                    calendar[date.Month()-1].InsertDay(date);
                    break;
                case    INSERT_APT  :
                    GetDate(date);
                    calendar[date.Month()-1].InsertApt(date);
                    break;
```

```
                            case DELETE_APT :
                                GetDate(date);
                                calendar[date.Month()-1].DeleteApt(date);
                                break;
                            case IS_FREE    :
                                GetDate(date);
                                if (calendar[date.Month()-1].IsFree(date))
                                    cout << "Time is free" << endl;
                                else
                                    cout << "Time is not free" << endl;
                                break;
                            case PRINT_DAY  :
                                GetDate(date);
                                calendar[date.Month()-1].PrintDay(outData,
                                                                 date);
                                break;
                            case QUIT    :
                                notQuit = false;
                                break;
                            case ERROR   :
                                throw UndefinedString();
                        }
                    }
                    catch ( UndefinedDay )
                    {
                        cout << "An operation has been defined on an "
                             << "undefined day" << endl;
                    }

                    catch ( DuplicateTime )
                    {
                        cout << "Entry with same time is already in the list"
                             << endl;
                    }

                    catch ( DuplicateDay )
                    {
                        cout << "Day with same date is already defined."
                             << endl;
                    }

                    catch ( UndefinedString )
                    {
                        cout << "Input string was not valid."
                             << endl
                             << "Read menu and try again."
```

```
                            << endl;
            }

        catch ( EntryListIsFull )
            {
                cout << "Entry list is full for this date" << endl;
        }
    outData.close();
    outList.close();
    return 0;

}


void GetDate(Date& date)
{
    int month;
    int day;
    int year;
    cout << "Enter month, day, and year in that order" << endl;
    cin >> month >> day >> year;
    date.Set(month, day, year);
}


void PrintMenu()
{
    cout << endl;
    cout << "Menu Options" << endl;
    cout << "      InsertDay sets up a new day " << endl;
    cout << "      InsertApt inserts a new entry" << endl;
    cout << "      DeleteApt deletes an entry " << endl;
    cout << "      IsFree checks to see if a time is free" << endl;
    cout << "      PrintDay prints all of the appointments "
         << " for a day" << endl;
    cout << "      Quit ends the processing" << endl;
    cout << "Type in the appropriate string " << endl << endl;
}


Operations Convert(string operation)
{
    if (operation == "InsertDay")
        return INSERT_DAY  ;
    else if (operation == "InsertApt")
        return INSERT_APT;
    else if (operation == "DeleteApt")
        return DELETE_APT;
    else if (operation == "IsFree")
```

```
                    return IS_FREE;
        else if (operation == "PrintDay")
            return PRINT_DAY;
        else if (operation == "Quit")
            return QUIT;
        else return ERROR;
}
```

TESTING   We can use the same test plan that we used in Chapter 16, but we need to attempt to insert a duplicate entry and insert into a full schedule. Should we use the new templated, linked SortedList ADT for the entry list or go back to the array-based one? Theoretically, it doesn't matter; however, practically it does. We have defined `NodeType` in `DayList` and in the linked sorted list; thus it is defined twice. Although there are ways to solve this problem, let's leave that to the Case Study Follow-Up exercises and use the array-based version.

Here is the output from the run that tests the new features.

```
Menu Options
        InsertDay sets up a new day
        InsertApt inserts a new entry
        DeleteApt deletes an entry
        IsFree checks to see if a time is free
        PrintDay prints all of the appointments  for a day
        Quit ends the processing
Type in the appropriate string

InsertDay
Enter month, day, and year in that order
1 3 2004
How many appointments can be made on this date?
2


. . .


InsertApt
Enter month, day, and year in that order
1 3 2004
Enter first name: Susy
Enter middle name: Sunshine
Enter last name: Smith
Enter hours (<= 23):
10
Enter minutes (<= 59):
30


. . .
```

```
InsertApt
Enter month, day, and year in that order
1 3 2004
Enter first name: Clara
Enter middle name: Cloudy
Enter last name: Clear
Enter hours (<= 23):
10
Enter minutes (<= 59):
30
Entry with same time is already in the list


...


InsertApt
Enter month, day, and year in that order
1 3 2004
Enter first name: Clara
Enter middle name: Cloudy
Enter last name: Clear
Enter hours (<= 23):
11
Enter minutes (<= 59):
30


...


InsertApt
Enter month, day, and year in that order
1 3 2004
Enter first name: Nora
Enter middle name: Night
Enter last name: Knight
Enter hours (<= 23):
12
Enter minutes (<= 59):
30
Entry list is full for this date


...


Quit
```

Testing and Debugging

When working with templates, it's important to remember that a generated template function or template class becomes an ordinary function or class and is subject to all the usual rules of syntax and semantics.

To test a template function or template class, you should start with a *nontemplate* version, using a specific data type such as `int` or whatever type is most appropriate to your needs. Apply the usual testing strategies we have outlined in previous chapters for algorithms and classes. After all errors have been noted and corrected, convert the function or class into a templatized form, and continue testing by supplying different data types as template arguments.

A program that handles exceptions must be tested to ensure that the exceptions are generated appropriately and then handled properly. Test cases must be included to cause exceptions to be thrown and to specify the expected results from handling them.

Testing and Debugging Hints

1. When declaring a template parameter, as in

   ```
   template<class AType>
   ```

   remember to use the word `class` (or `typename`). However, the template argument used when instantiating a template is *not* required to be the name of a C++ class. Any data type, built-in or user-defined, is allowed.

2. In the restricted form discussed in this book, template arguments are *data type names*, not variable names or expressions.

3. Template functions are usually called with implicit template arguments, but template classes *must* use explicit template arguments.

4. Just as with nontemplate functions, if template function definitions are physically placed after the code that calls the functions, then function prototypes (forward declarations) must precede the calling code.

5. With template classes, the member function definitions *must* be compiled together with the client code, not independently. One strategy is to group the class template and the member function definitions into a single file (the `.h` file). Another strategy is to place the class template into a `.h` file and the member function definitions into a `.cpp` file, with the `.h` file saying to `#include` the `.cpp` file. In the latter approach, if you are using an IDE (integrated development environment), do *not* list this `.cpp` file in your "project." Include *only* the client code file in the project.

6. It's a good idea to have the `main` function catch all exceptions, even if other functions perform partial exception handling. The `main` function can then decide whether to stop the program or keep executing.

7. Avoid using built-in types as exception types. Throw objects of a user-defined class or struct whose name suggests the nature of the error or exceptional event.

8. If `BadData` is the name of an exception class, be sure to throw an *object* of that class by writing

   ```
   throw BadData();   // Throw a constructed object
   ```

   rather than

   ```
   throw BadData;   // Syntax error
   ```

9. Make sure that all exceptions are caught. An uncaught exception results in program termination with a vague error message.

Summary

C++ templates are a powerful and convenient mechanism for implementing generic algorithms and generic data types. With a function template, we can define an entire family of functions that are the same except for the data types of the items they manipulate. With a class template, we can define an entire family of class types that differ only in the data types of their internal data representations. Class templates allow us to define structures such as lists of `int`s, lists of `float`s, and lists of `string`s, all in the same program.

A template is instantiated by placing the template argument in angle brackets next to the name of the function or class. In the examples shown in this chapter, a template argument is the name of a *data type*, not the name of a variable or expression. The compiler then generates a new function or class by substituting the template argument for the template parameter wherever the parameter appears in the template. With template classes, the template argument must be explicit in order for the compiler to instantiate the template. With template functions, the template argument is usually omitted, and the compiler deduces the template argument by examining the function's argument list.

An exception is an unusual, often unpredictable, event that requires special processing. The primary purpose of exception handling is to allow one part of a program to report an error to another part of the program if the error cannot be handled locally. C++ supports exception handling by means of the `throw` statement and the `try-catch` statement. A section of code that detects an error uses the `throw` statement to throw an exception, which in C++ is an object of some data type—often a class or struct. The thrown exception is said to be caught if the `try-catch` statement has a catch-clause (exception handler) with a formal parameter whose type matches that of the exception. If there is no matching exception handler, the enclosing function immediately returns and passes the exception up to its calling function. This process continues up the calling chain until either a matching exception handler is found or control reaches the `main` function. If `main` does not catch the exception, then the program terminates with a vague error message.

Quick Check

1. What kind of algorithm does a template enable us to write? (pp. 908–911)
2. What is an exception? (pp. 926–927)
3. Write a function template for a value-returning function `Thrice` that receives a parameter of any simple type and returns three times that value. (p. 911)
4. Write calling code that calls `Thrice` two times, once with an integer argument and once with a floating-point argument. (pp. 912–913)
5. Write a user-defined specialization of the `Thrice` template that, for a `char` parameter, outputs `"Can't triple a char value"` and returns the character `'x'`. (pp. 914–915)
6. In mathematics, an ordered pair is a pair of numbers written in the form (a, b). Rewrite the following `OrdPair` declaration as a class template so that clients can manipulate ordered pairs of any simple type, not just ordered pairs of `int`s. (pp. 918–920)

```
class OrdPair
{
public:
    int  First() const;    // Returns first component of the
                           //    pair
    int  Second() const;   // Returns second component of the
                           //    pair
    void Print() const;    // Outputs the pair
    OrdPair( int m, int n ); // Constructor. Creates ordered
                           //    pair (m,n)
private:
    int first;
    int second;
};
```

7. Given the `OrdPair` class template, write client code that declares three class objects named `pair1`, `pair2`, and `pair3` that represent the ordered pairs (5, 6), (2.95, 6.34), and ('+', '#'), respectively, and prints the ordered pairs represented by `pair1`, `pair2`, and `pair3`. (pp. 920–921)
8. Given the `OrdPair` class template, write function definitions for the member functions. (pp. 922–925)
9. a. Write the declaration of a user-defined exception type named `BadData`.
   b. Write a void function `GetAge` that prompts for and inputs the user's age (type `int`) from the keyboard. The function returns the user's age through the parameter list unless the input value is a negative number, in which case a `BadData` exception is thrown. (pp. 926–929)
10. Write a `try-catch` statement that calls the `GetAge` function of Question 7. If a `BadData` exception is thrown, print an error message and re-throw the exception to a caller; otherwise, execution should just continue. (pp. 929–935)

Answers

1. Generic algorithms.   2. An unusual, often unpredictable event that requires special processing.

3.
```
template<class SimpleType>
SimpleType Thrice( SimpleType val )
{
    return 3*val;
}
```

4.
```
cout << Thrice(75) << ' ' << Thrice(64.35);
```
   or
```
cout << Thrice<int>(75) << ' ' << Thrice<float>(64.35);
```

5.
```
template<>
char Thrice( char val )
{
    cout << "Can't triple a char value" << endl;
    return 'x';
}
```

6.
```
template<class SomeType>
class OrdPair
{
public:
    SomeType First() const;
    SomeType Second() const;
    void Print() const;
    OrdPair( SomeType m, SomeType n );
private:
    SomeType first;
    SomeType second;
};
```

7.
```
OrdPair<int>   pair1(5, 6);
OrdPair<float> pair2(2.95, 6.34);
OrdPair<char>  pair3('+', '#');

pair1.Print();
pair2.Print();
pair3.Print();
```

8.
```
template<class SomeType>
OrdPair<SomeType>::OrdPair( SomeType m, SomeType n )
// Constructor
{
    first = m;
    second = n;
}

template<class SomeType>
SomeType OrdPair<SomeType>::First() const
{
    return first;
}
```

```
template<class SomeType>
SomeType OrdPair<SomeType>::Second() const
{
    return second;
}

template<class SomeType>
void OrdPair<SomeType>::Print() const
{
    cout << '(' << first << ", " << second << ')' << endl;
}
```

9. a.
```
class BadData
{};                    // Don't forget the semicolon
```

  b.
```
void GetAge( int& age )
{
    cout << "Enter your age: ";
    cin >> age;
    if (age < 0)
        throw BadData();
}
```

10.
```
try
{
    GetAge(age);
}
catch ( BadData )
{
    cout << "Age must not be negative." << endl;
    throw;
}
```

Exam Preparation Exercises

1. In C++, two (nontemplate) functions can have the same name. True or False?
2. In C++, two (nontemplate) classes can have the same name. True or False?
3. Is the following a function template, a template function, or neither?

```
template<class T>
T OneLess( T var )
{
    return var-1;
}
```

4. In the statement

```
Group<char> oneGroup;
```

  a. is Group<char> a class template, a template class, or neither?
  b. is oneGroup a class template, a template class, or neither?

5. Define the following terms:

   instantiate (a template)   specialization (of a template)
   template parameter   user-defined specialization (of a template)
   template argument

6. Consider this function call:

   ```
   DoThis<float>(3.85)
   ```

   a. Which item is the template argument?
   b. Which item is the function argument?
   c. Could it be written as `DoThis(3.85)`?

7. What is the C++ control structure to use if you think an operation might throw an exception?
8. What is the C++ statement that raises an exception?
9. What part of the `try-catch` statement must be written with a formal parameter?
10. Mark the following statements True or False. If a statement is false, explain why.
    a. There can be only one catch-clause for each `try-catch` statement.
    b. A catch-clause is an exception handler.
    c. A `throw` statement must be located within a try-clause.
11. In the `WriteToFile` function of Section 17.3,
    a. what would happen if we deleted the `throw` statement in the exception handler?
    b. what would happen if we changed `throw` to `return`?
12. Consider the division-by-zero program at the end of Section 17.3. How would you change the `main` function so that the program terminates if a denominator is found to be 0?
13. What happens if you call a function that throws an exception, without placing the call in a *try-clause*?
14. What does the following statement do if it is written within an exception handler?

    ```
    throw;
    ```

15. What type of exception would be written as the parameter of a *catch-clause* if the try-clause is calling `new` and we want to check whether the free store has run out of space?

Programming Warm-Up Exercises

1. Write a function template for a `void` function that squares and outputs the value passed to its parameter. The type of the parameter is the template type.
2. Write statements that call the function in Exercise 1 for values of type `int`, `long`, and `float`.
3. Write a user specialization of the function in Exercise 1 that accepts a string argument and "squares" it by printing it twice with no intervening spaces.

4. We would like to have a value-returning function that returns twice the value of its incoming parameter.
   a. Using function overloading, write two C++ function definitions for such a function, one with an `int` parameter, and one with a `float` parameter.
   b. Write calling code that makes calls to both functions.

5. Write a function template for a function that returns the sum of all the elements in a one-dimensional array. The array elements can be of any simple numeric type, and the function has two parameters: the base address of the array and the number of elements in the array.

6. Write a function template for a void function, `GetData`, that receives a string through the parameter list, uses that string to prompt the user for input, reads a value from the keyboard, and returns that value (as a reference parameter) through the parameter list. The data type of the input value can be any type for which the `>>` operator is defined.

7. Assume you have an enumeration type

   ```
   enum AutoType {SEDAN, COUPE, OTHER};
   ```

   Write a user-defined specialization of the `GetData` template (see Exercise 6) that accommodates the `AutoType` type. For input, the user should type the character 's' for sedan, 'c' for coupe, and 'o' (or anything else) otherwise.

8. Consider the `GList` class template of Section 17.2.
   a. Write client code to instantiate the template twice, creating a list of `int`s and a list of `float`s.
   b. Assume that at some point in the client code the list of `int`s already contains values known to be in the range 10 through 80 and the list of `float`s is empty. Write client code that empties the list of `int`s as follows. As each item is removed from the list of `int`s, multiply it by 0.5 and insert the result into the list of `float`s.

9. Write a `MixedPair` class template that is similar to the `OrdPair` template of Quick Check Question 6 except that the pair of items can be of two different data types. *Hint:* Begin the template with

   ```
   template<class Type1, class Type2>
   ```

10. Given the `MixedPair` class template of Exercise 9, write client code that creates two class objects representing the pairs (5, 29.48) and ("Book", 36).

11. Given the `MixedPair` class template of Exercise 9, write function definitions for the class member functions.

12. a. Declare a user-defined exception class named `MathError`.
    b. Write a statement that throws an exception of type `MathError`.

13. Write a `try-catch` statement—assumed to be in the `main` function—that attempts to concatenate two `string` objects and prints an error message and terminates the program if an exception is thrown. You may wish to review Section 17.3 to see what exceptions are thrown by the `string` class.

14. Write a `Sum` function that returns the sum of its two nonnegative `int` parameters unless the sum would exceed `INT_MAX`, in which case it throws an excep-

tion. (*Caution:* You cannot check for overflow *after* adding the numbers. On most machines, integer overflow results in a change of sign, but you should not write code that depends on this fact.)

15. Write a `try-catch` statement that calls the `Sum` function of Exercise 14 and, if an exception is thrown, prints an error message and re-throws the exception to a caller.

Programming Problems

1. Programming Problem 1 in Chapter 9 asked you to output the ICAO word corresponding to each letter in a word. Change the function that converts a letter to the matching word so that it throws an exception if the letter is not in the alphabet, and add an exception handler to the program that outputs "Invalid letter" and the offending letter whenever the exception is thrown.

2. Programming Problem 2 in Chapter 9 asked you to compute a person's weight on a specified planet. Rewrite that program so that an erroneous planet name results in an exception being thrown by the input routine, and caught by the caller.

3. Programming Problem 2 in Chapter 12 asked you to write a simple database program for an art gallery. The problem required that a user be able to search the database using any of the values in a record for an art work. Rewrite the program using a template for the equality test function so that a single search function can be used for the different types of values in the database.

4. You're working for an observatory that keeps a database of stars. The most prominent stars are indexed by name (a string), less prominent stars are indexed by the name of the constellation in which they are found, and a sequentially assigned number (an int), and the least prominent stars are indexed by coordinates consisting of two floating point numbers. Each star record also contains a measurement of the star's brightness, called its magnitude (a float) and a letter indicating its color (a char).

    Write a C++ program that reads the star data from three files (`named.dat`, `numbered.dat`, and `coord.dat`) and places them all into a single list. The program should then allow the user to retrieve the data for any star using the different kinds of indexes. Use templates to simplify the coding of this application.

5. Programming Problem 5 in Chapter 9 asked you to write a program to input a time in numeric form and print it in English. Rewrite the program to check for entry of erroneous times in the input function, and throw an exception that is handled by the caller.

6. Develop a C++ class for a date that includes functions to construct a date, print a date, and compare two dates for equality. The function that constructs a date should check for different errors (invalid month, invalid day, invalid month-day combination such as April 31, and February 29 in a year that isn't a leap year). For each type of date error, the function should throw a different exception to the caller. Write a driver program that reads two dates, prints them out, and

indicates whether they are equal. The driver should catch any exceptions and output appropriate error messages as necessary.

Case Study Follow-Up

1. Why should there be a problem having `NodeType` defined in two places?
2. How might you solve the problem of duplicate identifiers?
3. Write a test plan for the enhanced version of the appointment calendar.
4. In the appointment calendar, classes `Entry` and `Time` have operations `Equal` and `LessThan`. Class `Name` and `Date` have operation `ComparedTo`. These classes should be consistent in their use of comparison functions. Rewrite `Entry` and `Time` to use a `ComparedTo` function.
5. Run the Entry driver program from the chapter using the classes altered in Exercise 4.

Recursion

Goals

Knowledge Goals

■ *To understand the distinction between the base case(s) and the general case in a recursive definition.*

Skill Goals

To be able to:

■ *Write a recursive algorithm for a problem involving only simple variables.*

■ *Write a recursive algorithm for a problem involving structured variables.*

■ *Write a recursive algorithm for a problem involving linked lists.*

In C++, any function can call another function. A function can even call itself! When a function calls itself, it is making a **recursive call**. The word *recursive* means "having the characteristic of coming up again, or repeating." In this case, a function call is being repeated by the function itself. Recursion is a powerful technique that can be used in place of iteration (looping).

> **Recursive call** A function call in which the function being called is the same as the one making the call.

Recursive solutions are generally less efficient than iterative solutions to the same problem. However, some problems lend themselves to simple, elegant, recursive solutions and are exceedingly cumbersome to solve iteratively. Some programming languages, such as early versions of FORTRAN, BASIC, and COBOL, do not allow recursion. Other languages are especially oriented to recursive algorithms—LISP is one of these. C++ lets us take our choice: We can implement both iterative and recursive algorithms.

Our examples are broken into two groups: problems that use only simple variables and problems that use structured variables. If you are studying recursion before reading Chapters 11–16 on structured data types, then cover only the first set of examples and leave the rest until you have completed the chapters on structured data types.

18.1 What Is Recursion?

You may have seen a set of gaily painted Russian dolls that fit inside one another. Inside the first doll is a smaller doll, inside of which is an even smaller doll, inside of which is yet a smaller doll, and so on. A recursive algorithm is like such a set of Russian dolls. It reproduces itself with smaller and smaller examples of itself until a solution is found—that is, until there are no more dolls. The recursive algorithm is implemented by using a function that makes recursive calls to itself.

In Chapter 8, we wrote a function named `Power` that calculates the result of raising an integer to a positive power. If X is an integer and N is a positive integer, the formula for X^N is

$$x^N = \underbrace{X \times X \times X \times X \times \ldots \times X}_{N \text{ times}}$$

We could also write this formula as

$$x^N = X \times \underbrace{(X \times X \times \ldots \times X)}_{(N-1) \text{ times}}$$

or even as

$$x^N = X \times X \times \underbrace{(X \times X \times \ldots \times X)}_{(N-2) \text{ times}}$$

In fact, we can write the formula most concisely as

$$X^N = X \times X^{N-1}$$

This definition of X^N is a classic recursive definition—that is, a definition given in terms of a smaller version of itself.

X^N is defined in terms of multiplying X times X^{N-1}. How is X^{N-1} defined? Why, as $X \times X^{N-2}$, of course! And X^{N-2} is $X \times X^{N-3}$; X^{N-3} is $X \times X^{N-4}$; and so on. In this example, "in terms of smaller versions of itself" means that the exponent is decremented each time.

When does the process stop? When we have reached a case for which we know the answer without resorting to a recursive definition. In this example, it is the case where N equals 1: X^1 is X. The case (or cases) for which an answer is explicitly known is called the base case. The case for which the solution is expressed in terms of a smaller version of itself is called the recursive or general case. A recursive algorithm is an algorithm that expresses the solution in terms of a call to itself, a recursive call. A recursive algorithm must terminate; that is, it must have a base case.

Figure 18–1 shows a recursive version of the Power function with the base case and the recursive call marked. The function is embedded in a program that reads in a number and an exponent and prints the result.

> **Recursive definition** A definition in which something is defined in terms of smaller versions of itself.
>
> **Base case** The case for which the solution can be stated non-recursively.
>
> **General case** The case for which the solution is expressed in terms of a smaller version of itself; also known as *recursive case*.
>
> **Recursive algorithm** A solution that is expressed in terms of (a) smaller instances of itself and (b) a base case.

Figure 18–1 *Power Function*

```
//***********************************************************
// Exponentiation program
//***********************************************************
#include <iostream>

using namespace std;

int Power( int, int );

int main()
{
    int number;            // Number that is being raised to power
    int exponent;          // Power the number is being raised to

    cin >> number >> exponent;
```

```
        cout << Power(number, exponent);   ←───────── // Nonrecursive call
        return 0;
}


//*********************************************************************

int Power( /* in */ int x,    // Number that is being raised to power
           /* in */ int n )   // Power the number is being raised to

// Computes x to the n power by multiplying x times the result of
// computing x to the n - 1 power

// Precondition:
//       x is assigned  &&  n > 0
// Postcondition:
//       Function value == x raised to the power n
// Note:
//       Large exponents may result in integer overflow

{
    if (n == 1)
        return x;   ←──────────────────────────── // Base case
    else
        return x * Power(x, n - 1);   ←─────────── // Recursive call
}
```

Each recursive call to Power can be thought of as creating a completely new copy of the function, each with its own copies of the parameters x and n. The value of x remains the same for each version of Power, but the value of n decreases by 1 for each call until it becomes 1.

Let's trace the execution of this recursive function, with number equal to 2 and exponent equal to 3. We use a new format to trace recursive routines: We number the calls and then discuss what is happening in paragraph form.

Call 1: Power is called by main, with number equal to 2 and exponent equal to 3. Within Power, the parameters x and n are initialized to 2 and 3, respectively. Because n is not equal to 1, Power is called recursively with x and n − 1 as arguments. Execution of Call 1 pauses until an answer is sent back from this recursive call.

Call 2: x is equal to 2 and n is equal to 2. Because n is not equal to 1, the function Power is called again, this time with x and n − 1 as arguments. Execution of Call 2 pauses until an answer is sent back from this recursive call.

Call 3: x is equal to 2 and n is equal to 1. Because n equals 1, the value of x is to be returned. This call to the function has finished executing, and the function return value (which is 2) is passed back to the place in the statement from which the call was made.

Call 2: This call to the function can now complete the statement that contained the recursive call because the recursive call has returned. Call 3's return value (which is 2) is multiplied by x. This call to the function has finished executing, and the function return value (which is 4) is passed back to the place in the statement from which the call was made.

Call 1: This call to the function can now complete the statement that contained the recursive call because the recursive call has returned. Call 2's return value (which is 4) is multiplied by x. This call to the function has finished executing, and the function return value (which is 8) is passed back to the place in the statement from which the call was made. Because the first call (the nonrecursive call in `main`) has now completed, this is the final value of the function `Power`.

This trace is summarized in Figure 18-2. Each box represents a call to the `Power` function. The values for the parameters for that call are shown in each box.

What happens if there is no base case? We have **infinite recursion**, the recursive equivalent of an infinite loop. For example, if the condition

| **Infinite recursion**   The situation in which a function calls itself over and over endlessly. |

```
if (n == 1)
```

were omitted, `Power` would be called over and over again. Infinite recursion also occurs if `Power` is called with n less than or equal to 0.

In actuality, recursive calls can't go on forever. Here's the reason. When a function is called, either recursively or nonrecursively, the computer system creates temporary storage for the parameters and the function's (automatic) local variables. This temporary storage is a region of memory called the *run-time stack*. When the function returns, its parameters

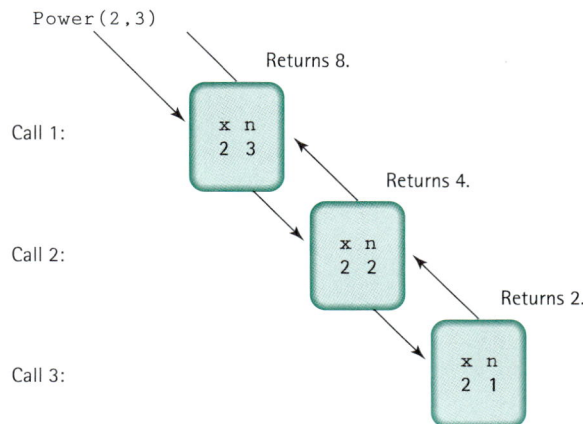

Power(2,3)

Returns 8.

Call 1:

x n
2 3

Returns 4.

Call 2:

x n
2 2

Returns 2.

Call 3:

x n
2 1

Figure 18-2   *Execution of* `Power(2, 3)`

and local variables are released from the run-time stack. With infinite recursion, the recursive function calls never return. Each time the function calls itself, a little more of the run-time stack is used to store the new copies of the variables. Eventually, all the memory space on the stack is used. At that point, the program crashes with an error message such as "RUN-TIME STACK OVERFLOW" (or the computer may simply hang).

18.2 Recursive Algorithms with Simple Variables

Let's look at another example: calculating a factorial. The factorial of a number N (written $N!$) is N multiplied by $N - 1$, $N - 2$, $N - 3$, and so on. Another way of expressing factorial is

$$N! = N \times (N - 1)!$$

This expression looks like a recursive definition. $(N - 1)!$ is a smaller instance of $N!$— that is, it takes one less multiplication to calculate $(N - 1)!$ than it does to calculate $N!$ If we can find a base case, we can write a recursive algorithm. Fortunately, we don't have to look too far: $0!$ is defined in mathematics to be 1.

Factorial (In: n)

```
IF n is 0
    Return 1
ELSE
    Return n * Factorial(n – 1)
```

This algorithm can be coded directly as follows.

```
int Factorial ( /* in */ int n )

// Precondition:
//      n >= 0
// Postcondition:
//      Function value == n!
// Note:
//      Large values of n may cause integer overflow

{
    if (n == 0)
        return 1;                              // Base case
    else
        return n * Factorial(n - 1);           // General case
}
```

Let's trace this function with an original n of 4.

Call 1: n is 4. Because n is not 0, the `else` branch is taken. The Return statement cannot be completed until the recursive call to `Factorial` with n − 1 as the argument has been completed.

Call 2: n is 3. Because n is not 0, the `else` branch is taken. The Return statement cannot be completed until the recursive call to `Factorial` with n − 1 as the argument has been completed.

Call 3: n is 2. Because n is not 0, the `else` branch is taken. The Return statement cannot be completed until the recursive call to `Factorial` with n − 1 as the argument has been completed.

Call 4: n is 1. Because n is not 0, the `else` branch is taken. The Return statement cannot be completed until the recursive call to `Factorial` with n − 1 as the argument has been completed.

Call 5: n is 0. Because n equals 0, this call to the function returns, sending back 1 as the result.

Call 4: The Return statement in this copy can now be completed. The value to be returned is n (which is 1) times 1. This call to the function returns, sending back 1 as the result.

Call 3: The Return statement in this copy can now be completed. The value to be returned is n (which is 2) times 1. This call to the function returns, sending back 2 as the result.

Call 2: The Return statement in this copy can now be completed. The value to be returned is n (which is 3) times 2. This call to the function returns, sending back 6 as the result.

Call 1: The Return statement in this copy can now be completed. The value to be returned is n (which is 4) times 6. This call to the function returns, sending back 24 as the result. Because this is the last of the calls to `Factorial`, the recursive process is over. The value 24 is returned as the final value of the call to `Factorial` with an argument of 4. Figure 18–3 summarizes the execution of the `Factorial` function with an argument of 4.

Let's organize what we have done in these two solutions into an outline for writing recursive algorithms.

1. Understand the problem. (We threw this in for good measure; it is always the first step.)

2. Determine the base case(s).

3. Determine the recursive case(s).

We have used the factorial and the power algorithms to demonstrate recursion because they are easy to visualize. In practice, one would never want to calculate either of these functions using the recursive solution. In both cases, the iterative solutions are simpler and much more efficient because starting a new iteration of a loop is a faster operation than calling a function. Let's compare the code for the iterative and recursive versions of the factorial problem.

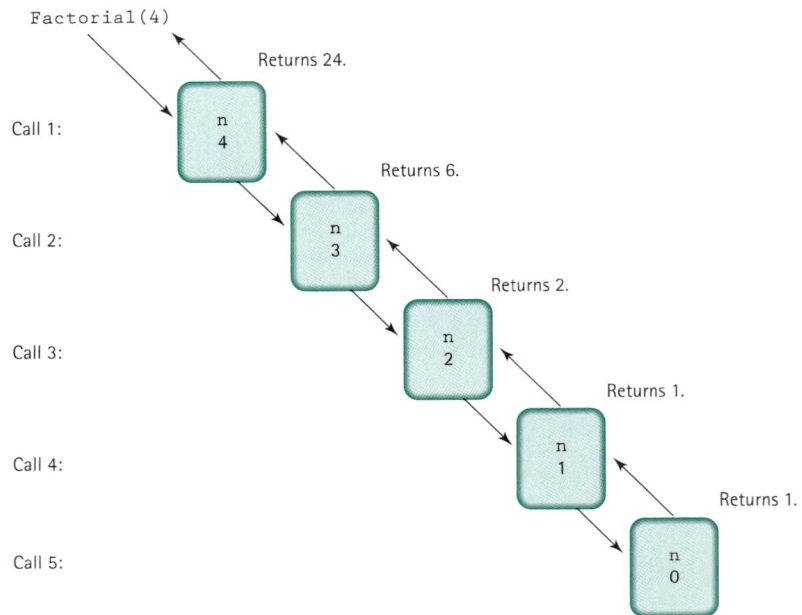

Figure 18–3   *Execution of* Factorial(4)

Iterative Solution

```
int Factorial ( /* in */ int n )
{
    int factor;
    int count;

    factor = 1;
    for (count = 2; count <= n; count++)
        factor = factor * count;
    return factor;
}
```

Recursive Solution

```
int Factorial ( /* in */ int n )
{
    if (n == 0)
        return 1;
    else
        return n * Factorial(n - 1);
}
```

The iterative version has two local variables, whereas the recursive version has none. There are usually fewer local variables in a recursive routine than in an iterative routine. Also, the iterative version always has a loop, whereas the recursive version always has a selection statement—either an If or a Switch. A branching structure is the main control structure in a recursive routine. A looping structure is the main control structure in an iterative routine.

In the next section, we examine a more complicated problem—one in which the recursive solution is not immediately apparent.

18.3 Towers of Hanoi

One of your first toys may have been three pegs with colored circles of different diameters. If so, you probably spent countless hours moving the circles from one peg to another. If we put some constraints on how the circles or discs can be moved, we have an adult game called the Towers of Hanoi. When the game begins, all the circles are on the first peg in order by size, with the smallest on the top. The object of the game is to move the circles, one at a time, to the third peg. The catch is that a circle cannot be placed on top of one that is smaller in diameter. The middle peg can be used as an auxiliary peg, but it must be empty at the beginning and at the end of the game.

To get a feel for how this might be done, let's look at some sketches of what the configuration must be at certain points if a solution is possible. We use four circles or discs. The beginning configuration is:

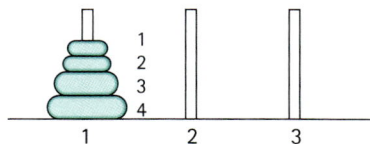

To move the largest circle (circle 4) to peg 3, we must move the three smaller circles to peg 2. Then circle 4 can be moved into its final place:

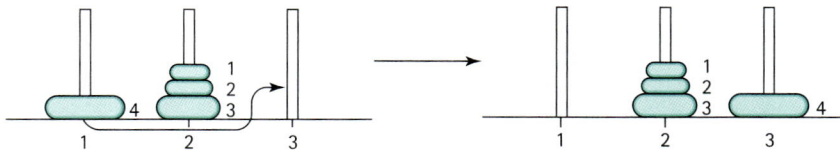

Let's assume we can do this. Now, to move the next largest circle (circle 3) into place, we must move the two circles on top of it onto an auxiliary peg (peg 1 in this case):

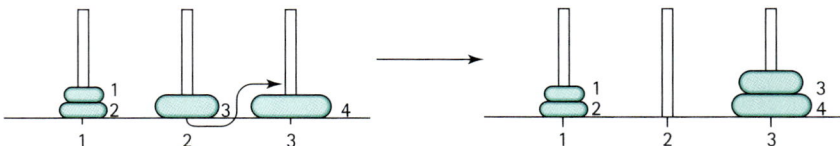

To get circle 2 into place, we must move circle 1 to another peg, freeing circle 2 to be moved to its place on peg 3:

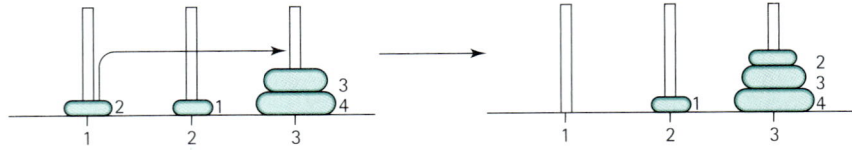

The last circle (circle 1) can now be moved into its final place, and we are finished:

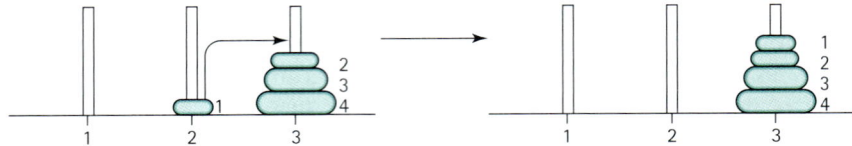

Notice that to free circle 4, we had to move three circles to another peg. To free circle 3, we had to move two circles to another peg. To free circle 2, we had to move one circle to another peg. This sounds like a recursive algorithm: To free the *n*th circle, we have to move $n - 1$ circles. Each stage can be thought of as beginning again with three pegs, but with one less circle each time. Let's see if we can summarize this process, using *n* instead of an actual number.

Get N Circles Moved from Peg 1 to Peg 3

> Get n 2 1 circles moved from peg 1 to peg 2
> Move nth circle from peg 1 to peg 3
> Get n 2 1 circles moved from peg 2 to peg 3

This algorithm certainly sounds simple; surely there must be more. But this really is all there is to it.

Let's write a recursive function that implements this algorithm. We can't actually move discs, of course, but we can print out a message to do so. Notice that the beginning peg, the ending peg, and the auxiliary peg keep changing during the algorithm. To make the algorithm easier to follow, we call the pegs `beginPeg`, `endPeg`, and `auxPeg`. These three pegs, along with the number of circles on the beginning peg, are the parameters of the function.

We have the recursive or general case, but what about a base case? How do we know when to stop the recursive process? The clue is in the expression "Get *n* circles moved." If we don't have any circles to move, we don't have anything to do. We are finished with that stage. Therefore, when the number of circles equals 0, we do nothing (that is, we simply return).

```cpp
void DoTowers(
    /* in */ int circleCount,    // Number of circles to move
    /* in */ int beginPeg,       // Peg containing circles to move
    /* in */ int auxPeg,         // Peg holding circles temporarily
    /* in */ int endPeg      )   // Peg receiving circles being moved
{
    if (circleCount > 0)
    {
        // Move n - 1 circles from beginning peg to auxiliary peg

        DoTowers(circleCount - 1, beginPeg, endPeg, auxPeg);
        cout << "Move circle from peg " << beginPeg
             << " to peg " << endPeg << endl;

        // Move n - 1 circles from auxiliary peg to ending peg

        DoTowers(circleCount - 1, auxPeg, beginPeg, endPeg);
    }
}
```

It's hard to believe that such a simple algorithm actually works, but we'll prove it to you. Following is a driver program that calls the `DoTowers` function. Output statements have been added so you can see the values of the arguments with each recursive call. Because there are two recursive calls within the function, we have indicated which recursive statement issued the call.

```cpp
//****************************************************************
// TestTowers program
// This program, a test driver for the DoTowers function, reads in
// a value from standard input and passes this value to DoTowers
//****************************************************************
#include <iostream>
#include <iomanip>    // For setw()

using namespace std;

void DoTowers( int, int, int, int );

int main()
```

```cpp
{
    int circleCount;      // Number of circles on starting peg

    cout << "Input number of circles: ";
    cin >> circleCount;
    cout << "OUTPUT WITH " << circleCount << " CIRCLES" << endl
         << endl;
    cout << "CALLED FROM  #CIRCLES" << setw(8) << "BEGIN"
         << setw(8) << "AUXIL." << setw(5) << "END"
         << "    INSTRUCTIONS" << endl
         << endl;
    cout << "Original    :";
    DoTowers(circleCount, 1, 2, 3);
    return 0;
}


//********************************************************************

void DoTowers(
    /* in */ int circleCount,      // Number of circles to move
    /* in */ int beginPeg,         // Peg containing circles to move
    /* in */ int auxPeg,           // Peg holding circles temporarily
    /* in */ int endPeg       )    // Peg receiving circles being moved

// This recursive function moves circleCount circles from beginPeg
// to endPeg.  All but one of the circles are moved from beginPeg
// to auxPeg, then the last circle is moved from beginPeg to endPeg,
// and then the circles are moved from auxPeg to endPeg.
// The subgoals of moving circles to and from auxPeg are what
// involve recursion

// Precondition:
//     All parameters are assigned  &&  circleCount >= 0
// Postcondition:
//     The values of all parameters have been printed
//  && IF circleCount > 0
//         circleCount circles have been moved from beginPeg to
//         endPeg in the manner detailed above
//     ELSE
//         No further actions have taken place

{
    cout << setw(6) << circleCount << setw(9) << beginPeg
         << setw(7) << auxPeg << setw(7) << endPeg << endl;
    if (circleCount > 0)
```

```
        {
            cout << "From  first:";
            DoTowers(circleCount - 1, beginPeg, endPeg, auxPeg);
            cout << setw(58) << "Move circle " << circleCount
                 << " from " << beginPeg << " to " << endPeg << endl;
            cout << "From second:";
            DoTowers(circleCount - 1, auxPeg, beginPeg, endPeg);
        }
    }
```

The output from a run with three circles follows. "Original" means that the parameters listed beside it are from the nonrecursive call, which is the first call to DoTowers. "From first" means that the parameters listed are for a call issued from the first recursive statement. "From second" means that the parameters listed are for a call issued from the second recursive statement. Notice that a call cannot be issued from the second recursive statement until the preceding call from the first recursive statement has completed execution.

OUTPUT WITH 3 CIRCLES

CALLED FROM	#CIRCLES	BEGIN	AUXIL.	END	INSTRUCTIONS
Original :	3	1	2	3	
From first:	2	1	3	2	
From first:	1	1	2	3	
From first:	0	1	3	2	
					Move circle 1 from 1 to 3
From second:	0	2	1	3	
					Move circle 2 from 1 to 2
From second:	1	3	1	2	
From first:	0	3	2	1	
					Move circle 1 from 3 to 2
From second:	0	1	3	2	
					Move circle 3 from 1 to 3
From second:	2	2	1	3	
From first:	1	2	3	1	
From first:	0	2	1	3	
					Move circle 1 from 2 to 1
From second:	0	3	2	1	
					Move circle 2 from 2 to 3
From second:	1	1	2	3	
From first:	0	1	3	2	
					Move circle 1 from 1 to 3
From second:	0	2	1	3	

18.4 Recursive Algorithms with Structured Variables

In our definition of a recursive algorithm, we said there were two cases: the recursive or general case, and the base case for which an answer can be expressed nonrecursively. In the general case for all our algorithms so far, an argument was expressed in terms of a smaller value each time. When structured variables are used, the recursive case is often in terms of a smaller structure rather than a smaller value; the base case occurs when there are no values left to process in the structure.

We examine a recursive algorithm for printing the contents of a one-dimensional array of *n* elements to show what we mean.

Print Array

IF more elements
    Print the value of the first element
    Print array of n − 1 elements

The recursive case is to print the values in an array that is one element "smaller"; that is, the size of the array decreases by 1 with each recursive call. The base case is when the size of the array becomes 0—that is, when there are no more elements to print.

Our arguments must include the index of the first element (the one to be printed). How do we know when there are no more elements to print (that is, when the size of the array to be printed is 0)? We know we have printed the last element in the array when the index of the next element to be printed is beyond the index of the last element in the array. Therefore, the index of the last array element must be passed as an argument. We call the indexes `first` and `last`. When `first` is greater than `last`, we are finished. The name of the array is `data`.

```cpp
void Print( /* in */ const int data[],    // Array to be printed
            /* in */          int first,   // Index of first element
            /* in */          int last  )  // Index of last element
{
    if (first <= last)
    {                                                   // Recursive case
        cout << data[first] << endl;
        Print(data, first + 1, last);
    }
    // Empty else-clause is the base case
}
```

Here is a code walk-through of the function call

```
Print(data, 0, 4);
```

using the pictured array.

   Call 1: first is 0 and last is 4. Because first is less than last, the value in data[first] (which is 23) is printed. Execution of this call pauses while the array from first + 1 through last is printed.

   Call 2: first is 1 and last is 4. Because first is less than last, the value in data[first] (which is 44) is printed. Execution of this call pauses while the array from first + 1 through last is printed.

   Call 3: first is 2 and last is 4. Because first is less than last, the value in data[first] (which is 52) is printed. Execution of this call pauses while the array from first + 1 through last is printed.

   Call 4: first is 3 and last is 4. Because first is less than last, the value in data[first] (which is 61) is printed. Execution of this call pauses while the array from first + 1 through last is printed.

   Call 5: first is 4 and last is 4. Because first is equal to last, the value in data[first] (which is 77) is printed. Execution of this call pauses while the array from first + 1 through last is printed.

   Call 6: first is 5 and last is 4. Because first is greater than last, the execution of this call is complete. Control returns to the preceding call.

   Call 5: Execution of this call is complete. Control returns to the preceding call.

   Calls 4, 3, 2, and 1: Each execution is completed in turn, and control returns to the preceding call.

   Notice that once the deepest call (the call with the highest number) was reached, each of the calls before it returned without doing anything. When no statements are executed after the return from the recursive call to the function, the recursion is known as **tail recursion**. Tail recursion often indicates that the problem could be solved more easily using iteration. We used the array example because it made the recursive process easy to visualize; in practice, an array should be printed iteratively.

> **Tail recursion**   A recursive algorithm in which no statements are executed after the return from the recursive call.

   Figure 18–4 shows the execution of the Print function with the values of the parameters for each call. Notice that the array gets smaller with each recursive call (data[first] through data[last]). If we want to print the array elements in reverse order recursively, all we have to do is interchange the two statements within the If statement.

data
[0] 23
[1] 44
[2] 52
[3] 61
[4] 77

Print(data, 0, 4)

data, which is the array, is not shown in the boxes

Call 1:

```
                first
                  0
data[0]         last
is printed        4
```

Call 2:

```
                first
                  1
data[1]         last
is printed        4
```

Call 3:

```
                first
                  2
data[2]         last
is printed        4
```

Call 4:

```
                first
                  3
data[3]         last
is printed        4
```

Call 5:

```
                first
                  4
data[4]         last
is printed        4
```

Call 6:

```
                first
                  5
                last
                  4
```

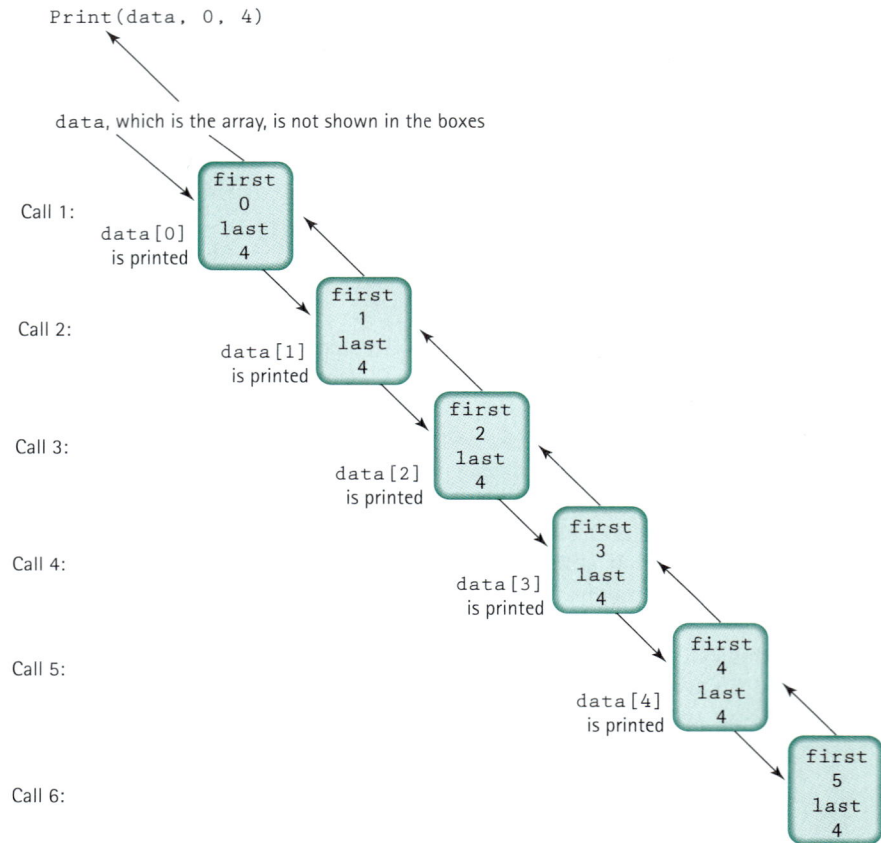

Figure 18–4   *Execution of* Print(data, 0, 4)

18.5 Recursion Using Pointer Variables

The previous recursive algorithm using a one-dimensional array could have been done much more easily using iteration. Now we look at two algorithms that cannot be done more easily with iteration: printing a linked list in reverse order and creating a duplicate copy of a linked list.

Printing a Dynamic Linked List in Reverse Order

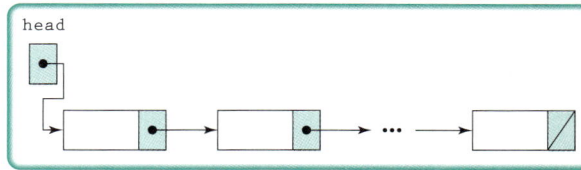

Printing a list in order from first to last is easy. We set a running pointer (ptr) equal to head and cycle through the list until ptr becomes NULL.

Print List (In: head)

```
Set ptr = head
WHILE ptr is not NULL
    Print ptr–>component
    Set ptr = ptr–>link
```

To print the list in reverse order, we must print the value in the last node first, then the value in the next-to-last node, and so on. Another way of expressing this is to say that we do not print a value until the values in all the nodes following it have been printed. We might visualize the process as the first node's turning to its neighbor and saying, "Tell me when you have printed your value. Then I'll print my value." The second node says to its neighbor, "Tell me when you have printed your value. Then I'll print mine." That node, in turn, says the same to its neighbor, and this continues until there is nothing to print.

Because the number of neighbors gets smaller and smaller, we seem to have the makings of a recursive solution. The end of the list is reached when the running pointer is NULL. When that happens, the last node can print its value and send the message back to the one before it. That node can then print its value and send the message back to the one before it, and so on.

RevPrint (In: head)

```
IF head is not NULL
    RevPrint rest of nodes in list
    Print current node in list
```

This algorithm can be coded directly as the following function:

```
void RevPrint( /* in */ NodePtr head )

// Precondition:
//      head points to a list node (or == NULL)
```

```
// Postcondition:
//      IF head != NULL
//          All nodes following *head have been output,
//          then *head has been output
//      ELSE
//          No action has taken place

{
    if (head != NULL)
    {
        RevPrint(head->link);                        // Recursive call
        cout << head->component << endl;
    }
    // Empty else-clause is the base case
}
```

This algorithm seems complex enough to warrant a code walk-through. We use the following list:

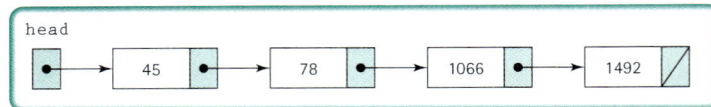

Call 1: head points to the node containing 45 and is not NULL. Execution of this call pauses until the recursive call with the argument head->link has been completed.

Call 2: head points to the node containing 78 and is not NULL. Execution of this call pauses until the recursive call with the argument head->link has been completed.

Call 3: head points to the node containing 1066 and is not NULL. Execution of this call pauses until the recursive call with the argument head->link has been completed.

Call 4: head points to the node containing 1492 and is not NULL. Execution of this call pauses until the recursive call with the argument head->link has been completed.

Call 5: head is NULL. Execution of this call is complete. Control returns to the preceding call.

Call 4: head->component (which is 1492) is printed. Execution of this call is complete. Control returns to the preceding call.

Call 3: head->component (which is 1066) is printed. Execution of this call is complete. Control returns to the preceding call.

Call 2: head->component (which is 78) is printed. Execution of this call is complete. Control returns to the preceding call.

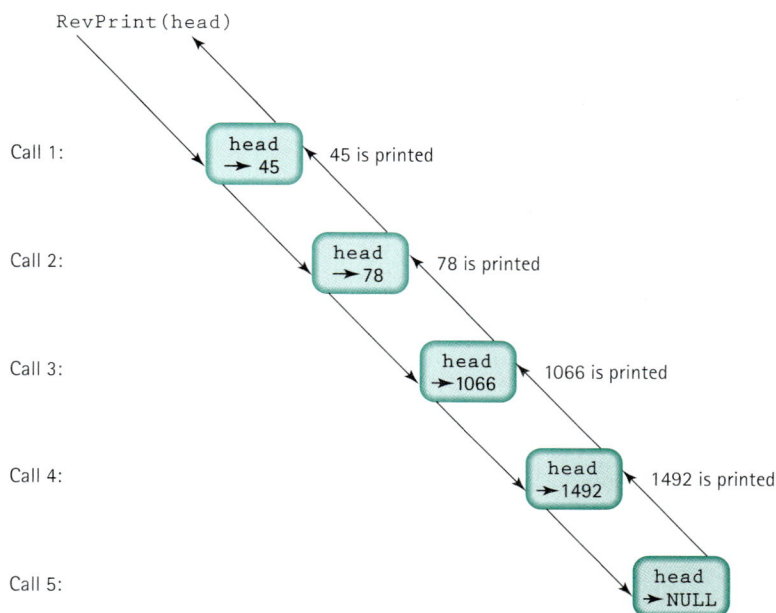

Figure 18-5   Execution of RevPrint(head)

Call 1: head->component (which is 45) is printed. Execution of this call is complete. Because this is the nonrecursive call, execution continues with the statement immediately following RevPrint(head).

Figure 18-5 shows the execution of the RevPrint function. The parameters are pointers (memory addresses), so we use → 45 to mean the pointer to the node whose component is 45.

Copying a Dynamic Linked List

When working with linked lists, we sometimes need to create a duplicate copy (a *clone*) of a linked list. For example, in Chapter 16, we wrote a copy-constructor for the Sort-edList2 class. This copy-constructor creates a new class object to be a clone of another class object, including its dynamic linked list.

Suppose that we want to write a value-returning function that receives the external pointer to a linked list (head), makes a clone of the linked list, and returns the external pointer to the new list as the function value. A typical call to the function would be the following:

```
NodePtr head;
NodePtr newListHead;
    ⋮
newListHead = PtrToClone(head);
```

Using iteration to copy a linked list is rather complicated. The following algorithm is essentially the same as the one used in the `SortedList2` copy-constructor.

PtrToClone (In: head)   // Iterative algorithm
    Out: Function value

```
IF head is NULL
    Return NULL

// Copy first node
Set fromPtr = head
Set cloneHead = new NodeType
Set cloneHead->component = fromPtr->component

// Copy remaining nodes
Set toPtr = cloneHead
Set fromPtr = fromPtr->link
WHILE fromPtr is not NULL
    Set toPtr->link = new NodeType
    Set toPtr = toPtr->link
    Set toPtr->component = fromPtr->component
    Set fromPtr = fromPtr->link
Set toPtr->link = NULL
Return cloneHead
```

A recursive solution to this problem is far simpler, but it requires us to think recursively. To clone the first node of the original list, we can allocate a new dynamic node and copy the component value from the original node into the new node. However, we cannot yet fill in the link member of the new node. We must wait until we have cloned the second node so that we can store its address into the link member of the first node. Likewise, the cloning of the second node cannot complete until we have finished cloning the third node. Eventually, we clone the last node of the original list and set the link member of the cloned node to NULL. At this point, the last node returns its own address to the next-to-last node, which stores the address into its link member. The next-to-last node returns its own address to the node before it, and so forth. The process completes when the first node returns its address to the first (nonrecursive) call, yielding an external pointer to the new linked list.

PtrToClone (In: fromPtr)   // Recursive algorithm
   Out: Function value

> IF fromPtr is NULL
>   Return NULL
> ELSE
>   Set toPtr = new NodeType
>   Set toPtr–>component = fromPtr–>component
>   Set toPtr–>link = PtrToClone(fromPtr–>link)
>   Return toPtr

Like the solution to the Towers of Hanoi problem, this looks too simple; yet, it is the algorithm. Because the argument that is passed to each recursive call is `fromPtr->link`, the number of nodes left in the original list gets smaller with each call. The base case occurs when the pointer into the original list becomes NULL. Below is the C++ function that implements the algorithm.

```cpp
NodePtr PtrToClone( /* in */ NodePtr fromPtr )

// Precondition:
//      fromPtr points to a list node (or == NULL)
// Postcondition:
//      IF fromPtr != NULL
//          A clone of the entire sublist starting with *fromPtr
//          is on the free store
//        && Function value == pointer to front of this sublist
//      ELSE
//          Return value == NULL

{
    NodePtr toPtr;       // Pointer to newly created node

    if (fromPtr == NULL)
        return NULL;                    // Base case
```

```
        else
        {                                           // Recursive case
            toPtr = new NodeType;
            toPtr->component = fromPtr->component;
            toPtr->link = PtrToClone(fromPtr->link);
            return toPtr;
        }
    }
```

Let's perform a code walk-through of the function call

```
newListHead = PtrToClone(head);
```

using the following list:

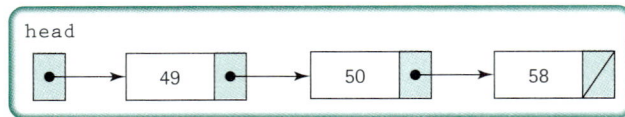

Call 1: `fromPtr` points to the node containing 49 and is not NULL. A new node is allocated and its `component` value is set to 49.

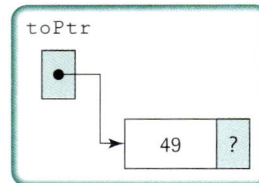

Execution of this call pauses until the recursive call with argument `fromPtr->link` has been completed.

Call 2: `fromPtr` points to the node containing 50 and is not NULL. A new node is allocated and its `component` value is set to 50.

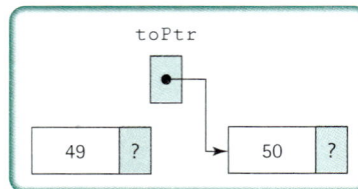

Execution of this call pauses until the recursive call with argument `fromPtr->link` has been completed.

Call 3: `fromPtr` points to the node containing 58 and is not NULL. A new node is allocated and its `component` value is set to 58.

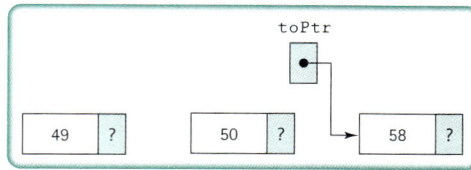

Execution of this call pauses until the recursive call with argument `fromPtr->link` has been completed.

Call 4: `fromPtr` is NULL. The list is unchanged.

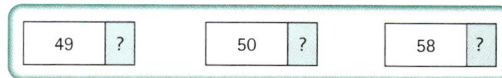

Execution of this call is complete. NULL is returned as the function value to the preceding call.

Call 3: Execution of this call resumes by assigning the returned function value (NULL) to `toPtr->link`.

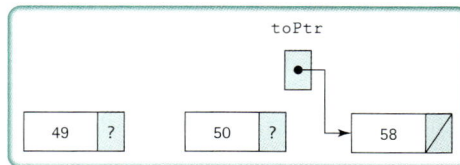

Execution of this call is complete. The value of `toPtr` is returned to the preceding call.

Call 2: Execution of this call resumes by assigning the returned function value (the address of the third node) to `toPtr->link`.

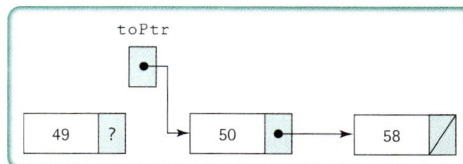

Execution of this call is complete. The value of `toPtr` is returned to the preceding call.

Call 1: Execution of this call resumes by assigning the returned function value (the address of the second node) to `toPtr->link`.

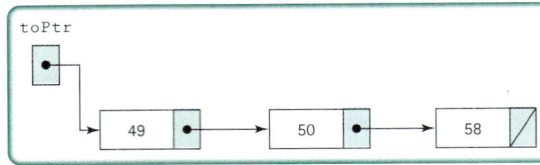

Execution of this call is complete. Because this is the nonrecursive call, the value of `toPtr` is returned to the assignment statement containing the original call. The variable `newListHead` now points to a clone of the original list.

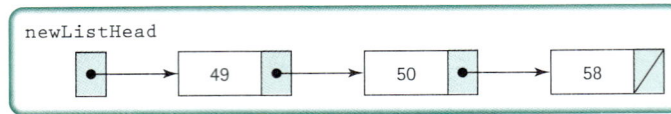

18.6 Recursion or Iteration?

Recursion and iteration are alternative ways of expressing repetition in a program. When iterative control structures are used, processes are made to repeat by embedding code in a looping structure such as a While, For, or Do-While. In recursion, a process is made to repeat by having a function call itself. A selection statement is used to control the repeated calls.

Which is better to use—recursion or iteration? There is no simple answer to this question. The choice usually depends on two issues: efficiency and the nature of the problem being solved.

Historically, the quest for efficiency, in terms of both execution speed and memory usage, has favored iteration over recursion. Each time a recursive call is made, the system must allocate stack space for all parameters and (automatic) local variables. The overhead involved in any function call is time-consuming. On early, slow computers with limited memory capacity, recursive algorithms were visibly—sometimes painfully—slower than the iterative versions. However, studies have shown that on modern, fast computers, the overhead of recursion is often so small that the increase in computation time is almost unnoticeable to the user. Except in cases where efficiency is absolutely critical, then, the choice between recursion and iteration more often depends on the second issue—the nature of the problem being solved.

Consider the factorial and power algorithms we discussed earlier in the chapter. In both cases, iterative solutions were obvious and easy to devise. We imposed recursive solutions on these problems only to demonstrate how recursion works. As a rule of thumb, if an iterative solution is more obvious or easier to understand, use it; it will be more efficient. However, there are problems for which the recursive solution is more obvious or easier to devise, such as the Towers of Hanoi problem. (It turns out that the Towers of Hanoi problem is surprisingly difficult to solve using iteration.) Computer science students should be aware of the power of recursion. If the definition of a problem is inherently recursive, then a recursive solution should certainly be considered.

Problem–Solving Case Study

QuickSort

PROBLEM   Throughout the last half of this book, we have worked with lists of items, both sorted and unsorted. At the logical level, sorting algorithms take an unsorted list and convert it into a sorted list. At the implementation level, sorting algorithms take an array and reorganize the data into some sort of order. We have used the straight selection algorithm to sort a list of numbers, and we have inserted entries into a list ordered by time. In this case study, we will create a function template that implements the Quicksort algorithm.

DISCUSSION   The Quicksort algorithm, developed by C. A. R. Hoare, is based on the idea that it is faster and easier to sort two small lists than one larger one. The name comes from the fact that, in general, quick sort can sort a list of data elements quite rapidly. The basic strategy of this sort is to divide and conquer.

If you were given a large stack of final exams to sort by name, you might use the following approach: Pick a splitting value, say L, and divide the stack of tests into two piles, A-L and M-Z. (Note that the two piles do not necessarily contain the same number of tests.) Then take the first pile and subdivide it into two piles, A-F and G-L. The A-F pile can be further broken down into A-C and D-F. This division process goes on until the piles are small enough to be easily sorted by hand. The same process is applied to the M-Z pile.

Eventually all the small sorted piles can be stacked one on top of the other to produce a sorted set of tests. (See Figure 18–6.)

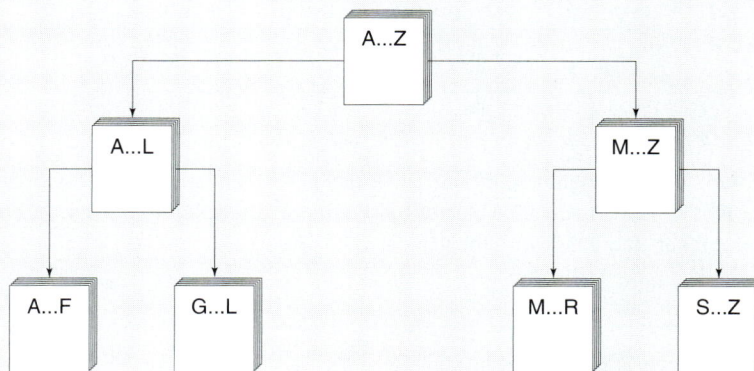

Figure 18–6   *Ordering a List Using the Quicksort Algorithm*

This strategy is based on recursion—on each attempt to sort the stack of tests the stack is divided and then the same approach is used to sort each of the smaller stacks (a smaller case). This process goes on until the small stacks do not need to be further divided (the base case). The parameter list of the Quicksort algorithm specifies the part of the list that is currently being processed. Be aware that we are sorting the list items *stored in the array,* not an abstract list about whose implementation we know nothing. To make this distinction clear, we call the array `data` rather than `list`.

Quicksort(In: first, last)

IF there is more than one item in data[first]..data[last]
Select splitVal
Split the data so that
    data[first]..data[splitPoint-1] <= splitVal
    data[splitPoint] = splitVal
    data[splitPoint+1]..data[last] > splitVal
Quicksort the left half
Quicksort the right half

How do we select splitVal? One simple solution is to use whatever value is in data[first] as the splitting value. Let's look at an example using data[first] as splitVal.

splitVal = 9

9	20	6	10	14	8	60	11
[first]							[last]

After the call to Split, all the items less than or equal to splitVal are on the left side of the data and all of those greater than splitVal are on the right side of the data.

smaller data			larger data				
9	8	6	10	14	20	60	11
[first]							[last]

The two "halves" meet at splitPoint, the index of the last item that is less than or equal to splitVal. Note that we don't know the value of splitPoint until the splitting process is complete. We can then swap splitVal (data[first]) with the value at data[split].

smaller data			larger data				
6	8	9	10	14	20	60	11
[first]		[splitPoint]					[last]

Our recursive calls to Quicksort use this index (splitPoint) to reduce the size of the problem in the general case.

Quicksort(first, splitPoint-1) sorts the left "half" of the data. Quicksort(splitPoint+1,last) sorts the right "half" of the data. (The "halves" are not necessarily the same size.) splitVal is already in its correct position in data[splitPoint].

What is the base case? When the segment being examined has only one item, we do not need to go on. So, "there is more than one item in data[first]..data[last]" translates into "if (first < last)". We can now code the function Quicksort.

```cpp
template<class ItemType>
void QuickSort(ItemType data[], int first, int last)

// Precondition:
//     ComparedTo has been defined on ItemType
// Postcondition:
//     data are sorted

{
    if (first < last)
    {
        int splitPoint;

        Split(data, first, last, splitPoint);
        // data[first]..data[splitPoint-1] <= splitVal
        // data[splitPoint] = splitVal
        // data[splitPoint+1]..data[last] > splitVal

        QuickSort(data, first, splitPoint-1);
        QuickSort(data, splitPoint+1, last);
    }
}
```

Now we must find a way to get all of the elements equal to or less than splitVal on one side of splitVal and the elements greater than splitVal on the other side. We do this by moving a pair of the indexes toward the middle of the data, looking for items that are on the wrong side of the split point. When we find pairs that are on the wrong side, we swap them and continue working our way into the middle of the data.

Figure 18–7a shows the initial state of the array to be sorted. We start out by moving first to the right, toward the middle, comparing data[first] to splitVal. If data[first] is less or equal to splitVal, we keep incrementing first; otherwise, we leave first where it is and begin moving last toward the middle. (See Figure 18–7b.)

Now data[last] is compared to splitVal. If it is greater, we continue decrementing last; otherwise we leave last in place (see Figure 18.7c). At this point it is clear that data[last] and data[first] are each on the wrong side of the array. Note that the elements to the left of data[first] and to the right of data[last] are not necessarily sorted; they are just on the correct side *with respect to splitVal*. To put data[first] and data[last] into their correct sides, we merely swap them, and then increment first and decrement last (see Figure 18–7d).

Now we repeat the whole cycle, incrementing first until we encounter a value that is greater than splitVal, and then decrementing last until we encounter a value that is less than or equal to splitVal (see Figure 18–7e).

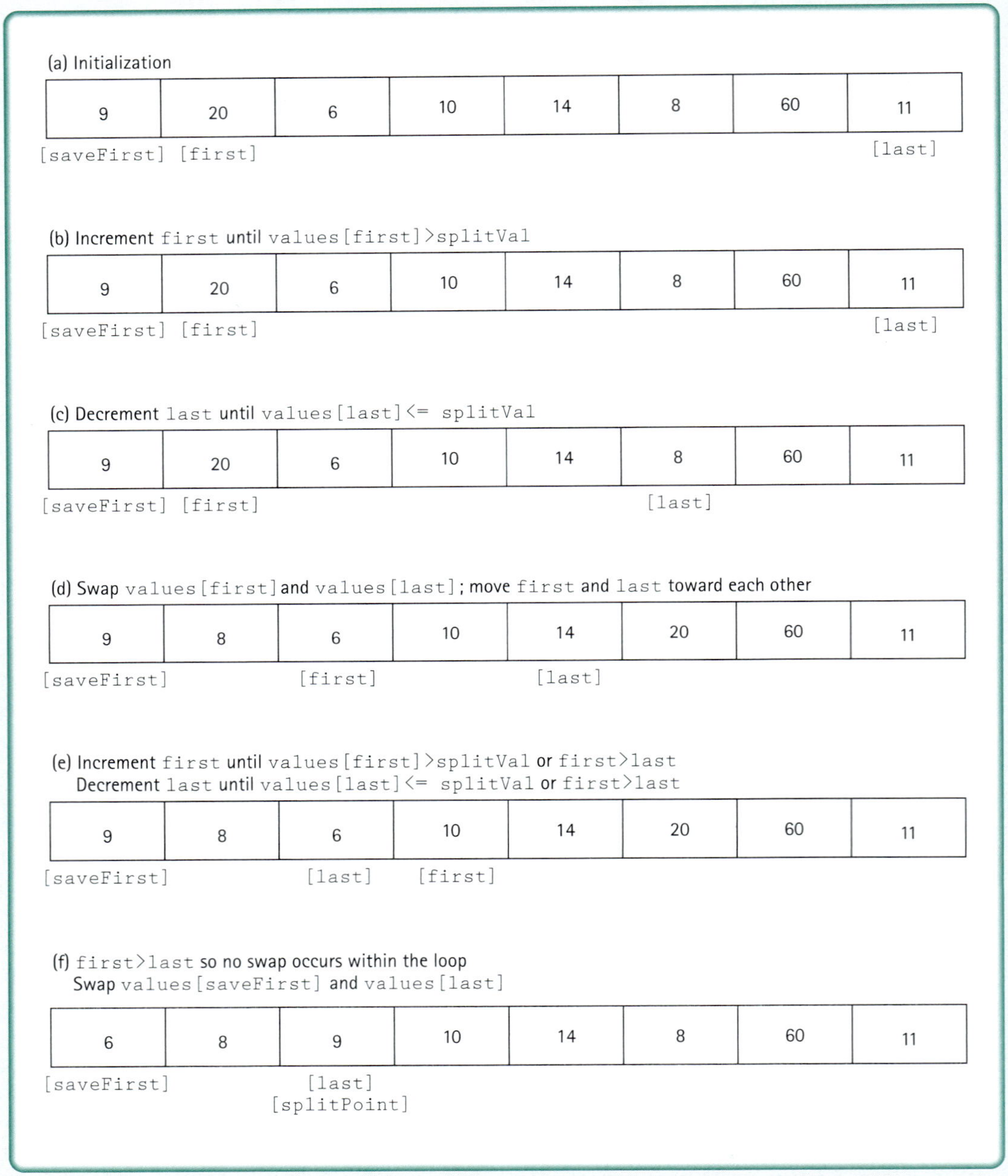

(a) Initialization

9	20	6	10	14	8	60	11

[saveFirst] [first] [last]

(b) Increment `first` **until** `values[first]>splitVal`

9	20	6	10	14	8	60	11

[saveFirst] [first] [last]

(c) Decrement `last` **until** `values[last]<= splitVal`

9	20	6	10	14	8	60	11

[saveFirst] [first] [last]

(d) Swap `values[first]` **and** `values[last]`; **move** `first` **and** `last` **toward each other**

9	8	6	10	14	20	60	11

[saveFirst] [first] [last]

(e) Increment `first` **until** `values[first]>splitVal` **or** `first>last`
Decrement `last` **until** `values[last]<= splitVal` **or** `first>last`

9	8	6	10	14	20	60	11

[saveFirst] [last] [first]

(f) `first>last` **so no swap occurs within the loop**
Swap `values[saveFirst]` **and** `values[last]`

6	8	9	10	14	8	60	11

[saveFirst] [last]
 [splitPoint]

Figure 18–7   *Function Split*

When does the process stop? When first and last meet each other, no further swaps are necessary. They meet at the splitPoint. This is the location where splitVal belongs, so we swap data[saveFirst], which contains splitVal, with the element at data[splitPoint] (Figure 18–7f). The index splitPoint is returned from the function, to be used by QuickSort to set up the next recursive call.

In order to make the Quicksort function template truly generic, let's assume that the items to be sorted can be compared with the ComparedTo function.

```
template<class ItemType>
void Swap(ItemType& item1, ItemType& item2)

// Postcondition:
//      item1 equals item2@entry AND item2 equals item1@entry

{
    ItemType tempItem;
    tempItem = item1;
    item1 = item2;
    item2 = tempItem;
}


template<class ItemType>
void Split(ItemType data[], int first, int last, int& splitPoint)
// Precondition:
//      ComparedTo has been defined on ItemType
// Postcondition:
//      All items greater than split value are to the left AND
//      all items less than or equal to split value are to the right
{
    ItemType splitVal = data[first];
    int saveFirst = first;
    bool onCorrectSide;

    first++;
    do
    {
        onCorrectSide = true;
        while (onCorrectSide)              // Move first toward last.
            switch (data[first].ComparedTo(splitVal))
            {
                case AFTER    : onCorrectSide = false;
                                break;
                case SAME     :
```

```
                    case BEFORE  : first++;
                                   onCorrectSide = (first <= last);
                                   break;
        }

    onCorrectSide = (first <= last);
    while (onCorrectSide)                // Move last toward first.
        switch (data[last].ComparedTo(splitVal))
        {
            case SAME     :
            case BEFORE   : onCorrectSide = false;
                            break;
            case AFTER    : last--;
                            onCorrectSide = (first <= last);
                            break;
        }

    if (first < last)
    {
        Swap(data[first], data[last]);
        first++;
        last--;
    }
    } while (first <= last);

    splitPoint = last;
    Swap(data[saveFirst], data[splitPoint]);
}
```

TESTING These three functions are placed in a single file and included into a driver to be tested. Class `Name` defines `ComparedTo`, so let's read in names, sort them, and print them. Here is the driver and the screen from the run.

```
//****************************************************************
//  Driver for the Quicksort algorithm.
//****************************************************************

#include <iostream>
#include <string>
#include "Name.h"
#include "Quicksort.h"
using namespace std;
```

```cpp
int main()
{
    Name data[15];
    Name name;

    // Read in 15 names
    for (int index = 0; index < 15; index++)
    {
        name.ReadName();
        data[index] = name;
    }

    // Sort 15 names
    Quicksort(data, 0, 14);

    // Print first and last name in sorted order
    for (int index = 0; index < 15; index++)
        cout << data[index].FirstName() << " "
             << data[index].LastName() << endl;

    return 0;
}
```

```
Enter first name: Sam
Enter middle name: S
Enter last name: Smith
Enter first name: Joe
Enter middle name: J
Enter last name: Jones
Enter first name: Bill
Enter middle name: B
Enter last name: Black
Enter first name: Jane
Enter middle name: J
Enter last name: Jones
Enter first name: Gray
Enter middle name: G
Enter last name: Green
Enter first name: Pansy
Enter middle name: P
Enter last name: Potter
Enter first name: Rose
Enter middle name: R
```

```
                    Enter last name: Red
                    Enter first name: Yellow
                    Enter middle name: Y
                    Enter last name: Yarn
                    Enter first name: Calvin
                    Enter middle name: C
                    Enter last name: Carson
                    Enter first name: Alfred
                    Enter middle name: A
                    Enter last name: Alred
                    Enter first name: Nell
                    Enter middle name: N
                    Enter last name: Night
                    Enter first name: Carol
                    Enter middle name: Carter
                    Enter last name: Carton
                    Enter first name: Zoe
                    Enter middle name: Z
                    Enter last name: Zebra
                    Enter first name: June
                    Enter middle name: May
                    Enter last name: July
                    Enter first name: Son
                    Enter middle name: S
                    Enter last name: Sunlight
Alfred Alred
Bill Black
Calvin Carson
Carol Carton
Gray Green
Jane Jones
Joe Jones
June July
Nell Night
Pansy Potter
Rose Red
Sam Smith
Son Sunlight
Yellow Yarn
Zoe Zebra
```

Testing and Debugging

Recursion is a powerful technique when used correctly. Improperly used, recursion can cause errors that are difficult to diagnose. The best way to debug a recursive algorithm is to construct it correctly in the first place. To be realistic, however, we give a few hints about where to look if an error occurs.

Testing and Debugging Hints

1. Be sure there is a base case. If there is no base case, the algorithm continues to issue recursive calls until all memory has been used. Each time the function is called, either recursively or nonrecursively, stack space is allocated for the parameters and automatic local variables. If there is no base case to end the recursive calls, the run-time stack eventually overflows. An error message such as "STACK OVERFLOW" indicates that the base case is missing.

2. Be sure you have not used a While structure. The basic structure in a recursive algorithm is the If statement. There must be at least two cases: the recursive case and the base case. If the base case does nothing, the else-clause is omitted. The selection structure, however, must be there. If a While statement is used in a recursive algorithm, the While statement usually should not contain a recursive call.

3. As with nonrecursive functions, do not reference global variables directly within a recursive function unless you have justification for doing so.

4. Parameters that relate to the size of the problem must be value parameters, not reference parameters. The arguments that relate to the size of the problem are usually expressions. Arbitrary expressions can be passed only to value parameters.

5. Use your system's debugger program (or use debug output statements) to trace a series of recursive calls. Inspecting the values of parameters and local variables often helps to locate errors in a recursive algorithm.

Summary

A recursive algorithm is expressed in terms of a smaller instance of itself. It must include a recursive case, for which the algorithm is expressed in terms of itself, and a base case, for which the algorithm is expressed in nonrecursive terms.

In many recursive problems, the smaller instance refers to a numeric argument that is being reduced with each call. In other problems, the smaller instance refers to the size of the data structure being manipulated. The base case is the one in which the size of the problem (value or structure) reaches a point for which an explicit answer is known.

In the example for finding the minimum using recursion, the size of the problem was the size of the array being searched. When the array size became 1, the solution was known. If there is only one array element, it is clearly the minimum (as well as the maximum).

In the Towers of Hanoi game, the size of the problem was the number of discs to be moved. When there was only one left on the beginning peg, it could be moved to its final destination.

Quick Check

1. Which case causes a recursive algorithm to end its recursion: the base case or the general case? (pp. 970–971)
2. In writing a recursive algorithm that computes the factorial of N, what would you use as the base case, and what would be the general case? (pp. 974–977)
3. In writing a recursive algorithm that outputs the values in an array, what would you use as the base case, and what would be the general case? (pp. 982–984)
4. In writing a recursive algorithm that outputs the values in linked list in reverse order, what would you use as the base case, and what would be the general case? (pp. 984–992)

Answers

1. The base case. 2. The base case would be that when N is zero, the result is one. The general case would be that when N is greater than zero, we multiply it by the product of the numbers from 1 to N-1, as returned from a recursive call. 3. The base case would be that if there are no elements remaining, we return. The general case would be that if there are elements remaining, we print the first one, then recurse to print the rest. 4. The base case would be that the link of the current node is NULL, and so we print it. The general case would be that if the link of the current node is not NULL, we print the remainder of the list before printing the current node.

Exam Preparation Exercises

1. Recursion is an alternative to:
   a. branching
   b. looping
   c. function invocation
   d. event handing
2. A recursive function can be void or value-returning? True or false?
3. When a function calls itself recursively, its parameters and local variables are saved on the run-time stack until it returns. True or false?
4. Tail recursion occurs when all of the processing happens at the end of the function, after the return from the recursive call. True or false?
5. Given the recursive formula $F(N) = F(N-2)$, with the base case $F(0) = 0$, what are the values of $F(4)$, $F(5)$, and $F(6)$? If any of the values are undefined, say so.
6. Given the recursive formula $F(N) = F(N - 1) * 2$, with the base case $F(0) = 1$, what are the values of $F(3)$, $F(4)$, and $F(5)$? If any of the values are undefined, say so.
7. What happens when a recursive function never encounters a base case?
8. What practical limitation prevents a function from calling itself recursively forever?

9. A tail-recursive function would be more efficiently implemented with a loop in most cases. True or false?

10. When you develop a recursive algorithm to operate on a simple variable, what does the general case typically make smaller with each recursive call?

   a. The data type of the variable
   b. The number of times the variable is referenced
   c. The value in the variable

10. When you develop a recursive algorithm to operate on a data structure, what does the general case typically make smaller with each recursive call?

   a. The number of elements in the structure
   b. The number of times the variable is referenced
   c. The distance to the end of the structure

12. Given the following input data:

```
10
20
30
```

what is output by the following program?

```cpp
#include <iostream>

using namespace std;

void Rev();

int main()
{
    Rev();
    return 0;
}

//********************

void Rev()
{
    int number;
    cin >> number;
    if (cin)
    {
        Rev();
        cout << number << endl;
    }
}
```

13. Repeat Exercise 12, replacing the Rev function with the following version.

```cpp
void Rev()
{
    int number;
    cin >> number;
    if (cin)
    {
        cout << number << endl;
        Rev();
        cout << number << endl;
    }
}
```

14. What is output by the following program?

```cpp
#include <iostream>

using namespace std;

void Rec(string word);

int main()
{
    Rec("abcde");
    return 0;
}

//********************

void Rec(string word)
{
    if (word.length() > 0)
    {
        cout << word.substr(0, 1);
        Rec(word.substr(1, word.length()-2));
        cout << word.substr(word.length()-1, 1) << endl;
    }
}
```

15. What does the program in Exercise 14 output if the initial call to Rec from main uses "abcdef" as the argument?

Programming Warm-Up Exercises

1. Write a value-returning recursive function that computes the sum of the digits in a given positive int argument. For example, if the argument is 12345, then the function returns 1 + 2 + 3 + 4 + 5 = 15.

2. Write a value-returning recursive function that uses the DigitSum function of Exercise 1 to compute the single digit to which the int argument's digits ultimately sum. For example, given the argument 999, the DigitSum would be 9 + 9 + 9 = 27, but the recursive digit sum would then be 2 + 7 = 9.

3. Write a recursive version of a binary search of a sorted array of int values that are in ascending order. The function's arguments should be the array, the search value, and the maximum and minimum indexes for the array. The function should return the index where the match is found, or else -1.

4. Write a recursive function that asks the user to enter a positive integer number each time it is called, until zero or a negative number is input. The function then outputs the numbers entered in reverse order. If the I/O dialog is the following:

```
Enter positive number, 0 to end: 10
Enter positive number, 0 to end: 20
Enter positive number, 0 to end: 30
Enter positive number, 0 to end: 0
```

the function outputs:

```
30
20
10
```

5. Extend the function of Exercise 4 so that it also outputs a running total of the numbers as they are entered. For example the I/O dialog might be the following:

```
Enter positive number, 0 to end: 10
Total: 10
Enter positive number, 0 to end: 20
Total: 30
Enter positive number, 0 to end: 30
Total: 60
Enter positive number, 0 to end: 0
```

and the function then outputs:

```
30
20
10
```

6. Extend the function of Exercise 5 so that it also outputs a running total as the numbers are printed out in reverse order. For example the I/O dialog might be the following:

```
Enter positive number, 0 to end: 10
Total: 10
Enter positive number, 0 to end: 20
Total: 30
Enter positive number, 0 to end: 30
Total: 60
Enter positive number, 0 to end: 0
```

and the function then outputs:

```
30 Total: 30
20 Total: 50
10 Total: 60
```

7. Extend the function of Exercise 4 so that it reports the greatest value entered, at the end of its output. If the I/O dialog is the following:

```
Enter positive number, 0 to end: 10
Enter positive number, 0 to end: 20
Enter positive number, 0 to end: 30
Enter positive number, 0 to end: 0
```

the function outputs:

```
30
20
10
The greatest is 30
```

8. Change the function of Exercise 7 so that it outputs the greatest number entered thus far, as the user is entering the data. For example, the I/O dialog might be the following:

```
Enter positive number, 0 to end: 10
Greatest: 10
Enter positive number, 0 to end: 30
Greatest: 30
Enter positive number, 0 to end: 20
Greatest: 30
Enter positive number, 0 to end: 0
```

and the function then outputs:

```
20
30
10
The greatest is 30
```

9. Change the function of Exercise 8 so that it also outputs the greatest number thus far, as it outputs the numbers in reverse order. For example, the I/O dialog might be the following:

```
Enter positive number, 0 to end: 10
Greatest: 10
Enter positive number, 0 to end: 30
Greatest: 30
Enter positive number, 0 to end: 20
Greatest: 30
Enter positive number, 0 to end: 0
```

and the function then outputs:

```
20 Greatest: 20
30 Greatest: 30
10 Greatest: 30
The greatest is 30
```

10. Given the following declarations:

```
struct NodeType;
typedef NodeType* PtrType;
struct NodeType
{
    int info;
    PtrType link;
};


PtrType head1;
PtrType head2;
```

Assume that the list pointed to by head1 contains an arbitrary number of nodes. Write a recursive function that makes a copy of this list in reverse order, which is pointed to by head2.

11. Given the declarations in Exercise 10, assume that the list pointed to by head1 contains an arbitrary number of nodes. Write a recursive function that makes a copy of this list in the same order, which is pointed to by head2.

12. Given the declarations in Exercise 10, assume that the list pointed to by head1 contains an arbitrary number of nodes. Write a recursive function that makes a single list containing two copies of the head1 list. The first copy will be in the same order and the second copy will be in reverse order. The new list is pointed to by head2.

Programming Problems

1. The greatest common divisor (GCD) of two positive integers is the largest integer that divides the numbers exactly. For example, the largest common factor of 14

and 21 is 7; for 13 and 22 it is 1; and for 45 and 27 it is 9. We can write a recursive formula for finding the GCD, given that the two numbers are called a and b, as:

GCD(a, b) = a, if b = 0
GCD(a, b) = LCF(b, a%b), if b > 0

Implement this recursive formula as a recursive C++ function, and write a driver program that allows you to test it interactively.

2. Write a C++ program to output the binary (base-2) representation of a decimal integer. The algorithm for this conversion is to repeatedly divide the decimal number by 2, until it is zero. Each division produces a remainder of 0 or 1, which becomes a digit in the binary number. For example, if we want the binary representation of decimal 13, we find it with the following series of divisions:

```
13/2 = 6     remainder 1
6/2 = 3      remainder 0
3/2 = 1      remainder 1
1/2 = 0      remainder 1
```

The binary representation of 13 is thus 1101. The only problem with this algorithm is that the first division generates the low-order binary digit, the next division generates the second-order digit, and so on, until the last division produces the high-order digit. Thus, if we output the digits as they are generated, they are in reverse order. You should use recursion to reverse the order of output.

3. Change the program for Problem 2 so that it works for any base up to 10. The user should enter the decimal number and the base, and the program outputs the number in the given base.

4. Write a C++ program using recursion to convert a number in binary (from 1 to 10) to a decimal number. The algorithm for this is that each successive digit in the number is multiplied by the base (two) raised to the power corresponding to its position in the number. The low-order digit is position 0. We sum together all of these products to get the decimal value. For example, if we have the binary number 111001, we convert it to decimal as follows:

$$1 * 2^0 = 1$$
$$0 * 2^1 = 0$$
$$0 * 2^2 = 0$$
$$1 * 2^3 = 8$$
$$1 * 2^4 = 16$$
$$1 * 2^5 = 32$$

Decimal value = 1 + 0 + 0 + 8 + 16 + 32 = 57

A recursive formulation of this can extract each digit and compute the corresponding power of the base by which to multiply. Once the base case (the last digit is extracted), the function can sum the products as it returns.

In C++ we can represent a binary number using integers. However, there is a danger—the user can enter an invalid number by typing a digit that's unrepresentable in the base. For example, the number 1011201 is an invalid binary number because 2 isn't allowed in the binary number system. Your program should check for invalid digits as they are extracted, and handle the error in a way that is appropriate (that is, it shouldn't output a numerical result), and provide an informative error message to the user.

5. Modify the program from Problem 4 to work for any number base in the range of 1 through 10. The user should enter a number and a base, and the program outputs the decimal equivalent. If the user enters a digit that is invalid for the base, the program should output an error message, and not display a numerical result.

6. A maze is to be represented by a 12 × 12 array composed of three values: Open, Wall, or Exit. There is one exit from the maze. Write a program to determine whether it is possible to exit the maze from each possible starting point (any open square can be a starting point). You may move vertically or horizontally to any adjacent open square. You may not move to a square containing a wall. The input consists of a series of 12 lines of 12 characters each, representing the contents of each square in the maze. The characters are O, W, or E. Your program should check that there is only one exit. As the data are entered, the program should make a list of all of the starting point coordinates. It can then run through this list, solving the maze for each starting point.

Case Study Follow-Up

1. What happens if the splitting value in the QuickSort is the largest or the smallest value in the segment? Explain.
2. What might be a better splitting value?
3. How could you use another splitting value without changing the algorithm?

Appendix A   Reserved Words

The following identifiers are *reserved words*—identifiers with predefined meanings in the C++ language. The programmer cannot declare them for other uses (for example, variable names) in a C++ program.

and	double	not	this
and_eq	dynamic_cast	not_eq	throw
asm	else	operator	true
auto	enum	or	try
bitand	explicit	or_eq	typedef
bitor	export	private	typeid
bool	extern	protected	typename
break	false	public	union
case	float	register	unsigned
catch	for	reinterpret_cast	using
char	friend	return	virtual
class	goto	short	void
compl	if	signed	volatile
const	inline	sizeof	wchar_t
const_cast	int	static	while
continue	long	static_cast	xor
default	mutable	struct	xor_eq
delete	namespace	switch	
do	new	template	

Appendix B   Operator Precedence

The following table summarizes C++ operator precedence. Several operators are not discussed in this book (typeid, the comma operator, ->*, and .*, for instance). For information on these operators, see Stroustrup's *The C++ Programming Language,* Third Edition (Addison-Wesley, 1997).

In the table, the operators are grouped by precedence level (highest to lowest), and a horizontal line separates each precedence level from the next-lower level.

In general, the binary operators group from left to right; the unary operators, from right to left; and the ?: operator, from right to left. Exception: The assignment operators group from right to left.

Precedence (highest to lowest)

Operator	Associativity	Remarks
`::`	Left to right	Scope resolution (binary)
`::`	Right to left	Global access (unary)
`()`	Left to right	Function call and function-style cast
`[]` `->` `.`	Left to right	
`++` `--`	Right to left	++ and - - as postfix operators
`typeid` `dynamic_cast`	Right to left	
`static_cast` `const_cast`	Right to left	
`reinterpret_cast`	Right to left	
`++` `--` `!` Unary `+` Unary `-`	Right to left	++ and - - as prefix operators
`~` Unary `*` Unary `&`	Right to left	
`(cast)` `sizeof` `new` `delete`	Right to left	
`->*` `.*`	Left to right	
`*` `/` `%`	Left to right	
`+` `-`	Left to right	
`<<` `>>`	Left to right	
`<` `<=` `>` `>=`	Left to right	
`==` `!=`	Left to right	
`&`	Left to right	
`^`	Left to right	
`|`	Left to right	
`&&`	Left to right	
`||`	Left to right	
`?:`	Right to left	
`=` `+=` `-=` `*=` `/=` `%=`	Right to left	
`<<=` `>>=` `&=` `|=` `^=`	Right to left	
`throw`	Right to left	
`,`	Left to right	The sequencing operator, not the separator

Appendix C   A Selection of Standard Library Routines

The C++ standard library provides a wealth of data types, functions, and named constants. This appendix details only some of the more widely used library facilities. It is a good idea to consult the manual for your particular system to see what other types, functions, and constants the standard library provides.

This appendix is organized alphabetically according to the header file your program must #include before accessing the listed items. For example, to use a mathematics routine such as sqrt, you would #include the header file cmath as follows:

```
#include <cmath>
using namespace std;
  ⋮
y = sqrt(x);
```

Note that every identifier in the standard library is defined to be in the namespace std. Without the using directive above, you would write

```
y = std::sqrt(x);
```

C.1   The Header File cassert

assert(booleanExpr)
Argument: A logical (Boolean) expression
Effect: If the value of booleanExpr is true, execution of the program simply continues. If the value of booleanExpr is false, execution terminates immediately with a message stating the Boolean expression, the name of the file containing the source code, and the line number in the source code.
Function return value: None (a void function)
Note: If the preprocessor directive #define NDEBUG is placed before the directive #include <cassert>, all assert statements are ignored.

C.2   The Header File cctype

isalnum(ch)
Argument: A char value ch
Function return value: An int value that is
- nonzero (true), if ch is a letter or a digit character ('A'–'Z', 'a'–'z', '0'–'9')
- 0 (false), otherwise

`isalpha(ch)`
Argument: A `char` value `ch`
Function return value: An `int` value that is
- nonzero (`true`), if `ch` is a letter ('A'-'Z', 'a'-'z')
- 0 (`false`), otherwise

`iscntrl(ch)`
Argument: A `char` value `ch`
Function return value: An `int` value that is
- nonzero (`true`), if `ch` is a control character (in ASCII, a character with the value 0–31 or 127)
- 0 (`false`), otherwise

`isdigit(ch)`
Argument: A `char` value `ch`
Function return value: An `int` value that is
- nonzero (`true`), if `ch` is a digit character ('0'-'9')
- 0 (`false`), otherwise

`isgraph(ch)`
Argument: A `char` value `ch`
Function return value: An `int` value that is
- nonzero (`true`), if `ch` is a nonblank printable character (in ASCII, '!' through '~')
- 0 (`false`), otherwise

`islower(ch)`
Argument: A `char` value `ch`
Function return value: An `int` value that is
- nonzero (`true`), if `ch` is a lowercase letter ('a'-'z')
- 0 (`false`), otherwise

`isprint(ch)`
Argument: A `char` value `ch`
Function return value: An `int` value that is
- nonzero (`true`), if `ch` is a printable character, including the blank (in ASCII, ' ' through '~')
- 0 (`false`), otherwise

`ispunct(ch)`
Argument: A `char` value `ch`
Function return value: An `int` value that is
- nonzero (`true`), if `ch` is a punctuation character (equivalent to `isgraph(ch) && !isalnum(ch)`)
- 0 (`false`), otherwise

`isspace(ch)`
Argument: A `char` value `ch`
Function return value: An `int` value that is
- nonzero (`true`), if `ch` is a whitespace character (blank, newline, tab, carriage return, form feed)
- 0 (`false`), otherwise

`isupper(ch)`
Argument: A `char` value `ch`
Function return value: An `int` value that is
- nonzero (`true`), if `ch` is an uppercase letter ('A'–'Z')
- 0 (`false`), otherwise

`isxdigit(ch)`
Argument: A `char` value `ch`
Function return value: An `int` value that is
- nonzero (`true`), if `ch` is a hexadecimal digit ('0'–'9', 'A'–'F', 'a'–'f')
- 0 (`false`), otherwise

`tolower(ch)`
Argument: A `char` value `ch`
Function return value: A character that is
- the lowercase equivalent of `ch`, if `ch` is an uppercase letter
- `ch`, otherwise

`toupper(ch)`
Argument: A `char` value `ch`
Function return value: A character that is
- the uppercase equivalent of `ch`, if `ch` is a lowercase letter
- `ch`, otherwise

C.3 The Header File `cfloat`

This header file supplies named constants that define the characteristics of floating-point numbers on your particular machine. Among these constants are the following:

`FLT_DIG`   Approximate number of significant digits in a `float` value on your machine
`FLT_MAX`   Maximum positive `float` value on your machine
`FLT_MIN`   Minimum positive `float` value on your machine
`DBL_DIG`   Approximate number of significant digits in a `double` value on your machine
`DBL_MAX`   Maximum positive `double` value on your machine
`DBL_MIN`   Minimum positive `double` value on your machine

LDBL_DIG	Approximate number of significant digits in a `long double` value on your machine
LDBL_MAX	Maximum positive `long double` value on your machine
LDBL_MIN	Minimum positive `long double` value on your machine

C.4   The Header File `climits`

This header file supplies named constants that define the limits of integer values on your particular machine. Among these constants are the following:

CHAR_BITS	Number of bits in a byte on your machine (8, for example)
CHAR_MAX	Maximum `char` value on your machine
CHAR_MIN	Minimum `char` value on your machine
SHRT_MAX	Maximum `short` value on your machine
SHRT_MIN	Minimum `short` value on your machine
INT_MAX	Maximum `int` value on your machine
INT_MIN	Minimum `int` value on your machine
LONG_MAX	Maximum `long` value on your machine
LONG_MIN	Minimum `long` value on your machine
UCHAR_MAX	Maximum `unsigned char` value on your machine
USHRT_MAX	Maximum `unsigned short` value on your machine
UINT_MAX	Maximum `unsigned int` value on your machine
ULONG_MAX	Maximum `unsigned long` value on your machine

C.5   The Header File `cmath`

In the `math` routines listed below, the following notes apply.

1. Error handling for incalculable or out-of-range results is system dependent.
2. All arguments and function return values are technically of type `double` (double-precision floating-point). However, single-precision (`float`) values may be passed to the functions.

`acos(x)`
Argument: A floating-point expression x, where $-1.0 \le x \le 1.0$
Function return value: Arc cosine of x, in the range 0.0 through π

`asin(x)`
Argument: A floating-point expression x, where $-1.0 \le x \le 1.0$
Function return value: Arc sine of x, in the range $-\pi/2$ through $\pi/2$

`atan(x)`
Argument: A floating-point expression x
Function return value: Arc tangent of x, in the range $-\pi/2$ through $\pi/2$

`ceil(x)`
   Argument: A floating-point expression x
   Function return value: "Ceiling" of x (the smallest whole number $\geq$ x)

`cos(angle)`
   Argument: A floating-point expression `angle`, measured in radians
   Function return value: Trigonometric cosine of `angle`

`cosh(x)`
   Argument: A floating-point expression x
   Function return value: Hyperbolic cosine of x

`exp(x)`
   Argument: A floating-point expression x
   Function return value: The value e(2.718...) raised to the power x

`fabs(x)`
   Argument: A floating-point expression x
   Function return value: Absolute value of x

`floor(x)`
   Argument: A floating-point expression x
   Function return value: "Floor" of x (the largest whole number $\leq$ x)

`log(x)`
   Argument: A floating-point expression x, where x > 0.0
   Function return value: Natural logarithm (base e) of x

`log10(x)`
   Argument: A floating-point expression x, where x > 0.0
   Function return value: Common logarithm (base 10) of x

`pow(x, y)`
   Arguments: Floating-point expressions x and y. If x = 0.0, y must be positive; if x $\leq$ 0.0, y must be a whole number
   Function return value: x raised to the power y

`sin(angle)`
   Argument: A floating-point expression `angle`, measured in radians
   Function return value: Trigonometric sine of `angle`

`sinh(x)`
   Argument: A floating-point expression x
   Function return value: Hyperbolic sine of x

```
sqrt(x)
```
Argument: A floating-point expression x, where x ≥ 0.0
Function return value: Square root of x

```
tan(angle)
```
Argument: A floating-point expression `angle`, measured in radians
Function return value: Trigonometric tangent of `angle`

```
tanh(x)
```
Argument: A floating-point expression x
Function return value: Hyperbolic tangent of x

C.6 The Header File `cstddef`

This header file defines a few system-dependent constants and data types. From this header file, the only item we use in this book is the following symbolic constant:

NULL   The null pointer constant 0

C.7 The Header File `cstdlib`

```
abs(i)
```
Argument: An `int` expression i
Function return value: An `int` value that is the absolute value of i

```
atof(str)
```
Argument: A C string (null-terminated `char` array) `str` representing a floating point number, possibly preceded by whitespace characters and a '+' or '−'
Function return value: A `double` value that is the floating-point equivalent of the characters in `str`
Note: Conversion stops at the first character in `str` that is inappropriate for a floating-point number. If no appropriate characters were found, the return value is system dependent.

```
atoi(str)
```
Argument: A C string (null-terminated `char` array) `str` representing an integer number, possibly preceded by whitespace characters and a '+' or '−'
Function return value: An `int` value that is the integer equivalent of the characters in `str`

Note:	Conversion stops at the first character in `str` that is inappropriate for an integer number. If no appropriate characters were found, the return value is system dependent.

`atol(str)`

Argument:	A C string (null-terminated `char` array) `str` representing a long integer, possibly preceded by whitespace characters and a '+' or '–'
Function return value:	A `long` value that is the long integer equivalent of the characters in `str`
Note:	Conversion stops at the first character in `str` that is inappropriate for a `long` integer number. If no appropriate characters were found, the return value is system dependent.

`exit(exitStatus)`

Argument:	An `int` expression `exitStatus`
Effect:	Program execution terminates immediately with all files properly closed
Function return value:	None (a void function)
Note:	By convention, `exitStatus` is 0 to indicate normal program completion and is nonzero to indicate an abnormal termination.

`labs(i)`

Argument:	A `long` expression `i`
Function return value:	A `long` value that is the absolute value of `i`

`rand()`

Argument:	None
Function return value:	A random `int` value in the range 0 through RAND_MAX, a constant defined in `cstdlib` (RAND_MAX is usually the same as INT_MAX)
Note:	See `srand` below.

`srand(seed)`

Argument:	An `int` expression `seed`, where `seed` ≥ 0
Effect:	Using `seed`, the random number generator is initialized in preparation for subsequent calls to the `rand` function.
Function return value:	None (a void function)
Note:	If `srand` is not called before the first call to `rand`, a seed value of 1 is assumed.

`system(str)`

Argument:	A C string (null-terminated `char` array) `str` representing an operating system command, exactly as it would be typed by a user on the operating system command line
Effect:	The operating system command represented by `str` is executed.
Function return value:	An `int` value that is system dependent
Note:	Programmers often ignore the function return value, using the syntax of a void function call rather than a value-returning function call.

C.8   The Header File `cstring`

The header file `cstring` (not to be confused with the header file named `string`) supports manipulation of C strings (null-terminated `char` arrays).

`strcat(toStr, fromStr)`

Arguments:	C strings (null-terminated `char` arrays) `toStr` and `fromStr`, where `toStr` must be large enough to hold the result
Effect:	`fromStr`, including the null character '\0', is concatenated (joined) to the end of `toStr`.
Function return value:	The base address of `toStr`
Note:	Programmers usually ignore the function return value, using the syntax of a void function call rather than a value-returning function call.

`strcmp(str1, str2)`

Arguments:	C strings (null-terminated `char` arrays) `str1` and `str2`
Function return value:	An `int` value < 0, if `str1` < `str2` lexicographically
	The `int` value 0, if `str1` = `str2` lexicographically
	An `int` value > 0, if `str1` > `str2` lexicographically

`strcpy(toStr, fromStr)`

Arguments:	`toStr` is a `char` array and `fromStr` is a C string (null-terminated `char` array), and `toStr` must be large enough to hold the result
Effect:	`fromStr`, including the null character '\0', is copied to `toStr`, overwriting what was there.
Function return value:	The base address of `toStr`
Note:	Programmers usually ignore the function return value, using the syntax of a void function call rather than a value-returning function call.

`strlen(str)`

Argument: A C string (null-terminated `char` array) `str`

Function return value: An `int` value ≥ 0 that is the length of `str` (excluding the '\0')

C.9   The Header File `string`

This header file supplies a programmer-defined data type (specifically, a *class*) named `string`. Associated with the `string` type are a data type `string::size_type` and a named constant `string::npos`, defined as follows:

`string::size_type`   An unsigned integer type related to the number of characters in a string

`string::npos`   The maximum value of type `string::size_type`

There are dozens of functions associated with the `string` type. Below are several of the most important ones. In the descriptions, `s` is assumed to be a variable (an *object*) of type `string`.

`s.c_str()`

Arguments: None

Function return value: The base address of a C string (null-terminated `char` array) corresponding to the characters stored in `s`

`s.find(arg)`

Argument: An expression of type `string` or `char`, or a C string (such as a literal string)

Function return value: A value of type `string::size_type` that gives the starting position in `s` where `arg` was found. If `arg` was not found, the return value is `string::npos`.

Note: Positions of characters within a string are numbered starting at 0.

`getline(inStream, s)`

Arguments: An input stream `inStream` (of type `istream` or `ifstream`) and a `string` object `s`

Effect: Characters are input from `inStream` and stored into `s` until the newline character is encountered. (The newline character is consumed but not stored into s.)

Function return value: Although the function technically returns a value (which we do not discuss here), programmers usually invoke the function as though it were a void function.

`s.length()`
    Arguments: None
    Function return value: A value of type `string::size_type` that gives the number of characters in the string

`s.size()`
    Arguments: None
    Function return value: The same as `s.length()`

`s.substr(pos, len)`
    Arguments: Two unsigned integers, `pos` and `len`, representing a position and a length. The value of `pos` must be less than `s.length()`.
    Function return value: A temporary `string` object that holds a substring of at most `len` characters, starting at position `pos` of s. If `len` is too large, it means "to the end" of the string in s.
    Note: Positions of characters within a string are numbered starting at 0.

C.10   The Header File `sstream`

This header file supplies various classes derived from `iostream` that enable the user to apply stream-like operations to strings instead of files. In this text, we use only the `ostringstream` class, which enables us to convert numeric types to formatted string values. We can apply the insertion operator (`<<`) to an `ostringstream` object to append values to it, and then read back its contents in string form, using the `str` member function. In the following, `oss` is an `ostringstream` object.

`ostringstream()`
    Argument: None
    Return value: An empty `osstringstream` object

`ostringstream(arg)`
    Argument: A string
    Return value: An `ostringstream` object initialized to the argument string

`<<`
    Left argument: An `ostringstream` object
    Right argument: An expression that can be converted to a string, including output manipulators.
    Return value: An `ostringstream` object
    Evaluated: Left to right

```
oss.str()
```
   Argument: None
   Return value: A string containing whatever has been appended to `oss`

```
oss.str(arg)
```
   Argument: A string
   Effect: Assigns the value of the argument to `oss`. Using the empty string as the argument effectively sets the content of the `ostringstream` object to be empty.

Appendix D   Using This Book with a Prestandard Version of C++

D.1   The `string` Type

Prior to the ISO/ANSI C++ language standard, the standard library did not provide a `string` data type. Compiler vendors often supplied their own programmer-defined types with names like `String`, `StringType`, and so on. The syntax and semantics of string operations often varied from vendor to vendor.

For readers with prestandard compilers, the authors of this book have created a data type named `StrType` that mimics a subset of the standard `string` type. The subset is sufficient to match the string operations displayed throughout this book.

The files related to `StrType` are available for download from the publisher's Web site (www.jbpub.com). Among the files is one called `README.TXT`, which explains how to compile the source code and link it with the programs you write. Another file is the header file `strtype.h`, which contains important declarations that define the `StrType` type. Programs that use `StrType` must #include this header file:

```
#include "strtype.h"
```

In the #include directive, you cannot place the file name in angle brackets (< >), which tell the preprocessor to look for the file in the standard include directory. Instead, you enclose the file name in double quotes (" "). The double quotes tell the preprocessor to look for the file in the programmer's current directory. Therefore, to use `StrType` in your program, you must (a) verify that the file `strtype.h` is in the directory in which you are currently working on your program, and (b) make sure your program uses the directive

```
#include "strtype.h"
```

Additional directions are given in `README.TXT`.

Throughout this book you can use `StrType` instead of the `string` data type as follows. First, in your variable declarations, substitute the word `StrType` for `string` as the name of the data type. Second, change the directive `#include <string>` to `#include "strtype.h"`. For example, instead of

```
#include <string>
      ⋮
string lastName;
```

you would write

```
#include "strtype.h"
      ⋮
StrType lastName;
```

Finally, there is a restriction on performing input into `StrType` variables. Chapter 4 discusses the use of the `>>` operator and the `getline` function to input characters into a `string` variable. Using `>>` with `StrType` variables, at most 1023 characters can be read and stored into one variable. In practice, however, this isn't much of a restriction. It would be extremely rare for an input string to consist of that many characters. Input using `getline` is also restricted to 1023 characters. In the function call

```
getline(cin, myString);
```

in which `myString` is a `StrType` variable, the `getline` function does not skip leading white-space characters and continues until it either has read 1023 characters or it reaches the newline character '\n', whichever comes first. That is, `getline` reads and stores an entire input line (to a maximum of 1023 characters), embedded blanks and all. Note that for an input line of 1023 characters or less, the newline character *is* consumed (but is not stored into `myString`).

D.2   Standard Header Files and Namespaces

Historically, the standard header files in both C and C++ had file names ending in `.h` (meaning "header file"). Certain header files—for example, `iostream.h`, `iomanip.h`, and `fstream.h`—related specifically to C++. Others, such as `math.h`, `stddef.h`, `stdlib.h`, and `string.h`, were carried over from the C standard library and were available to both C and C++ programs. When you used an `#include` directive such as

```
#include <math.h>
```

near the beginning of your program, all identifiers declared in `math.h` were introduced into your program in global scope (as discussed in Chapter 8). With the advent of the *namespace* mechanism in ISO/ANSI standard C++ (see Chapter 2 and, in more detail, Chapter 8), all of the standard header files were modified so that identifiers are declared within a namespace called std. In standard C++, when you #include a standard header file, the identifiers therein are not automatically placed into global scope.

To preserve compatibility with older versions of C++ that still need the original files iostream.h, math.h, and so forth, the new standard header files are renamed as follows: The C++-related header files have the .h removed, and the header files from the C library have the .h removed *and* the letter *c* inserted at the beginning. Here is a list of the old and new names for some of the most commonly used header files.

Old Name	New Name
iostream.h	iostream
iomanip.h	iomanip
fstream.h	fstream
assert.h	cassert
ctype.h	cctype
float.h	cfloat
limits.h	climits
math.h	cmath
stddef.h	cstddef
stdlib.h	cstdlib
string.h	cstring

Be careful: The last entry in the list above refers to the C language concept of a string and is unrelated to the string type defined in the C++ standard library.

If you are working with a prestandard compiler that does not recognize the new header file names or namespaces, simply substitute the old header file names for the new ones as you encounter them in the book. For example, where we have written

```
#include <iostream>
using namespace std;
```

you would write

```
#include <iostream.h>
```

For compatibility, C++ systems are likely to retain both versions of the header files for some time to come.

D.3 The `fixed` and `showpoint` Manipulators

Chapter 3 introduces five manipulators for formatting the output: `endl`, `setw`, `fixed`, `showpoint`, and `setprecision`. If you are using a prestandard compiler with the header file `iostream.h`, the `fixed` and `showpoint` manipulators may not be available.

In place of the following code shown in Chapter 3,

```
#include <iostream>
using namespace std;
  ⋮
cout << fixed << showpoint;        // Set up floating-pt.
                                   //    output format
```

you can substitute the following code:

```
#include <iostream.h>
  ⋮
cout.setf(ios::fixed, ios::floatfield);
cout.setf(ios::showpoint);
```

These two statements employ some advanced C++ notation. Our advice is simply to use the statements just as you see them and not worry about the details. Here's the general idea. `setf` is a void function associated with the `cout` stream. (Note that the dot, or period, between `cout` and `setf` is required.) The first function call ensures that floating-point numbers are always printed in decimal form rather than scientific notation. The second function call specifies that the decimal point should always be printed, even for whole numbers. In other words, these two function calls accomplish the same effect as the `fixed` and `showpoint` manipulators.

Note: If your compiler complains about the syntax `ios::fixed`, `ios::floatfield`, or `ios::showpoint`, you may have to replace `ios` with `ios_base` as follows:

```
cout.setf(ios_base::fixed, ios_base::floatfield);
cout.setf(ios_base::showpoint);
```

D.4 The `bool` Type

Before the ISO/ANSI C++ language standard, C++ did not have a `bool` data type. Some prestandard compilers implemented the `bool` type before the standard was approved, but others did not. If your compiler does not recognize the `bool` type, the following discussion will assist you in writing programs that are compatible with those in this book.

In versions of C++ without the `bool` type, the value 0 represents *false*, and any nonzero value represents *true*. It is customary in pre–standard C++ to use the `int` type to represent Boolean data:

```
int dataOK;
   ⋮
dataOK = 1;   // Store "true" into dataOK
   ⋮
dataOK = 0;   // Store "false" into dataOK
```

To make the code more self-documenting, many pre–standard C++ programmers define their own Boolean data type by using a *Typedef statement*. This statement allows you to introduce a new name for an existing data type:

```
typedef int bool;
```

All this statement does is tell the compiler to substitute the word `int` for every occurrence of the word `bool` in the rest of the program. Thus, when the compiler encounters a statement such as

```
bool dataOK;
```

it translates the statement into

```
int dataOK;
```

With the Typedef statement and declarations of two named constants, `true` and `false`, the code at the beginning of this discussion becomes the following:

```
typedef int bool;
const int true = 1;
const int false = 0;
   ⋮
bool dataOK;
   ⋮
dataOK = true;
   ⋮
dataOK = false;
```

Throughout the book, our programs use the words `bool`, `true`, and `false` when manipulating Boolean data. If your compiler recognizes `bool` as a built-in type, there is nothing you need to do. Otherwise, here are three steps you can take.

1. Use your system's editor to create a file containing the following lines:

```
#ifndef BOOL_H
#define BOOL_H
typedef int bool;
const int true = 1;
const int false = 0;
#endif
```

   Don't worry about the meaning of the first, second, and last lines. They are explained in Chapter 14. Simply type the lines as you see them above.

2. Save the file you created in step 1, giving it the name `bool.h`. Save this file into the same directory in which you work on your C++ programs.

3. Near the top of every program in which you need `bool` variables, type the line

```
#include "bool.h"
```

   Be sure to surround the file name with double quotes, not angle brackets (< >). The quotes tell the preprocessor to look for `bool.h` in your current directory rather than the C++ system directory.

   With `bool`, `true`, and `false` defined in this fashion, the programs in this book run correctly, and you can use `bool` in your own programs, even if it is not a built-in type.

Appendix E   Character Sets

The following charts show the ordering of characters in two widely used character sets: ASCII (American Standard Code for Information Interchange) and EBCDIC (Extended Binary Coded Decimal Interchange Code). The internal representation for each character is shown in decimal. For example, the letter *A* is represented internally as the integer 65 in ASCII and as 193 in EBCDIC. The space (blank) character is denoted by a "□".

Left Digit(s)	Right Digit	ASCII									
		0	*1*	*2*	*3*	*4*	*5*	*6*	*7*	*8*	*9*
0		NUL	SOH	STX	ETX	EOT	ENQ	ACK	BEL	BS	HT
1		LF	VT	FF	CR	SO	SI	DLE	DC1	DC2	DC3
2		DC4	NAK	SYN	ETB	CAN	EM	SUB	ESC	FS	GS
3		RS	US	□	!	"	#	$	%	&	'
4		(	)	*	+	,	−	.	/	0	1
5		2	3	4	5	6	7	8	9	:	;
6		<	=	>	?	@	A	B	C	D	E
7		F	G	H	I	J	K	L	M	N	O
8		P	Q	R	S	T	U	V	W	X	Y
9		Z	[	\	]	^	_	`	a	b	c
10		d	e	f	g	h	i	j	k	l	m
11		n	o	p	q	r	s	t	u	v	w
12		x	y	z	{	|	}	~	DEL		

Codes 00–31 and 127 are the following nonprintable control characters:

NUL	Null character	VT	Vertical tab	SYN	Synchronous idle
SOH	Start of header	FF	Form feed	ETB	End of transmitted block
STX	Start of text	CR	Carriage return	CAN	Cancel
ETX	End of text	SO	Shift out	EM	End of medium
EOT	End of transmission	SI	Shift in	SUB	Substitute
ENQ	Enquiry	DLE	Data link escape	ESC	Escape
ACK	Acknowledge	DC1	Device control one	FS	File separator
BEL	Bell character (beep)	DC2	Device control two	GS	Group separator
BS	Back space	DC3	Device control three	RS	Record separator
HT	Horizontal tab	DC4	Device control four	US	Unit separator
LF	Line feed	NAK	Negative acknowledge	DEL	Delete

Left Digit(s)	Right Digit	EBCDIC									
		0	1	2	3	4	5	6	7	8	9
6						□					
7						¢	.	<	(	+	|
8		&									
9		!	$	*	)	;		¬	-	/	
10								^	,	%	-
11		>	?								
12			`	:	#	@	'	=	"		a
13		b	c	d	e	f	g	h	i		
14							j	k	l	m	n
15		o	p	q	r						
16			~	s	t	u	v	w	x	y	z
17									\	{	}
18		[	]								
19					A	B	C	D	E	F	G
20		H	I								J
21		K	L	M	N	O	P	Q	R		
22								S	T	U	V
23		W	X	Y	Z						
24		0	1	2	3	4	5	6	7	8	9

In the EBCDIC table, nonprintable control characters—codes 00–63, 250–255, and those for which empty spaces appear in the chart—are not shown.

Appendix F   Program Style, Formatting, and Documentation

Throughout this text, we encourage the use of good programming style and documentation. Although the programs you write for class assignments may not be looked at by anyone except the person grading your work, outside of class you will write programs that will be used by others.

Useful programs have very long lifetimes, during which they must be modified and updated. When maintenance work must be done, either you or another programmer will have to do it. Good style and documentation are essential if another programmer is to understand and work with your program. You will also discover that after not working with your own program for a few months, you'll be amazed at how many of the details you've forgotten.

F.1   General Guidelines

The style used in the programs and fragments throughout this text provides a good starting point for developing your own style. Our goals in creating this style were to make it simple, consistent, and easy to read.

Style is of benefit only for a human reader of your program—differences in style make no difference to the computer. Good style includes the use of meaningful variable names, comments, and indentation of control structures, all of which help others to understand and work with your program. Perhaps the most important aspect of program style is consistency. If the style within a program is not consistent, then it becomes misleading and confusing.

Sometimes, a particular style is specified for you by your instructor or by the company you work for. When you are modifying someone else's code, you should use his or her style in order to maintain consistency within the program. However, you will also develop your own, personal programming style based on what you've been taught, your own experience, and your personal taste.

F.2   Comments

Comments are extra information included to make a program easier to understand. You should include a comment anywhere the code is difficult to understand. However, don't overcomment. Too many comments in a program can obscure the code and be a source of distraction.

In our style, there are four basic types of comments: headers, declarations, in-line, and sidebar.

Header comments appear at the top of the program and should include your name, the date that the program was written, and its purpose. It is also useful to include sections describing input, output, and assumptions. Think of the header comments as the reader's introduction to your program. Here is an example:

```
// This program computes the sidereal time for a given date and
// solar time.
//
// Written By: Your Name
//
// Date Completed: 4/8/05
//
// Input: A date and time in the form MM DD YYYY HH MM SS
//
// Output: Sidereal time in the form HH MM SS
//
// Assumptions: Solar time is specified for a longitude of 0
//     degrees (GMT, UT, or Z time zone)
```

Header comments should also be included for all user-defined functions (see Chapters 7 and 8).

Declaration comments accompany the constant and variable declarations in the program. Anywhere that an identifier is declared, it is helpful to include a comment that explains its purpose. In programs in the text, declaration comments appear to the right of the identifier being declared. For example:

```
const float E = 2.71828;      // The base of the natural logarithms

float deltaX;                 // The difference in the x direction
float deltaY;                 // The difference in the y direction
```

Notice that aligning the comments gives the code a neater appearance and is less distracting.

In-line comments are used to break long sections of code into shorter, more comprehensible fragments. These are often the names of modules in your algorithm design, although you may occasionally choose to include other information. It is generally a good idea to surround in-line comments with blank lines to make them stand out. For example:

```
// Prepare file for reading

scoreFile.open("scores.dat");

// Get data

scoreFile >> test1 >> weight1;
scoreFile >> test2 >> weight2;
scoreFile >> test3 >> weight3;

// Print heading

cout << "Test Score   Weight" << endl;
```

Even if comments are not used, blank lines can be inserted wherever there is a logical break in the code that you would like to emphasize.

Sidebar comments appear to the right of executable statements and are used to shed light on the purpose of the statement. Sidebar comments are often just pseudocode statements from the lowest levels of your design. If a complicated C++ statement requires some explanation, the pseudocode statement should be written to the right of the C++ statement. For example:

```
while (file1 && file2)     // While neither file is empty...
{
    ⋮
```

In addition to the four main types of comments that we have discussed, there are some miscellaneous comments that we should mention. After the `main` function, we recommend using a row of asterisks (or dashes or equal signs or ...) in a comment before and after each function to help it to stand out. For example:

```
//*****************************************************************

void PrintSecondHeading()
{
    ⋮
}

//*****************************************************************
```

In this text, we use C++'s alternative comment form

```
/* Some comment */
```

to document the flow of information for each parameter of a function:

```
void GetData( /* out */ int age,         // Patient's age
              /* out */ int weight )     // Patient's weight
{
    ⋮
}

void Print( /* in */      float val,     // Value to be printed
            /* inout */ int&  count )    // Number of lines printed
                                         //   so far
{
    ⋮
}
```

(Chapter 7 describes the purpose of labeling each parameter as /* in */, /* out */, or /* inout */.)

Programmers sometimes place a comment after the right brace of a block (compound statement) to indicate which control structure the block belongs to:

```
while (num >= 0)
{
    ⋮

    if (num == 25)
    {
        ⋮
    } // if
} // while
```

Attaching comments in this fashion can help to clarify the code and aid in debugging mismatched braces.

F.3 Identifiers

The most important consideration in choosing a name for a data item or function in a program is that the name convey as much information as possible about what the data item is or what the function does. The name should also be readable in the context in which it is used. For example, the following names convey the same information but one is more readable than the other:

```
datOfInvc        invoiceDate
```

Identifiers for types, constants, and variables should be nouns, whereas names of void functions (non-value-returning functions) should be imperative verbs or phrases containing imperative verbs. Because of the way that value-returning functions are invoked, their names should be nouns or occasionally adjectives. Here are some examples:

Variables	`address, price, radius, monthNumber`
Constants	`PI, TAX_RATE, STRING_LENGTH, ARRAY_SIZE`
Data types	`NameType, CarMakes, RoomLists, Hours`
Void functions	`GetData, ClearTable, PrintBarChart`
Value-returning functions	`CubeRoot, Greatest, Color, AreaOf, IsEmpty`

Although an identifier may be a series of words, very long identifiers can become quite tedious and can make the program difficult to read.

The best approach to designing an identifier is to try writing out different names until you reach an acceptable compromise—and then write an especially informative declaration comment next to the declaration.

Capitalization is another consideration when choosing an identifier. C++ is a case-sensitive language; that is, uppercase and lowercase letters are distinct. Different programmers use different conventions for capitalizing identifiers. In this text, we begin each variable name with a lowercase letter and capitalize the beginning of each successive English word. We begin each function name and data type name with a capital letter and, again, capitalize the beginning of each successive English word. For named constants, we capitalize the entire identifier, separating successive English words with underscore (_) characters. Keep in mind, however, that C++ reserved words such as `main`, `if`, and `while` are always lowercase letters, and the compiler will not recognize them if you capitalize them differently.

F.4 Formatting Lines and Expressions

C++ allows you to break a long statement in the middle and continue onto the next line. (However, you cannot split a line in the middle of an identifier, a literal constant, or a string.) When you must split a line, it's important to choose a breaking point that is logical and readable. Compare the readability of the following code fragments.

```
cout << "For a radius of " << radius << " the diameter of the cir"
    << "cle is " << diameter << endl;
```

```
cout << "For a radius of " << radius
     << " the diameter of the circle is " << diameter << endl;
```

When you must split an expression across multiple lines, try to end each line with an opera-tor. Also, try to take advantage of any repeating patterns in the expression. For example,

```
meanOfMaxima = (Maximum(set1Value1, set1Value2, set1Value3) +
                Maximum(set2Value1, set2Value2, set2Value3) +
                Maximum(set3Value1, set3Value2, set3Value3)) / 3.0;
```

When writing expressions, also keep in mind that spaces improve readability. Usually you should include one space on either side of the = operator and most other operators. Occasionally, spaces are left out to emphasize the order in which operations are performed. Here are some examples:

```
if (x+y > y+z)
    maximum = x + y;
else
    maximum = y + z;
hypotenuse = sqrt(a*a + b*b);
```

F.5 Indentation

The purpose of indenting statements in a program is to provide visual cues to the reader and to make the program easier to debug. When a program is properly indented, the way the statements are grouped is immediately obvious. Compare the following two program fragments:

```
while (count <= 10)            while (count <= 10)
{                             {
cin >> num;                       cin >> num;
if (num == 0)                     if (num == 0)
{                                 {
count++;                              count++;
num = 1;                              num = 1;
}                                 }
cout << num << endl;              cout << num << endl;
cout << count << endl;           cout << count << endl;
}                             }
```

As a basic rule in this text, each nested or lower-level item is indented by four spaces. Exceptions to this rule are parameter declarations and statements that are split across two or more lines. Indenting by four spaces is a matter of personal preference. Some people prefer to indent by three, five, or even more than five spaces.

In this book, we indent the entire body of a function. Also, in general, any statement that is part of another statement is indented. For example, the If-Then-Else contains two parts, the then-clause and the else-clause. The statements within both clauses are indented four spaces beyond the beginning of the If-Then-Else statement. The If-Then statement is indented like the If-Then-Else, except that there is no else-clause. Here are examples of the If-Then-Else and the If-Then:

```cpp
if (sex == MALE)
{
    maleSalary = maleSalary + salary;
    maleCount++;
}
else
    femaleSalary = femaleSalary + salary;

if (count > 0)
    average = total / count;
```

For nested If-Then-Else statements that form a generalized multiway branch (the If-Then-Else-If, described in Chapter 5), a special style of indentation is used in the text. Here is an example:

```cpp
if (month == JANUARY)
    monthNumber = 1;
else if (month == FEBRUARY)
    monthNumber = 2;
else if (month == MARCH)
    monthNumber = 3;
else if (month == APRIL)
    :
else
    monthNumber = 12;
```

The remaining C++ statements all follow the basic indentation guideline mentioned previously. For reference purposes, here are examples of each.

```cpp
while (count <= 10)
{
    cin >> value;
    sum = sum + value;
    count++;
}

do
{
    GetAnswer(letter);
    PutAnswer(letter);
} while (letter != 'N');

for (count = 1; count <= numSales; count++)
    cout << '*';
```

```
for (count = 10; count >= 1; count--)
{
    inFile >> dataItem;
    outFile << dataItem << ' ' << count << endl;
}

switch (color)
{
    RED     : cout << "Red";
              break;
    ORANGE  : cout << "Orange";
              break;
    YELLOW  : cout << "Yellow";
              break;
    GREEN   :
    BLUE    :
    INDIGO  :
    VIOLET  : cout << "Short visible wavelengths";
              break;
    WHITE   :
    BLACK   : cout << "Not valid colors";
              color = NONE;
}
```

GLOSSARY

Abstract data type   A data type whose properties (domain and operations) are specified independently of any particular implementation.

Abstract step   A step for which some implementation details remain unspecified.

Abstraction barrier   The invisible wall around a class object that encapsulates implementation details. The wall can be breached only through the public interface.

Aggregate operation   An operation on a data structure as a whole, as opposed to an operation on an individual component of the data structure.

Algorithm   A step-by-step procedure for solving a problem in a finite amount of time.

Anonymous type   A type that does not have an associated type identifier.

Argument   A variable or expression listed in a call to a function; also called *actual argument* or *actual parameter*.

Argument list   A mechanism by which functions communicate with each other.

Arithmetic/logic unit (ALU)   The component of the central processing unit that performs arithmetic and logical operations.

Array   A collection of components, all of the same type, ordered on N dimensions ($N \geq 1$). Each component is accessed by N indexes, each of which represents the component's position within that dimension.

Assembler   A program that translates an assembly language program into machine code.

Assembly language   A low-level programming language in which a mnemonic is used to represent each of the machine language instructions for a particular computer.

Assignment expression   A C++ expression with (1) a value and (2) the side effect of storing the expression value into a memory location.

Assignment statement   A statement that stores the value of an expression into a variable.

Automatic variable A variable for which memory is allocated and deallocated when control enters and exits the block in which it is declared.

Auxiliary storage device A device that stores data in encoded form outside the computer's main memory.

Base address The memory address of the first element of an array.

Base case The case for which the solution can be stated nonrecursively.

Base class (superclass) The class being inherited from.

Binary operator An operator that has two operands.

Black box An electrical or mechanical device whose inner workings are hidden from view.

C string In C and C++, a null-terminated sequence of characters stored in a `char` array.

Catch To process a thrown exception. (The catching is performed by an exception handler.)

Central processing unit (CPU) The part of the computer that executes the instructions (program) stored in memory; made up of the arithmetic/logic unit and the control unit.

Class A structured type in a programming language that is used to represent an abstract data type.

Class member A component of a class. Class members may be either data or functions.

Class object (class instance) A variable of a `class` type.

Class template A C++ language construct that allows the compiler to generate multiple versions of a class by allowing parameterized data types.

Client Software that declares and manipulates objects of a particular class.

Communication complexity A measure of the quantity of data passing through a module's interface.

Compiler A program that translates a high-level language into machine code.

Complexity A measure of the effort expended by the computer in performing a computation, relative to the size of the computation.

Composition (containment) A mechanism by which the internal data (the state) of one class includes an object of another class.

Computer A programmable device that can store, retrieve, and process data.

Computer program A sequence of instructions to be performed by a computer.

Computer programming The process of planning a sequence of steps for a computer to follow.

Concrete step A step for which the implementation details are fully specified.

Constructor An operation that creates a new instance (variable) of an ADT.

Control abstraction The separation of the logical properties of an action from its implementation.

Control structure A statement used to alter the normally sequential flow of control.

Control unit The component of the central processing unit that controls the actions of the other components so that instructions (the program) are executed in the correct sequence.

Count-controlled loop A loop that executes a specified number of times.

Dangling pointer A pointer that points to a variable that has been deallocated.

Data Information in a form a computer can use.

Data abstraction The separation of a data type's logical properties from its implementation.

Data flow The flow of information from the calling code to a function and from the function back to the calling code.

Data representation The concrete form of data used to represent the abstract values of an abstract data type.

Data type A specific set of data values, along with a set of operations on those values.

Declaration A statement that associates an identifier with a data object, a function, or a data type so that the programmer can refer to that item by name.

Deep copy An operation that not only copies one class object to another but also makes copies of any pointed-to data.

Demotion (narrowing) The conversion of a value from a "higher" type to a "lower" type according to a programming language's precedence of data types. Demotion may cause loss of information.

Derived class (subclass) The class that inherits.

Direct addressing Accessing a variable in one step by using the variable name.

Documentation The written text and comments that make a program easier for others to understand, use, and modify.

Driver A simple `main` function that is used to call a function being tested. The use of a driver permits direct control of the testing process.

Dynamic binding The run-time determination of which function to call for a particular object.

Dynamic data Variables created during execution of a program by means of special operations. In C++, these operations are `new` and `delete`.

Dynamic data structure A data structure that can expand and contract during execution.

Dynamic linked list A linked list composed of dynamically allocated nodes that are linked together by pointers.

Editor An interactive program used to create and modify source programs or data.

Encapsulation Hiding a module implementation in a separate block with a formally specified interface.

Enumeration type A user-defined data type whose domain is an ordered set of literal values expressed as identifiers.

Enumerator One of the values in the domain of an enumeration type.

Evaluate To compute a new value by performing a specified set of operations on given values.

Event counter A variable that is incremented each time a particular event occurs.

Event-controlled loop A loop that terminates when something happens inside the loop body to signal that the loop should be exited.

Exception An unusual, often unpredicatable event, detectable by software or hardware, that requires special processing; also, in C++, a variable or class object that represents an exceptional event.

Exception handler A section of program code that is executed when a particular exception occurs.

Expression An arrangement of identifiers, literals, and operators that can be evaluated to compute a value of a given type.

Expression statement A statement formed by appending a semicolon to an expression.

External (head) pointer A pointer variable that points to the first node in a dynamic linked list.

External representation The printable (character) form of a data value.

Field (member, in C++) A component of a record.

File A named area in secondary storage that is used to hold a collection of data; the collection of data itself.

Flow of control The order in which the computer executes statements in a program.

Free store (heap) A pool of memory locations reserved for allocation and deallocation of dynamic data.

Function A subprogram in C++.

Function call (function invocation) The mechanism that transfers control to a function.

Function call (to a void function) A statement that transfers control to a void function. In C++, this statement is the name of the function, followed by a list of arguments.

Function definition A function declaration that includes the body of the function.

Function overloading The use of the same name for different C++ functions, distinguished from each other by their parameter lists.

Function prototype A function declaration without the body of the function.

Function template A C++ language construct that allows the compiler to generate multiple versions of a function by allowing parameterized data types.

Function value type The data type of the result value returned by a function.

Functional cohesion A property of a module in which all concrete steps are directed toward solving just one problem, and any significant subproblems are written as abstract steps. Also, the principle that a module should perform exactly one abstract action.

Functional decomposition A technique for developing software in which the problem is divided into more easily handled subproblems, the solutions of which create a solution to the overall problem.

Functional equivalence A property of a module that performs exactly the same operation as the abstract step it defines. A pair of modules are also functionally equivalent to each other when they perform exactly the same operation.

General case The case for which the solution is expressed in terms of a smaller version of itself; also known as *recursive case*.

Generic algorithm An algorithm in which the actions or steps are defined but the data types of the items being manipulated are not.

Generic data type A type for which the operations are defined but the data types of the items being manipulated are not.

Hardware   The physical components of a computer.

Hierarchical record   A record in which at least one of the components is itself a record.

Identifier   A name associated with a function or data object and used to refer to that function or data object.

Inaccessible object   A dynamic variable on the free store without any pointer pointing to it.

Indirect addressing   Accessing a variable in two steps by first using a pointer that gives the location of the variable.

Infinite recursion   The situation in which a function calls itself over and over endlessly.

Information   Any knowledge that can be communicated.

Information hiding   The encapsulation and hiding of implementation details to keep the user of an abstraction from depending on or incorrectly manipulating these details.

Inheritance   A mechanism by which one class acquires the properties—the data and operations—of another class.

Input/output (I/O) devices   The parts of the computer that accept data to be processed (input) and present the results of that processing (output).

Interactive system   A system that allows direct communication between user and computer.

Interface   A connecting link at a shared boundary that permits independent systems to meet and act on or communicate with each other. Also, the formal description of the purpose of a subprogram and the mechanism for communicating with it.

Internal representation   The form in which a data value is stored inside the memory unit.

Iteration   An individual pass through, or repetition of, the body of a loop.

Iteration counter   A counter variable that is incremented with each iteration of a loop.

Iterator   An operation that allows us to process—one at a time—all the components in an instance of an ADT.

Length   The number of values currently stored in a list.

Lifetime   The period of time during program execution when an identifier has memory allocated to it.

Linked list   A list in which the order of the components is determined by an explicit link member in each node, rather than by the sequential order of the components in memory.

List   A variable-length, linear collection of homogeneous components.

Literal value   Any constant value written in a program.

Local variable   A variable declared within a block and not accessible outside of that block.

Loop   A control structure that causes a statement or group of statements to be executed repeatedly.

Loop entry   The point at which the flow of control reaches the first statement inside a loop.

Loop exit   The point at which the repetition of the loop body ends and control passes to the first statement following the loop.

Loop test   The point at which the While expression is evaluated and the decision is made either to begin a new iteration or skip to the statement immediately following the loop.

Machine language   The language, made up of binary-coded instructions, that is used directly by the computer.

Member selector   The expression used to access components of a struct or class variable. It is formed by using the struct or class variable name and the member name, separated by a dot (period).

Memory leak   The loss of available memory space that occurs when dynamic data is allocated but never deallocated.

Memory unit   Internal data storage in a computer.

Metalanguage   A language that is used to write the syntax rules for another language.

Mixed type expression   An expression that contains operands of different data types; also called *mixed mode expression.*

Module   A self-contained collection of steps that solves a problem or subproblem; can contain both concrete and abstract steps.

Name precedence   The precedence that a local identifier in a function has over a global identifier with the same name in any references that the function makes to that identifier; also called *name hiding.*

Named constant (symbolic constant)   A location in memory, referenced by an identifier, that contains a data value that cannot be changed.

Named type   A user-defined type whose declaration includes a type identifier that gives a name to the type.

Nonlocal identifier   With respect to a given block, any identifier declared outside that block.

Object-oriented design (OOD)   A technique for developing software in which the solution is expressed in terms of objects—self-contained entities composed of data and operations on that data.

Object-oriented programming (OOP)   The use of data abstraction, inheritance, and dynamic binding to construct programs that are collections of interacting objects.

Object program   The machine language version of a source program.

Observer   An operation that allows us to observe the state of an instance of an ADT without changing it.

One-dimensional array   A structured collection of components, all of the same type, that is given a single name. Each component (array element) is accessed by an index that indicates the component's position within the collection.

Operating system   A set of programs that manages all of the computer's resources.

Out-of-bounds array index   An index value that, in C++, is either less than 0 or greater than the array size minus 1.

Parameter   A variable declared in a function heading; also called *formal argument* or *formal parameter.*

Peripheral device   An input, output, or auxiliary storage device attached to a computer.

Pointer type A simple data type consisting of an unbounded set of values, each of which addresses or otherwise indicates the location of a variable of a given type. Among the operations defined on pointer variables are assignment and testing for equality.

Polymorphic operation An operation that has multiple meanings depending on the type of the object to which it is bound at run time.

Postcondition An assertion that should be true after a module has executed.

Precision The maximum number of significant digits.

Precondition An assertion that must be true before a module begins executing.

Programming Planning or scheduling the performance of a task or an event.

Programming language A set of rules, symbols, and special words used to construct a computer program.

Promotion (widening) The conversion of a value from a "lower" type to a "higher" type according to a programming language's precedence of data types.

Range of values The interval within which values of a numeric type must fall, specified in terms of the largest and smallest allowable values.

Record (structure, in C++) A structured data type with a fixed number of components that are accessed by name. The components may be heterogeneous (of different types).

Recursive algorithm A solution that is expressed in terms of (a) smaller instances of itself and (b) a base case.

Recursive call A function call in which the function being called is the same as the one making the call.

Recursive definition A definition in which something is defined in terms of smaller versions of itself.

Reference parameter A parameter that receives the location (memory address) of the caller's argument.

Reference type A simple data type consisting of an unbounded set of values, each of which is the address of a variable of a given type. The only operation defined on a reference variable is initialization, after which every appearance of the variable is implicitly dereferenced.

Representational error Arithmetic error that occurs when the precision of the true result of an arithmetic operation is greater than the precision of the machine.

Reserved word A word that has special meaning in C++; it cannot be used as a programmer-defined identifier.

Scope The region of program code where it is legal to reference (use) an identifier.

Scope rules The rules that determine where in the program an identifier may be accessed, given the point where that identifier is declared.

Self-documenting code Program code containing meaningful identifiers as well as judiciously used clarifying comments.

Semantics The set of rules that determines the meaning of instructions written in a programming language.

Shallow copy An operation that copies one class object to another without copying any pointed-to data.

Short-circuit (conditional) evaluation Evaluation of a logical expression in left-to-right order with evaluation stopping as soon as the final truth value can be determined.

Side effect Any effect of one function on another that is not a part of the explicitly defined interface between them.

Significant digits Those digits from the first nonzero digit on the left to the last nonzero digit on the right (plus any 0 digits that are exact).

Simple (atomic) data type A data type in which each value is atomic (indivisible).

Software Computer programs; the set of all programs available on a computer.

Software engineering The application of traditional engineering methodologies and techniques to the development of software.

Software piracy The unauthorized copying of software for either personal use or use by others.

Sorting Arranging the components of a list into order (for instance, words into alphabetical order or numbers into ascending or descending order).

Source program A program written in a high-level programming language.

Static binding The compile-time determination of which function to call for a particular object.

Static variable A variable for which memory remains allocated throughout the execution of the entire program.

Structured data type A data type in which each value is a collection of components and whose organization is characterized by the method used to access individual components. The allowable operations on a structured data type include the storage and retrieval of individual components.

Structured (procedural) programming The construction of programs that are collections of interacting functions or procedures.

Stub A dummy function that assists in testing part of a program. A stub has the same name and interface as a function that actually would be called by the part of the program being tested, but it is usually much simpler.

Switch expression The expression whose value determines which switch label is selected. It cannot be a floating-point or string expression.

Syntax The formal rules governing how valid instructions are written in a programming language.

Tail recursion A recursive algorithm in which no statements are executed after the return from the recursive call.

Termination condition The condition that causes a loop to be exited.

Test plan A document that specifies how a program is to be tested.

Test plan implementation Using the test cases specified in a test plan to verify that a program outputs the predicted results.

Testing the state of a stream The act of using a C++ stream object in a logical expression as if it were a Boolean variable; the result is `true` if the last I/O operation on that stream succeeded, and `false` otherwise.

Throw To signal the fact that an exception has occurred; also called *raise.*

Transformer An operation that builds a new value of the ADT, given one or more previous values of the type.

Two-dimensional array   A collection of components, all of the same type, structured in two dimensions. Each component is accessed by a pair of indexes that represent the component's position in each dimension.

Type casting   The explicit conversion of a value from one data type to another; also called type conversion.

Type coercion   The implicit (automatic) conversion of a value from one data type to another.

Unary operator   An operator that has just one operand.

Value parameter   A parameter that receives a copy of the value of the corresponding argument.

Value-returning function   A function that returns a single value to its caller and is invoked from within an expression.

Variable   A location in memory, referenced by an identifier, that contains a data value that can be changed.

Virus   A computer program that replicates itself, often with the goal of spreading to other computers without authorization, and possibly with the intent of doing harm.

Void function (procedure)   A function that does not return a function value to its caller and is invoked as a separate statement.

Answers to Selected Exercises

Chapter 1   Exam Preparation Exercises

2. Analysis and specification, general solution (algorithm), verify.
4. The analysis and specification step within the problem-solving phase.
6. **a.** vi, **b.** ii, **c.** v, **d.** i, **e.** vii, **f.** iv.
8. The control unit directs the actions of the other components in the computer to execute program instruction in the proper order.
10. False. Peripheral devices are external to the CPU and its main memory.
12. **a.** ii, **b.** v, **c.** iii, **d.** vii, **e.** i, **f.** vi, **g.** iv.

Chapter 1   Programming Warm-Up Exercises

2. Follow separate algorithm for filling glass with water and placing on counter
    If right-handed,
      pick up toothpaste tube in left hand and unscrew cap by turning counter-clockwise
      place toothpaste cap on counter
      transfer toothpaste tube to right hand and pick up toothbrush in left hand, holding it by its handle
      place open end of toothpaste tube against tips of brush bristles and squeeze toothpaste tube just enough to create a 0.5-inch-long extrusion of toothpaste on brush
      pull toothpaste tube away from brush and place tube on counter
      transfer toothbrush to right hand, holding it by its handle
      open mouth and insert brush, placing toothpaste-covered bristles against one tooth
      scrub tooth with brush by moving brush up and down 10 times
      reposition brush to an unscrubbed tooth
      repeat previous two steps until all teeth have been brushed
      spit toothpaste into sink

    put toothbrush in sink
    pick up glass in right hand
    fill mouth with water from glass
    swish water in mouth for five seconds
    spit water from mouth into sink
    repeat previous three steps three times
  Otherwise (if left-handed)
    pick up toothpaste tube in right hand and unscrew cap by turning counter-clockwise
    place toothpaste cap on counter
    transfer toothpaste tube to left hand and pick up toothbrush in right hand, holding it by its
      handle
    place open end of toothpaste tube against tips of brush bristles and squeeze toothpaste tube
      just enough to create a 0.5-inch-long extrusion of toothpaste on brush
    pull toothpaste tube away from brush and place tube on counter
    transfer toothbrush to left hand, holding it by its handle
    open mouth and insert brush, placing toothpaste-covered bristles against one tooth
    scrub tooth with brush by moving brush up and down 10 times
    reposition brush to an unscrubbed tooth
    repeat previous two steps until all teeth have been brushed
    spit toothpaste into sink
    put toothbrush in sink
    pick up glass in left hand
    fill mouth with water from glass
    swish water in mouth for five seconds
    spit water from mouth into sink
    repeat previous three steps three times
  Place glass on counter
  Follow separate algorithm for cleaning up after brushing teeth

4. Change step u to:
   u. Repeat step t nine times.

Chapter 2 Exam Preparation Exercises

2. **a.** vi, **b.** ix, **c.** iv, **d.** v, **e.** vii, **f.** ii, **g.** i, **h.** x, **i.** iii, **j.** viii.
4. The template allows an identifier to begin with a digit. Identifiers can begin with a letter or an underscore, and digits may appear only in the second character position and beyond.
6. True.
8. Note that the second line concatenates two words without a separating space.

```
Four score and
seven years agoour fathers
brought forth on this
continent a new nation...
```

10. By preceding it with a backslash character (\").

12. The `//` form of comment cannot span more than one line. It also cannot be inserted into the middle of a line of code because everything to the right of `//` becomes a comment.

14. No. The `endl` identifier is a manipulator, and is not a string value.

16. `std::cout << "Hello everybody!" << std::endl;`

18. By splitting it into pieces that fit on a line, and joining them with the concatenation operator.

Chapter 2   Programming Warm-Up Exercises

2. Note that the `\"` escape sequence is needed in six places here:

```
cout << "He said, \"How is that possible?\"" << endl
     << "She replied, \"Using manipulators.\"" << endl
     << "\"Of course,\" he exclaimed!" << endl;
```

4.
```
const string FIRST = "Your first name inserted here";
const string LAST = "Your last name inserted here";
// Insert your middle initial in place of A:
const char MIDDLE = 'A';
```

6. `PART1 + PART2 + PART1 + PART3`

8.
```
#include <iostream>
#include <string>

using namespace std;

const string TITLE = "Rev.";
const char FIRST = 'H';
const char MID 'G';
const char DOT = '.';

int main()
{
    cout << TITLE << FIRST << DOT << MID << DOT
         << " Jones";
}
```

Chapter 3   Exam Preparation Exercises

2. `char, short, int, long.`

4. E signifies an exponent in scientific notation. The digits to the left of the E are multiplied by 10 raised to the power given by the digits to the right of the E.

6. Integer division with an integer result, and floating division with a floating result.

8. `()    unary -    [ *  /  % ]    [ +  - ]`

10. a. vi, b. ii, c. vii, d. iv, e. i, f. v, g. iii.

12. You write the name of a data type, followed by an expression enclosed in parentheses.

14. `215.00`

16. `string::size_type`
18. It tells the stream to print floating-point numbers without using scientific notation.

Chapter 3   Programming Warm-Up Exercises

2. a. `days / 7`
   b. `days % 7`
4. `float(dollars * 100 + quarters * 25 + dimes * 10 +`
   `     nickels * 5 + pennies) / 100.0`
6. a. `3 * X + Y`
   b. `A * A + 2 * B + C`
   c. `((A + B)/(C - D)) * (X / Y)`
   d. `((A * A + 2 * B + C)/D) / (X * Y)`
   e. `sqrt(fabs(A - B))`
   f. `pow(X, -cos(Y))`
8. `startOfMiddle = name.find(' ') + 1;`
10. `cout << setprecision(5) << setw(15) << distance;`
12.
```
//*********************************************
// Celsius program
// This program outputs the Celsius temperature
// corresponding to a given Fahrenheit temperature
//*********************************************

#include <iostream>

using namespace std;

int main()
{
    const float FAHRENHEIT = 72.0;
    float celsius;

    celsius = 5/9 * (FAHRENHEIT - 32);
    cout << fixed << "Celsius equivalent of Fahrenheit "
        << FAHRENHEIT << " is " << celsius << " degrees.";
    return 0;
}
```

Chapter 4   Exam Preparation Exercises

2. a. The insertion operator cannot be used with `cin`.
   b. The extraction operator cannot be used with `cout`.
   c. The right operand of the extraction operator must be a variable.
   d. The arguments are in reverse order.
   e. The function name should not have a capital L, and the arguments are reversed.

4. a = 70, b = 80, c = 30, d = 0, e = 20, f = 30.
6. **a.** `string1 = "January 25, 2005"`
   b. The reading marker is at the start of the next line.
8. It returns \n.
10. Some variation in the answer is acceptable, as long as it is clear that the prompt for the inexperienced user is much more detailed.
   a. `cout << "Enter a date in the format of mm/dd/yyyy."`
   `            << " For example, for October 18, 1989, enter 10/18/1989.";`
   b. `cout << "Enter date, format mm/dd/yyyy.";`
12. `ifstream` and `ofstream`.
14. The correction is to convert the name into a C string.

```
ifstream inData;
string name;

cout << "Enter the name of the file: ");
cin >> name;
infile.open(name.c_str());
```

16. False. The file immediately enters the fail state, and I/O operations on it are simply ignored.
18. The answer can vary, but should at least include vehicle, customer, and agency. A little more thought might add garage, repair shop, contract, and so on.
20. **a.** A step for which the implementation details are fully specified.
   b. A step for which some implementation details remain to be specified.
   c. A self-contained series of steps that solves a given problem or subproblem.
   d. A module that performs the same operation as the abstract step it defines.
   e. A property of a module in which the concrete steps are all directed to solving just one problem, and any significant subproblems are written as abstract steps.
22. **a.** no, **b.** yes, **c.** yes, **d.** no, **e.** no.

Chapter 4   Programming Warm-Up Exercises

2. ```
cout << "Enter a name in the format: first middle last:";
cin >> first >> middle >> last;
```

4. ```
float number1;
float number2;
float number3;
float average;

cout << "Enter the first number and press return: ";
cin >> number1;
cout << "Enter the second number and press return: ";
cin >> number2;
cout << "Enter the third number and press return: ";
```

```
cin >> number3;
average = (number1 + number2 + number3) / 3.0;
cout << "The average is: " << average << endl;
```

6. The names of the variables may differ from those shown here. Instead of using the ignore function to skip a single character, reading into a dummy char variable may also be used.

a.
```
int int1;
char char1;
float float1;

cin >> int1 >> char1 >> float1;
```

b.
```
string string1;
string string2;
int int1;
int int2;

cin >> string1 >> int1 >> string2 >> int2;
```

c.
```
int int1;
int int2;
float float1;

cin >> int1;
cin.ignore(1, ',');
cin >> int2;
cin.ignore(1, ',');
cin >> float1;
```

d.
```
char char1;
char char2;
char char3;
char char4;

cin >> char1;
cin.ignore(1, ' ');
cin >> char2;
cin.ignore(1, ' ');
cin >> char3;
cin.ignore(1, ' ');
cin >> char4;
cin.ignore(1, ' ');
```

e.
```
float float1;

cin.ignore(1, '$');
cin >> float1;
```

8. ```
   #include <fstream>
   fstream temps;
   temps.open("temperatures.dat");
   ```

10. ```
    #include <iostream>
    #include <fstream>


    using namespace std;

    fstream inData;
    fstream outData;
    const float PI = 3.14159265;
    float radius;
    float circumference;
    float area;

    int main()
    {
      inData.open("indata.dat");
      outData.open("outdata.dat");
      inData >> radius;
      circumference = radius * 2 * PI;
      area = radius * radius * PI;
      cout << "For the first circle, the circumference is "
           << circumference << " and the area is " << area << endl;
      outData << radius << " " << circumference << " " << area << endl;
      inData >> radius;
      circumference = radius * 2 * PI;
      area = radius * radius * PI;
      cout << "For the second circle, the circumference is "
           << circumference << " and the area is " << area << endl;
      outData << radius << " " << circumference << " " << area << endl;
    }
    ```

12. `inFile >> int1 >> int2 >> int3;`

14.

Top level:

Write letter
Mail letter

Write letter   **Level 2**

Write return address and date
Write company address
Write salutation
Write body of letter
Write closing
Sign letter

Mail letter

Address envelope
Write return address
Attach stamp to envelope
Fold letter in thirds
Insert letter in envelope
Seal envelope
Place envelope in mail box

Chapter 5   Exam Preparation Exercises

2. False. They are predefined constants.
4. Because, in the collating sequence of the character set, the uppercase letters all come before the lowercase letters.
6. **a.** true
   b. true
   c. true
   d. true
   e. true
   f. false
   g. false
8. True.
10. It outputs "The data doesn't make sense."
12. Nothing.
14. It outputs Very good
16. Add braces to enclose the If-Then statement.
18. There is no limit, although a human reader finds it difficult to follow too many levels.

Chapter 5   Programming Warm-Up Exercises

2. `!inFile1 && !inFile2`
4.
```
if (year1 < year2 && month1 < month2 && day1 < day2)
    cout << month1 << "/" << day1 << "/" year1
        << " comes before "
        << month2 << "/" << day2 << "/" << year2;
```

```
    else
        cout << month1 << "/" << day1 << "/" year1
            << " does not come before "
            << month2 << "/" << day2 << "/" << year2;
```

6. `bool1 || bool2 && !(bool1 && bool2)`

8.
```
if (score < 0 || score > 100)
    cout << "Score is out of range";
else
{
    scoreTotal = scoreTotal + score;
    scoreCount++;
}
```

10.
```
if (score > 100)
    cout << "Duffer.";
else if (score > 80)
    cout << "Weekend regular.";
else if (score > 72)
    cout << "Competitive player.";
else if (score > 68)
    cout << "Turn pro!";
else
    cout << "Time to go on tour!";
```

12. The conditional tests are using = instead of ==. Both branches have the error, but the second one doesn't output the message because the result of the assignment expression is 0, which is treated as false by the branch.

```
maximum = 75;
minimum = 25;
if (maximum == 100)
    cout << "Error in maximum: " << maximum << endl;
if (minimum == 0)
    cout << "Error in minimum: " << minimum << endl;
```

14. Values of temp that should be tried are: 213, 212, 211, 33, 32, 31.

Chapter 6   Exam Preparation Exercises

2. False.

4. a. ii, b. ix, c. iv, d. viii, e. vi, f. i, g. v, h. vii, i. iii.

6. Twelve times.

```
0, 1, 2, 3, 4, 5, 6, 7, 8, 9, 10, 11,
```

8. The output is:

```
      @
     @@
    @@@
   @@@@
  @@@@@
 @@@@@@
@@@@@@@
@@@@@@@@
@@@@@@@@@
@@@@@@@@@@
@@@@@@@@@@
```

10. The code fails to process the first value on the file. The corrected code is:

```
sum = 0;
indata >> number;
while (indata)
{
    sum = sum + number;
    indata >> number;
}
```

12. The output is:

```
3 5 7 9 11 13 15 17 19
```

The corrected code is:

```
number = 0;
while (number < 10)
{
    cout << number * 2 - 1 << " ";
    number++;
}
```

14. What is the condition that ends the loop? How should the condition be initialized? How should the condition be updated? What is the process being repeated? How should the process be initialized? How should the process by updated? What is the state of the program on exiting the loop?

Chapter 6   Programming Warm-Up Exercises

2.
```
count = 1;
sum = 0;
while (sum <= 10000)
{
    sum = sum + count;
```

```
        count++;
    }
    cout << count - 1;
4.  count = 0;
    getline(chapter6, line);
    while (chapter6)
    {
        if (line.find("code segment") < string::npos)
          count++;
        getline(chapter6, line);
    }
    cout << "The string was found " << count << " times."
6.  cout << "Sun   Mon   Tue   Wed   Thu   Fri   Sat" << endl;
    count = 1;
    while (count <= startDay)   //Print blanks in first week
    {
        cout << "    ";
        count++;
    }
    dayNumber = 1;
    while (dayNumber <= days)   //Print day numbers for month
    {
        while (count <= 7)       //Print for one week in month
        {
            if (dayNumber <= days)
                cout << setw(3) << dayNumber << "  ";
            count++;
            dayNumber++;
        }
        cout << endl;
        count = 1;
    }
8.  char oneChar;
    int eCount;
    int charCount;
    eCount = 0;
    textData >> oneChar;
    charCount = 0;
    while (textData)
    {
        charCount++;
        if (oneChar == 'z')
            eCount++;
```

```
        textData >> oneChar;
    }
    cout << "Percentage of letter 'z': "
        << float(eCount) / charCount * 100;
```

10.
```
    first = 1;
    second = 1;
    cout << first << endl << second << endl;
    while (second < 30000)
    {
        next = first + second;
        first = second;
        second = next;
        cout << second << endl;
    }
```

12.
```
    cout << "Enter number of stars: ";
    cin >> number;
    count = 1;
    while (count <= number)
    {
        cout << '*';
        count++;
    )
    cout << endl;
```

14.
```
    indata >> number;
    while (indata)
    {
        count = 1;
        while (count <= number)
        {
            cout << '*';
            count++;
        }
        cout << endl;
        indata >> number;
    }
```

Chapter 7   Exam Preparation Exercises

2. False. The parameter name is optional.
4. a. v, b. iii, c. vi, d. i, e. iv, f. viii, g. ii, h. vii.
6. The call must have six arguments, unless default parameters are used (we do not cover their use in this book, but they are mentioned).

8. The type must come before the name of each parameter instead of after it. The & should be appended to the type instead of to the parameter name. The prototype should end with a semicolon.

10. Hiding a module implementation in a separate block with a formally specified interface.

12. It should not contain a return statement.

14. The result is not passed back to the caller—result should be a reference parameter instead of a value parameter.

16. False. Like any other variable declaration, it can be accessed only by statements within the block that follows its declaration.

18. That the file contains valid data (only integers), and that it has at least one value (the mean is undefined for an empty data set).

Chapter 7   Programming Warm-Up Exercises

2.
```cpp
void Max (int, int, int&);
```

4.
```cpp
void GetLeast (/* inout */ ifstream& infile,
               /* out */   int&       lowest)
```

6.
```cpp
void GetLeast (/* inout */ ifstream& infile,
               /* out */   int&       lowest)
{
    int number;
    infile >> number;       // Get a number
    lowest = INT_MAX;        // Initially use greatest int
    while (infile)
    {
        if (number < lowest)
            lowest = number;    // Remember lower number
        infile >> number;       // Get next number
    }
}
```

8.
```cpp
void Reverse ( /* in */   string  original,
              /* out */  string& lanigiro )
```

10.
```cpp
void Reverse ( /* in */   string  original,
              /* out */  string& lanigiro )
{
    int count;
    count = 1;
    lanigiro = "";
    while (count <= original.length())
    {
        lanigiro = lanigiro +
            original.substr(original.length() - count, 1);
        count++;
    }
)
```

```
12. void LowerCount ( /* out */ int& count)
    {
        char inChar;
        count = 0;
        cin >> inChar;
        while (cin && inChar != '\n')
        {
          if (islower(inChar))
              count++;
          cin >> inChar;
        }
    }

14. void GetNonemptyLine ( /* inout */ ifstream& infile,
                           /* out */   string&   line)
    {
        getline(infile, line);
        while (infile && line == "")
            getline(infile, line);
    }

16. void TimeAdd ( /* inout */ int& days,
                   /* inout */ int& hours,
                   /* inout */ int& minutes,
                   /* in */    int  addDays,
                   /* in */    int  addHours,
                   /* in */    int  addMinutes)
    {
        int extraHour;
        int extraDay;
        minutes = (minutes + addMinutes) % 60;
        extraHour = (minutes + addMinutes) / 60;
        hours = (hours + addHours + extraHour) % 24;
        extraDay = (hours + addHours + extraHour) / 24;
        days = days + addDays + extraDay;
    }

18. void SeasonPrint (/* in */ int month,
                      /* in */ int day)
    {
        if (month == 12 && day >= 21)
            cout << "Winter";
        else if ((month == 9 and day >= 21) || month > 9)
            cout << "Fall";
        else if ((month == 6 and day >= 21) || month > 6)
            cout << "Summer";
```

```
    else if ((month == 3 and day >= 21) || month > 3)
        cout << "Spring";
    else
        cout << "Winter";
}
```

Chapter 8   Exam Preparation Exercises

2. False. It is local to the function's body.
4. True.
6. The combination of `param2` being a reference parameter and the erroneous use of an assignment expression instead of an equality test in the first If statement results in the argument to `param2` being assigned the value in `param1` every time the function is called.
8. The namespace is in global scope.
10. a. Static, b. Automatic, c. Static.
12. It is initialized once, when control first reaches the statement.
14. False.
16. The `return` expression is of type `float`, and the return type of the function is `int`.
18. It makes a side effect error more likely.

Chapter 8   Programming Warm-Up Exercises

```
2. bool Equals (/* in */ float x,
               /* in */ float y)
```

```
4. bool Equals (/* in */ float x,
               /* in */ float y)
   {
       return abs(x - y) < 0.00000001;
   }
```

```
6. float ConeVolume (/* in */ float radius,
                     /* in */ float height);
   {
       return 1.0/3.0 * 3.14159265 * radius * radius * height;
   }
```

```
8. string Reverse (/* in */  string  original)
   {
       string lanigiro;
       int count;
       count = 1;
       lanigiro = "";
       while (count <= original.length())
       {
           lanigiro = lanigiro +
```

```
                           original.substr(original.length() - count, 1);
                    count++;
               }
               return lanigiro;
         )
```

10.
```
   float SquareKm (/* in */ float length,
                   /* in */ float width);
   {
        return length * 1.6 * width * 1.6;
   }
```

12.
```
   string MonthAbbrev (/* in */ int month)
   {
        if (month == 12) return "Dec";
        else if (month == 11) return "Nov";
        else if (month == 10) return "Oct";
        else if (month == 9) return "Sep";
        else if (month == 8) return "Aug";
        else if (month == 7) return "Jul";
        else if (month == 6) return "Jun";
        else if (month == 5) return "May";
        else if (month == 4) return "Apr";
        else if (month == 3) return "Mar";
        else if (month == 2) return "Feb";
        else return "Jan";
   }
```

14.
```
   float RunningAvg (/* in */ float value)
   {
        static float total = 0.0;
        static int count = 0;
        total = total + value;
        count++;
        return total/float(count);
   }
```

Chapter 9   Exam Preparation Exercises

2. False. It has local scope.
4. False. Both Break and Continue are allowed in any of the looping statements.
6. Control jumps to the `case` matching the `switch` expression, but then proceeds to execute the remaining statements in all of the succeeding `cases`.
8. 1000 times.
10. A While statement would be the best choice.
12. August

14. 2
   1
   0
   3
   2
   1
   4
   3
   2

16. How now brown cow?

18. 12

Chapter 9   Programming Warm-Up Exercises

2.
```
switch (day)
{
    case 0 : cout << "Sunday"; break;
    case 1 : cout << "Monday"; break;
    case 2 : cout << "Tuesday"; break;
    case 3 : cout << "Wednesday"; break;
    case 4 : cout << "Thursday"; break;
    case 5 : cout << "Friday"; break;
    case 6 : cout << "Saturday"; break;
    default: cout << "Error";
}
```

4.
```
for (int day = 6, day >= 0, day--)
    cout << DayOfWeek(day) << endl;
```

6.
```
char response;
do
{
    cout << "Please enter 'Y' or 'N': ";
    cin >> response;
    if (response != 'Y' && response != 'N')
        cout << "Invalid response. ";
} while (response != 'Y' && response != 'N');
```

8.
```
for (int row = 1; row <= 10; row++)
{
    for (int col = 1; col <= 10; col++)
        cout << setw(5) << row * col;
    cout << endl;
}
```

10.
```
int line;
int star;
line = 1;
do
{
    star = 1;
    do
    {
        cout << '*';
        star++;
    } while (star <= line);
    cout << endl;
    line++;
} while (line <= 10);
```

12.
```
void Rectangle (/* in */ int height,
                /* in */ int width)
{
    for (int col = 1; col <= width; col++)
        cout << '*';
    cout << endl;
    for (int row = 2; row <= height - 1; row++)
    {
        cout << '*';
        for (int col = 2; col < width - 1; col++)
            cout << ' ';
        cout << '*' << endl;
    }
    for (int col = 1; col <= width; col++)
        cout << '*';
    cout << endl;
}
```

14.
```
int startHour = 3;
int endHour = 7;
int startMin = 15;
int endMin = 30;
int beginMin;
int lastMin;

for (int hour = startHour; hour <= endHour; hour++)
{
    if (hour == startHour)
        beginMin = startMin;
    else
        beginMin = 0;
```

```
    if (hour == endHour)
        lastMin = endMin;
    else
        lastMin = 59;

    for (int min = beginMin; min <= lastMin; min++)
        for (int sec = 0; sec <= 59; sec++)
            cout << hour << ':' << min << ':' << sec << endl;
}
```

Chapter 10   Exam Preparation Exercises

2. True.
4. True.
6. char, short, int, long, bool.
8. The assignment operators.
10. When the type name is not a single word, as in unsigned int.
12. 'g'
14. Absolute error is a fixed value of allowable error, whereas relative error multiplies the allowable error by one of the values being compared.
16. The value of the expression is 3.
18. Because we must use the same type name for arguments, parameters, and function prototypes. If the type doesn't have a name, we can't use it in this context.

Chapter 10   Programming Warm-Up Exercises

2. a. 3.14159265F
   b. 3.14159265
   c. 3.14159265L
   d. 3.14159265E0
4. sizeof(long) * 8
6. cin >> charIn;
   if (isdigit(charIn))
      numIn = charIn - '0';

8.
```
int MonthNum (/* in */ string month)
{
    switch (tolower(month[0]))
    {
        case 'a': switch (tolower(month[1]))
            {
                case 'p': return 4;
                case 'u': return 8;
                default : return 0;
            }
```

```
              case 'd': return 12;
              case 'f': return 2;
              case 'j': switch (tolower(month[3]))
                       {
                              case 'e': return 6;
                              case 'u': return 1;
                              case 'y': return 7;
                              default : return 0;
                       }
              case 'm': switch (tolower(month[2]))
                       {
                              case 'r': return 3;
                              case 'y': return 5;
                              default : return 0;
                       }
              case 'n': return 11;
              case 'o': return 10;
              case 's': return 9;
              default : return 0;
          }
      }
```

10. `abs(balance - audit) <= 0.001`
12. `enum Planets {MERCURY, VENUS, EARTH, MARS,`
    `          JUPITER, SATURN, URANUS, NEPTUNE, PLUTO};`

14.
```
string PlanetToString (/* in */ Planet sphere)
{
    switch (sphere)
    {
        case MERCURY: return "Mercury";
        case VENUS: return "Venus";
        case EARTH: return "Earth";
        case MARS: return "Mars";
        case JUPITER: return "Jupiter";
        case SATURN: return "Saturn";
        case URANUS: return "Uranus";
        case NEPTUNE: return "Neptune";
        case PLUTO: return "Pluto";
        default : return "Error";
    }
}
```

Chapter 11   Exam Preparation Exercises

2. True.
4. True.
6. Assignment, passing as a parameter, return value from a function.
8. **a.** `sally.studentName.first = "Sally";`
   `sally.studentName.middle = "Ellen";`
   `sally.studentName.last = "Strong";`

   b. `sally.gradeNumber = 7;`

   c. `spring = sally.grades[3]`

10. **a.** Makes the type of `grade` be `char`, and inputs a `char` to `grade`.
    b. Compares the value in `grade` to see if it is in the range of 'A' through 'D'.
    c. Computes the integer equivalent of the letter grade, changes the type of `grade` to `int`, and assigns the numeric value to it.
12. The data representation is a concrete form of the domain, expressed in terms of structures and types supported by the programming language.
14. `current.plus(period);`
16. By matching the number, order, and types of the arguments with the parameter list.
18. It is written with a tilde before the name.

Chapter 11   Programming Warm-Up Exercises

2. `someTime.minutes = 6;`
   `someTime.seconds = 54;`

4. `Song mySong;`

   `mySong.title = "Long Run for a Collie Dog";`
   `mySong.album = "Timmy's Nightmare"`
   `mySong.artist = "Rebekah MacIntash";`
   `mySong.playTime = someTime;`
   `mySong.type = BLUES;`

6. ```
   union Temporal
   {
       string asString;
       int asInteger;
       Time asTime;
   }
   ```

8. ```
   //****************************************
   // SPECIFICATION FILE (Period)
   // This file gives the specification of a
   // class for geologic time periods
   //****************************************
   ```

```
class Period
{
public:
    enum PeriodName { PRECAMBRIAN, CAMBRIAN, ORDOVICIAN,
                      SILURIAN, DEVONIAN, CARBONIFEROUS,
                      PERMIAN, TRIASSIC, JURASSIC,
                      CRETACEOUS, TERTIARY, QUATERNARY};

    Period();
    // Default constructor
    // Creates object with value PRECAMBRIAN

    Period(PeriodName);
    // Constructor
    // Creates object with value specified

    String ToString() const;
    // Observer
    // Returns name of object as a string

    int ToInt() const;
    // Observer
    // Returns value of object as an int, 0 = PRECAMBRIAN

    float StartDate() const;
    // Observer
    // Returns starting date of period in millions of years ago

    void Increment();
    // Transformer
    // Advances value of object to next most recent period
    // Won't advance past QUATERNARY

private:

    PeriodName thisPeriod;

}
```

10.
```
Period::Period()
// Default constructor
// Creates object with value PRECAMBRIAN
{
    PeriodName = PRECAMBRIAN;
}
```

```cpp
Period::Period(/* in */ PeriodName aPeriod)
// Constructor
// Creates object with value specified
{
    thisPeriod = aPeriod;
}
```

12. The file would be called `Period.h`.

14.
```cpp
//****************************************
// SPECIFICATION FILE (Money)
// This file gives the specification of a
// class for representing money as dollars
// and cents using integers.
//****************************************

class Money
{
public:

    Money();
    // Default constructor
    // Creates object with value $0.00

    Money(int, int);
    // Constructor
    // Creates object with value specified
    // in dollars and cents

    int Dollars() const;
    // Observer
    // Returns dollars portion of object as an int

    int Cents() const;
    // Observer
    // Returns cents portion of object as an int

    float Amount() const;
    // Observer
    // Returns money value as a float

    void Add(Money);
    // Transformer
    // Adds value of money object in parameter
```

```
    void Sub(Money);
    // Transformer
    // Subtracts value of money object in parameter

private:

    int dollars;
    int cents;
}
```

16. The file name would be Money.h.

18. ```
float Money::Amount() const
// Observer
// Returns money value as a float
{
    return float(dollars) + float(cents)/100.0;
}
```

## Chapter 12    Exam Preparation Exercises

2. True.

4. True.

6. C++ does not report an out-of-bounds access as an error. The program accesses the location preceding the first element of the array, which may be a completely unrelated value in memory.

8. The base address is the memory location of the first element of an array. It is the value that is passed to a reference parameter in a function call.

10. The inner loop would increment the column index, keeping the row constant. The outer loop would increment the row index to move to the next row after each row is processed.

12. The For loop runs from 1 to 100 instead of 0 to 99. The last iteration will assign zero to an out-of-bounds location.

14. Functions cannot return array types.

16. Because the index value is input and then used without any checking, an out-of-bounds array access is likely.

18. ```
*  **
*  *
 *  **
*  *
 *  **
```

20. ```
* * *
 * *
* * *
 * *
* * *
```
```

Chapter 12   Programming Warm-Up Exercises

2.
```
typedef float DataSet[5];
DataSet input;
DataSet output;
DataSet working;
```

4.
```
for (int row = 0; row < 3; row++)
    for (int col = 0; col < 5; col++)
        set[row][col] = 0.0;
```

6.
```
bool Equals (/* in */ const DataSet first,
             /* in */ const DataSet second)
{
    for(int index = 0; index < 5; index++)
        if (first[index] != second[index])
            return false;
    // Only reaches end of loop if all are equal
    return true;
}
```

8. **a.** `currentList[36]`
   b. `currentList[11].title`
   c. `currentList[84].size.width`
   d. `currentList[119].room`
   e. `currentList[77].artist[0]`

10.
```
float total = 0.0;
for (int index = 0; index < numPieces; index++)
    total = total + currentList[index].price;
```

12.
```
float total = 0.0;
for (int index = 0; index < numPieces; index++)
    if(currentList[index].medium == OIL)
        if (currentList[index].size.width *
                currentList[index].size.height > 400)
            total = total + currentList[index].price;
```

14.
```
for (int octave = 0; octave < 8; octave++)
    for (Notes note = A; note <= GSHARP; note = Notes(note + 1))
        cin >> scale[octave][note];
```

16.
```
for (int octave = 0; octave < 8; octave++)
    cout << scale[octave][C] << endl;
```

18.
```
void Reset (float humidity[10][52][50][3])
{
    for (int year = 0; year < 10; year++)
        for (int week = 0; week < 52; week++)
            for (int state = 0; state < 50; state++)
```

```
                        for (Type type = MAX; type <= AVERAGE;
                              type = Type(type + 1));
                           humidity = 0.0;
     }
20. for (int year = 5; year < 10; year++)
        for (int week = 0; week < 52; week++)
            cout << humidity[year][week][22][AVERAGE] << endl;
```

Chapter 13   Exam Preparation Exercises

2. That all of the components have the same type.
4. `while (index < length && fabs(item -data[index]) >= EPSILON)`
   We need to change it because floating point numbers cannot be compared reliably for exact equality.
6. It has identified the smallest value in the portion of the list that remains to be sorted.
8. True.
10. 5
12. Two iterations. Middle is initially 7, then location 11 (which holds the 12th value) becomes middle.

Chapter 13   Programming Warm-Up Exercises

2.
```
void List::Insert( /* in */ ItemType item)

// Inserts item into list without duplication

{
    if (!IsPresent(item))
    {
        data[length] = item;
        length++;
    }
}
```

4.
```
void DeleteAll( /* in */ ItemType item);
    // Precondition:
    //      NOT IsEmpty()
    //      && item is assigned
    // Postcondition:
    //      IF item is present in list
    //          All occurrences of item are deleted from list
    //          && Length() ==
    //              Length()@entry - number of occurrences of item
    //      ELSE
    //          List is unchanged
```

6. ```
   void Replace( /* in */ ItemType item,
                 /* in */ ItemType newItem);
   // Precondition:
   //       NOT IsEmpty()
   //       && oldItem is assigned
   //       && newItem is assigned
   // Postcondition:
   //       IF oldItem is present in list
   //          First occurrence of oldItem is replaced by newItem
   //       ELSE
   //          List is unchanged
   ```

8. The `Insert` and `BinSearch` functions must be changed to enable descending order. We don't have to change `IsPresent` or `Delete`, because they both use `BinSearch` to locate the item.

10. ```
    void SortedList::DeleteAll( /* in */ ItemType item)

    // Deletes all occurrences of item from the list

    {
        int first;
        int index = 0;
        while (index < length && item != data[index])
            index++;
        first = index;
        while (index < length && item == data[index])
            index++;
        for (int position = index; position < length; position++)
            data[first + position - index] = data[position];
        length = length - (index - first);
    }
    ```

12. ```
    SortedList inData;
    ifstream unsorted;
    ItemType oneItem;

    unsorted >> oneItem;
    while (unsorted && !inData.IsFull())
    {
        inData.Insert(oneItem);
        unsorted >> oneItem;
    }
    ```
    ```

Chapter 14   Exam Preparation Exercises

2. True.

4. True.

6. Declaration of a class data member to be an object of the class that we want to compose into the new class being defined.

8. The class declaration for `DerivedClass` doesn't specify that it is making the members of `BaseClass` public, so they are not available to the client code. The heading should be changed to:

```
class DerivedClass : public BaseClass
```

10. **a.** The `BaseClass` constructor is called first.

    b. The `DerivedClass` constructor is called last.

12. The `virtual` designation should be used only with the base class declaration of `BaseAlpha`.

14. c.

Chapter 14   Programming Warm-Up Exercises

2.
```cpp
#include "testscore.h"
#include <iostream>
#include <string>

using namespace std;

TestScore::TestScore(
    /* in */ string name,
    /* in */ int score)
{
    studentName = name;
    studentScore = score;
}

TestScore::string GetName() const
{
    return studentName;
}

TestScore::int GetScore() const
{
    return studentScore;
}
```

4.
```cpp
#include "idscore.h"

class Exam
{
```

```
  public:
    SetScore(
        /* in */ int location,
        /* in */ IDScore score );
    IDScore GetScore(
        /* in */ int location ) const;

  private:
      IDScore examList[100];
  }
```

6.
```
class InternPhone : public Phone
{
public
    InternPhone
        ( /* in */ int newCountry,
          /* in */ int newAreaCode,
          /* in */ int newNumber,
          /* in */ PhoneType newType );
    void Write () const;
private:
    int country;
}
```

8.
```
void InternPhone::Write() const
{
    cout << country;
    Phone::Write();
    cout << endl;
}
```

10.
```
class InstallRecord : public Computer
{
public:
    InstallRecord(
        /* in */ string newName,
        /* in */ string newBrand,
        /* in */ string newModel,
        /* in */ int    newSpeed,
        /* in */ string newSerial,
        /* in */ int    newNumber,
        /* in */ string newLocation,
        /* in */ SimpleDate newDate );
    void Write() const;
```

```
        string getNewLocation();
        SimpleDate getSimpleDate();

    private:
        string location;
        SimpleDate installDate;
    };
```

12.
```
    InstallRecord::InstallRecord(
        /* in */ string newName,
        /* in */ string newBrand,
        /* in */ string newModel,
        /* in */ int    newSpeed,
        /* in */ string newSerial,
        /* in */ int    newNumber,
        /* in */ string newLocation,
        /* in */ SimpleDate newDate )
      : Computer( newName, newBrand, newModel,
                  newSpeed, newSerial, newNumber )
    {
        location = newLocation;
        installDate = newDate;
    }
```

14.
```
    void InstallRecord::Write() const;
    {
        Computer::Write();
        cout << location << endl;
        installDate.Write();
    }
```

Chapter 15   Exam Preparation Exercises

2. a. ii, b. i, c. iii, d. v, e. vi, f. iv.
4. True.
6. True.
8. The pointer(s) are deleted but the pointed-to data is not. It thus becomes inaccessible, and contributes to memory leakage.
10. It creates and references a dangling pointer in `germanShortHair`.
12. b.
14. `faxLog`
16. A destructor.
18. `*libraryRecord`

Chapter 15   Programming Warm-Up Exercises

2.
```
char* charArrPointer;
char[4] initials;
charArrPointer = initials;
charArrPointer[1] = 'A';
charArrPointer[2] = 'E';
charArrPointer[3] = 'W';
```

4.
```
struct Phone
{
    int country;
    int area;
    int number;
}
Phone newPhone;
Phone& structReference = newPhone;
structReference.country = 1;
structReference.area = 888;
structReference.number = 5551212;
```

6.
```
bool DeepCompare
    ( /* in */ structPointer first,
      /* in */ structPointer second )
{
    return (first->country == second->country &&
            first->area    == second->area &&
            first->number  == second->number);
}
```

8.
```
int Greatest(
    ( /* inout */ int data[],
      /* in */    int size )
{
    static max = data[0];
    for(int index = 1; index < size; index++)
        if (data[index] > max)
            max = data[index];
    delete [] data;
    return max;
}
```

10.
```
~Circuit()
{
    delete [] source;
    delete [] sink;
}
```

12. `if (oldValue != newValue)`
       `delete oldValue;`

Chapter 16   Exam Preparation Exercises

2. False.

4. a. The address of the next node in the list.
  b. The data in the current node.
  c. The data in the next node in the list.
  d. The address of the node after the next node.
  e. The data in the node after the next node.
  f. The data in the fourth node in the list.

6. a. An empty list. **b.** That processing has reached the end of the list.

8. Set a temporary pointer equal to the link field of the current node, set the current node link field equal to the link field of its successor, and delete the data pointed to by the temporary pointer.

10. A direct array representation keeps the elements physically adjacent in the array. A linked list implemented with an array allows elements to be in any physical order in the array, and connects them logically using a link field in each element.

12. a. An array—the list is small and bounded, and searches are done frequently.
  b. A linked list—the list varies unpredictably in size, and does not require frequent searching.
  c. A linked list—the list is unbounded, and deletion is at the head.

Chapter 16   Programming Warm-Up Exercises

2. a. `head->component`
  b. `currPtr = currPtr->link`
  c. `(currPtr->link)->link`
  d. `((currPtr->link)->link)->link`

4.
```
newNodePtr = new NodeType;
newNodePtr->component = 212;
currPtr->link = newNodePtr;
currPtr = newNodePtr;
```

6.
```
NodePtr savePtr;
savePtr = head;
head = currPtr->link;
head->link = savePtr;
currPtr->link = currPtr->link->link;
```

8.
```
auxPtr = currPtr;
if (auxPtr != NULL)
    if (auxPtr->link == NULL)
        auxPtr = NULL;
    else
```

```
    {
        while (auxPtr->link != NULL)
            auxPtr= currPtr->link;
        auxPtr->NULL;
    }
```

10.
```
CopyReverse(NodeType* head, NodeType*& headR)
{
    headR = NULL;       // head of new list

    NodePtr newNode;
    NodePtr tempPtr = head;             // used for traversal
    while (tempPtr != NULL)
    {
        newNode = new NodeType;
        newNode->component = tempPtr->component;

        newNode->link = headR;
        headR = newNode;
        tempPtr = tempPtr->link
    }
}
```

Chapter 17   Exam Preparation Exercises

2. False.
4. a. Template class, b. Neither (it's a class object)
6. a. float, b. 3.85, c. Yes.
8. The Throw statement.
10. a. False. There can be many Catch clauses, as long as their parameters are different.
    b. True.
    c. False. A Throw statement can appear anywhere. A Throw statement often is located in a function that is called from a Try clause.
12. In the Catch clause, insert return 1; after the output statement.
14. It rethrows the exception.

Chapter 17   Programming Warm-Up Exercises

2.
```
PrintSquare<int>(10);
PrintSquare<long>(10L);
PrintSquare<float>(10.0);
```

or

```
PrintSquare(10);
PrintSquare(10L);
PrintSquare(10.0);
```

4. **a.**
```
int Twice( int num )
{
    return 2*num;
}
float Twice( float num )
{
    return 2.0*num;
}
```
b.
```
cout << Twice(someInt) << ' ' << Twice(someFloat) << endl;
```

6.
```
template<class SomeType>
void GetData( string promptStr, SomeType& data )
{
    cout << promptStr << ' ';
    cin >> data;
}
```

8. **a.**
```
GList<int>   intList;
GList<float> floatList;
```
b.
```
i = 10;
while (i <= 80 && !intList.IsEmpty())
{
    // Below, use "while", not "if", because
    // duplicates are allowed in a list

    while (intList.IsPresent(i))
    {
        intList.Delete(i);
        floatList.Insert(0.5 * float(i));
    }
    i++;
}
```

10.
```
MixedPair<int, float>  pair1(5, 29.48);
MixedPair<string, int> pair2("Book", 36);
```

12. **a.**
```
class MathError
{};                        // Don't forget the semicolon
```
b.
```
throw MathError();   // Don't forget the parentheses
```
14.
```
class SumTooLarge   // Exception class
{};
  ⋮
int Sum( int int1, int int2 )
{
    if (int1 > INT_MAX - int2)
        throw SumTooLarge();
```

```
        return int1 + int2;
    }
```

16. **a.**
```
    class OpenFailed     // Exception class
    {};

    void OpenForInput( /* inout */ ifstream& someFile )

    // Prompts the user for the name of an input file
    // and attempts to open the file

    // Postcondition:
    //      The user has been prompted for a file name
    //   && IF the file could not be opened
    //             An error message has been printed
    //          && An OpenFailed exception has been thrown

    {
        string fileName;     // User-specified file name

        cout << "Input file name: ";
        cin >> fileName;

        someFile.open(fileName.c_str());
        if ( !someFile )
        {
            cout << "** Can't open " << fileName << " **" << endl;
            throw OpenFailed();
        }
    }
```

b. Note that the calling code below does not print an error message. The error message has already been printed by OpenForInput, as advertised by its postcondition.

```
    ifstream inFile;

    try
    {
        OpenForInput(inFile);
    }
    catch ( OpenFailed )
    {
        return 1;
    }
        // Success keep executing
```

Chapter 18   Exam Preparation Exercises

2. True.
4. False. Tail recursion occurs when nothing is done after the return from the recursive call.
6. F(3) = 8, F(4) = 16, F(5) = 32.
8. It will run out of space on the run time stack.
10. c. The value in the variable.
12. 30
    20
    10

14. abcc
    d
    e

Chapter 18   Programming Warm-Up Exercises

2.
```
int OneDigit (int number)
{
    if (number <= 9)
        return number;
    else
        return OneDigit(DigitSum(number));
}
```

4.
```
void Ex4()
{
    int number;
    cout << "Enter a positive number, 0 to end: ";
    cin >> number;

    if (number != 0)
    {
        cout << number << endl;
        Ex4();
        cout << number << endl;
    }
}
```

6.
```
void Ex6(int sum, int& revSum)
{
    int number;
    cout << "Enter a positive number, 0 to end: ";
    cin >> number;
```

```
        if (number != 0)
        {
            cout << "Total: " << sum + number <<endl;
            Ex6(sum + number, revSum);
            revSum = revSum + number;
            cout << number << " Total: " << revSum << endl;
        }
    }
```

8.
```
    void Ex8(int& greatest)
    {
        int number;
        cout << "Enter a positive number, 0 to end: ";
        cin >> number;

        if (number > greatest)
            greatest = number;

        if (number != 0)
        {
            cout << "Greatest: " << greatest << endl;
            Ex8(greatest);
            cout << number << endl;
        }

    }
```

The greatest must be written immediately following the call.

10.
```
    void CopyReverse(PtrType head1, PtrType& head2)
    // Assumption:  head2 is originally NULL
    {
        PtrType tempPtr;
        if (head1 != NULL)
        {
            tempPtr = new NodeType;
            tempPtr->info = head1->info;
            tempPtr->link = head2;
            head2 = tempPtr;
            CopyReverse(head1->link, head2);

        }
    }
```

12.
```
void CopyDouble(PtrType head1, PtrType& head2)
// Assumption:  head2 is originally NULL
{

    PtrType tempPtr;
    if (head1 != NULL)
    {
        tempPtr = new NodeType;
        tempPtr->info = head1->info;
        tempPtr->link = head2;
        head2 = tempPtr;
        CopyReverse(head1->link, head2);
        if (head1 != NULL)
        {
            tempPtr = new NodeType;
            tempPtr->info = head1->info;
            tempPtr->link = head2;
            head2 = tempPtr;
            Copy(head1->link, head2->link);
        }
    }
}
```

or

```
void CopyDouble(PtrType head1, PtrType& head2)
{
    CopyReverse(head1, head2);
    Copy(head1, head2);
}
```

Outstanding New Titles:

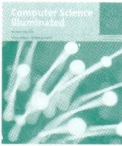

Computer Science Illuminated, Second Edition
Nell Dale and John Lewis
ISBN: 0-7637-0799-6
©2004

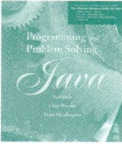

Programming and Problem Solving with C++, Fourth Edition
Nell Dale and Chip Weems
ISBN: 0-7637-0798-8
©2004

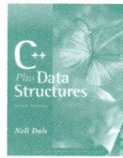

Programming and Problem Solving with Java
Nell Dale, Chip Weems,
and Mark R. Headington
ISBN: 0-7637-0490-3
©2003

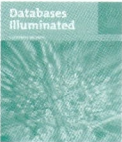

C++ Plus Data Structures, Third Edition
Nell Dale
ISBN: 0-7637-0481-4
©2003

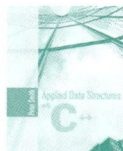

Databases Illuminated
Catherine Ricardo
ISBN: 0-7637-3314-8
©2004

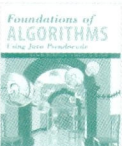

Applied Data Structures with C++
Peter Smith
ISBN: 0-7637-2562-5
©2004

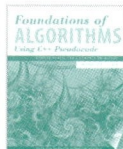

Foundations of Algorithms Using Java Pseudocode
Richard Neapolitan and Kumarss Naimipour
ISBN: 0-7637-2129-8
©2004

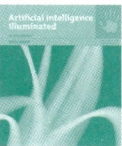

Foundations of Algorithms Using C++ Pseudocode, Third Edition
Richard Neapolitan and Kumarss Naimipour
ISBN: 0-7637-2387-8
©2004

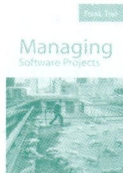

Artificial Intelligence Illuminated
Ben Coppin
ISBN: 0-7637-3230-3
©2004

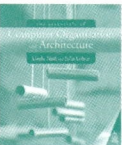

Managing Software Projects
Frank Tsui
ISBN: 0-7637-2546-3
©2004

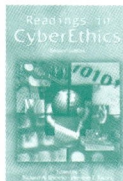

The Essentials of Computer Organization and Architecture
Linda Null and Julia Lobur
ISBN: 0-7637-0444-X
©2003

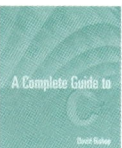

Readings in CyberEthics, Second Edition
Richard Spinello and Herman Tavani
ISBN: 0-7637-2410-6
©2004

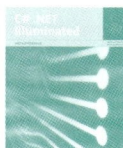

A Complete Guide to C#
David Bishop
ISBN: 0-7637-2249-9
©2004

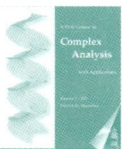

C#.NET Illuminated
Art Gittleman
ISBN: 0-7637-2593-5
©2004

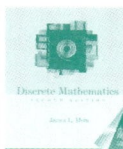

A First Course in Complex Analysis with Applications
Dennis G. Zill and Patrick Shanahan
ISBN: 0-7637-1437-2
©2003

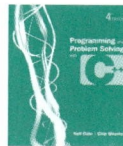

Discrete Mathematics, Second Edition
James L. Hein
ISBN: 0-7637-2210-3
©2003

http://www.jbpub.com/

JONES AND BARTLETT
PUBLISHERS
BOSTON   TORONTO   LONDON   SINGAPORE

1.800.832.0034

Take Your Courses to the Next Level

Turn the page to preview new and forthcoming titles in Computer Science and Math from Jones and Bartlett…

Providing solutions for students and educators in the following disciplines:

- Introductory Computer Science
- Java
- C++
- Databases
- C#
- Data Structures

- Algorithms
- Network Security
- Software Engineering
- Discrete Mathematics
- Engineering Mathematics
- Complex Analysis

Please visit http://computerscience.jbpub.com/ and http://math.jbpub.com/ to learn more about our exciting publishing programs in these disciplines.

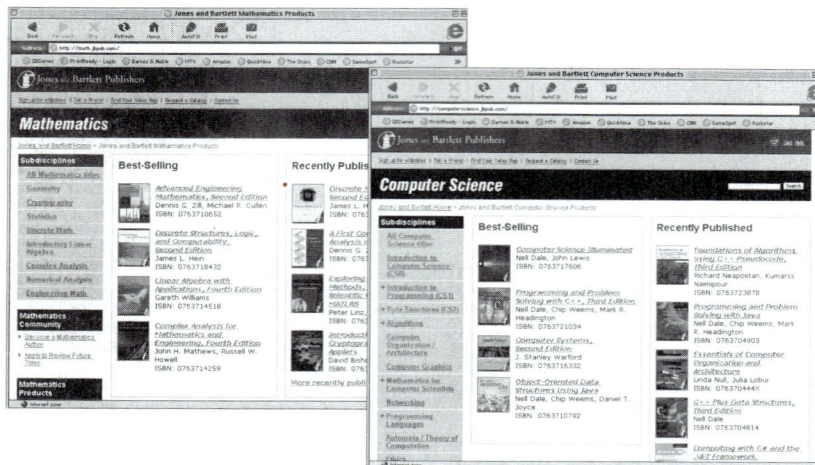